Clinical Neuropathology

TEXT AND COLOR ATLAS

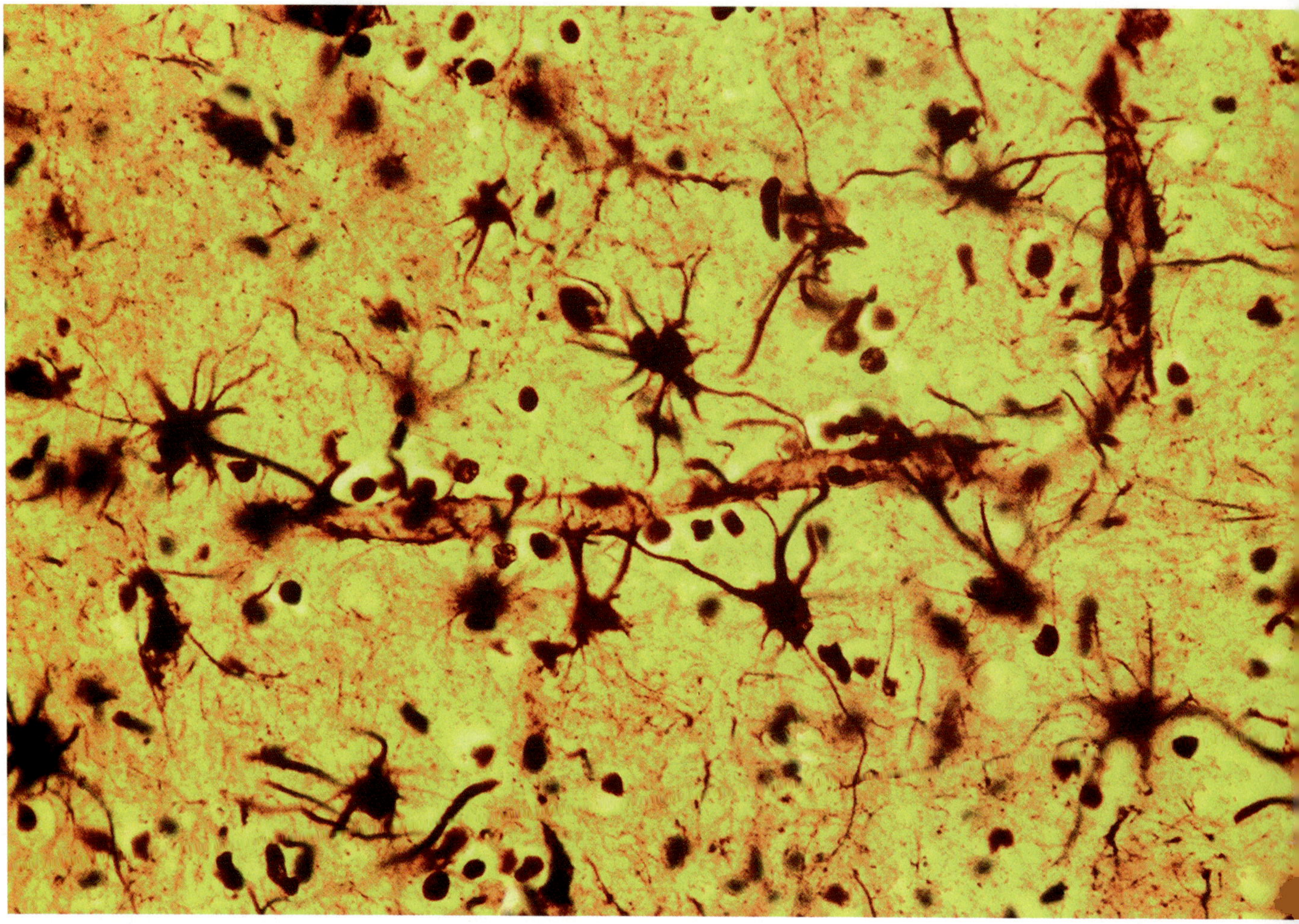

CATHERINE HABERLAND, MD

The Chicago Medical School at
Rosalind Franklin University
Departments of Neurology and Pathology
and
Section of Neurology
and
Neuropathology Laboratory at the
Veterans Administration Medical
Center at North Chicago, Illinois

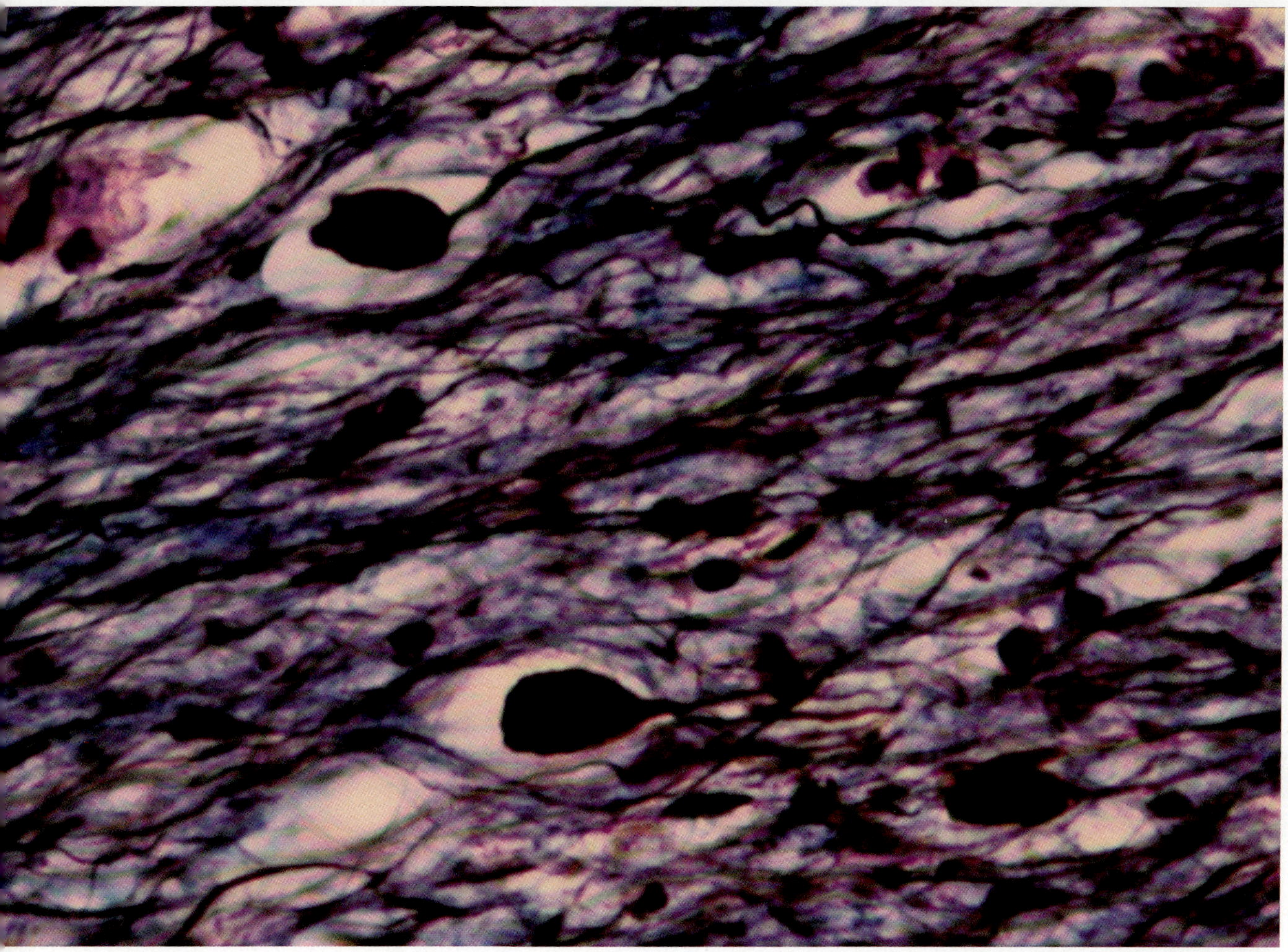

Clinical Neuropathology

TEXT AND COLOR ATLAS

Demos

DEMOS MEDICAL PUBLISHING, LLC
386 Park Avenue South
New York, New York 10016

Visit our website at www.demosmedpub.com

Senior Editor: Craig Percy

LIBRARY OF CONGRESS CATALOGING-IN-PUBLICATION DATA
Haberland, Catherine.
Clinical neuropathology : text and color atlas / Catherine Haberland.
p. ; cm.
Includes bibliographical references and index.
ISBN-13: 978-1-888799-97-2 (softcover)
ISBN-10: 1-888799-97-8 (softcover)
1. Nervous system—Diseases—Atlases. I. Title.
[DNLM: 1. Nervous System Diseases—pathology—Atlases.
WL 17 H114c 2007]
RC347.H33 2007
616.8—dc22
2006020445

Text designed by Steven Pisano
Cover designed by Cathleen Elliott

MANUFACTURED IN THE UNITED STATES OF AMERICA

06 07 08 09 10 5 4 3 2 1

Contents

Preface ix
Acknowledements xi

CHAPTER 1
Introduction to Clinical Neuropathology

Bibliography 4
Review Questions 4

CHAPTER 2
Basics of Neuropathology

Reactions of Neural Tissue to Diseases 7
Types of Degenerations in the Central Nervous System 19
Cerebral Edema 21
Cerebral Changes Associated With Intracranial Expanding Mass Lesions 22
Clinical Manifestations of Intracranial Expanding Mass Lesions and Rising Intracranial Pressure 25
Hydrocephalus 26
Cerebral Changes in Physiologic Aging 27
Artificial Cerebral Changes 29
Bibliography 30
Review Questions 30

CHAPTER 3
Cerebral Hypoxia

Etiology 33
Pathology 34
Clinical Features 36
Permanent Global Ischemia: Brain Death 37
Cerebral Pathology in Chronic Epilepsy 37
Bibliography 41
Review Questions 41

CHAPTER 4
Cerebrovascular Diseases

Etiology, Pathology, and Clinical Aspects of Stroke 43
Various Stroke Etiologies: Stroke in the Young 66

Cerebral Pathology in Arteriolosclerosis: Vascular Dementia 77
Bibliography 80
Review Questions 80

CHAPTER 5
Neurodegenerative Diseases

Dementias 84
Motor Neuron Diseases 97
Extrapyramidal Diseases 100
Cerebellar and Spinocerebellar Degenerations 109
Multiple System Atrophy 112
Bibliography 116
Review Questions 117

CHAPTER 6
Infectious Diseases

Bacterial Infections 120
Viral Infections 124
Mycotic Infections 136
Syphilitic Infections 138
Parasitic Infections 142
Miscellaneous Infections 147
Bibliography 148
Review Questions 148

CHAPTER 7
Prion Diseases: Transmissible Spongiform Encephalopathies

Animal Prion Diseases 152
Human Prion Diseases 152
Bibliography 155
Review Questions 156

CHAPTER 8
Demyelinating Diseases

Diseases with Autoimmune Pathogenesis 157
Diseases with Probable Autoimmune Pathogenesis 166
Bibliography 167
Review Questions 167

CHAPTER 9
Hereditary Neurometabolic Diseases

Lysosomal Diseases 170
Peroxisomal Diseases 179
Leukodystrophies 182
Mitochondrial Diseases 186
Amino Acid Metabolic Diseases 189
Carbohydrate Metabolic Diseases 190
Copper Metabolic Diseases 192
Neuroaxonal Dystrophies 193
Miscellaneous Neurometabolic Diseases 194
Bibliography 196
Review Questions 196

CHAPTER 10
Acquired Neurometabolic Diseases

Vitamin Deficiencies 199
Metabolic Encephalopathies 202
Calcium Metabolic Disorders 205
Neurologic Complications of Chronic Alcoholism 205
Toxic Diseases of the Nervous System 210
Bibliography 210
Review Questions 211

CHAPTER 11

Tumors of the Central Nervous System

General Aspects **213**
Tumors of the Neuroepithelium **216**
Tumors of the Meninges **231**
Tumors of the Pituitary Gland and Sellar Region **235**
Germ Cell Tumors **237**
Tumors of the Cranial and Spinal Nerves **238**
Maldevelopmental Tumors and Cysts **240**
Hemangiomas **244**
Lymphomas and Hematopoietic Tumors **245**
Primary Central Nervous System Lymphomas **246**
Metastatic Tumors **246**
Tumors of the Spinal Cord, Nerve Roots, and Meninges **249**
Tumors of the Cranium and the Spine **251**
Primary Intracranial Tumors in Children **251**
Hereditary Tumor Syndromes **253**
Nervous System Complications of Radiation and Chemotherapy **255**
Paraneoplastic Diseases **256**
Bibliography **257**
Review Questions 257

CHAPTER 12

Traumatic Injuries of the Central Nervous System

Blunt Head Injuries **261**
Missile Head Injuries **267**
Secondary Injuries **267**
Clinical Presentation of Cerebral Injuries **268**
Spinal Cord Injuries **269**
Other Injuries **269**
Bibliography **270**
Review Questions 271

CHAPTER 13

Congenital Malformations of the Central Nervous System

Neural Tube Defects: Dysraphic Disorders **274**
Malformation of the Prosencephalon: Holoprosencephaly **277**
Malformations of the Cerebral Hemispheres **279**
Malformations of the Midline Structures and Ventricles **284**
Malformations of the Cerebellum **285**
Malformations of the Brainstem **287**
Disorders of Brain Weight **287**
Meningeal and Vascular Anomalies **288**
Phakomatoses: Ectomesodermal Dysgenetic Syndromes **288**
Congenital and Neonatal Hydrocephalus **291**
Chromosomal Disorders **295**
Bibliography **296**
Review Questions 297

CHAPTER 14

Fetal and Perinatal Cerebral Pathology

Pathology of Vascular Insults **299**
Late Sequelae of Vascular Injuries **301**
Metabolic and Toxic Diseases **304**
Congenital and Neonatal Infections **305**
Sudden Infant Death Syndrome **307**
Bibliography **307**
Review Questions 307

Appendix: Answers to Review Questions 309
Index 313

Preface

This book, *Clinical Neuropathology*, is particularly aimed at neurologists, pathologists-in-training, and medical students involved in clinical neurosciences and pathology. It also addresses psychiatrists and those practitioners interested in diseases of the nervous system.

Over the last decade, a wealth of information has accumulated, impacting practically all disciplines of neurology. Numerous studies have enriched our knowledge of the molecular and genetic basis of neurodegenerative diseases, the genetics of neoplasms, and the molecular biology of inherited neurometabolic diseases, to mention a few. Some studies prompted new classifications, some opened new therapeutic strategies, and some still await elucidation.

The intent of this book is twofold:

- To provide a solid background in the structural alterations of common and less common but important nervous system diseases, along with their clinical manifestations.
- To incorporate into this background new information selected from the vast number of studies on molecular pathology and the pathogenesis of major nervous system diseases.

The reader thus finds easy access to recent developments in basic and clinical neurology.

For psychiatrists, this book presents material on the neuropathologic aspects of psychiatric disorders and on the molecular pathology of several dementing diseases. Pathologists-in-training who, due to a regrettable decline in autopsies, lack personal experience of postmortem examination of neurologic diseases, will find useful material here. Medical students can easily access the essential elements of neuropathology, and those with special interests can find sufficient material for their particular needs.

The material is divided into 14 chapters. The first chapter deals with the goals of neuropathologic examination. It includes representative pictures of the brain and spinal cord and tables of histologic methods. The second chapter presents characteristic histologic reactions of neural tissue to diseases and pathologic conditions particular to the nervous system. The following chapters deal with major disease categories. Each category contains an overview of general pathologic and clinical characteristics; descriptions of the gross and histologic features of individual diseases, along with their clinical features; and data on the pathogenetic mechanism in particular diseases. Brief case histories and neuroimaging accompany many pathologic illustrations. Tables summarize the characteristic clinical and pathologic features of particular diseases and point out distinctive features of other related diseases. A number of review questions follow each chapter. The answers are presented in an addendum following the last chapter. The bibliography is limited to the latest and most pertinent references.

It is hoped that *Clinical Neuropathology* will meet the educational needs of the reader.

Acknowledgments

My thanks to the histologic technicians, photographers, and secretaries for their valuable contribution to this work. I am indebted to Tariq I. Hassan, M.D., Associate Professor of Neurology at the Chicago Medical School at Rosalind Franklin University and Chief of Staff at the Veterans Administration Medical Center at North Chicago for his continuous support for the Neuropathology Laboratory. My special thanks to Frederick Sierles, Professor of Psychiatry at the Chicago Medical School at Rosalind Franklin University for his invaluable comments and advice. I gratefully acknowledge the patience and the tireless assistance of Mrs. Janice Weber-Rasmussen, B.S., at the Neuropathology Laboratory of the Veterans Administration Medical Center at North Chicago in the technical preparation of the manuscript. And I thank Mr. Craig Percy, Senior Editor of Demos Medical Publishing, and his staff.

Gratitude is also due to the late Percival Bailey, M.D., who initiated and supported the Neuropathology Laboratory at the Illinois State Psychiatric Institute and the Illinois State Pediatric Institute. M. Perou, M.D., performed the autopsies at Dixon State School and A. Pedroso, M.D., at Chicago State Hospital.

And last, my special thanks to the late Kálmán Sántha, M.D., Chairman of the Department of Neurology and Neurosurgery at the Medical School in Debrecen, Hungary for introducing me to the captivating and rewarding field of Neuropatholgy.

CHAPTER 1

Introduction to Clinical Neuropathology

The objectives of the neuropathologic examination are twofold: First, to identify and localize any lesion(s), interpret histologic changes and ultimately, formulate a diagnosis. Second, to correlate the location and histopathologic features of the lesion(s) with the clinical presentation. Fulfilling these goals requires familiarity with the anatomy and histology of the nervous system. For this purpose, photographs of representative brain and spinal cord slices and myelin-stained sections are provided (Figs. 1.1 through 1.5).

Knowledge of the normal structure of neural tissue enables the student to recognize pathologic alterations. Thus, Chapter 2 gives a brief description of the histology of neural tissue components, along with their pathologic reactions.

The histologic examination requires, in addition to conventional stains, the application of specific stains for each constituent of the neural tissue: neuron, axon, myelin, glial cells, blood vessels, and meninges. Familiarity with staining methods is necessary to select the appropriate stains for the study of a particular disease. Histochemical stains are valuable for the study of neurometabolic diseases, and immunohistologic stains are essential for diagnosing tumors and defining neurodegenerative diseases (Tables 1.1 through 1.3). Electron microscopic examination is performed to define tumors and delineate inherited metabolic diseases.

The examination of the histologic sections begins first by identifying the pathologic alterations of each tissue component involved, then combining them into an orderly whole—that is, formulating a diagnosis. The final correlation of the pathologic features with the clinical features becomes a learning experience.

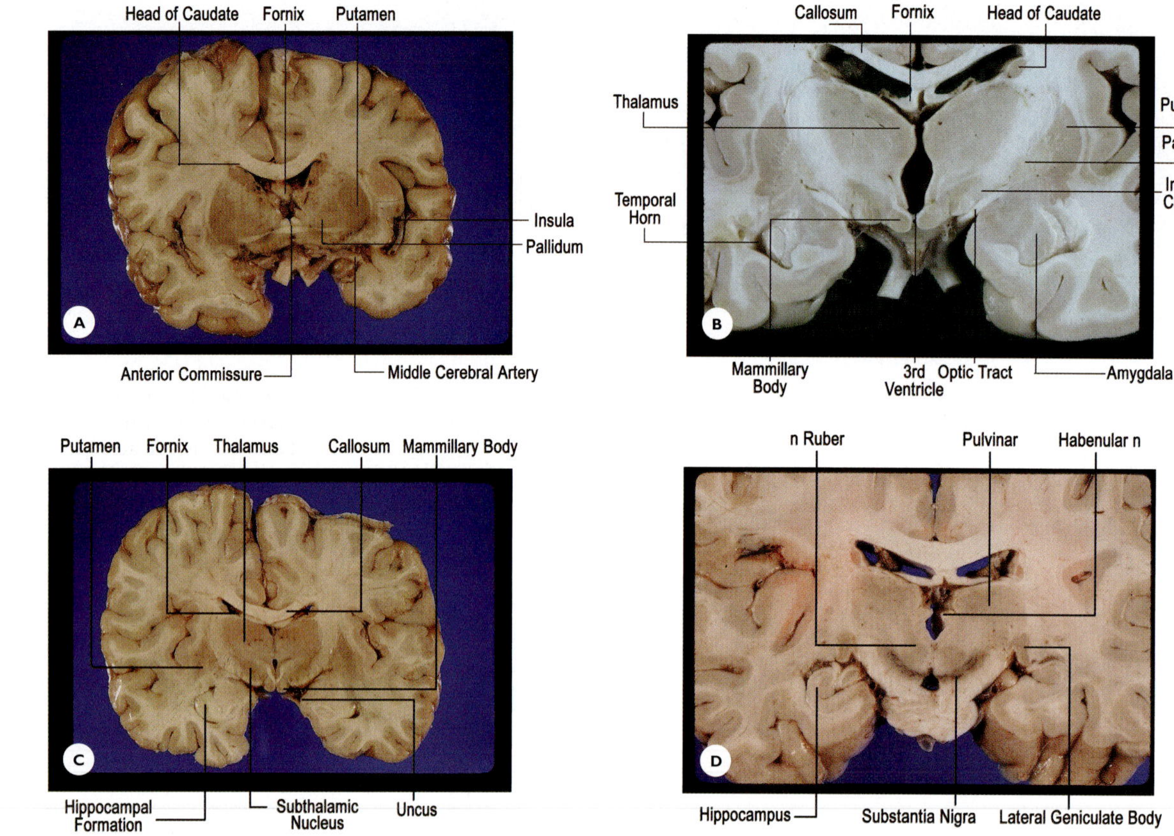

FIGURE 1.1
Transverse slices of the brain.

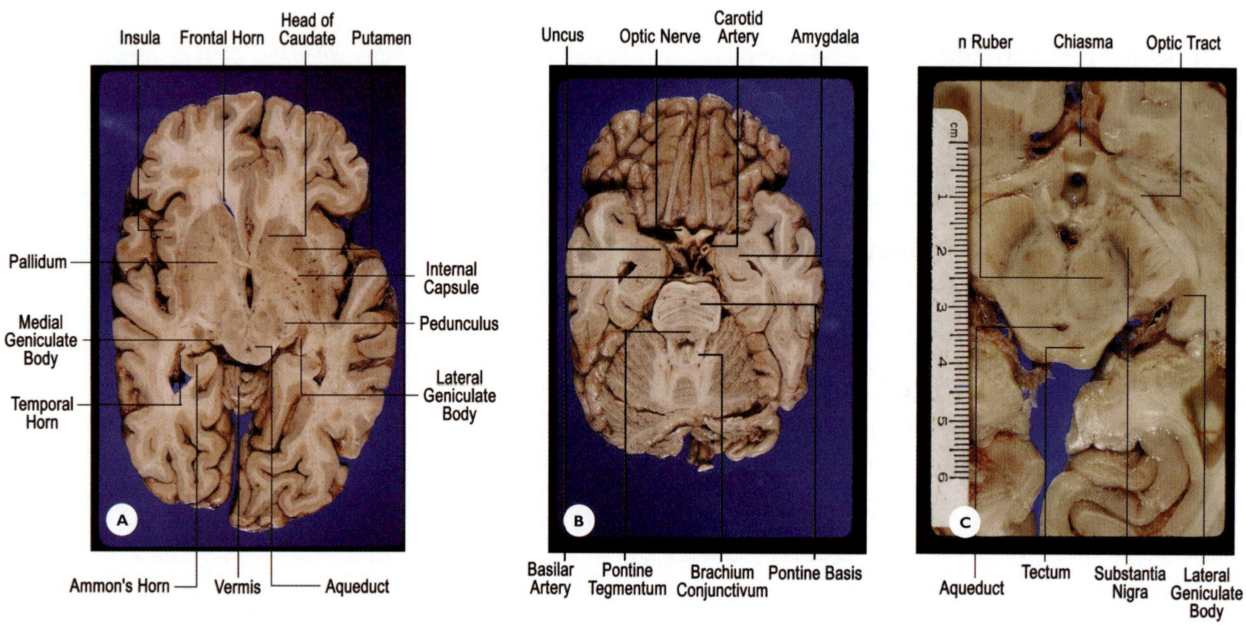

FIGURE 1.2
Horizontal slices of the brain.

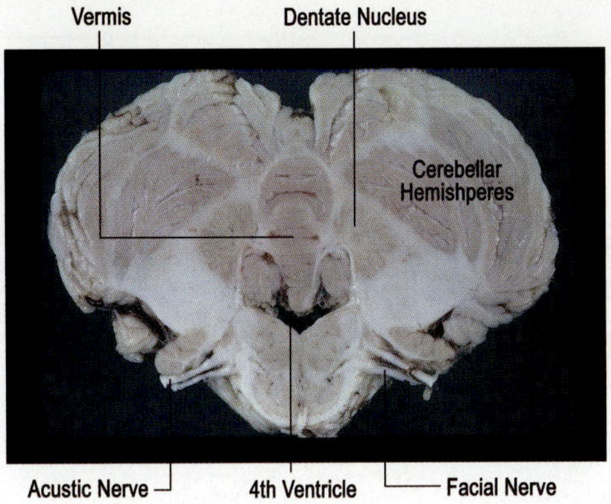

FIGURE 1.3
Transverse slice of the cerebellum.

TABLE 1.1.
Common Neurohistologic Stains

Tissue Components	*Stains*
Neurons/glial nuclei	Nissl: thionin, toluidine blue
	Klüver-Barrerra: cresyl violet
Nerve fibers	Bielschowsky: silver nitrate
Neurofibrillary tangles	Bodian: protargol
Neuritic plaques	Gallyas: silver nitrate
	Glees and Marsland: silver nitrate
Myelin	Woelcke: iron hematoxylin
	Loyez: iron aluminum
	Klüver-Barrera: Luxol fast blue
Neuron/myelin	Klüver-Barrera: Luxol fast blue-cresyl violet
Nerve fiber/myelin	Holmes
Astrocytes	Cajal: gold chloride
	Hortega: lithium carbonate
	Holzer: crystal violet
	Phosphotungstic acid/ hematoxylin (PTAH)
Oligodendrocytes	Penfield: silver nitrate
Microglia	Hortega: silver carbonate
Meninges/blood vessels	van Gieson
	Masson: trichrome
Reticulin fibers	Gömöri: silver nitrate
Elastic fibers	Verhoeff: hematoxylin
General stain	Hematoxylin-eosin

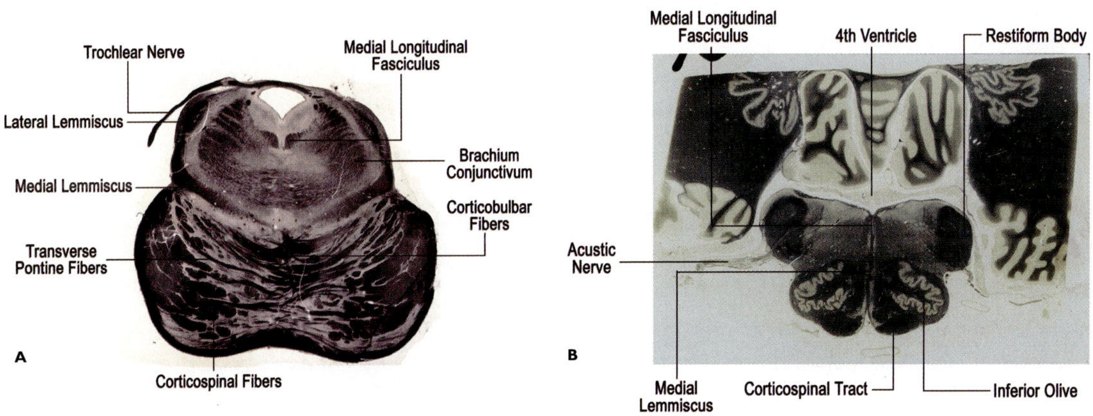

FIGURE 1.4
Myelin-stained section of the **A.** Pons and. **B.** Medulla.

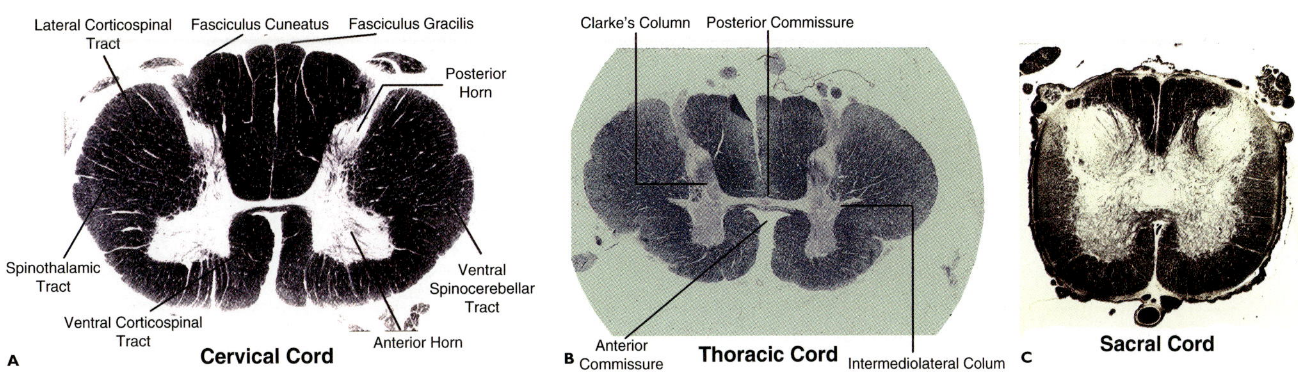

FIGURE 1.5
Myelin-stained sections of the spinal cord.

TABLE 1.2.
Common Histochemical Stains

Substance	*Stains*	*Results*
Lipid*	Oil-red O	Red
	Sudan III, IV	Orange-red, orange
	Sudan B-Black	Blue-black
Carbohydrate	Periodic acid Schiff (PAS) with and without diastase	Bright rose red
Glycogen	Best carmine	Bright red
Amyloid	Congo-red	Deep pink red
	Congo-red in polarized light	Green refringence
	Thioflavine S in fluorescent light	Yellow-yellow green
Calcium	Von Kossa	Black
Ferrous iron	Turnbull blue	Blue
Ferric iron	Prussian blue	Blue

*Frozen section

TABLE 1.3.
Basic Immunohistologic Stains

Markers	*Cell/Tissue*
NFP, NeuN, Synaptophysin, S-100 protein, NSE	Neuron
GFAP	Astrocyte
APP	Axonal degeneration
CD3	T cells
CD20	B cells
CD68	Macrophages
Cytokeratin	Epithelial filament
Desmin, Vimentin	Fibroblast
Desmin, Vimentin	Endothelial cell
Aβ peptide	Amyloid
MBP	Myelin
α-Synuclein, TAU, Ubiquitin	Neuronal/glial inclusions

NFP: neurofilament protein, Neu N: neuronal nucleus, NSE: neuron-specific enolase, GFAP: glial fibrillary acidic protein, APP: amyloid precursor protein, MBP: myelin basic protein. *For tumor-related immunohistologic stains, see Chapter 11.

BIBLIOGRAPHY

Arslan, O. (2001). *Neuroanatomical basis of clinical neurology*. New York: The Parthenon Publishing Group.

Esiri, M. M., and Perl, D. (2006). *Oppenheimer's diagnostic neuropathology: a practical manual*, 3rd ed. London: Hodder-Arnold.

REVIEW QUESTIONS

1. You are examining an atrophic brain. The patient's clinical diagnosis is dementia, probably Alzheimer's disease. Which of the following stains is most appropriate to confirm the diagnosis?
   A. Klüver-Berrera stain
   B. Hematoxylin-eosin
   C. Cajal stain
   D. Bielschowsky stain
   E. Oil-red O

2. Gross section of the pons shows a large infarct destroying parts of the basis and tegmentum. To identify the fiber tracts and neurons involved, which is the most appropriate stain?
   A. Periodic acid Schiff (PAS)
   B. Klüver-Berrera stain
   C. Holzer stain
   D. Nissl stain
   E. Gallyas stain

3. You are examining a tumor in a hematoxylin-eosin–stained section and would like to identify the cells of astrocytic origin. Which stain would you choose?
   A. PAS stain
   B. Vimentin
   C. S-100 protein
   D. GFAP
   E. Bodian stain

4. You are examining a large brain. The patient's clinical diagnosis is psychomotor regression, probably lipid storage disease. Which is the most appropriate stain to confirm the diagnosis?
   A. Best carmine
   B. Congo red
   C. Phosphotungstic acid hematoxylin (PTAH)
   D. Oil-red O
   E. Von Kossa stain

5. All of the following stains are useful to demonstrate pathology of axons *except*:

   A. Bielschowsky stain
   B. Klüver-Berrera stain
   C. Amyloid precursor protein (APP)
   D. Gallyas stain
   E. Bodian stain

(Answers are provided in the Appendix.)

CHAPTER 2

Basics of Neuropathology

Reactions of Neural Tissue to Diseases
Types of Degenerations in the Central Nervous System
Cerebral Edema
Cerebral Changes Associated with Intracranial Expanding Mass Lesions
Clinical Manifestations of Intracranial Expanding Mass Lesions and Rising Intracranial Pressure
Hydrocephalus
Cerebral Changes in Physiologic Aging
Artificial Cerebral Changes

The human nervous system performs greatly varied and highly complex functions: It oversees the functions of all bodily organs; it receives and integrates information from all senses; it initiates and coordinates motor activities; and notably, it processes our thoughts, generates our emotions, and stores our memories. Billions of cells are organized, categorized, and specialized to carry out these functions. The neurons are the executives, the glial cells provide adequate environment, the blood vessels furnish nutrients, and the meninges protect from injuries. The neurons, glial cells, blood vessels, and meninges each has a distinct morphology and displays characteristic changes in diseases.

This chapter presents the characteristic reactions of neural tissue to diseases, along with a brief description of their normal histology, and the pathologic conditions particular to the nervous system.

REACTIONS OF NEURAL TISSUE TO DISEASES

Neurons

The neurons, derivatives of the epithelium of the embryonic neural tube, greatly vary in appearance. In the cerebral cortex, most neurons are pyramidalshaped, whereas those in the spinal ganglia are round. The largest pyramidal cells in the motor cortex (Betz cells) measure up to 100 microns, whereas the granular cells of the cerebellar cortex measure only 5 microns. A neuron consists of (a) the cell body, or soma; (b) the dendrites, and (c) the axon (nerve fiber) (Fig. 2.1).

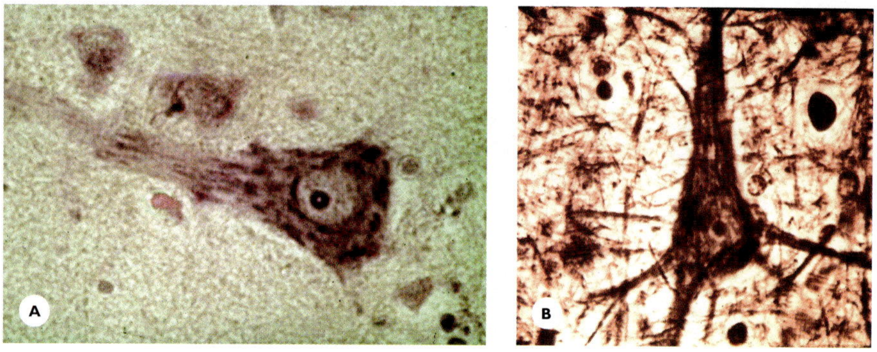

FIGURE 2.1
Cortical pyramidal neuron as seen in section stained with (**A**) cresyl violet and (**B**) silver.

Cell Body

The cell body contains the nucleus and the perikaryon (cytoplasm). The nucleus has a prominent nucleolus and a variable amount of chromatin. The perikaryon comprises the Nissl bodies and the argyrophilic fibrils (see Fig 2.1). The neurons in the compact zone of the substantia nigra, locus ceruleus, and dorsal nucleus of vagus contain melanin pigments. The perikaryon, at ultrastructural level, contains a variety of subcellular organelles: a rough endoplasmic reticulum with ribosomes (Nissl bodies in light microscopy), a smooth endoplasmic reticulum, Golgi apparatus, mitochondria, peroxisomes, lysosomes, and cytoskeletal organelles. Three major classes of cytoskeletal organelles are the microtubules, the intermediate filaments, and the microfilaments, all associated with proteins. The microtubules are associated with tau proteins, the neurofilaments (argyrophilic fibrils in light microscopy) with neuron-specific peptides, and the microfilaments with actin.

TABLE 2.1.
Major Neurotransmitters

Acetylcholine	Amino acids
Catecholamines	γ-Aminobutyric acid (GABA)
Dopamine	Glutamate
Norepinephrine	Aspartate
Epinephrine	Glycine
Serotonin	
Neuropeptides	
Opioids	
Neurohypophyseal peptides	
Substance P	
Enkephalin	

Dendrites

The dendrites, or cytoplasmic processes, are structurally similar to the perikaryon. They gradually divide into thinner processes, eventually terminating in small spines.

Axons

The axon, conductor of nervous impulses, arises from the axon hillock of the perikaryon, an area lacking Nissl bodies. Mitochondria and cytoskeletal organelles are the major axonal components. Two types of axons are Golgi type 1, which are long myelinated axons carrying nervous impulses to distant neurons, and Golgi type 2, which are short unmyelinated axons connecting local neurons.

Synapses

The neurons communicate with each other at the synapses through chemical substances collectively referred to as *neurotransmitters* (Table 2.1). The contact between two neurons occurs at the axon of one neuron and the axon, dendrites, or soma of the other neuron. A neurotransmitter, released at the axonal terminal of a presynaptic neuron, exerts an excitatory or an inhibitory effect on a postsynaptic neuron or on an end organ (muscle, gland).

Pathology of the Neurons

The reactions of neurons to disease manifest in alterations in the size, shape, and staining properties of the

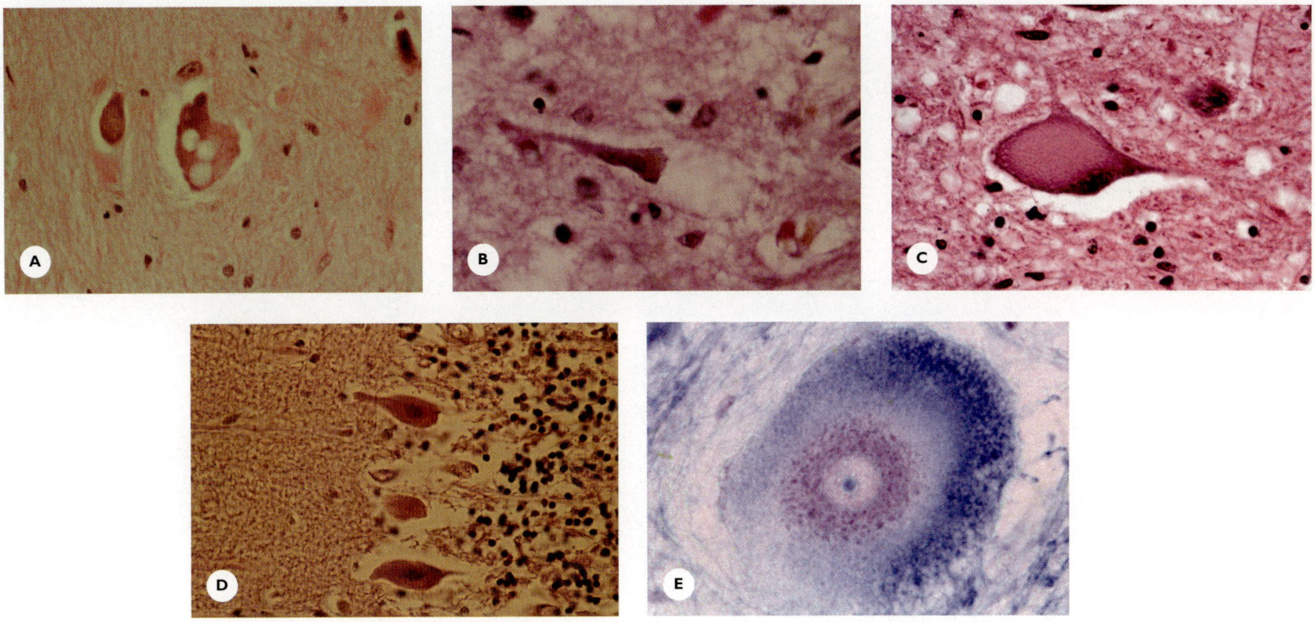

FIGURE 2.2
Neuronal alterations. **A.** Vacuolated swollen motor neuron in medulla. **B.** Chronic atrophy of pyramidal neuron: The perikaryon is shrunken, the dendrites are corkscrew-like, and the nucleus is densely basophilic. **C.** Axonal or retrograde changes in hypoglossal neuron caused by tumorous infiltration of the nerve roots. The swollen perikaryon is rounded, the dendrites are retracted, the Nissl bodies are partially dissolved, and remaining ones are clustered around the peripherally displaced nucleus (hematoxylin-eosin [HE] stain). **D.** Ischemic Purkinje cells in the cerebellar cortex showing eosinophilic shrunken perikaryons and homogenous basophilic nuclei (HE). **E.** Spinal motor storage neuron in Tay-Sachs disease; the cytoplasm is markedly distended and the nucleus displaced to the periphery (LFB-CV).

perikaryon and nucleus, and in reduction or loss of the Nissl bodies and dendrites. Some alterations are nonspecific, whereas others characterize particular diseases (Figs. 2.2 and 2.3; Table 2.2).

Acute Changes

Swelling, vacuolation of the perikaryon, dissolution of the Nissl bodies (chromatolysis), and shrinkage of the nucleus appear in a variety of acute infectious, toxic, vascular, and metabolic diseases.

Chronic Changes

Atrophic neurons with shrunken cell bodies, corkscrew-like dendrites, and shrunken and intensely basophilic nuclei are common in degenerative diseases.

Lipofuscin accumulation consists of small golden brown pigments that are deposited in the perikaryon of the neurons during normal aging.

Specific Neuronal Changes

Axonal or Retrograde Neuronal Changes

Axonal changes develop in response to a transection of their axon. The cytoplasm swells and becomes rounded with retracted dendrites. The Nissl bodies partially dissolve and some of the remaining Nissl bodies surround the eccentrically displaced nucleus.

Hypoxic-Ischemic Changes (Red Neurons)

The shrunken perikaryon, partially or totally devoid of Nissl bodies, stains brightly red with eosin, and the pyknotic triangular- shaped nucleus stains uniformly blue with hematoxylin.

Ferrugination of the Neurons

Ferrugination in chronic ischemic-hypoxic lesions results from the deposition (incrustation) of basophilic calcium and iron granules on the dendrites and cytoplasm of dead neurons.

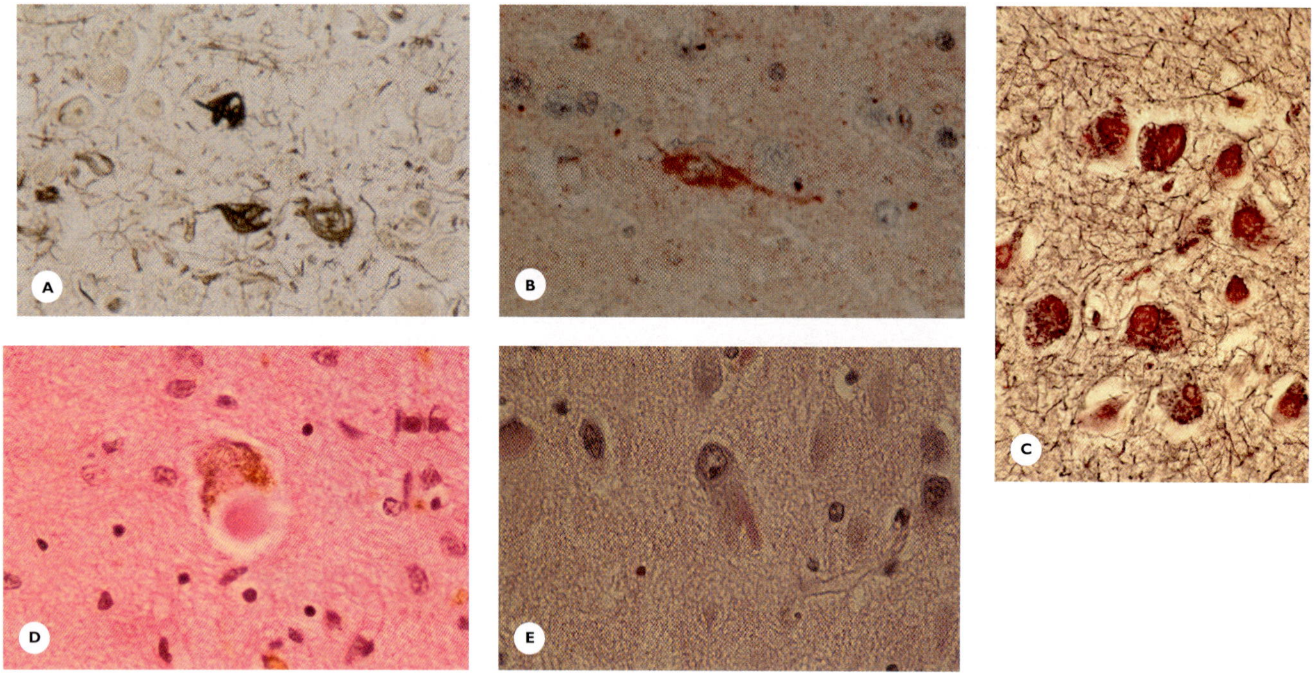

FIGURE 2.3
Neuronal inclusions. **A.** Neurofibrillary tangles in Alzheimer's disease (Gallyas silver stain), showing (**B**) positive immunostaining for tau protein, (**C**) Pick bodies in pyramidal neurons of hippocampus (Bodian silver stain), (**D**) Lewy body in substantia nigra in Parkinson's disease (HE), and (**E**) Hirano body in pyramidal neuron of hippocampus (HE).

TABLE 2.2.
Pathology of Neurons

Pathology of Neurons
Acute swelling, chromatolysis
Chronic atrophy
Axonal/retrograde reaction
Hypoxic-ischemic changes
Ferrugination
Distension in storage diseases
Ballooned achromasia
Granulovacuolar degeneration
Inclusion bodies
Degenerative
Viral
Neoplastic transformation

Distended Storage Neurons

Distended storage neurons in neurometabolic diseases are markedly swollen and pear-shaped, with the nucleus and the Nissl bodies displaced toward the apical dendrite. Histochemical stains reveal the composition of the substances stored within the perikaryon.

Ballooned Achromatic Neurons

Ballooned neurons seen in corticobasal dementia display enlarged palely stained perikaryon, a lack of Nissl bodies, and argyrophilic fibrillary structures.

Granulo-Vacuolar Degeneration

This degenerative change manifests small basophilic granules within vacuoles in the pyramidal neurons of the hippocampus. It is found both in Alzheimer's disease and normal aging.

Neuronal Inclusion Bodies in Degenerative Diseases

Neuronal cytoplasmic inclusion bodies are the distinguishing features of several important neurodegenerative diseases. Some are identified in hematoxylin-eosin (HE)–stained sections, others only in silver-stained sections, and still others with immunohistologic stains (see Fig. 2.3). The molecular components of these inclusions are identified using immunohistochemical stains. Some

TABLE 2.3.

Neuronal Cytoplasmic Inclusions in Degenerative Diseases

Inclusions	*Proteins*
Neurofibrillary tangle	Tau protein
Pick body	Tau protein
Lewy body	α-Synuclein
Hirano body	Actin
Bunina body	Cystatin C
Skein-like inclusions	Ubiquitin

TABLE 2.4.

Diseases with Neurofibrillary Tangles

Alzheimer's disease
Down's syndrome
Parkinson-Dementia-ALS complex of Guam
Progressive supranuclear palsy
Postencephalitic parkinsonism
Dementia pugilistica
Subacute sclerosing panencephalitis
Tuberous sclerosis
Niemann-Pick disease, type C
Gerstmann-Sträussler-Scheinker disease

inclusions immunoreact for tau, a microtubule-associated protein, others for α-synuclein, a synaptic protein, and still others for ubiquitin, a stress protein (Table 2.3).

Intranuclear inclusions derived from the proteins of polyglutamate tracts characterize trinucleotide repeat diseases.

Neurofibrillary tangles, a histologic hallmark of Alzheimer's disease, are argyrophilic torch- and basket-shaped or globose filamentous cytoplasmic structures that immunoreact for tau protein. They also are found in normal aging and in a variety of diseases (Table 2.4).

Pick bodies, histologic hallmarks of Pick's disease, are argyrophilic, round, homogenous structures in the swollen perikaryons of cortical and subcortical neurons. They immunoreact for tau protein.

Lewy bodies are eosinophilic, round inclusions in the melanin-containing neurons of the substantia nigra and locus ceruleus in idiopathic Parkinson's disease and in the cortical neurons of the diffuse Lewy body dementia. They immunoreact for α-synuclein and ubiquitin.

Hirano bodies are rod-shaped or ovoid eosinophilic structures within or adjacent to the pyramidal neurons of the hippocampus in Alzheimer's disease, and they are also found in normal aging. They immunoreact for actin.

Bunina bodies are small, eosinophilic granules in the cytoplasm of motor neurons in amyotrophic lateral sclerosis (ALS). They immunoreact for cystatin C.

Skein-like inclusions in ALS immunoreact for ubiquitin.

Lafora bodies in Lafora disease with myoclonus epilepsy are round, basophilic cytoplasmic inclusions containing polyglucosans that stain strongly with PAS reagent.

Neuronal Inclusions in Viral Infections

In viral diseases, the inclusions are commonly intranuclear, except that in rabies they occur in the cytoplasm of the Purkinje cells and the pyramidal neurons of the Ammon's horn.

Neoplastic Transformation

Transformation of the neurons into neurocytomas, neuroblastomas, and gangliogliomas are relatively rare but may occur from infancy to old age.

Pathology of the Dendrites

The *reduction and loss of dendritic processes* in cortical neurons occur in neurodegenerative diseases, chiefly in Alzheimer's disease, prion diseases, and HIV encephalitis.

Cactus formation refers to a focal enlargement of the dendrites of the Purkinje cells in Menkes kinky hair disease, storage diseases, and granular cell aplasia of the cerebellum.

Pathology of the Axons

Degeneration of the axons occurs in a number of diseases: traumatic, demyelinating, infectious, metabolic, and ischemic. The injured axons swell, become fusiform, and disintegrate into small argyrophilic fragments that are gradually removed by macrophages. Early degeneration of axons is readily detected with immunohistologic stain using antibodies against β-amyloid precursor protein (β-APP) (Fig. 2.4).The β-APP- immunoreactivity of damaged axons precedes changes observed in conventional histologic stain.

Axonal spheroids are round, homogenous, or slightly granular eosinophilic and argyrophilic structures commonly found in traumatic shearing injuries and at the edge of infarcts. They consist of axoplasm extruded from the disrupted ends of the axons (see Fig. 2.4).

Axonal torpedo, a fusiform enlargement of the proximal portion of the Purkinje cell axon, frequently occurs in cerebellar cortical degenerations (see Fig. 2.4).

Dystrophic axonal spheroids are distinctive histologic features of infantile neuroaxonal dystrophy. They also may occur in congenital biliary atresia, mucoviscidosis of children, and in nucleus gracilis of elderly subjects.

Death of the Neurons

Neurons die in one of two ways: through apoptosis or necrosis. *Apoptosis*, or programmed cell death, is genetically regulated and commonly occurs in degenerative diseases. During brain development, the apoptosis of excess neurons is physiologic. In apoptotic cell death, the nuclear chromatin condenses into masses of various sizes and shapes, the nuclear membrane buds and fragments. These nuclear buds, along with cytoplasmic buds, form the apoptotic bodies, which then are phagocytosed by macrophages or neighboring cells. An apoptotic cell in HE-stained section appears as a round, dense, strongly eosinophilic mass. Apoptosis occurs rapidly, usually affects individual neurons, and elicits no inflammatory response.

Necrosis is initiated by a variety of exogenous factors: toxins, infectious pathogens, metabolic disorders and, chiefly, by hypoxia and ischemia. The nucleus undergoes pyknosis, fragmentation, and lysis. The cytoplasm loses its organelles, becomes strongly eosinophilic and, ultimately, by enzymatic digestion, dissolves.

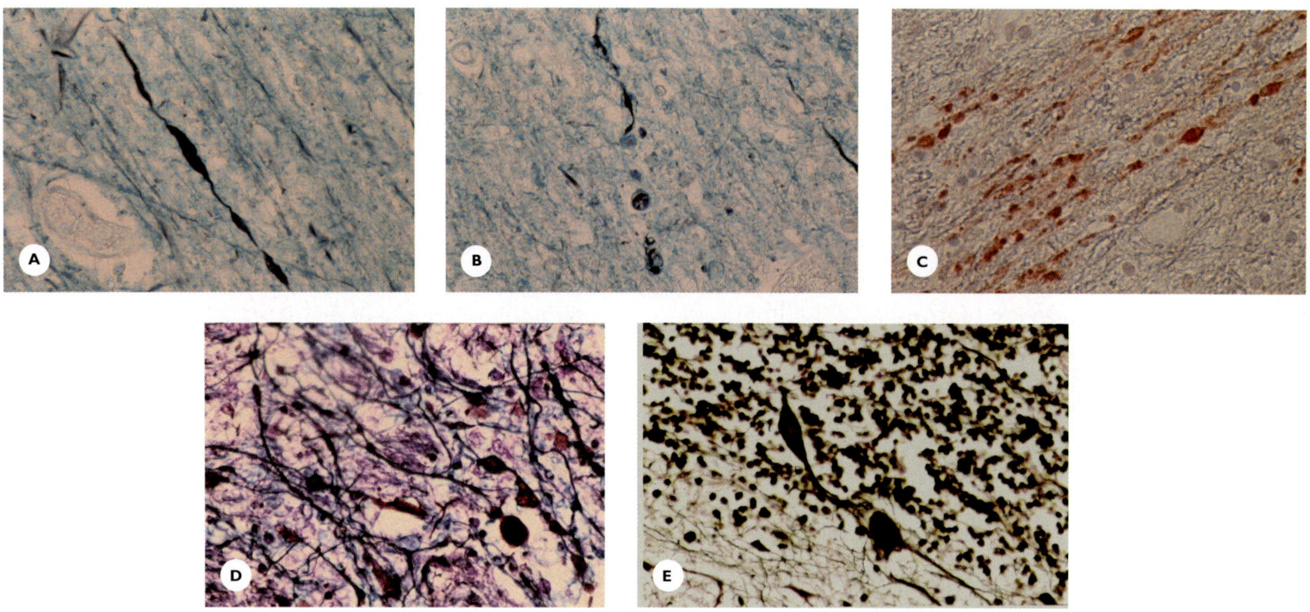

FIGURE 2.4
Axonal degeneration. (**A**) Fusiform swelling and (**B**) disintegration of axon into small argyrophilic fragments (Holmes stain). **C.** Beta-amyloid precursor protein (β-APP) immunoreaction of injured axons (immunostain). **D.** Axonal spheroids in traumatic injury (Holmes stain) **E.** Fusiform enlargement of the axon (torpedo) of a degenerated Purkinje cell (Bodian stain).

Necrosis usually affects a group of neurons and is accompanied by an inflammatory response.

Glial Cells

Astrocytes, oligodendrocytes, and ependymal cells originate, as do neurons, from the primitive neuroepithelium of the neural tube, whereas microglial cells originate from bone marrow–derived monocytes.

Glial cells play important roles in both physiologic and pathologic conditions:

- They maintain an environment appropriate for the efficient functioning of the neurons.
- They respond to diseases by removing tissue debris, repairing damaged tissue, and taking the place of lost tissue.
- They are specifically implicated in a number of degenerative, infectious, and metabolic diseases. By displaying cytoplasmic inclusions, glial cells are important in defining several neurodegenerative diseases. Infected glial cells are pathologic markers for certain viral diseases. Furthermore, glial changes are the diagnostic features of several metabolic diseases.
- Glial cells are capable of proliferating into a variety of gliomas, which constitute the largest group of primary intracranial tumors.

Astrocytes

The role of astrocytes begins during brain development, when the radial astrocytes guide the migrating neurons. After birth, the astrocytes are important in a number of physiologic processes: They provide support and nutrients to the neurons, protect them from excitotoxic neurotransmitters, contribute to the blood–brain barrier, and maintain homeostasis in the extracellular compartment.

Astrocytes are star-shaped. In HE-stained section, only the nucleus is visible; it is medium-sized, round or oval, with a moderate amount of chromatin and one or two nucleoli. Astrocytic processes and fibrils are visualized with specific stains. A longer process is attached to the capillary walls or the pial surface by a foot-plate. The fibrils contain glial fibrillary acidic protein (GFAP), an important astrocytic marker (Fig. 2.5).

The two types of astrocytes are protoplasmic and fibrillary. *Protoplasmic astrocytes*, predominantly in the cortex and subcortical gray structures, display shorter processes and less fibrils. *Fibrillary astrocytes*, predominantly in the white matter, contain abundant fibrils. In diseases, protoplasmic astrocytes may convert to fibrillary.

Pathology

The pathology of astrocytes is summarized in Table 2.5. *Swelling* is an early reaction to a variety of injuries,

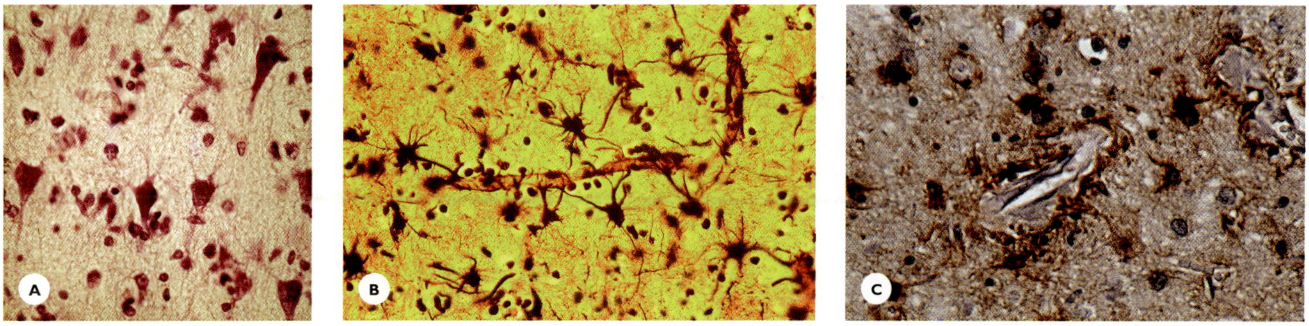

FIGURE 2.5

Astrocytes. **A.** Protoplasmic astrocytes. Cerebral cortex shows oval and round astrocytic nuclei with moderate amount of chromatin and prominent nucleoli (Cresyl violet). **B.** Fibrillary astrocytes display numerous short, fine processes and one long process attached to the capillary wall with a foot plate (Cajal gold stain). **C.** Positive immunostaining for glial fibrillary acidic protein (GFAP).

TABLE 2.5.
Pathology of Glial Cells

Astrocytes	*Oligodendrocytes*
Swelling	Swelling
Hypertrophy/hyperplasia	Satellitosis
Gemistocytic astrocytes	Inclusions
Fibrillary gliosis	Argyrophilic
Alzheimer type 1 and 2 glia	Viral
Rosenthal fibers	Neoplastic transformation
Corpora amylacea	
Inclusions	
Argyrophilic	
Viral	
Neoplastic transformation	
Ependymal glia	***Microglia***
Atrophy–tearing	Rod-shaped activated microglia
Granular ependymitis	Multinucleated giant cell
Viral inclusions	Macrophage
Neoplastic transformation	

chiefly hypoxia, and results from an influx of fluid and electrolytes into the cytoplasm (cellular edema). In histologic preparations, the swollen cytoplasm appears clear, and the nucleus is prominent.

Hypertrophy and hyperplasia. In acute and chronic diseases, astrocytes commonly increase in size and number. A *gemistocytic* or hypertrophied astrocyte displays a large, round cytoplasm with short fibrillated processes and a vesicular, eccentrically displaced nucleus. The cytoplasm stains intensely with eosin and immunoreacts strongly with GFAP (Fig. 2.6).

Fibrillary gliosis. Astrocytes are capable of replacing destroyed tissue by producing more and more fibrils and ultimately forming a dense fibrillary gliosis or *glial scar.* A glial scar is isomorphic when the astrocytic fibers conform to the pattern of the original structures, or is anisomorphic when the pattern is haphazard (see Fig. 2.6).

Alzheimer's type 1 and type 2 astrocytes. Alzheimer's type 2 astrocytes have large, round or lobulated vesicular nuclei with scanty chromatin condensed at the margin of well-defined nuclear membranes (see Fig. 2.6). They are characteristic findings in hepatic and other metabolic encephalopathies and Wilson disease, and are commonly found in the cerebral cortex, pallidum, and dentate nucleus. Alzheimer's type 1 astrocytes, also found in metabolic encephalopathies, have large lobulated nuclei and large slightly granular cytoplasms.

Rosenthal fibers. These alterations in astrocytic processes appear as homogenous oval, round, elongated, or carrot-shaped eosinophilic structures. They are found in the walls of cystic cavities, fibrillary gliosis, and astrocytic tumors, and are the diagnostic hallmark of Alexander's leukodystrophy (see Fig. 2.6).

Corpora amylacea. Corpora amylacea are the degenerative products of astrocytic processes. They are round, basophilic and argyrophilic structures, 20 to 50 microns in diameter. They commonly occur beneath the pia mater and around the ventricles and blood vessels. They contain polyglucosans, are PAS positive, and immunoreact for ubiquitin. Corpora amylacea are found in variable amounts in brains after the age of 40 to 45 years, and are particularly abundant in chronic degenerative diseases (see Fig. 2.6).

Cytoplasmic argyrophilic and tau positive inclusions. These features are characteristic of several neurodegenerative diseases collectively referred to as tauopathies (see Fig. 2.6).

Viral nuclear inclusions. These inclusions are found in herpes simplex encephalitis, subacute sclerosing panencephalitis, and in progressive multifocal leukoencephalopathy, in which the astrocytes are transformed into large atypical cells.

Neoplastic transformation. Astrocytes have the capacity to proliferate into a variety of relatively benign or malignant astrocytomas constituting the most common glial tumors.

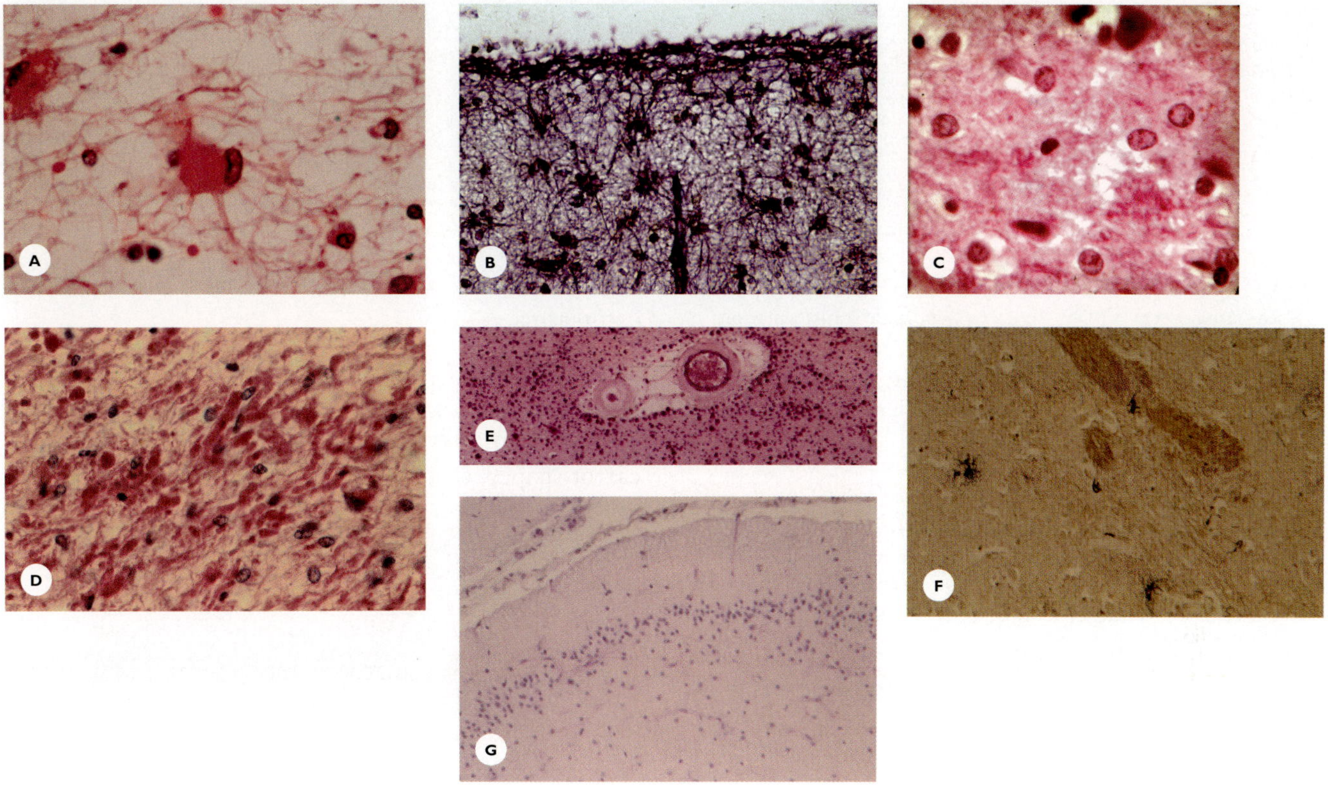

FIGURE 2.6
Pathology of astrocytes. **A.** Gemistocytic (reactive) astrocytes display a large eosinophilic glassy cytoplasm with short processes and a peripherally displaced nucleus (HE). **B.** Fibrillary astrogliosis beneath the pia mater. Fibrous astrocytes showing numerous fine fibrillated processes (Holzer stain). **C.** Alzheimer's type 2 astrocytes display a large vesicular nucleus with scanty chromatin and a prominent nucleolus (HE). **D.** Rosenthal fibers in an astrocytoma appear as eosinophilic rod-shaped, homogenous structures (HE). **E.** Corpora amylacea around blood vessels (HE). **F.** Argyrophilic astrocytic plaque in cortical basal degeneration (Gallyas). **G.** Bergmann astrocytes replace degenerated Purkinje cells in cerebellar cortex (HE).

Oligodendrocytes

In standard preparations, oligodendrocytes are recognized by their small, round, dark nuclei, rich in chromatin. The small perikaryons, with few and short processes, are visualized using silver stains. In the gray matter, oligodendrocytes serve as satellite cells around the neurons and regulate the perineuronal environment. In the white matter, oligodendrocytes are aligned along the myelin sheaths as interfascicular glia (Fig. 2.7). The major function of interfascicular oligodendrocytes is the formation of myelin during brain development and its maintenance thereafter. The myelin–oligodendrocyte entity plays an important role in autoimmune-mediated myelin diseases and in some viral diseases. Reactions of oligodendrocytes to injury are few.

Pathology

The pathology of oligodendrocytes is summarized in Table 2.5.

Swelling occurs in a variety of diseases, and it appears in HE-stained section as a clear halo of cytoplasm around the nucleus.

Satellitosis, an increase in number of satellite cells, indicates neuronal injury.

Cytoplasmic argyrophilic inclusions are markers of several neurodegenerative diseases. Cap-, flame-, or sickle-shaped inclusions are the histologic hallmarks of

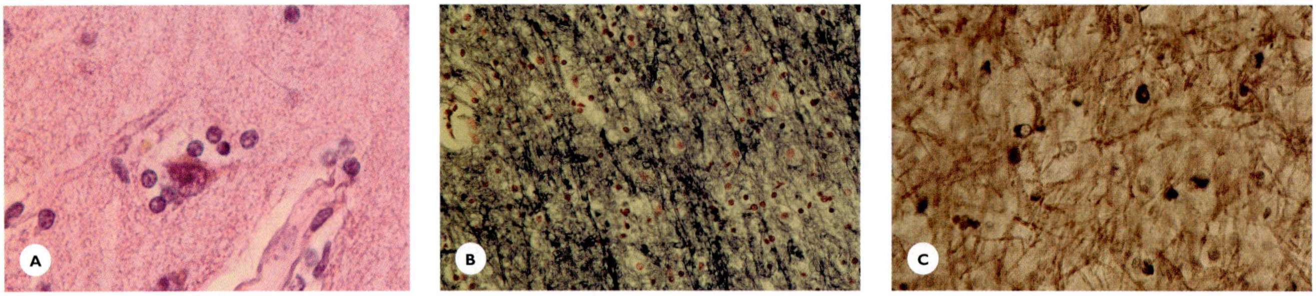

FIGURE 2.7
Oligodendrocytes. **A.** Satellite oligodendrocytes around cortical neurons (HE). **B.** Interfascicular oligodendrocytes along myelin sheaths (LFB-CV). Oligodendrocytes showing (C) argyrophilic cytoplasmic inclusions in multiple system atrophy (Gallyas stain).

multiple system atrophy (see Fig. 2.7). These inclusions are distinguished by positive immunostaining for ubiquitin, α-synuclein and α-β crystalline. Argyrophilic coiled bodies occur in progressive supranuclear palsy, corticobasal dementia, and argyrophilic grain dementia.

Viral nuclear inclusions in large, monster-like oligodendrocytes are characteristic of progressive multifocal leukoencephalopathy. They contain virions of JC virus of the papova virus group.

Neoplastic transformation. Oligodendrocytes commonly proliferate into slowly growing neoplasms.

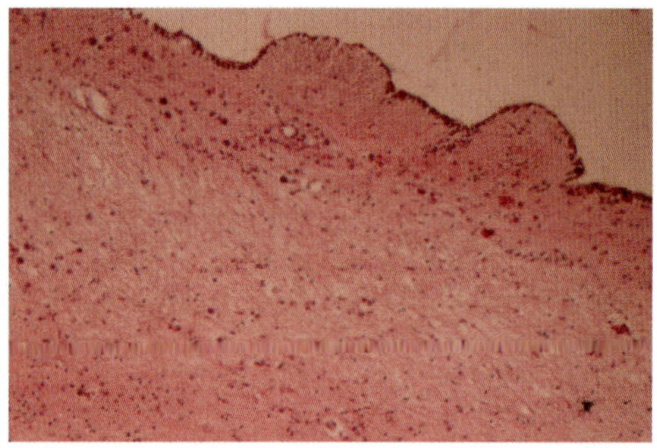

FIGURE 2.8
Ependymal glia. Cuboidal epithelial cells cover the ventricular surface and small nodules of proliferated astrocytes project into the ventricular lumen (granular ependymitis) (HE).

Ependymal Glia

Ependymal glia, columnar or cuboidal ciliated epithelial cells, line the surface of the ventricles and the spinal canal (Fig. 2.8). They react to a variety of pathologic insults.

Pathology

The pathology of ependymal glia is summarized in Table 2.5.

Atrophy, tearing, and *discontinuity* commonly occur in chronic hydrocephalus. *Ependymitis,* caused by a variety of pathogens, consists of necrosis, breaking up of the ependymal lining, and subependymal inflammatory infiltrations.

Subependymal gliosis, or *granular ependymitis,* develops in syphilitic and various other infectious, toxic, metabolic, and vascular diseases. Grossly, tiny nodules from the ventricular surface project into the lumen. Histologically, these nodules are proliferated subependymal fibrillary astrocytes. Some are covered with continuous or disrupted ependymal layer and others are denuded. Occasionally, these nodules may enlarge enough to obstruct the aqueduct of Sylvius and cause hydrocephalus (see Fig. 2.8).

Nuclear and cytoplasmic viral inclusions in enlarged ependymal cells are characteristic of cytomegalovirus infection.

Neoplastic Transformation

Ependymal cells are capable of proliferating into neoplasms that may grow into the parenchyma or project into the ventricle.

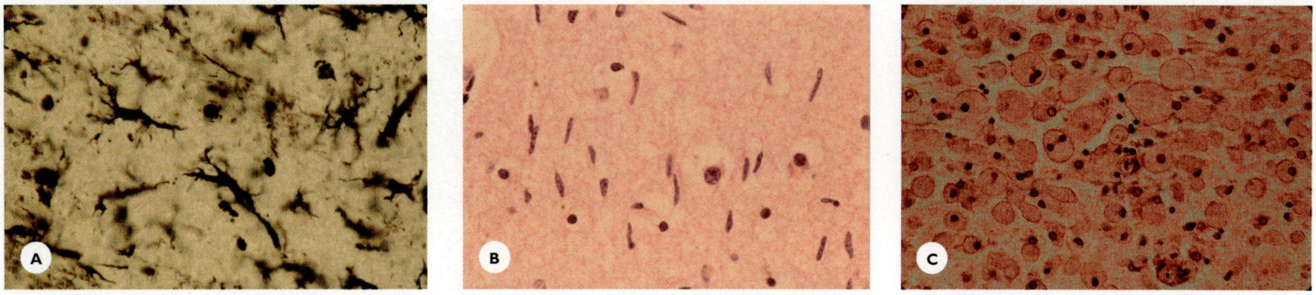

FIGURE 2.9
Microglia. **A.** Resting microglia showing small elongated nucleus, scanty cytoplasm, and bipolar processes (Hortega silver stain). **B.** Activated rod-shaped microglia in encephalitis. **C.** Macrophages showing large, round, foamy cytoplasms and small eccentric nuclei (HE).

Microglia

Microglial cells, derived from bone marrow monocytes, enter the nervous tissue during early brain development. They proliferate, migrate, and mature into resident or resting microglia. A major function of microglia is the surveillance of and participation in immunologic processes.

Resident microglia are distributed in gray and white matter around neurons as satellite cells and around blood vessels. Their small, round, or elongated nuclei are not readily recognizable in HE preparation. Silver stain discloses a triangular perikaryon with two or more branching processes (Fig. 2.9). Pathologic states rapidly activate the microglial cells, which then are easily identifiable.

Pathology

The pathology of microglial cells is summarized in Table 2.5.

Activated microglia. *Rod cells*, prominent in viral diseases and parenchymal neurosyphilis, are distinguished by conspicuously hypertrophied rod-shaped nuclei. They are diffusely distributed in gray and white matter and are almost perpendicularly oriented to the cortical surface (see Fig. 2.9). Rod-, crescent-, and kidney–shaped microglial cells occur around neuritic plaques in Alzheimer's disease.

Microglial nodules. Nodules commonly are found in viral diseases, in which they cluster around infected neurons, invade and digest them (neuronophagia), and eventually replace them with residual nodules. Loose collections of microglial cells (shrubs) are occasionally found in the molecular layer of the cerebellar cortex.

Multinucleated giant cells. These giant cells, derived from microglia and macrophages, are distinctive features of HIV encephalitis.

Macrophages. Macrophages with phagocytic activity are scavengers of the neural tissue. They are prominent in vascular infarcts, acute demyelinating diseases, leukodystrophies, hemorrhages, and traumatic lesions. Distinguished by large, rounded, foamy cytoplasms and small eccentric nuclei, the macrophages engulf and remove degraded myelin, necrotic tissue debris, and hemosiderin pigments (see Fig. 2.9).

Myelin

Myelin ensheathes the nerve fibers in a spiral lamellar fashion, promoting a faster and more effective conduction of nervous impulses along the nerve fibers. It is produced by the oligodendrocytes during development of the brain and spinal cord and maintained by them after completion of myelination (Fig. 2.10). The major chemical components of myelin are lipids, which constitute about 70% to 85%. The sphingolipids and cholesterol are the most important of these. The remaining 15% to 30% of myelin consists of proteins; among them, myelin basic protein, proteolipid protein, and

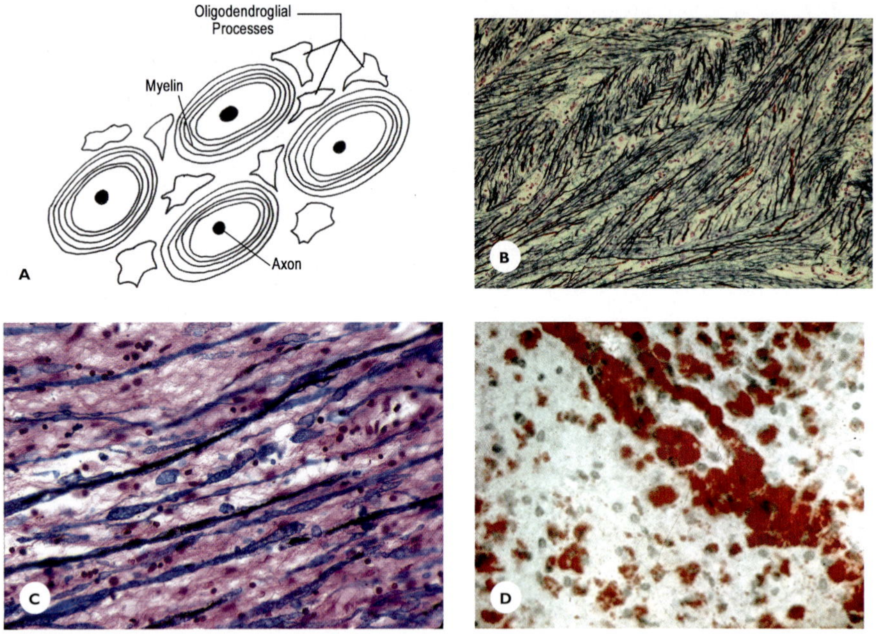

FIGURE 2.10
Myelin. **A.** Schematic drawing of axons, myelin sheaths, and oligodendrocytes. **B.** Light microscopic picture showing longitudinally oriented myelin sheaths (stained blue) along nerve fibers (stained black; Holmes stain). **C.** Swelling and breaking up of myelin sheaths (LFB-eosin). **D.** Disintegration of myelin into small oil-red O-positive lipid globules.

TABLE 2.6.
Chemical Composition of Central Myelin

Lipids 70%–85%
Sphingolipids:
Sphingomyelin: phospholipid
Cerebroside: glycolipid (galactose)
Sulfatide: cerebroside sulfate ester
Cholesterol
Proteins 15%–30%
Myelin basic protein
Myelin proteolipid protein
Myelin-associated glycoprotein
Myelin oligodendrocyte-glycoprotein

myelin oligodendrocyte-glycoprotein are particularly important because of their antigenic role in autoimmune diseases (Table 2.6).

Pathology

Degeneration

Myelin is primarily involved in immune- and virus-mediated diseases, hereditary and acquired metabolic diseases, and various toxic disorders. It is also affected in vascular, infectious, and traumatic disorders, and in wallerian degeneration of the axons. The pattern of myelin degeneration is the same regardless of the cause. The myelin sheath swells, becomes irregular, and breaks down first into larger, and then smaller and smaller globules, which contain cholesterol ester and triglycerides. These globules are phagocytosed and gradually removed by macrophages to the perivascular and subarachnoid spaces (see Fig. 2.10).

Meninges

The brain and spinal cord are covered with three membranes: (a) *the dura mater*, a thick outer fibrous membrane, containing large venous sinuses and separating the cranial cavity into a supratentorial and an infratentorial compartment; (b) *the arachnoid*, beneath the dura, a thin avascular membrane covered with mesothelial cells; the arachnoid villi (granulations) are tufts of arachnoidal (meningothelial) cells that project into the venous sinuses and veins; and (c) *the pia mater*, a thin, inner fibrous membrane attached to the surface of the brain and spinal cord and connected to the arachnoid by delicate fibrous trabeculae. The arachnoid and the pia together form the *leptomeninges*. Between them is the subarachnoid space, filled with cerebrospinal fluid (CSF). The CSF is absorbed into the venous sinuses at the arachnoid villi. The pia mater contains blood vessels, accompanying them into the neural parenchyma and forming the perivascular or Virchow-Robin spaces filled with CSF. The Virchow-Robin spaces usually end at the

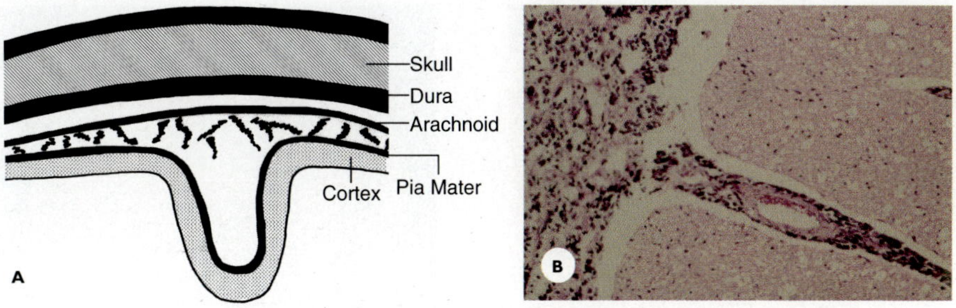

FIGURE 2.11
Meninges. **A.** Schematic drawing of the anatomic relationship between the dura, arachnoid, and pia. **B.** Leptomeningeal carcinomatosis extends into the cerebral cortex along the Virchow-Robin spaces (HE).

level of transition of arterioles to capillaries. They provide a route for the extension of inflammation or neoplasm from the subarachnoid space into the parenchyma (Fig. 2.11).

Pathology

The meninges are involved in traumatic, infectious, hemorrhagic, and neoplastic diseases. The epidural and the subdural spaces are common sites of traumatic hemorrhages. The subarachnoid space is the site of exudate from leptomeningeal inflammation, of hemorrhage from rupture of a berry aneurysm, and of neoplastic infiltration from primary or metastatic neoplasms. Postinflammatory and posthemorrhagic fibrosis of the leptomeninges and arachnoid villi interferes with the circulation and absorption of CSF, ultimately leading to hydrocephalus.

Blood Vessels

Vascular supply of the brain and the pathology of arteries are presented in Chapter 4. A few distinct features are mentioned here.

Cerebral arteries differ from systemic arteries by having only one elastic layer.

Capillaries are distinguished by the presence of (a) tight junctions between endothelial cells, (b) basement membrane, and (c) astrocytic foot-plates attached to the adventitia. These three features provide a barrier between the blood and the brain. This blood–brain barrier (BBB) can prevent harmful substances from reaching the nervous parenchyma, but it can also prevent therapeutic agents from crossing to the parenchyma.

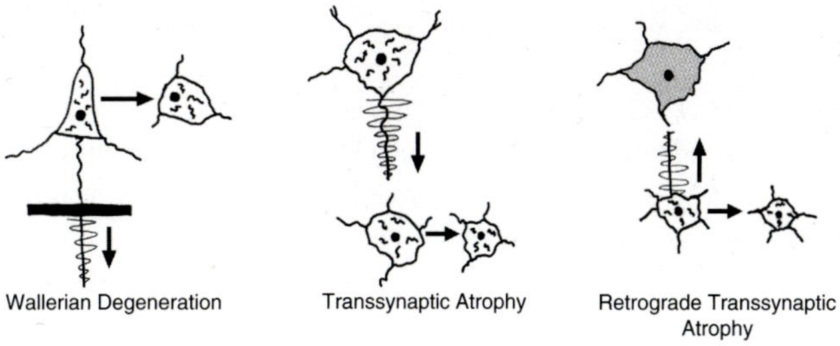

FIGURE 2.12
Types of degenerations in the central nervous system: schematic drawing.

TYPES OF DEGENERATIONS IN THE CENTRAL NERVOUS SYSTEM

Anterograde Degeneration

Anterograde (wallerian) degeneration results from transection of the axons commonly by infarcts, hemorrhages, tumors, and trauma. Distal to the injury, first the axons break down into small argyrophilic fragments, then their myelin sheaths break down into neutral lipid globules. The neurons of the injured axons undergo retrograde degeneration: The cytoplasm swells, the dendrites retract, the Nissl bodies dissolve, and the nucleus is peripherally displaced (Figs. 2.12 through 2.14).

Trans-Synaptic Degeneration

In trans-synaptic degeneration or transneuronal atrophy, those neurons that lose their chief or only afferent connection (that is, their synaptic input) atrophy. Particular sites of trans-synaptic neuronal atrophy are (a) the lateral geniculate bodies following degeneration of the ganglion cells of the retina, optic nerve, or optic tract;

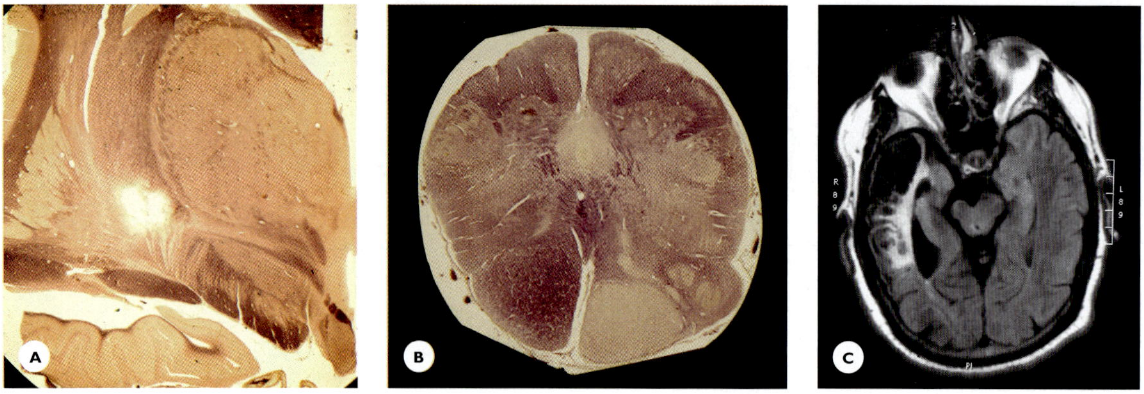

FIGURE 2.13
Anterograde or Wallerian degeneration. **A.** Lacunar infarct in the internal capsule. **B.** Degeneration of the ipsilateral pyramidal tract in the medulla (myelin stain). **C.** MRI of a 68-year-old man showing an old infarct in distribution of middle cerebral artery. Note the atrophy of the ipsilateral pedunculus due to wallerian degeneration of the descending corticopontine and pyramidal tracts.

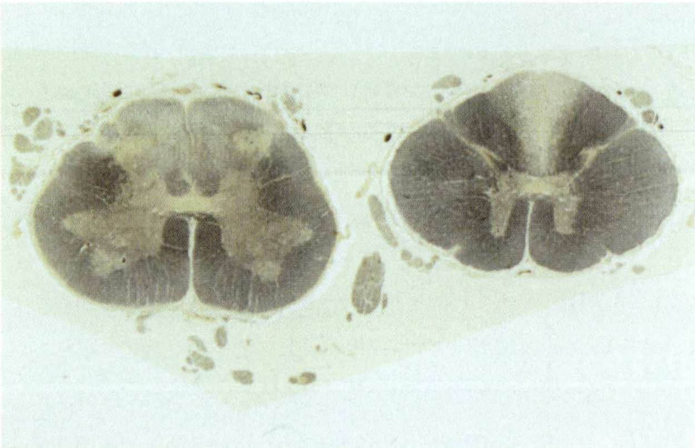

FIGURE 2.14
Wallerian degeneration. Degeneration of the fasciculus gracilis from compression of the sensory nerve roots by a metastatic carcinoma in the lumbar spine (myelin stain).

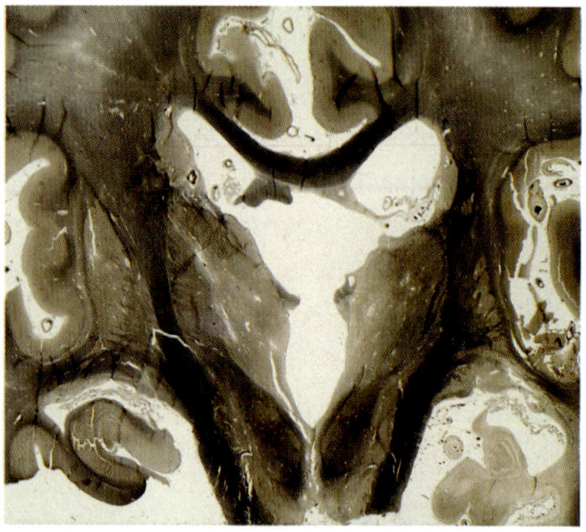

FIGURE 2.15
Trans-synaptic atrophy of the mammillary body. A 58-year-old known hypertensive man suffered a stroke 7 years prior to his death. **A.** Transverse section reveals a large infarct in the right Ammon horn, hippocampus, and fusiform gyrus. The right fornix, the most prominent efferent connection to the mammillary body, is degenerated (wallerian degeneration). The right mammillary body, not included in the picture, is severely atrophic (trans-synaptic atrophy; myelin stain).

(b) the mammillary body following degeneration of the fornix (Fig. 2.15); and (c) the neurons of the gracile and cuneate nuclei of the medulla following degeneration of the posterior columns in the spinal cord.

Retrograde Trans-Synaptic Degeneration

Retrograde trans-synaptic degeneration develops in those neurons that project to neurons that have already degenerated. For example, the neurons of the inferior olivary nuclei atrophy when the Purkinje cells in the contralateral cerebellar cortex have degenerated.

Dying-Back Degeneration

Degeneration of the axons begins in their distal ends and progresses toward the neurons of their origin. It occurs in systemic degenerative diseases.

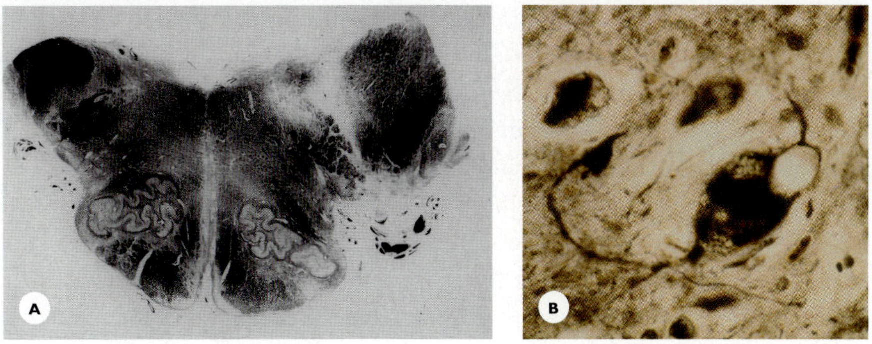

FIGURE 2.16
Pseudohypertrophic degeneration of the inferior olivary nuclei in a 45-year-old man with bilateral palatal myoclonus and a large malignant glioma infiltrating the dentate nuclei and the upper midbrain. **A.** Medulla showing hypertrophy of both inferior olivary nuclei (myelin stain). **B.** The neurons are enlarged, their cytoplasms vacuolated, and the processes thickened and fragmented (Bodian stain).

Pseudohypertrophic Degeneration of the Inferior Olives

Pseudohypertrophic degeneration of the inferior olivary nucleus is a particular type of trans-synaptic degeneration (Fig. 2.16). It is associated with lesions either in the ipsilateral central tegmental tract or the contralateral dentate nucleus of the cerebellum. The olivary neurons enlarge and display cytoplasmic vacuoles, peripherally displaced nucleus, and thick, rich, dendritic arborization.

CEREBRAL EDEMA

Cerebral edema is the abnormal accumulation of fluid within brain tissue resulting in an *increase in brain volume*. Brain edema is always a serious, often life threatening complication of diverse conditions: expanding mass lesion, ischemic or hemorrhagic stroke, head injury, infection, and ischemic-hypoxic, metabolic, toxic, and hypertensive encephalopathies.

General Aspects

Intracranial pressure (ICP), the pressure of the CSF, remains within physiologic range (90 to 180 mm H_2O) as long as the volume of the brain, circulating blood, and CSF remain constant. An increase in brain volume initially is compensated for by a decrease in blood flow and CSF volume. When the edema persists and progresses, however, this compensatory mechanism fails; subsequently, the intracranial pressure rises. When it exceeds 200 mm H_2O, clinical symptoms develop: headache, nausea, vomiting, altered mentation, visual impairment, and papilledema. A computed tomography (CT) scan readily reveals the edema, showing obliteration of the sulci and cisterns, hypodensity of the white matter with fingerlike projections, and compression of the ventricles.

As the brain volume continues to increase, hippocampal and cerebellar tonsillar herniations with brainstem and medullary compressions occur. When the intracranial pressure reaches the level of the systemic blood pressure, the circulation ceases and death occurs.

Types of Edema

Three types of edema are vasogenic, cellular, and interstitial. *Vasogenic edema*, the most common, is generally associated with mass lesion, infarction, hematoma, and traumatic and inflammatory lesions. The edema, generalized or focal, results from a breakdown of the blood–brain barrier and escape of fluid and protein into the intercellular space, chiefly into the white matter.

Cellular (cytotoxic) edema results from an accumulation of fluid in the cytoplasm of the neurons, glial cells, and capillary endothelium, which swell and may suffer irreparable damage. Cellular edema develops in a wide range of disorders: ischemic-hypoxic states, hypo-osmolality states associated with dilutional hyponatremia, inappropriate antidiuretic hormone secretion, osmotic dysequilibrium syndrome of hemodialysis, head injuries, diabetic ketoacidosis, and Reye syndrome.

Interstitial edema is associated with chronic hydrocephalus. Fluid infiltrates the periventricular white matter around the frontal and occipital horns through a disrupted ependymal layer.

CEREBRAL CHANGES ASSOCIATED WITH INTRACRANIAL EXPANDING MASS LESIONS

Vasogenic Edema

Intracranial expanding mass lesions, such as neoplasms, abscesses, granulomas, and hematomas, induce a vasogenic edema, which, if not resolved, leads to herniations, vascular lesions, and bony erosions (Table 2.7). Herniations and vascular lesions are particularly important, because they create serious clinical situations, and death can ensue. Initially, the edema surrounds the mass lesion then gradually propagates further along the fiber tracts, ultimately becoming generalized. The severity of edema is usually proportional to the rate of growth of the mass: It is most extensive around fast-growing lesions.

Pathology

Grossly, the edematous brain is voluminous and heavy. The convolutions are broadened and flattened, and the sulci are shallow or obliterated (Fig. 2.17). On cut sections, the edematous white matter is soft and yellowish. The ventricle adjacent to the mass lesion is compressed and, in severe edema, the midline is shifted to the opposite side (see Fig. 2.17).

TABLE 2.7.

Pathologic Consequences of Intracranial Expanding Mass Lesions

Herniations	*Vascular Lesions*
Transtentorial uncal/ hippocampal	Infarcts
	Mesiotemporal
Central	Occipital
Cerebellar tonsillar	Frontal
Cerebellar transtentorial	Superior cerebellar
Subfalcial cingular	Brainstem hemorrhage
	Pituitary necrosis
Bony Erosion	
Dorsum sellae	
Post clinoid process	

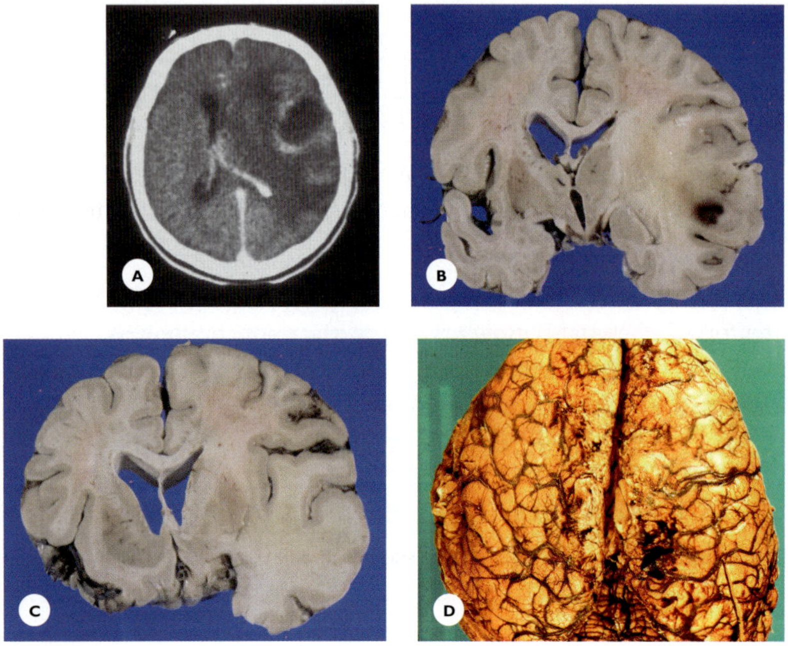

FIGURE 2.17
Cerebral edema. **A.** CT scan showing massive edema and mass effect around a malignant neoplasm with ring-like enhancement. The ipsilateral ventricle is obliterated. B and **C.** Focal swelling of the white matter around a large temporal lobe glioblastoma: The ipsilateral ventricle is compressed and the third ventricle is shifted to the opposite side. **D.** Generalized edema associated with a large temporal lobe glioma. Dorsal view shows diffuse enlargement, broadened convolutions, and obliterated sulci.

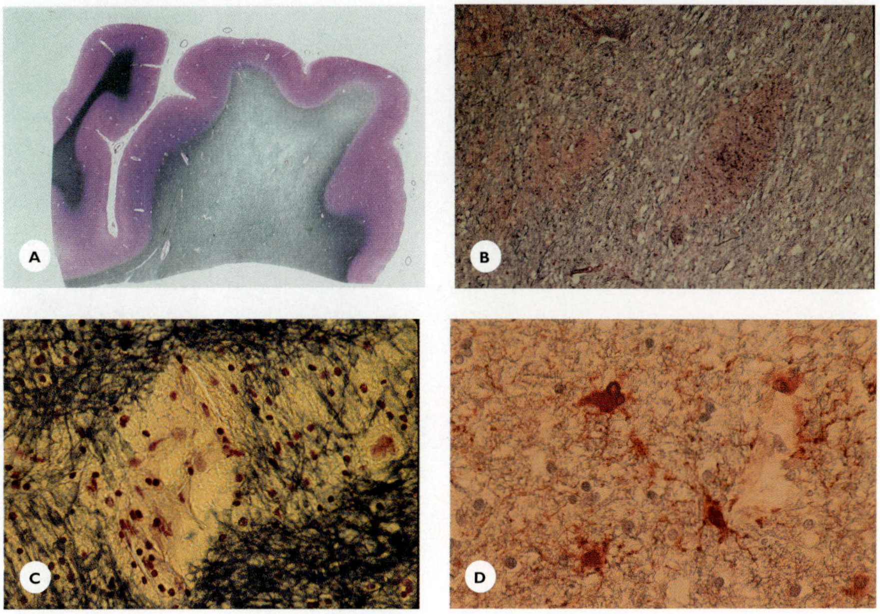

FIGURE 2.18
Histology of vasogenic edema. **A.** Macrosection of the hemispheric white matter shows loss of affinity of myelin for Luxol fast blue. The arcuate fibers are relatively preserved. **B.** Extravasated plasma infiltrates the white matter and the pericapillary spaces. **C.** The white matter is vacuolated and spongy, and the myelin sheaths are separated from each other and are broken up (LFB-CV). **D.** Hypertrophied GFAP-positive astrocytes are noted in spaces between the myelin sheaths (immunostains).

Histologically, the edematous white matter stains pale with Luxol fast blue, except for the arcuate fibers, which are relatively well preserved. Lakes of sera fill the pericapillary spaces (Fig. 2.18). The myelin sheaths are swollen, beaded, and separated from each other. Hypertrophied astrocytes and a few macrophages are scattered in the spaces between them.

Herniations

The infant's cranium is expandable; separation of the sutures and enlargement of the head compensate for increasing brain volume. Because the adult's cranium has rigid bony walls, a gradual increase in brain volume displaces certain structures from one compartment into another (Fig. 2.19; see also Table 2.7).

Transtentorial Uncal and Hippocampal Herniation

A hemispheric mass lesion displaces the uncus and all or part of the hippocampus through the tentorial opening. Subsequently, the oculomotor nerve-roots are pressed against the rigid tentorial edge or the petroclinoid ligament. The rostral brainstem with the aqueduct is compressed and displaced to the opposite side. This displacement allows the tentorial edge to lacerate the pyramidal fibers in the opposite pedunculus, producing the Kernohan's notch (see the section Localizing Features).

Central Herniation

Bilateral anterior hemispheric or centrally situated mass lesions displace the diencephalon and/or upper midbrain downward into the tentorial opening.

Cerebellar Tonsillar Herniation

A mass lesion in the posterior fossa or in the supratentorial compartment thrusts the cerebellar tonsils downward through the foramen magnum, compressing the medulla and obliterating the cisterna magna. The cerebellar tonsils then may undergo necrosis.

Cerebellar Transtentorial Herniation

A posterior fossa mass lesion displaces the superior vermis and hemispheres upward through the tentorial opening.

Subfalcial Herniation

A frontocentral mass lesion displaces the cingular gyrus under the falx.

Vascular Lesions

Herniations, by pressing the cerebral arteries against the surrounding structures, produce pale or hemorrhagic infarcts (Fig. 2.20; see also Table 2.7).

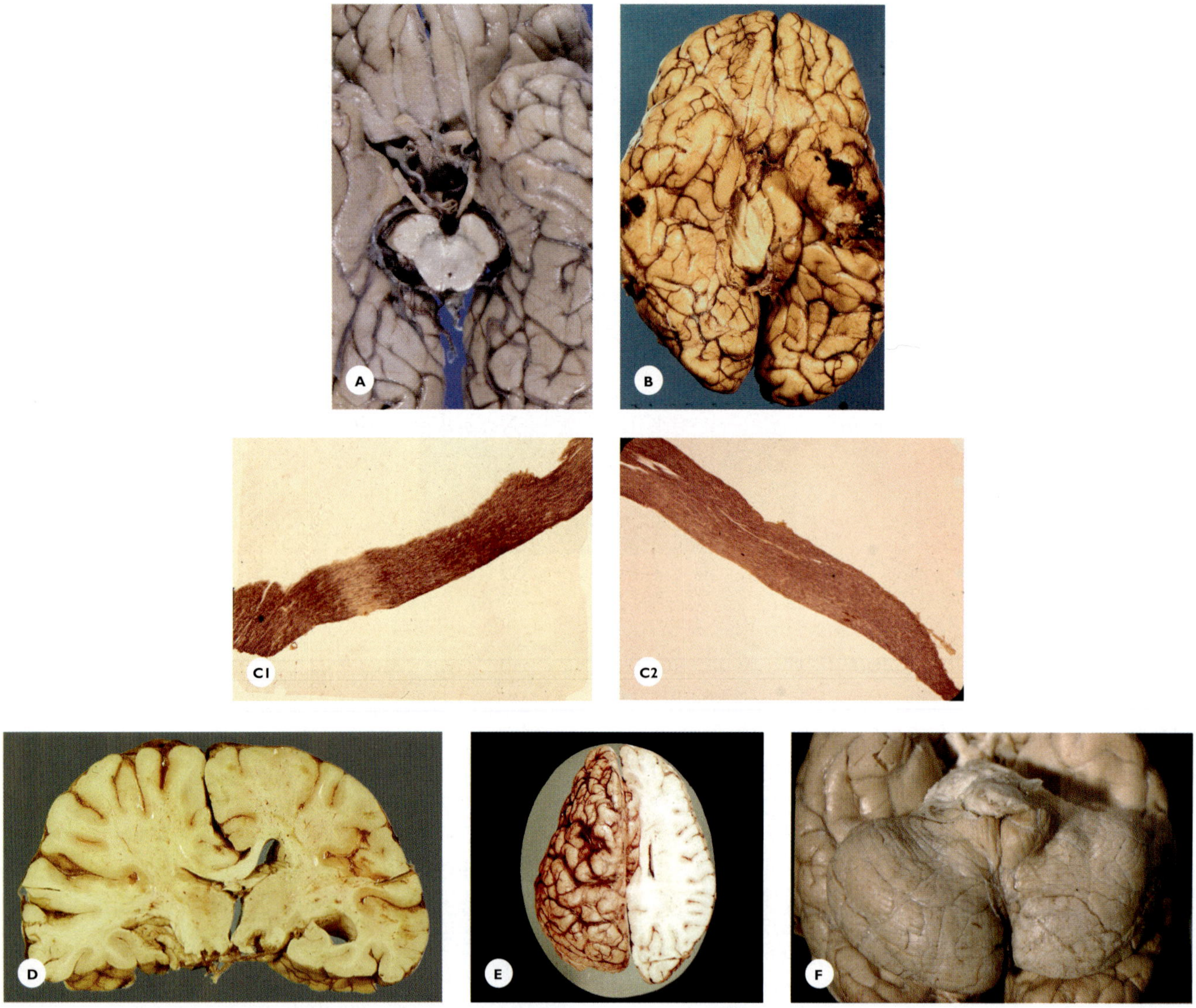

FIGURE 2.19

Types of cerebral herniations. **A.** Anatomic specimen showing the structures in the tentorial opening. Note the relationship between the midbrain, oculomotor nerves, posterior cerebral arteries, uncus, and parahippocampal gyrus. **B.** Transtentorial herniation of the left uncus and parahippocampal gyrus in an acute subdural hematoma. Note the deep groove around the herniated gyri caused by the rigid tentorial edge. The midbrain and the aqueduct are compressed and displaced to the right. **C1.** A transverse band of pallor in the myelin-stained left oculomotor nerve likely corresponds to the site of compression against the tentorial edge. **C2.** The right oculomotor nerve is normal. **D.** Right peduncular notch associated with a left temporal mass lesion. Displacement of the midbrain to the right pressed the pedunculus against the tentorial edge, which resulted in a notch (Kernohan's notch). Note also the herniation of the cingular gyrus and compression of the ventricle. **E.** Subfalcial herniation. Dorsal view of herniated cingular gyrus associated with a frontal mass lesion. **F.** Cerebellar tonsillar herniation associated with a hemispheric carcinoma metastasis. Note the deep groove around the tonsils caused by their downward thrust through the foramen magnum.

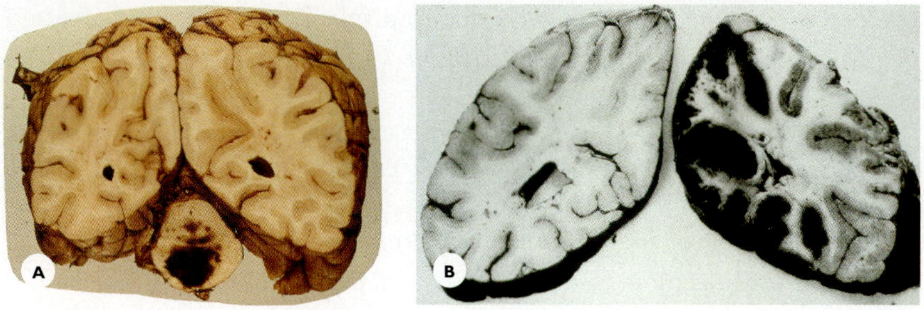

FIGURE 2.20
Vascular lesions associated with mass lesions and raised intracranial pressure. **A.** Massive pontine hemorrhage (Düret hemorrhage). **B.** Occipital hemorrhagic infarct.

Mesial temporal and occipital infarct results when the herniated hippocampus compresses the posterior cerebral artery against the tentorial edge.

Anterior cerebral artery infarct occurs with the subfalcial herniation of the cingulum, when the artery is pressed against the rigid falx.

Superior cerebellar infarct occurs in upward cerebellar herniation and results from compression of the artery against the tentorial edge.

Brainstem hemorrhage (Düret hemorrhage) occurs when displacement of the brainstem stretches, angulates, or tears the branches of the basilar artery, thus leading to multiple confluent petechial hemorrhages. Hemorrhages also can result from impairment of venous drainage into the vein of Galen.

Pituitary necrosis results from the impairment of circulation in the hypophyseal portal blood vessels.

Bony erosions result from long-standing edema. Common sites are the dorsum sellae and the posterior clinoid process.

CLINICAL MANIFESTATIONS OF INTRACRANIAL EXPANDING MASS LESIONS AND RISING INTRACRANIAL PRESSURE

Intracranial expanding lesions and a rising intracranial pressure produce characteristic symptoms and signs; some provide important diagnostic clues and others warn of a deteriorating and life threatening situation. They are divided into (a) general features, (b) localizing features, and (c) signs of herniations.

General Features

Headaches, variable in nature, present often at night or on awakening. Intermittent at onset, they gradually increase in frequency, severity, and duration. They often are localized to the vicinity of the mass lesion, but with rising intracranial pressure, become more diffuse.

Nausea and vomiting occur with or without headaches and are more common with posterior fossa mass lesions.

Seizures, partial or generalized, may be the presenting symptom and, for months or even years, the only manifestations of a slow-growing mass.

Papilledema is the most important diagnostic sign of increased intracranial pressure, but is not always present. It presents with a gradual decrease of visual acuity, constriction of the visual field, and enlargement of the blind spot.

Alteration in level of alertness, progressing from lethargy and obtundation to stupor and coma, indicates rising intracranial pressure and is usually associated with signs of herniation.

Mental symptoms are manifold; decline of cognitive functions, loss of spontaneity and initiative, affective disorders, behavioral changes, hallucinations and, occasionally, psychotic behavior have been associated with mass lesions. Some relate to rising intracranial pressure and others are reactions of the personality to an impaired cerebral function.

Localizing Features

Neurologic symptoms and signs indicate the location of the lesions.

Psychiatric symptoms of localizing significance are most likely associated with lesions in the frontal lobe and temporomesial region.

A *false localizing sign* is a hemiparesis on the side of a hemispheric mass lesion, which results from a contralateral peduncular notch associated with hippocampal herniation.

Isolated abducens nerve palsy due to displacement of the brainstem and stretching of the nerve roots has no localizing significance.

Signs of Herniations

Transtentorial uncal-hippocampal herniation manifests with ipsilateral occulomotor nerve palsy, dilated pupil, nonreactive to light, and ptosis.

Central diencephalic-rostral midbrain herniation manifests with small pupils, nonreactive to light and changing to midsize, respiratory changes, and decorticate posturing.

Cerebellar tonsillar herniation, or *pressure cone syndrome*, manifests with rising systolic and diastolic blood pressure, bradycardia, and irregular breathing, culminating in respiratory arrest.

Brainstem hemorrhage is a terminal event manifested by coma, small nonreactive pupils, bilateral pyramidal signs, and decerebrate posturing.

HYDROCEPHALUS

Hydrocephalus (Greek *hydros*, water and *cephaly*, head) denotes an excessive accumulation of the CSF that considerably enlarges the ventricles.

Hydrocephalus may result from (a) obstruction to CSF circulation, (b) overproduction of CSF, and (c) failure of CSF absorption at the arachnoid granulations (Table 2.8). Hydrocephalus is classified as obstructive, nonobstructive, and other.

Obstructive Hydrocephalus

Obstructive hydrocephalus is the most common type. Obstruction to CSF circulation may occur within the ventricles or within the subarachnoid space. If the obstruction is within the ventricles, the hydrocephalus is noncommunicating; that is, the ventricles do not communicate with the subarachnoid space. If the obstruction is within the subarachnoid space, the hydrocephalus is communicating.

Common causes of obstructive hydrocephalus are congenital malformations and acquired pathologic lesions.

Congenital Obstructive Hydrocephalus

Obstruction to CSF circulation commonly occurs at the aqueduct of Sylvius due to atresia or severe stenosis. Less often, the obstruction is at the outlet foramina of the fourth ventricle, as occurs in the Arnold-Chiari and the Dandy Walker malformations (see Chapter 12).

TABLE 2.8.
Hydrocephalus

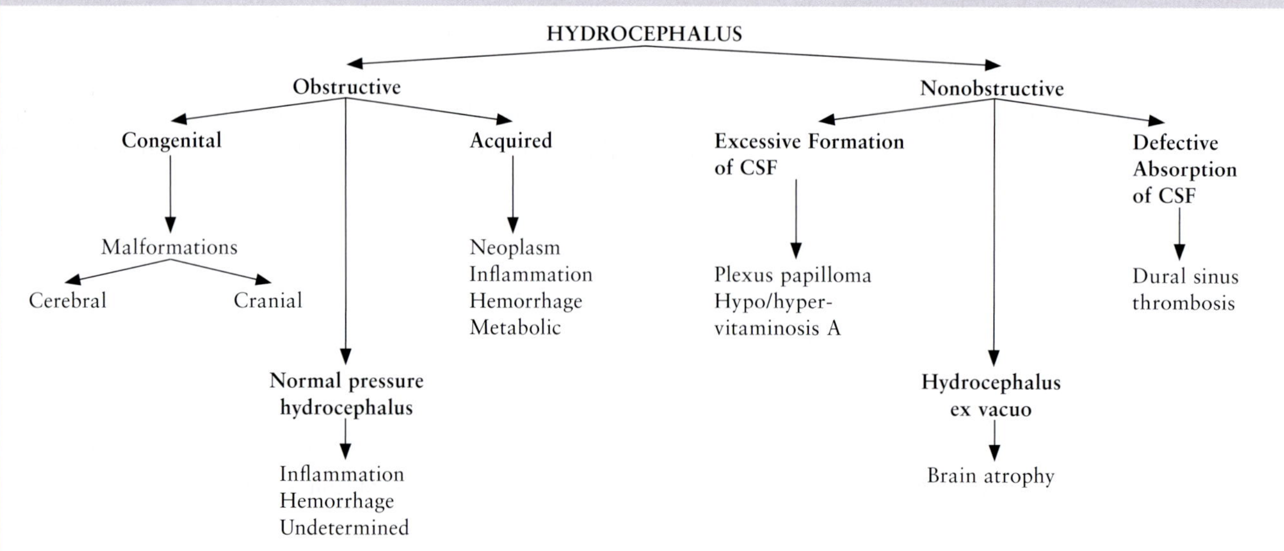

Acquired Obstructive Hydrocephalus

Acquired obstructive hydrocephalus may occur at any age and from various causes. Intracerebral mass lesions, especially tumors, may obstruct the flow of the CSF at any point within the ventricles. The ventricles dilate proximal to the block and remain of normal size distal to it. Acute obstruction within the subarachnoid space results from meningitis and subarachnoid hemorrhage. Chronic obstruction results from postinflammatory and posthemorrhagic fibrosis of the leptomeninges, neoplastic infiltration, and fibrous thickening of the leptomeninges in some neurometabolic diseases (e.g., mucopolysaccharidosis).

Nonobstructive Hydrocephalus

Nonobstructive hydrocephalus results from an overproduction of CSF by a choroid plexus papilloma or from failure of absorption at the arachnoid villi due to a thrombotic or neoplastic occlusion of the superior sagittal sinus.

Other Forms of Hydrocephalus

Normal Pressure Hydrocephalus

Normal pressure hydrocephalus (NPH), a particular form of obstructive hydrocephalus, is distinguished by a progressive enlargement of the ventricles without clinical evidence of raised intracranial pressure. The CSF flow is obstructed in the subarachnoid space or at the arachnoid villi. In a few cases, the history discloses previous head trauma, meningitis, or subarachnoid hemorrhage; however, in a large percentage of cases, no cause is evident.

Clinical Features

NPH occurs in individuals 60 to 70 years of age or older. The clinical criteria include the triad of progressive gait disorder, often the presenting symptom; dementia; and urinary incontinence. The gait disorder manifests with short shuffling steps and postural instability (frontal gait apraxia). The dementia has components of frontal lobe dysfunction: psychomotor slowing, loss of initiative, and apathy. Spasticity in the legs and the appearance of Babinski sign may develop due to stretching of the descending corticospinal fibers around the anterior horns. The clinical diagnosis is supported by magnetic resonance imaging (MRI), which shows markedly enlarged ventricles and a normal or variably obliterated subarachnoid space (Fig. 2.21). NPH is one of the few treatable causes of dementias, provided it is diagnosed early. The removal of a large quantity of CSF by lumbar puncture usually improves the gait. The improvement is considered a good prognostic sign and an indication for shunting the CSF from the lateral ventricle to the jugular vein or peritoneal cavity.

Pathologic Features

The leptomeninges appear normal or variably thickened. The ventricles are markedly enlarged. The ependymal lining often is disrupted, and the subependymal glia is proliferated. The cerebral cortex is normal or mildly atrophic.

Hydrocephalus Ex Vacuo

Hydrocephalus ex vacuo (passive hydrocephalus) results from a reduction of the brain volume, mostly of the hemispheric white matter. It commonly occurs in neurodegenerative diseases, hereditary metabolic diseases, chronic infectious diseases, chronic postanoxic encephalopathies, and following head injuries. On CT scan and MRI, the subarachnoid space is widened due to convolutional atrophy.

Grossly, the cerebral cortex is variably thin, and the white matter is reduced in amount. The lateral ventricles and the third ventricle are enlarged, whereas the aqueduct and fourth ventricle usually remain normal (see Fig. 2.21).

CEREBRAL CHANGES IN PHYSIOLOGIC AGING

Aging is an inescapable natural biologic process affecting all organ systems of the body. This process, regulated by genetic factors (longevity genes) and influenced by environmental factors, begins after age 50 to 60 years or later. Aging of the central nervous system primarily

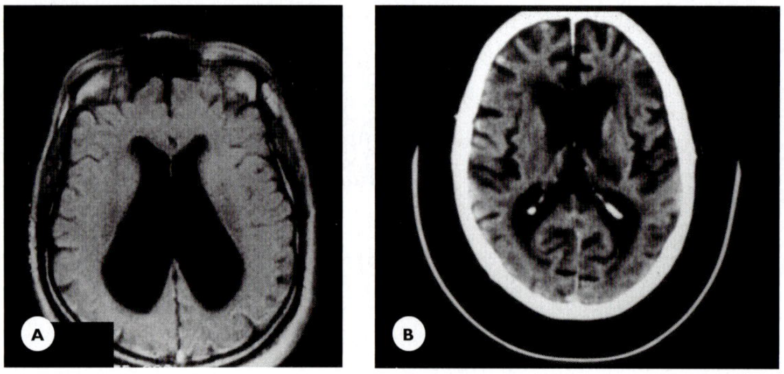

FIGURE 2.21
A. Normal pressure hydrocephalus in a 60-year-old man with "gait difficulties over the years" and memory decline. MRI shows enormously enlarged ventricles and only mildly enlarged subarachnoid space. **B.** Hydrocephalus ex vacuo in a 70-year-old demented patient. CT scan shows enlarged ventricles and significantly widened subarachnoid space.

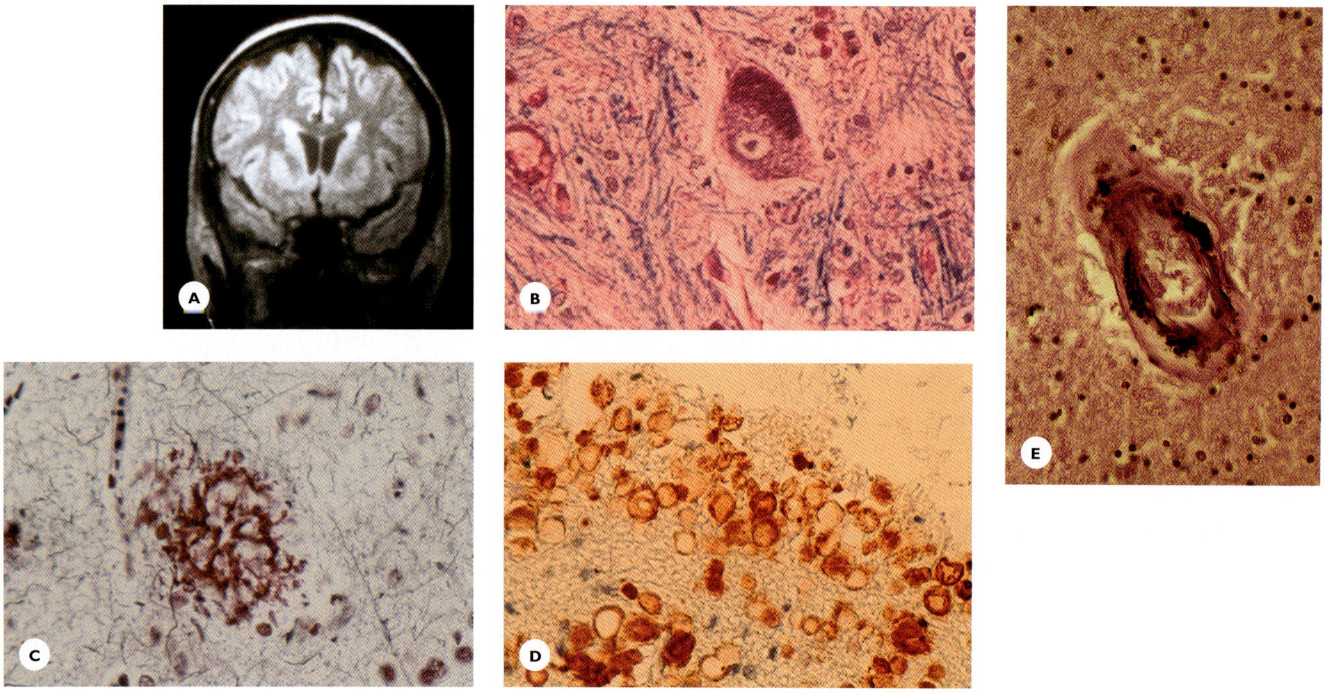

FIGURE 2.22
Cerebral changes in physiologic aging. **A.** MRI showing periventricular caps around the anterior horns. **B.** Lipofuscin accumulation in thalamic neuron in the brain of a 73-year-old man (HE). **C.** Neuritic plaque in hippocampus (Bodian stain). **D.** Abundance of corpora amylacea in the pia matter (immunostain for ubiquitin). **E.** Siderocalcinosis of small blood vessel in basal ganglia (HE).

manifests with cerebral atrophy—a reduction of brain volume. The morphologic changes are clinically undiscovered for some time. The appearance of neurologic decline, chiefly motor dysfunction, and of cognitive decline, chiefly memory impairment, varies greatly among individuals.

CT scan and MRI demonstrate the atrophy as a widening of the subarachnoid space and cisterns, reduction of hemispheric white matter, and enlargement of lateral ventricles. Frequent, incidental age-related findings are periventricular caps and rims corresponding to periventricular ischemic demyelination (Fig. 2.22).

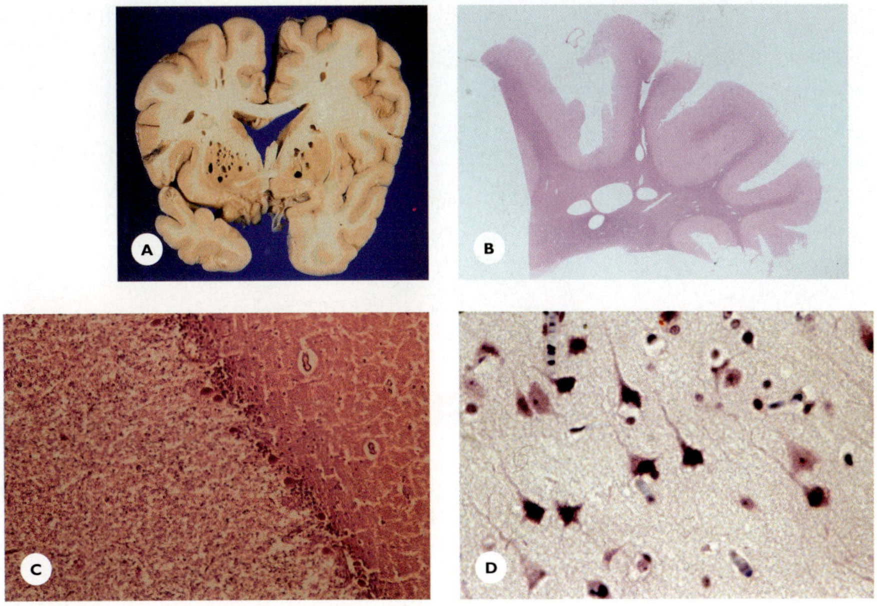

FIGURE 2.23
Cerebral artifacts. "Swiss cheese" brain showing **A.** multiple smooth-walled cavities, **B.** corresponding to empty holes lacking tissue reaction (HE). Artificial histologic changes. **C.** Dissolution of granule cells in cerebellar cortex. **D.** Spiky neurons in surgical specimen (HE).

The pathomechanism of cerebral aging is complex. Mitochondria play a central role in the aging process. With advancing age, the amount of mitochondria-derived free oxygen radicals increases, damaging cellular lipids and proteins and the mitochondrial DNA. This oxidative stress is not effectively countered due to a decline in antioxidant defense mechanisms. It is noteworthy that aging increases the risk for neurodegenerative diseases, vascular diseases, and malignancies, all leading causes of death in the elderly.

Pathology

Grossly, the brain volume diminishes by about 2% to 3% per decade after age 50, resulting in convolutional and white matter atrophy and enlargement of the subarachnoid space and lateral ventricles. The leptomeninges thicken, with prominent arachnoid granulations. Histologically, lipofuscin, a yellowish-brown pigment (the wear-and-tear pigment), accumulates in the perikaryon of the neurons. The neuronal density may be reduced in the hippocampus, the frontal cortex, and the cerebellum. The number of fibrous astrocytes and microglial cells increases. Corpora amylacea accumulate around the blood vessels and beneath the ependyma and pia mater. The pyramidal neurons of the hippocampus may display a small number of neuritic plaques, neurofibrillary tangles, granulovacuolar degeneration, and Hirano bodies (see Fig. 2.22). The spinal cord may display small, thin calcified plaques attached to the leptomeninges.

ARTIFICIAL CEREBRAL CHANGES

Artificial changes, gross and histologic, result from postmortem autolysis, insufficient fixation and prolonged histological processing. "Swiss cheese" changes are multiple smooth-walled cavities caused postmortem by gas-producing organisms. Tissue reactions are typically absent, and microorganisms may clog the lumens of small blood vessels (Fig. 2.23).

Among histologic changes, the dissolution of granular cells in the cerebellar cortex results from postmortem autolysis. Buscaino bodies—round, mucinous structures in the white matter—result from postmortem myelin degradation. Prolonged histologic processing shrinks the parenchyma, producing dilated perivascular and pericellular spaces. Dark, spiky neurons with corkscrew dendrites are seen at the edge of surgical specimens (see Fig. 2.23).

BIBLIOGRAPHY

Kurosinski, P., & Götz, J. (2002). Glial cells under physiologic and pathologic conditions. *Arch Neurol*, *59*, 1524–1528.

Ludwin, S. K. (1997). The pathobiology of the oligodendrocytes. *J Neuropath Exp Neurol*, *56*, 111–127.

Mattson, M. P. (2001). Molecular biology of the aging nervous system. In S. Duckett, J.C. De La Torre (Eds.), *Pathology of the aging human nervous system*, 2nd edition (pp. 16–41). New York: Oxford University Press.

Medana, I. M., & Esiri, M. M. (2003). Axonal damage: a key predictor of outcome in human CNS diseases. *Brain*, *126*, 515–530.

Norenberg, M. D. (1994). Astrocyte responses to CNS injury. *J Neuropath Exp Neurol*, *53*, 213–220.

Sarnat, H. B. (1995). Ependymal reactions to injury. A review. *J Neuropath Exp Neurol*, *54*, 1–15.

REVIEW QUESTIONS

1. Neurofibrillary tangles are encountered in:
   - A. Normal aging
   - B. Down syndrome
   - C. Postencephalitic parkinsonism
   - D. None of these
   - E. All of these

2. Lewy bodies are diagnostic of:
   - A. Amyotrophic lateral sclerosis
   - B. Idiopathic Parkinson's disease
   - C. Peroxisomal diseases
   - D. Progressive supranuclear palsy
   - E. Arteriosclerotic parkinsonism

3. Axonal spheroids:
   - A. Result from swelling of Golgi type 2 axons
   - B. Occur in hippocampus
   - C. Characterize viral diseases
   - D. Result from shearing injuries of axons
   - E. Are fixation artifacts

4. A glial scar is produced by:
   - A. Oligodendrocytes
   - B. Alzheimer's type 2 astrocytes
   - C. Fibrillary astrocytes
   - D. Rosenthal fibers
   - E. Schwann cells

5. The major function of oligodendrocytes is:
   - A. Phagocytosis of tissue debris
   - B. Replacement of lost tissue
   - C. Protection against bacterial invasion
   - D. Formation of blood–brain barrier
   - E. Formation of myelin

6. The term Wallerian degeneration in the CNS refers to:
   - A. Degeneration of axons beginning in their distal ends
   - B. Degeneration of axons and their myelin sheaths proximal to transection
   - C. Degeneration of axons and their myelin sheaths distal to transection
   - D. Degeneration of neurons that have lost their synaptic connections
   - E. Degeneration of neurons that project to denervated neurons

7. All of the following statements concerning vasogenic edema are correct *except*:
   - A. It is associated with dilutional hyponatremia.
   - B. It results from the breakdown of the blood–brain barrier.
   - C. It is associated with expanding mass lesions.
   - D. It causes herniations.
   - E. It affects chiefly the white matter.

8. Increased intracranial pressure associated with a mass lesion can cause all of the following *except*:
   - A. Cerebellar tonsillar herniation
   - B. Pituitary necrosis
   - C. Isolated abducens nerve palsy
   - D. Hydrocephalus ex-vacuo
   - E. Hippocampal herniation

9. If a 40-year-old woman, diagnosed with an acute right subdural hematoma, suddenly develops a right ptosis with a dilated pupil nonreactive to light, the most likely cause is:

   A. Acute hydrocephalus
   B. Occipital lobe infarct
   C. Laceration of ipsilateral pedunculus
   D. Laceration of contralateral pedunculus
   E. Transtentorial hippocampal herniation

10. All of the following statements concerning normal pressure hydrocephalus are correct *except*:

    A. It manifests with gait disorder.
    B. It can develop after purulent meningitis.
    C. It can complicate a subarachnoid hemorrhage.
    D. MRI shows normal ventricles and enlarged subarachnoid space.
    E. MRI shows large ventricles and normal or mildly enlarged subarachnoid space.

11. All of the following statements concerning cerebral changes in physiologic aging are correct *except*:

    A. Lipofuscin accumulates in the perikaryon of the neurons.
    B. A few cortical neurons display neurofibrillary tangles.
    C. Pyramidal neurons in hippocampus display Hirano bodies.
    D. Neurons of dentate gyrus display Pick bodies.
    E. A few neuritic plaques occur in the Ammon's horn.

12. Artificial cerebral changes include all of the following *except*:

    A. Dissolution of the granular cell layer in the cerebellar cortex
    B. Dilated pericellular spaces
    C. Spiky neurons
    D. "Swiss-cheese" brain
    E. Corpora amylacea

(Answers are provided in the Appendix.)

CHAPTER 3

Cerebral Hypoxia

Etiology
Pathology
Clinical Features
Permanent Global Ischemia: Brain Death
Cerebral Pathology in Chronic Epilepsy

Adequate oxygen (O_2) supply, approximately 6 mL/100 g/min for the gray matter and less for the white matter, is vital for normal functioning of the nervous tissue; insufficient O_2 supply leads to cerebral hypoxia.

ETIOLOGY

The major causes of cerebral hypoxia are (a) hypoxemia, (b) anemia, (c) histotoxicity, and (d) ischemia (stagnant cerebral blood flow).

Hypoxemic hypoxia develops when the blood oxygen tension falls below 40 mm Hg, which may occur in acute respiratory arrest, chronic obstructive pulmonary disease, alveolar hypoventilation, airway obstruction, near-drowning, diminished oxygen concentration in the air, weakness of respiratory muscles, and status epilepticus.

Anemic hypoxia develops when the oxygen-carrying hemoglobin falls to half its normal concentration, as occurs in severe blood loss and chronic anemia.

Histotoxic hypoxia is caused by toxic substances, such as carbon monoxide, cyanide, and sulfide, which prevent utilization of oxygen by the neural tissue.

Ischemic (stagnant) hypoxia develops when the blood flow falls below 18 mL/100 g tissue/min. This drop may be regional, confined to an arterial territory (see Chapter 4), or global, leading to generalized cerebral hypoperfusion. Global cerebral ischemia, transient or permanent, may occur in a variety of clinical settings: cardiac arrest, cardiac arrhythmias, sudden hypotension from myocardial infarct, and severe rise of intracranial pressure. Unlike in hypoxemic and anemic hypoxias, in ischemic hypoxia, the brain is deprived of all blood constituents, most importantly of glucose; moreover, the harmful metabolites such as lactic acid are not eliminated.

In certain clinical situations, different types of hypoxias are combined; in cardiopulmonary arrest ischemia and hypoxemia occur concurrently.

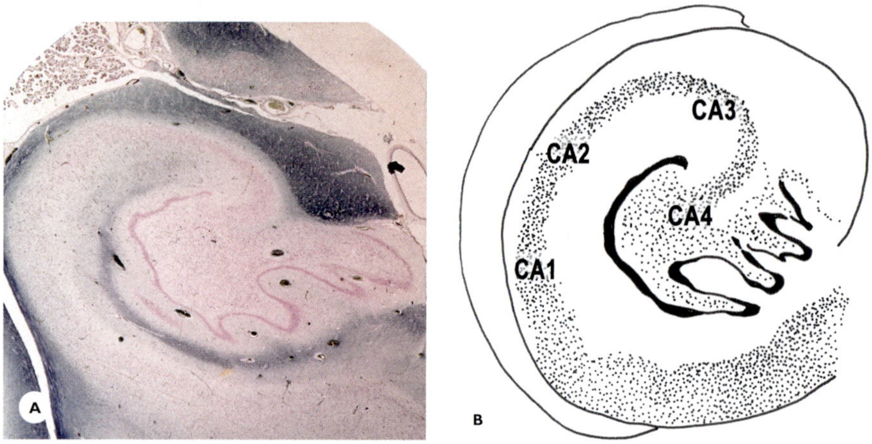

FIGURE 3.1
Ammon's horn (Cornu Ammonis CA) **A.** histologic section (LFB-CV). **B.** Schematic drawing showing the sections of CA.

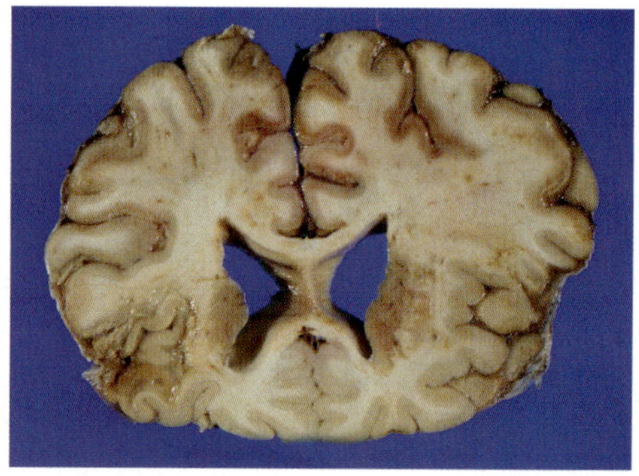

FIGURE 3.2
Acute ischemic–hypoxia. A few days' survival following myocardial infarct and cardiac arrest in a 62-year-old man. Coronal section shows patchy congestion in the cerebral cortex.

PATHOLOGY

General Aspects

The severity and extent of the pathologic process depends chiefly on the severity and duration of the hypoxic event, on the body temperature, and on the blood glucose concentration. Hyperglycemia aggravates the ischemic damage whereas hypothermia protects the brain.

The cerebral pathology is distinguished by (a) selective neuronal necrosis and (b) selective regional vulnerability.

In selective neuronal necrosis, a lack of oxygen from any cause affects first, and usually, only the neurons. Necrosis of the glial cells, axons, and myelin (pannecrosis) occurs in severe and protracted hypoxic-ischemic events.

Selective regional vulnerability determines the *anatomic distribution of* the lesions. Most vulnerable are the hippocampus, the neocortex, the cerebellar cortex, the thalamus, and the basal ganglia. The hypothalamus, the brainstem, and the spinal cord are the least vulnerable. In the hippocampus, the pyramidal neurons in the CA1 zone (Sommer's sector) are primarily affected (Fig. 3.1); in the neocortex, laminae 3, 5, and 6; in the cerebellum, the Purkinje cells;. in the thalamus, the anterior and dorsomedial nuclei; and, in the basal ganglia, the spiny neurons. Carbon monoxide poisoning has an affinity for the iron-rich globus pallidus and the reticular zone of the substantia nigra.

Gross features range from patchy congestions of gray structures in the very acute stage, through soft, spongy cortex in the subacute stage, to atrophic sclerotic cortex in the chronic stage. The deep gray structures and the hemispheric white matter are variably atrophic, and the ventricles are dilated in chronic cases (Figs 3.2. 3.5, 3.7, 3.8 and 3.9).

Histologic Features

Neuronal Necrosis

Red neurons, the histologic hallmarks of hypoxic-ischemic injuries, display bright eosinophilia of the perikaryon, loss of Nissl substance, and shrunken basophilic homogenous nucleus (Fig 3.3). Other neurons appear as ghost neurons, displaying faintly stained perikaryon and nucleus, or as dark neurons, displaying condensed, darkly stained perikaryon and corkscrew-

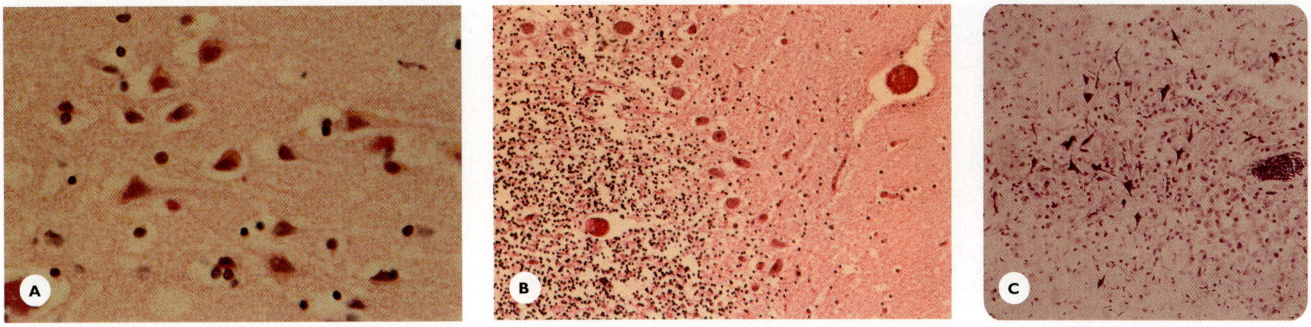

FIGURE 3.3
Hypoxic-ischemic neurons in (**A**) Ammon's horn and (**B**) cerebellar cortex. The perikaryon, shrunken and devoid of Nissl substance, stains intensely red. The condensed pyknotic nucleus stains deeply blue. **C.** Chronic mineralized (ferruginated) dead neurons in cerebral cortex, hematoxylin-eosin (HE).

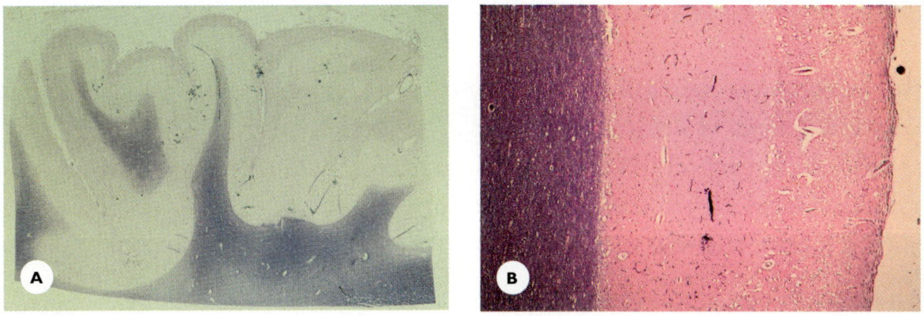

FIGURE 3.4
Acute cortical multilaminar necrosis (case in Fig 3.2). **A** and **B.** The faintly stained ischemic laminae are sharply demarcated from the relatively spared external laminae and are depleted of neurons and glial cells (LFB-HE; HE).

like dendrites. Irreversibly damaged neurons gradually disintegrate and disappear. Some remaining dead neurons become incrusted with calcium and iron salts (ferrugination) (Fig. 3.3). Death of the cortical neurons, particularly those in the hippocampus, may be delayed hours to days following a short episode of global ischemia. This delayed neuronal death, or maturation phenomenon, may account for a delay in a patient's deterioration, affording a short time for therapeutic intervention.

Cortical Laminar Neuronal Necrosis

Neuronal necrosis in the cerebral cortex typically occurs in a laminar fashion, seldom in multiple small foci. The neuronal necrosis may involve one or several laminae, or even the whole width of the cortex. With time, a dense astrocytic fibrillary gliosis forms at the site of lost neurons. In the cerebellum, Bergmann astrocytosis replaces the Purkinje cells.

Cortical Laminar Pan-Necrosis

A severe and prolonged hypoxic-ischemic insult affects not only the neurons but also the oligodendrocytes, the astrocytes, the myelin, and the axons, all of which undergo necrosis (infarction). This may occur in one or several laminae, or throughout the entire width of the cortex. The capillaries, least vulnerable to hypoxia, show prominent endothelial swelling and proliferation. Macrophages derived from microglial cells and blood monocytes gradually remove the tissue debris. Meanwhile, at the edge of the necrosis, the astrocytes proliferate into large gemistocytic astrocytes, separating the cortex from the healthy white matter. Ultimately, a loose mesoglial network replaces the cerebral cortex (see Figs. 3.4, 3.5, 3.7, and 3.8).

Hypoxic-Ischemic Leukoencephalopathy

Hypoxic-ischemic leukoencephalopathy, a rare condition, results from less severe but prolonged hypotension

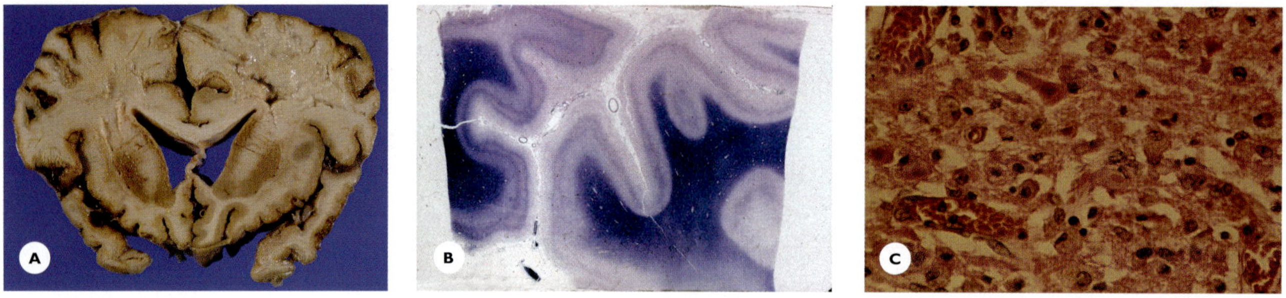

FIGURE 3.5
Subacute cortical pan-necrosis. A 52-year-old man survived 12 days in a coma following a cardiorespiratory arrest of approximately 28 minutes. **A.** Transverse section of cerebral hemispheres shows reddish-brown discoloration of the cerebral cortex and softening of the white matter. **B.** The cerebral cortex is outlined by a darkly stained outer and a faintly stained inner layer. **C.** The outer layer contains necrotic tissue densely packed with macrophages. A few ischemic neurons are entrapped among macrophages (HE).

and cerebral hypoperfusion. It is characterized by multiple small areas of demyelination in the cerebral hemispheric white matter (Fig. 3.6). Within these areas, axonal changes vary in severity, macrophages are absent, and astrocytic reaction is insignificant.

Pathomechanism of Hypoxic-Ischemic Neuronal Necrosis

Hypoxic-ischemic neurons die of the excitotoxic effects of the neurotransmitter glutamate and its analogs that accumulate in excess in ischemic tissue. These excitatory neurotransmitters depolarize the neuronal membrane, allowing excessive influx of sodium, chloride, water, and calcium into the neuronal compartment. Subsequent swelling, metabolic dysfunction, and disruption of the cellular membrane ultimately lead to the disintegration of the neurons.

Why neurons in certain regions are more vulnerable to hypoxia-ischemia than are those in other regions has not been elucidated fully. Regional differences in vascular architecture seem not to be a satisfactory explanation. Regional differences among neurons possessing specific receptors for locally released excitatory neurotransmitters are a more likely explanation. Hence, regions with the highest concentration of neurons that possess glutamate-sensitive receptors are the most vulnerable to hypoxia-ischemia.

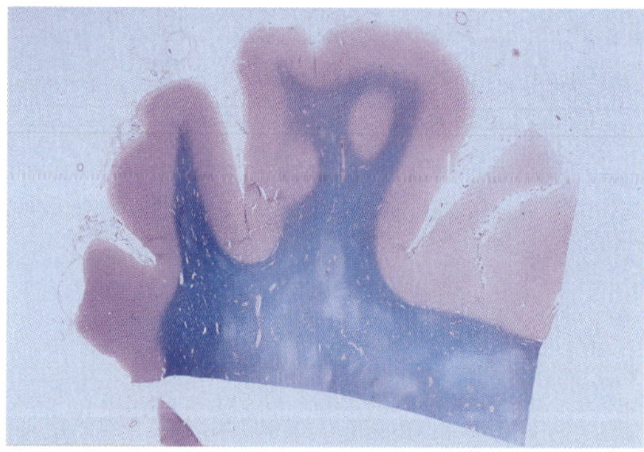

FIGURE 3.6
Hypoxic-ischemic leukoencephalopathy. Twelve days prior to his death, a 66-year-old man with chronic obstructive lung disease suffered a severe acute exacerbation, which failed to respond to intensive therapy. Macrosection from the cerebral hemisphere shows small focal areas of myelin pallor (LFB-HE).

CLINICAL FEATURES

Syncope, the momentary loss of consciousness, results from transient global ischemia of a few seconds duration.

Hypoxic and ischemic encephalopathy results from a mild to moderate continuous hypoxia that produces a variety of symptoms, including headaches, confusion, memory and cognitive impairment, seizures, myoclonus, and motor and sensory deficits. Severe hypoxia, when it lasts 10 minutes or more, produces diffuse and profound cerebral damage manifested by alterations of consciousness ranging from lethargy to deep coma, seizures, myoclonic jerks, changes of muscle tone, and pathologic reflexes.

Late sequelae comprise a broad spectrum of neurologic and mental symptoms. At one extreme is full recovery and, at the other, irreversible coma, persistent vegetative state, or dementia (Figs. 3.7, 3.8 and 3.9; Tables 3.1 and 3.2). A variety of temporary or permanent symptoms may occur between these extremes: seizures, action myoclonus, parkinsonian features; cerebellar ataxia; visual, motor, and sensory deficits; variable degrees of cognitive and memory impairment; affective disorders; and behavioral changes.

PERMANENT GLOBAL ISCHEMIA: BRAIN DEATH

The difference between the mean systemic arterial blood pressure and the intracranial pressure (ICP) (pressure of the CSF) maintains the cerebral perfusions pressure (CPP). A drop in arterial blood pressure or an increase in ICP depresses blood perfusion. When the CPP suddenly drops below a critical value (about 40 mm Hg), cerebral circulation gradually ceases. If blood flow is not restored, the nonperfused brain suffers total and irreversible damage, eventually leading to irreversible cessation of all functions of the brain, in both the cerebral hemispheres and the brainstem. *Brain death* is defined clinically as irreversible coma, apnea, and loss of all brainstem reflexes. Cardiorespiratory functions can be temporarily maintained with mechanical support and vasopressor agents.

Pathologic Features

The term *respirator brain* is considered inappropriate, because the pathologic changes relate not to the use of mechanical ventilation but to permanent nonperfusion. The changes due to *in vivo* autolysis become noticeable within 12 to 24 hours. Grossly, the brain is congested, swollen, soft, and mushy (Fig. 3.10). The hippocampus and the cerebellar tonsils are herniated and necrotic. The cortex is dusky, and the white matter pinkish and soft due to incomplete fixation. Histologically, the neural tissue stains faintly: The neurons are pale, ghost-like, or brightly eosinophilic; the glial nuclei are shrunken; the astrocytes and the blood vessels show no reactive changes; and the pituitary gland is necrotic (Fig. 3.10).

CEREBRAL PATHOLOGY IN CHRONIC EPILEPSY

Hypoxic-ischemic lesions often are encountered in the brains of patients who suffer from epilepsy with generalized tonic-clonic seizures and status epilepticus. The lesions result from respiratory and circulatory

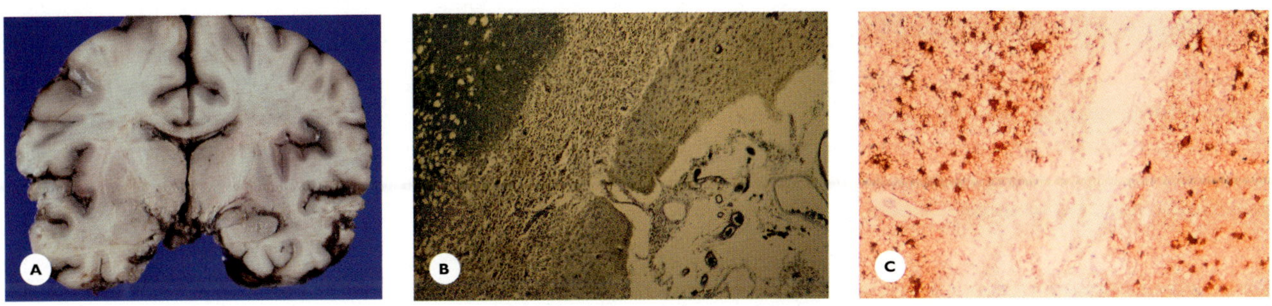

FIGURE 3.7
Prolonged coma following cardiac arrest. Chronic cortical pan-necrosis. Three-month survival in a 69-year-old man. **A.** Transverse section of the cerebral hemispheres shows thinning and sponginess of the cortex, necrosis of the basal ganglia, and focal softening of the white matter. The cerebral cortex shows (**B**) ischemic necrosis of the entire width of the cortex (LFB-CV) and (**C**) intense perinecrotic astrocytic reaction (GFAP).

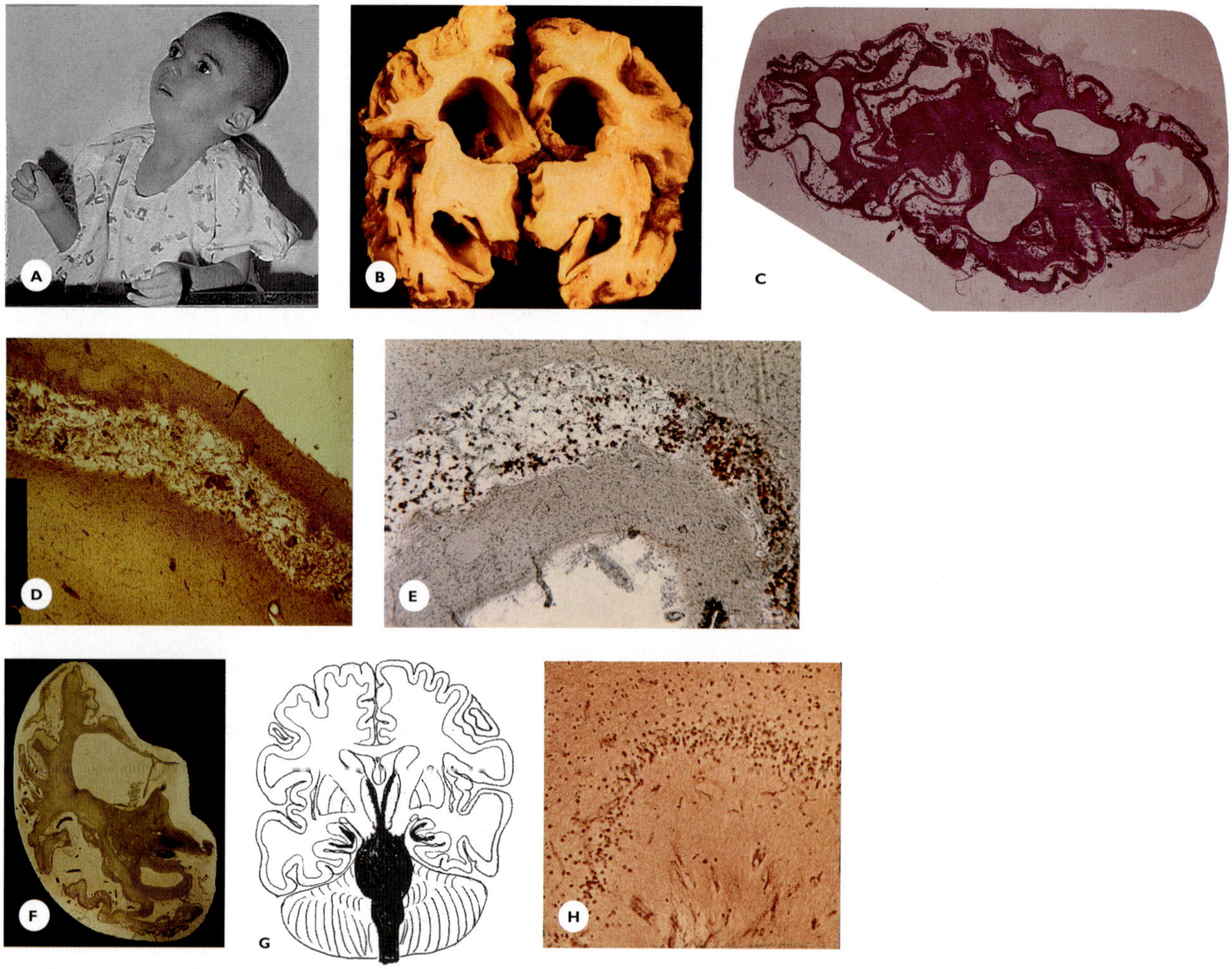

FIGURE 3.8
Persistent vegetative state following cardiac arrest with 4.5-year survival. Chronic cortical pan-necrosis. At 7 months of age, a previously healthy baby girl suffered a cardiac arrest for 10 minutes during anesthesia for repair of a diaphragmatic hernia. After 40 minutes, the heart rate returned to normal. The child remained in a permanent vegetative state until her death at age 5 years. **A.** On examination, at 5 years of age, her eyes were open and moved around but she did not react to visual or verbal stimuli and made no spontaneous movements. Her extremities were spastic, atrophic, and deformed. She slept through the night and also for a few hours during the day. **B.** On transverse section, the cerebral cortex is thin and spongy, the gray structures are atrophic, the hemispheric white matter is reduced, and the ventricles are enlarged. **C.** The cortex from the frontal to the occipital lobes underwent cystic necrosis (HE). **D.** It is replaced by a glial mesodermal network (van Gieson), **E.** which contains lipid-laden macrophages (oil-red O). **F.** The hemispheric white matter is devoid of myelin (Weil stain). **G.** Schematic representation of the sites of the surviving neurons: hypothalamus, brainstem, and parts of hippocampus. **H.** The cerebellar cortex is totally depleted of Purkinje cells, basket fibers and granule cells; it is outlined by a prominent Bergmann astrocytic layer (Bodian stain).

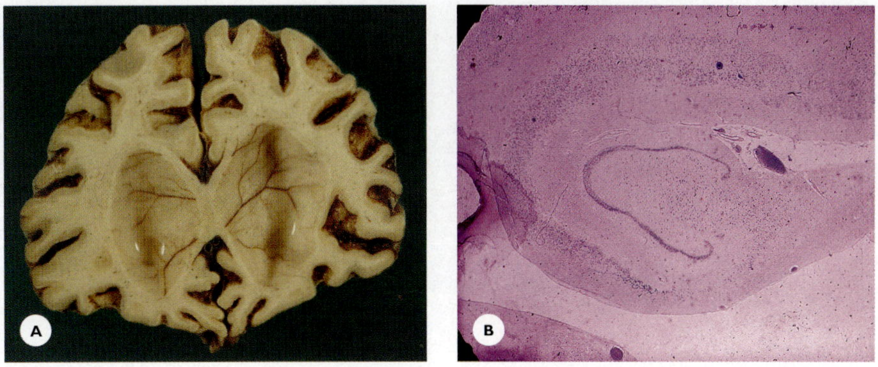

FIGURE 3.9
Post-hypoxic dementia. Following resuscitation from ventricular fibrillation and cardiac arrest, a 23-year-old man became severely demented. Thirteen years later, at age 36 years, he died. **A.** Multifocal thinning of the cerebral cortex, atrophy of the white matter, and enlargement of the anterior horns. **B.** Loss of neurons in hippocampal gyrus.

TABLE 3.1.
Comparison Between Clinical Presentation of Prolonged Coma and Persistent Vegetative State

Clinical Presentation	*Prolonged Coma*	*Persistent Vegetative State*
Consciousness	Lost	Awareness of self and environment lost, wakefulness retained
Motor activity	Lost	Markedly reduced
Speech	Lost	Reduced to sound, screaming, moaning, groaning
Sleep-wake cycle	Lost	Retained
Respiration	Altered	Intact
Autonomic functions	Altered	Retained

TABLE 3.2.
Comparison Between Anatomic Sites of Pathology in Prolonged Coma and Persistent Vegetative State

Anatomic Sites of Pathology	
Prolonged Coma	*Persistent Vegetative State*
Widespread bi-hemispheric cortical and/or white matter	Widespread bi-hemispheric cortical and/or white matter
Diencephalon	Bi-thalami
Rostral brainstem	

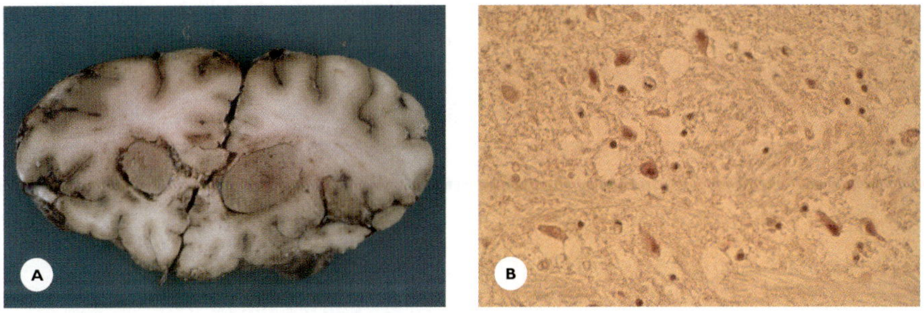

FIGURE 3.10
Permanent global ischemia: Brain death. A 72-year-old man suffered a cardiopulmonary arrest and survived 11 days with the assistance of mechanical ventilation. **A.** Transverse section of the cerebral hemispheres shows break-up of neural tissue in the basal ganglia and white matter and patchy, dusky discoloration of the cortex. **B.** Ghost neurons in the brainstem and lack of glial and vascular reactions (HE).

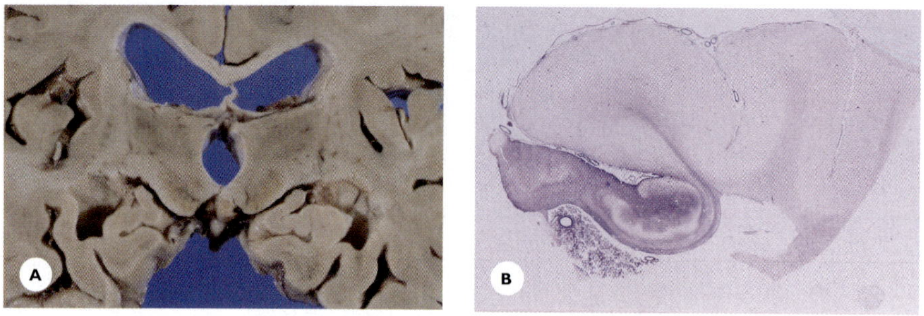

FIGURE 3.11
Ammon's horn sclerosis in a 28-year-old woman with generalized tonic-clonic seizures. **A.** The Ammon's horns are atrophic, and the temporal horns are enlarged. **B.** Thinning of the Sommer's sector from neuronal losses and dense diffuse astrogliosis in another chronic epileptic patient (Holzer stain).

impairments that occur during and after the seizures. Two characteristic lesions are Ammon's horn sclerosis and cerebellar cortical atrophy.

Ammon's Horn Sclerosis

Grossly, the Ammon's horn is atrophic, gray, and firm, and the adjacent temporal horn is variably dilated. Histologically, severe or total loss of pyramidal neurons and astrocytic gliosis are present in CA1 zone (Sommer's sector). The lesion may extend beyond the Sommer's sector to involve the entire Ammon's horn (hippocampal sclerosis) and also may extend into the parahippocampal regions and amygdala (mesial temporal sclerosis) (Fig. 3.11).

Cerebellar Cortical Atrophy

Grossly, the cerebellar folia are atrophic, often in a lobular pattern, the atrophy being more prominent at the depth and walls of the folia than at the crest. Histologically, the cortex shows Purkinje cell losses and replacement Bergmann astrocytosis. The lobular pattern results from edema that develops during the seizures and compromises the blood flow, first at the depths of sulci (Fig. 3.12).

Scattered laminar and small focal neuronal losses and astrogliosis in the neocortex, amygdala, and thalamus variably occur.

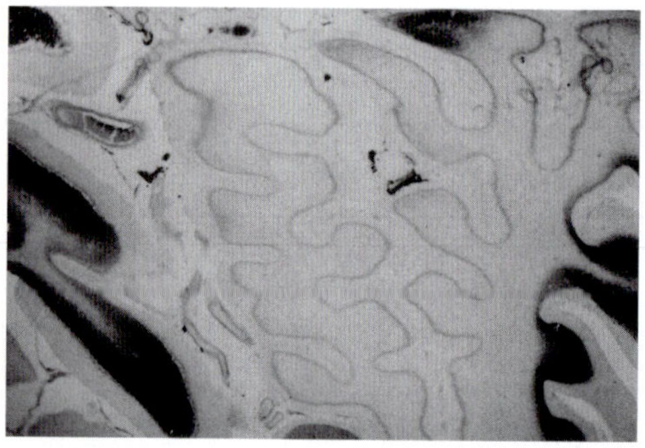

FIGURE 3.12
Cerebellar cortical lobular atrophy in a child with intractable tonic-clonic seizures. Loss of Purkinje cells and granule cells. The cortex is outlined by a prominent Bergmann astrocytic layer (cresyl violet).

Ammon's Horn Sclerosis in Temporal Lobe Epilepsy

Ammon's horn sclerosis has been identified in a significant number of surgically resected mesio-temporal lobes from patients with a history of intractable or drug-resistant complex partial seizures. Some patients also suffered from generalized tonic-clonic seizures (Fig. 3.13).

A causal relationship between Ammon's horn sclerosis and temporal lobe seizures has often been raised. Ammon's horn sclerosis may develop in a variety of clinical conditions complicated by severe hypoxia: birth injuries, febrile seizures, and vascular, infectious, and

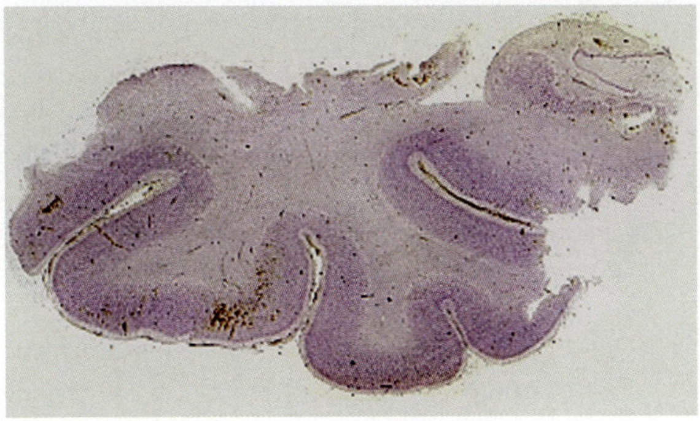

FIGURE 3.13
Ammon's horn sclerosis in temporal lobe epilepsy (cresyl violet stain). Surgically resected right temporal lobe specimen from a 28-year-old woman. At age 11 years, she had a few generalized tonic-clonic seizures. Temporal lobe seizures began at age 23 years.

traumatic injuries. It is conceivable that Ammon's horn sclerosis, when acquired early in life, may, in time, become epileptogenic, capable of triggering complex partial seizures.

BIBLIOGRAPHY

Bernat, J. L. (1997). Systemic hypoperfusion brain injury In K. M. A. Welch, D. J. Caplan, et al. (Eds.) *Primer on cerebrovascular diseases* (pp. 289–292). San Diego: Academic Press.

Ginsberg, M. D., Hedley-Whyte, E. T., & Richardson, E. P., Jr. (1976). Hypoxic-ischemic leukoencephalopathy in man. *Arch Neurol, 33*, 5–14.

Hogan, R. E. (2001). Mesial temporal sclerosis Clinicopathological correlations. *Arch Neurol, 58*, 1484–1486.

Kinney H. C., Samuels, M. A. (1994). Neuropathology of the persistent vegetative state. A review. *J Neuropathol Exp Neurol, 53*, 548–558.

Leestma, J. E. (2001). Neuropathology of brain death. In E. F. M. Wijdicks (Ed.). *Brain death* (pp. 45–60). Philadelphia: Lippincott–Wilkins.

Multi-Society Task Force on PVS, The. Medical aspects of the persistent vegetative state. (1994). *N Engl J Med, 330*, 1499–1508.

Plum, F. & Posner, J. B. (1980). *The diagnosis of stupor and coma*, 3rd ed. Philadelphia: FA Davis Company.

REVIEW QUESTIONS

1. Ischemic neurons reveal:
   A. Swollen cytoplasm
   B. Pale staining with eosin
   C. Bright eosinophilia in hematoxylin-eosin–stained sections
   D. Enlarged nucleus
   E. Bluish discoloration of cytoplasm in hematoxylin-eosin–stained sections

2. The characteristic pattern of cortical neuronal losses in cerebral hypoxia is:
   A. Haphazard
   B. Laminar
   C. Perivascular
   D. None of these
   E. All of these

3. The neural tissue elements most vulnerable to hypoxia are:
   A. Oligodendrocytes
   B. Astrocytes
   C. Neurons
   D. Axons
   E. Myelin

4. The cerebral regions most vulnerable to hypoxia are:
   A. Hippocampus
   B. Neocortex
   C. Purkinje cells
   D. All of these
   E. None of these

5. In delayed death from carbon monoxide, the site of cerebral pathology is the:

   A. Putamen
   B. Pallidum
   C. Ammon's horn
   D. Thalamus
   E. Red nucleus

6. All of the following statements concerning brain death are correct *except*:

   A. It is caused by permanent cerebral global ischemia.
   B. Lack of response to noxious stimuli is present.
   C. Brainstem reflexes are present.
   D. EEG is isoelectric.
   E. Patient is apneic.

7. The zone of the hippocampus most vulnerable to hypoxia is:

   A. CA1 (Sommer's sector) of Ammon's horn
   B. CA2 zone
   C. CA4 zone
   D. Presubiculum

8. Cerebral changes encountered in the brains of patients who had suffered from chronic epilepsy are:

   A. Purkinje cell degeneration
   B. Ammon's horn sclerosis
   C. Astrocytic gliosis in cerebral cortex
   D. None of these
   E. All of these

9. All of the following statements concerning cerebral hypoxia are correct *except*:

   A. It develops during an acute cardiorespiratory arrest.
   B. Histotoxic hypoxia can be caused by cyanide.
   C. Ischemic hypoxia develops when the blood flow falls below 18 mL/100 g/min.
   D. Hypothermia aggravates ischemic brain damage.
   E. Hyperglycemia aggravates ischemic brain damage.

10. The brains of patients kept for some time on mechanical ventilation show all of the following *except*:

    A. Poor fixation
    B. Dusky discoloration
    C. Myelin pallor
    D. Pituitary necrosis
    E. Leukocytic infiltration

(Answers are provided in the Appendix.)

CHAPTER 4

Cerebrovascular Diseases

Etiology, Pathology, and Clinical Aspects of Stroke
Various Stroke Etiologies: Stroke in the Young
Cerebral Pathology in Arteriolosclerosis: Vascular Dementia

ETIOLOGY, PATHOLOGY, AND CLINICAL ASPECTS OF STROKE

The incidence and mortality of stroke are high. An estimated 500,000 to 700,000 new cases occur every year. Despite early identification and treatment of risk factors, it remains the third leading cause of death in Western countries. The most disabling neurologic disease of the elderly, stroke commonly affects individuals over 55 years of age, and the incidence increases with advancing age. It is more common among men and among African Americans. Importantly, stroke also occurs among younger subjects, even children, in whom etiologies comprise a broader spectrum.

Stroke presents with a sudden onset and rapid progression of focal neurologic symptoms and signs, culminating within minutes or hours—at most within 24 to 48 hours. It results from a sudden alteration of cerebral blood flow in an arterial territory (regional cerebral blood flow, rCBF). This alteration occurs in one of two ways: A reduction of rCBF causes ischemia and eventually an infarction, or B bleeding into the brain parenchyma or into the subarachnoid space causes a massive intracerebral hematoma or a subarachnoid hemorrhage.

Thus, a stroke is either *ischemic* or *hemorrhagic*; its pathologic substrate is either an infarct or a hemorrhage.

Ischemic Stroke

Cerebral Infarction

The brain requires a constant and adequate blood flow to supply oxygen and glucose essential for its high energy metabolism. A constant blood flow is assured by an autoregulatory mechanism of arteries and arterioles; they constrict in response to rising systemic blood pressure and dilate in response to falling systemic blood pressure. This mechanism operates while the arterial pressure remains between 50 and 160 mm Hg. One-

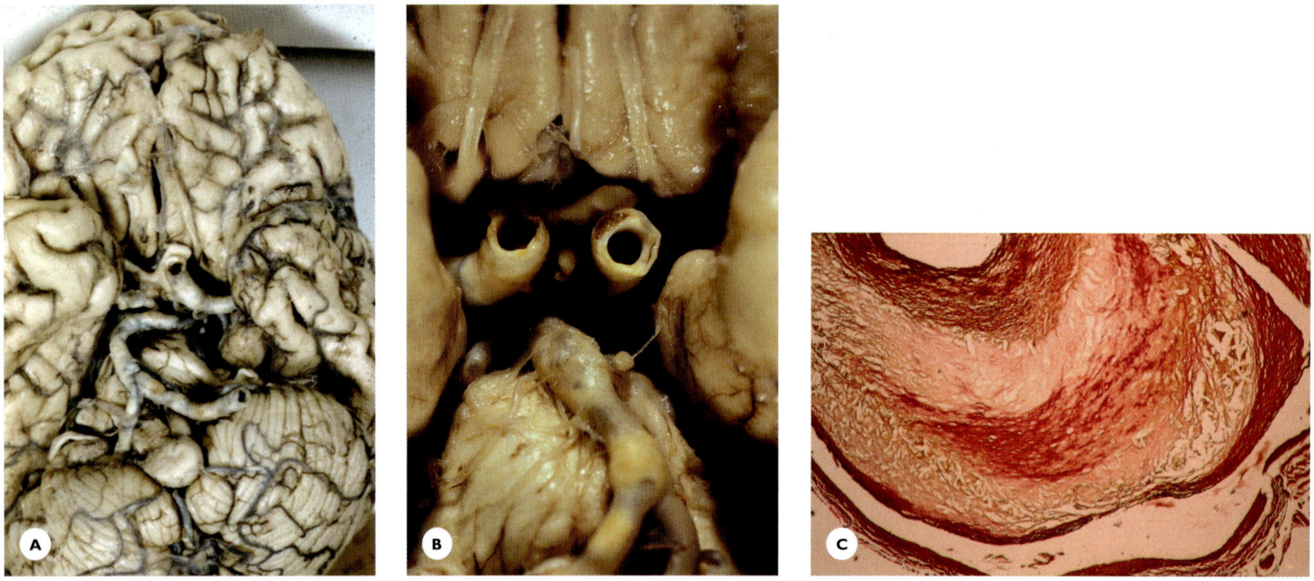

FIGURE 4.1
Atherosclerosis of cerebral arteries. **A.** Severe atheromatosis of basal arteries. Confluent yellow atheromatous plaques occur in the arterial walls. The basilar artery is elongated and stiff, and the lumen is distended. The sclerotic right carotid presses on the optic nerve. **B.** The atheromatous basilar artery displays focal dilation and narrowing of the lumen and presses on the pontine basis. The rigid walls of the carotids press on the optic nerves. **C.** Atheromatous plaque in the wall of the basilar artery shows focal subintimal cholesterol clefts, disruption of the elastic lamina, and marked intimal proliferation severely reducing the lumen (van Gieson).

fourth of the cardiac output is to the brain—an average blood flow of 700 to 800 mL/min (55 to 65 mL/100 g/min). A reduction of blood supply to 15 to 20 mL/100 g/min for a few minutes produces ischemia and neurologic deficits. A prolonged fall to 8 to 10 mL/100 g/min results in ischemic necrosis, that is, an infarction.

Etiologies

Arteriosclerosis of the cervicocranial arteries and diseases of the heart are primary causes of infarctions in the elderly. A group of less common but important etiologies affect chiefly younger individuals and are presented in the section, Various Stroke Etiologies.

Arteriosclerosis of cervicocranial arteries. *Atherosclerosis* affects chiefly the large arteries: the extracranial cerebral arteries and their major intracranial branches. Preferential sites are the bifurcations of common carotid arteries, origins of internal carotids, and vertebral arteries. Intracranially, atheromatosis commonly develops in the cavernous segment and syphon of carotids, and at the points of junction, proximal segments, and bifurcations of major arteries. The atherosclerotic artery is rigid, elongated, or tortuous. The lumen is distended or reduced, and the wall contains multiple, often confluent yellow atheromatous plaques (Fig. 4.1).

Potential consequences of atherosclerosis. Atherosclerosis promotes infarction in several ways (Fig. 4.2): (a) It predisposes to local thrombus formation and luminal occlusion; (b) it is a potential source of fibrinoplatelet and cholesterol emboli to the brain; and (c) it can critically reduce the vascular lumen by 70% or more, thus rendering the arterial territory vulnerable to systemic circulatory insufficiency.

Arteriolosclerosis affects the small parenchymal arteries and arterioles. Several pathologic forms exist, such as fibrosis, hyalinosis, mural lipid deposits, micro-

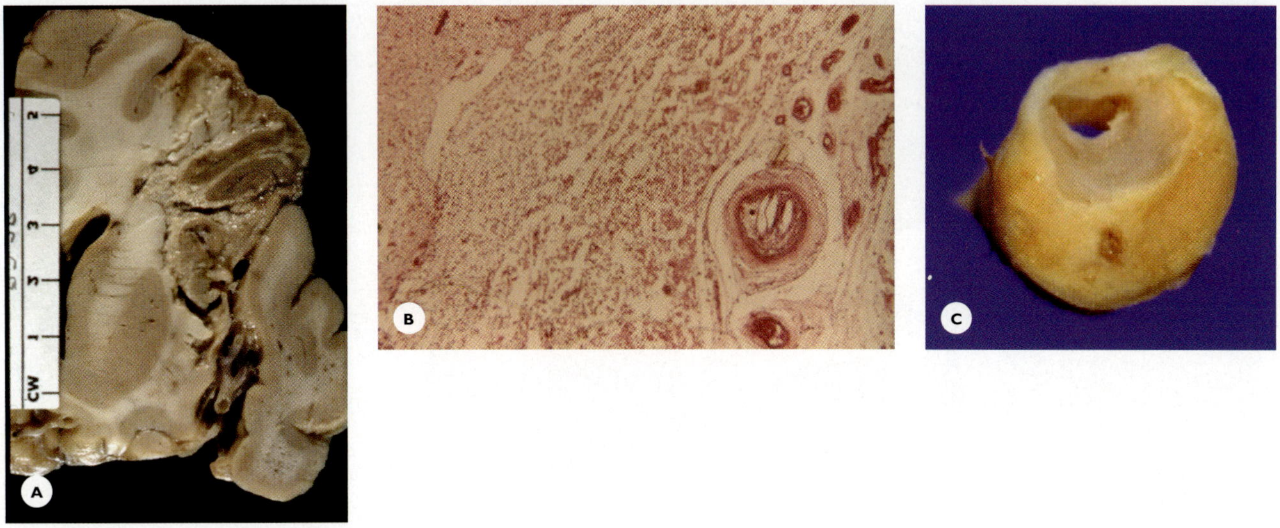

FIGURE 4.2
Consequences of atherosclerosis. **A.** Thrombotic occlusion of MCA in the Sylvian fissure causing a large infarct. **B.** Cholesterol embolus in a small leptomeningeal artery overlying a cortical infarct, hematoxylin-eosin (HE) **C.** Hemodynamically significant (greater than 75%) stenosis in a carotid endarterectomy specimen.

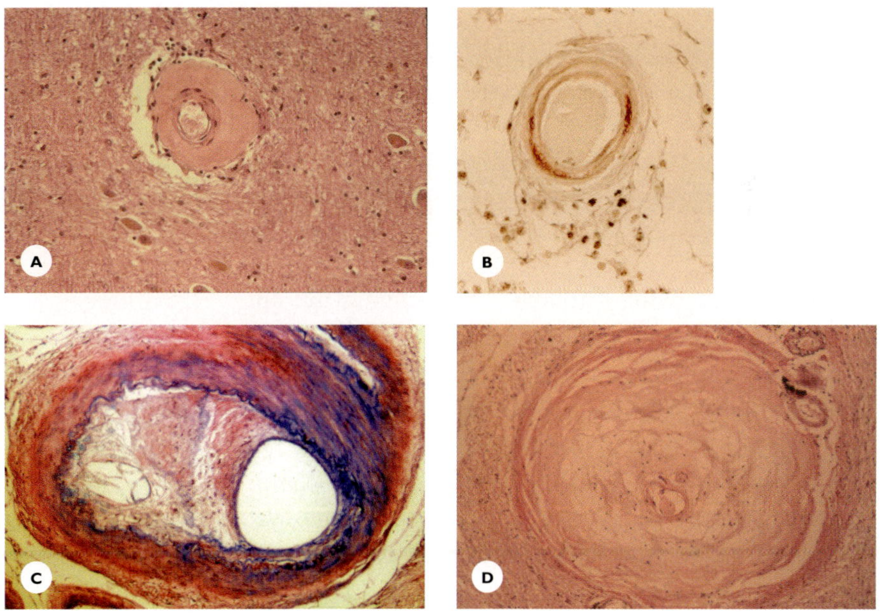

FIGURE 4.3
Pathologic forms of arteriolosclerosis. **A.** Fibrohyalinosis with mural thickening and luminal stenosis (HE), **B.** Mural lipid deposits (oil-red-O). **C.** Eccentric microatheroma (LFB-HE). **D.** Markedly thickened, structureless fibrotic wall and virtually nonexisting lumen (HE).

atheroma, and fibrinoid necrosis (Fig. 4.3). These changes are commonly associated with chronic hypertension and are important in the etiology of lacunar infarcts.

Diseases of the heart. Most cardiac diseases are potential sources of emboli to the brain. The most important are chronic atrial fibrillation, sick sinus syndrome, mitral and aortic valvular diseases, and myocardial

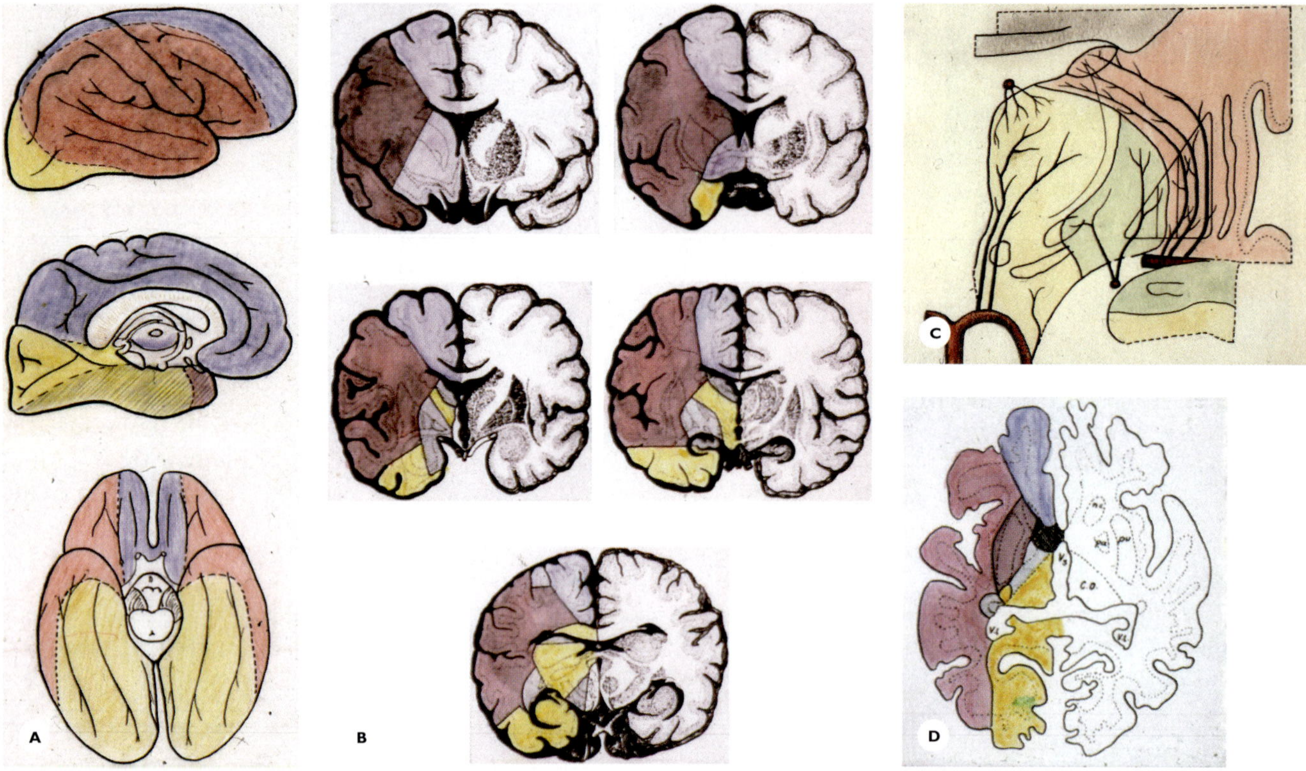

FIGURE 4.4
Arterial supply of the brain. Schematic drawings of territorial supplies of major cerebral arteries on (**A**) lateral, median, and basal surfaces; (**B**) and (**C**) on transverse planes; and (**D**) on horizontal plane. Blue, anterior cerebral artery (ACA); red, middle cerebral artery (MCA); yellow, posterior cerebral artery (PCA); green, anterior choroidal artery (AchA).

infarct with overlying thrombus. Arrhythmias are apt to dislodge platelet or fibrin fragments and calcium flecks from a mural thrombus or from the valves. A left atrial myxoma is a rare source of emboli. An atrial septal defect (right–left shunt) opens the way to emboli from deep venous thrombi to the brain (paradoxical emboli). Heart failure with systemic hypotension or hypovolemia is another important cause of focal ischemia in the territory of a severely stenotic artery.

Less common etiologies. This group comprises various vasculopathies and vasculitis, hematologic diseases, iatrogenic complications, illicit substance abuse–related diseases, and some inherited metabolic diseases (see section, Various Stroke Etiologies).

Pathology

Gross features. The assessment should include the type, age, size, and arterial territory (Fig. 4.4; Table 4.1):

- Type of infarct. A *bland infarct* is pale over the entire area, and a *hemorrhagic infarct* contains confluent petechial hemorrhages in the cortex and subcortical gray structures (Fig. 4.5). Emboli are an important cause of a hemorrhagic infarct. The bleeding occurs through damaged capillary walls, following fragmentation and migration of the embolus. Bleeding distally to the occlusion through retrograde collateral circulation is an alternative mechanism. A sudden rise in blood pressure can precipitate such a situation.
- Age of infarct. An infarct evolves through three stages: necrosis, liquefaction, and cavitation (Fig. 4.6). During

the acute stage, which occurs approximately the first week following stroke, the ischemic tissue undergoes necrosis. During the first 24 hours, it swells, appears somewhat pale, and is slightly soft. After 24 to 48 hours, it becomes friable, breaks up, and is demarcated from the surrounding healthy tissue by artificial cracks.

- During the acute stage, ischemic necrosis invariably is associated with edema (cellular and vasogenic), which reaches its peak by the fifth or sixth day. Cellular edema affects chiefly the gray matter, and vasogenic edema affects the white matter. Importantly, extensive edema, by increasing the brain volume, leads to herniations with brainstem and medullary compression. These subject the patient to serious risk of deterioration and even death.
- By the end of the first week, the subacute stage begins, as the necrotic tissue breaks down and liquefies, which may take 2 to 3 weeks. Gradually, the edema resolves, the tissue debris is removed, the infarcted area shrinks, and ultimately is transformed into a cystic cavity. This chronic stage of cavitation may take several weeks or months, depending on the size of the infarct.
- Size and arterial territories. Infarcts are situated within territorial boundaries of the arteries subjected to ischemic insults. A *large infarct* occupies all or part of the supply territory of a cervical or large intracranial artery; a large infarct is commonly caused by atherothrombotic or thromboembolic occlusion. It is more common in the carotid than in the vertebral arterial territory (Figs. 4.7 through 4.10). The most common site is the territory of the middle cerebral artery (MCA).

TABLE 4.1.
Gross Assessment of Arterial Infarcts

Type:	Pale Hemorrhagic
Arterial territory:	Carotid Vertebrobasilar
Size:	Large—macrovessels Lacune—microvessels
Age:	Acute—ischemic necrosis Subacute—liquefaction Chronic—cavitation

A *watershed* or *border-zone infarct* is situated between the terminal branches of adjacent major arteries (Fig. 4.11). Likely causes are embolus or a sudden drop in blood pressure, which first compromises the blood flow in the terminal branches (hemodynamic failure). A *small* or *lacunar infarct* is a cystic cavity with irregular margins, measuring 0.5 to 1 cm (rarely, 1.5–2 cm [giant lacune]), which results from the removal of necrotic tissue. It is associated with arteriolosclerosis of the deep penetrating basal arteries and the cortical (medullary) arteries, and it occurs commonly in the basal ganglia, internal capsule, thalamus, and pons (Fig. 4.12). In the white matter, the site of predilection is the watershed zone between the cortical and basal penetrating arteries—the corona radiata, the outer angle of the

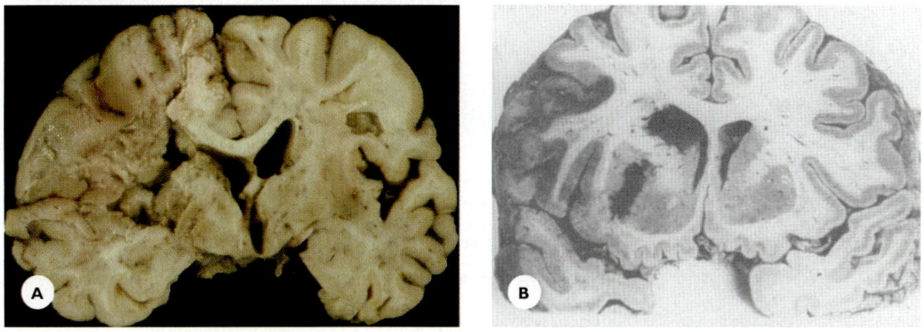

FIGURE 4.5
Types of infarcts. **A.** Pale, bland infarct in carotid territory (MCA and ACA). **B.** Hemorrhagic infarct in MCA territory. Petechial hemorrhages are confined to the gray structures.

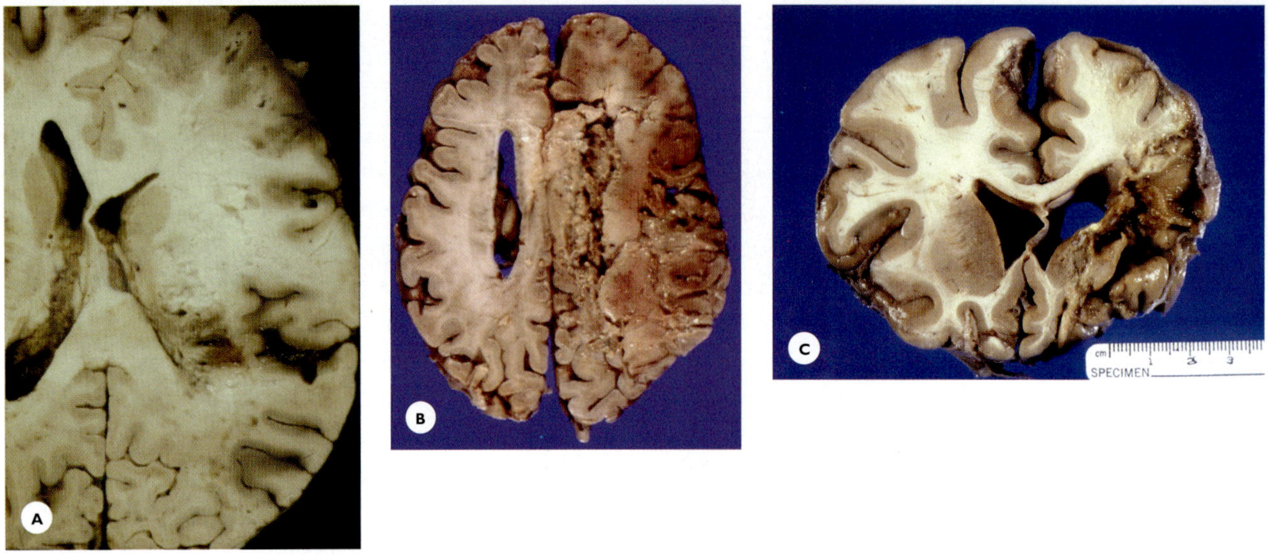

FIGURE 4.6
Morphologic evolution of infarcts in MCA territory. **A.** Ischemic necrosis. Note the swelling of ischemic territory and compression of adjacent ventricle. **B.** Liquefaction of ischemic tissue. **C.** Cavitation following removal of tissue debris. Note the enlargement of adjacent ventricle, indicating chronicity of the lesion.

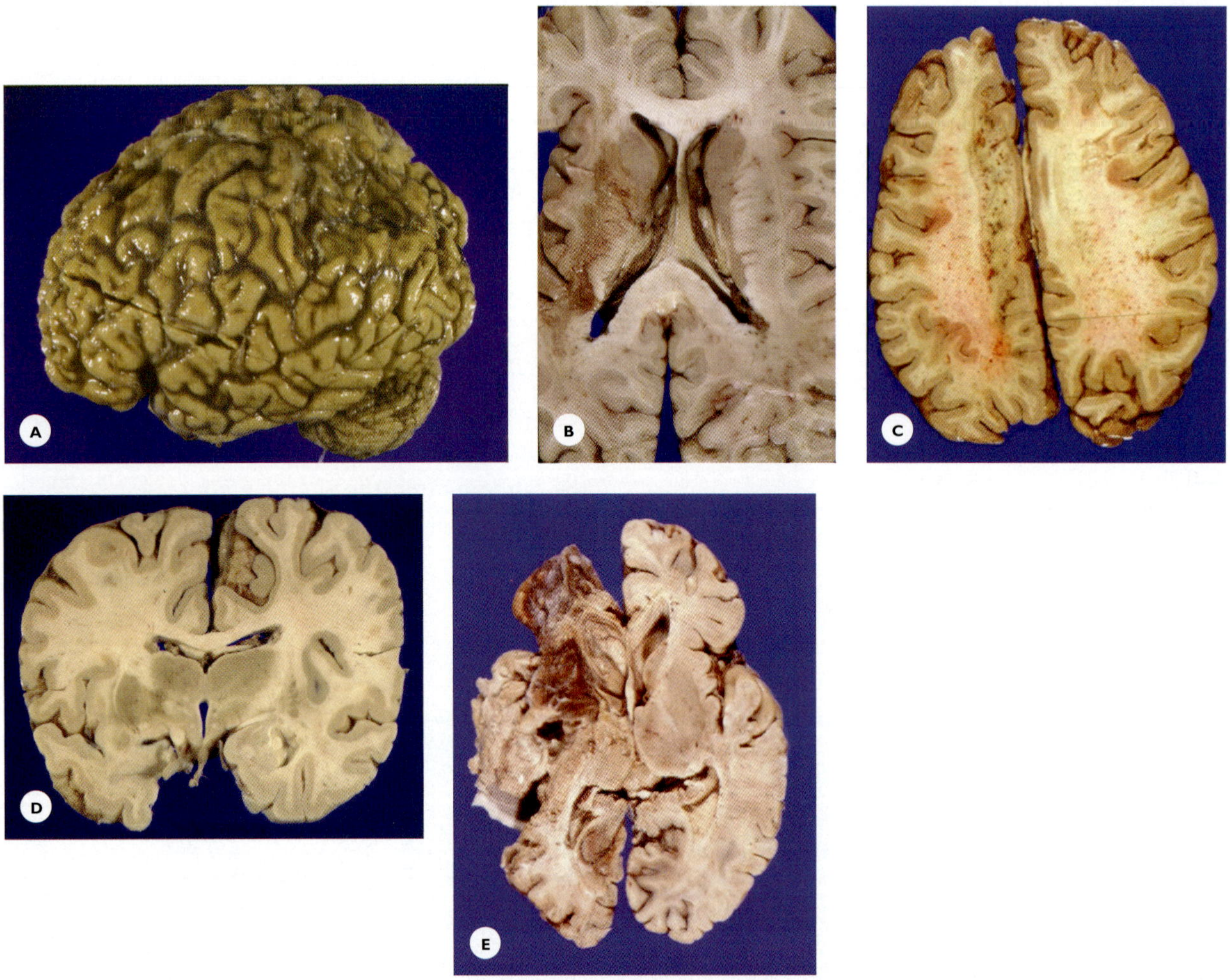

FIGURE 4.7
Infarcts in carotid arterial territories. MCA infarcts: **A.** cortical (parietal artery). **B.** basal ganglia (lenticulostriate artery). **C.** ACA infarct. **D.** AchA infarct. E. MCA and ACA infarct.

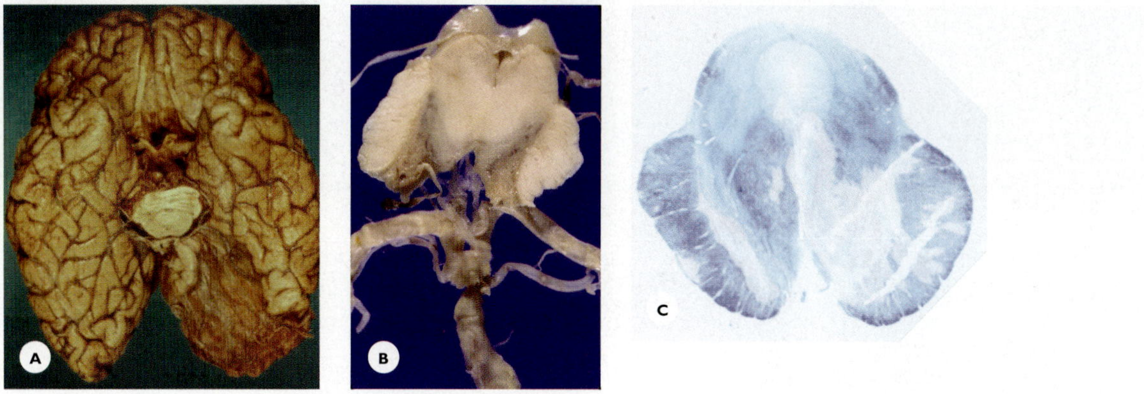

FIGURE 4.8
Infarcts in vertebrobasilar arterial territories. **A.** PCA infarct. **B** and **C.** Bilateral midbrain infarcts (LFB-CV) (peduncular branches of PCA and BA).

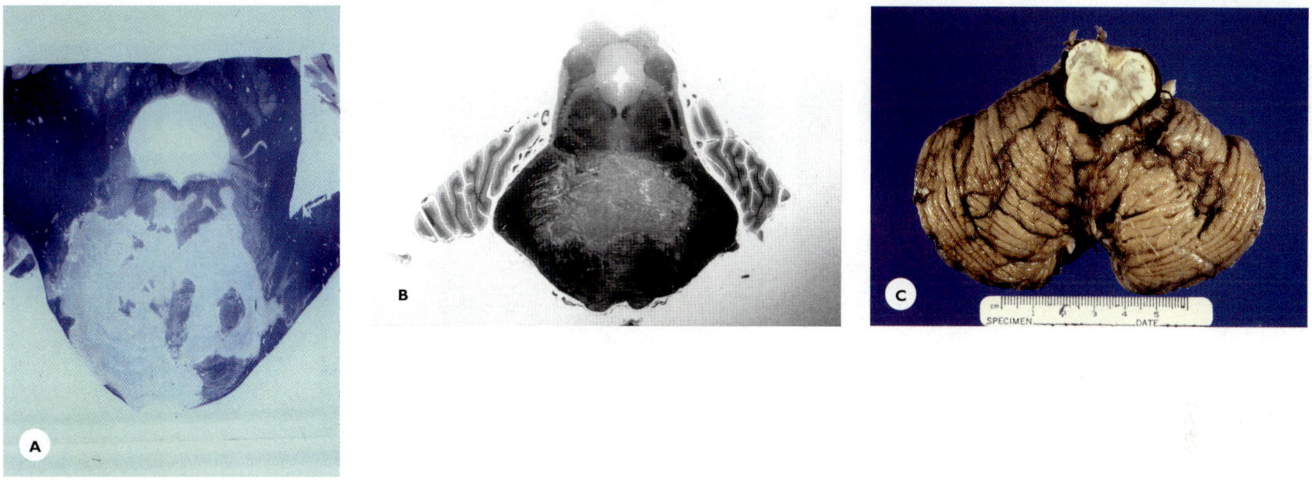

FIGURE 4.9
Basilar artery infarcts. **A.** Extensive thrombotic infarct involves the basis and tegmentum of the pons. **B.** Pontine basis infarct (myelin stain). **C.** Cerebellar infarct (SCA territory).

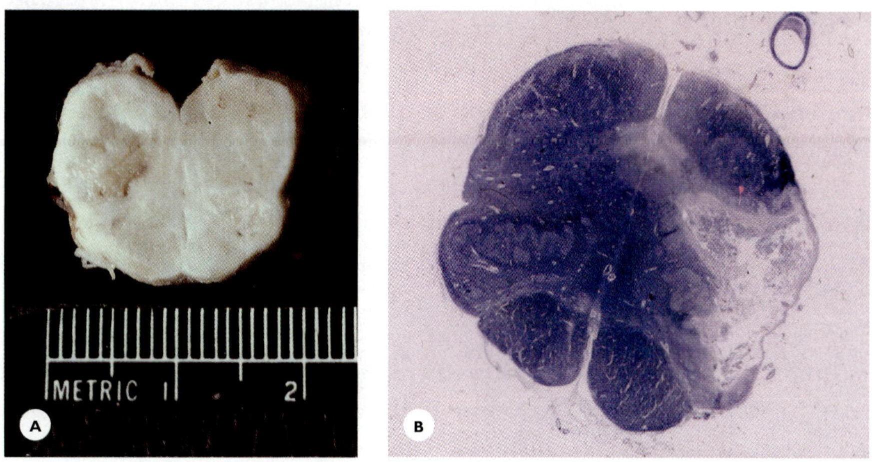

FIGURE 4.10
Vertebral artery infarcts. A and B. Gross and histologic picture of lateral medullary infarct (LFB-CV), the territory of the posterior inferior cerebellar artery, (PICA).

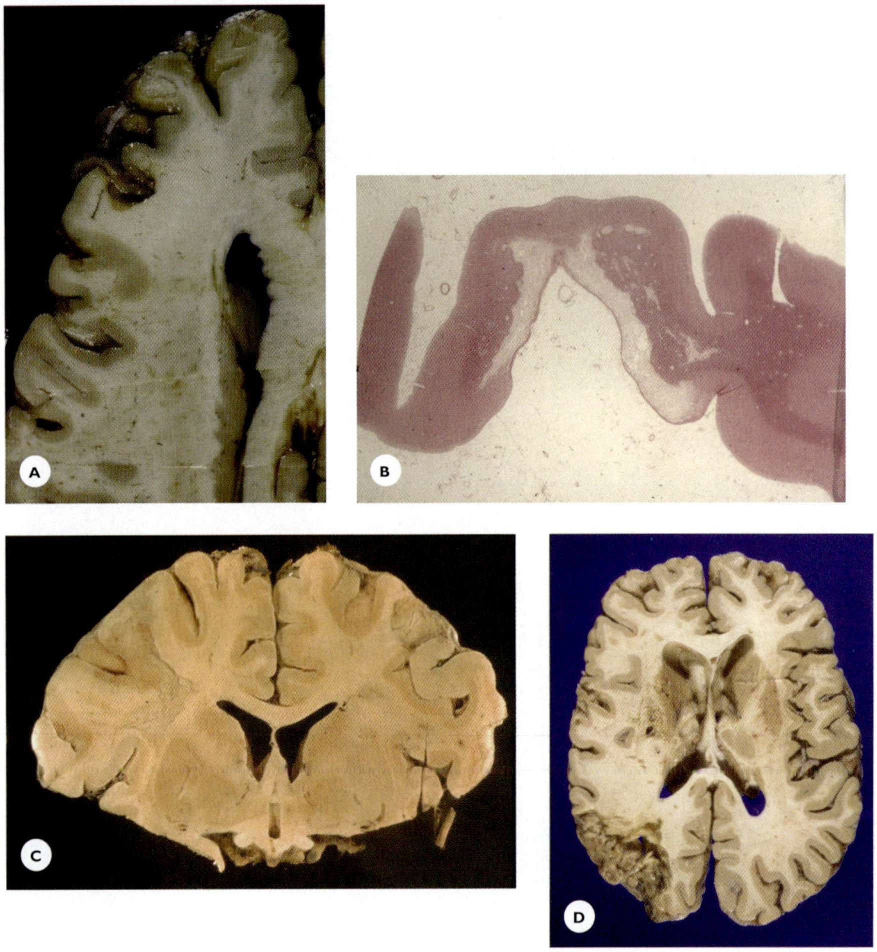

FIGURE 4.11
Watershed infarcts. **A.** Cortical infarct in the border zone between ACA and MCA showing **B.** laminar cortical pannecrosis (the external cortical layer is spared (HE). **C.** Bilateral cortical–subcortical infarcts in the border zones between ACAs and MCAs. **D.** Cortical–subcortical infarct in the border zone between MCA and PCA.

lateral ventricle, and the subinsular region (Fig. 4.13). Systemic hypoperfusion due to cardiac failure, hypotension, or hypovolemia, plays a primary role in the pathogenesis. Alternate mechanisms are atheromatous occlusion, microembolus, and, less often, stenosis of extracranial or large intracranial arteries. *Multiple infarcts* may occur within the carotid or vertebrobasilar territories, or within both.

Concomitant infarct and hemorrhage. It is not unusual to find within one brain recent or old infarcts and hemorrhages together (Fig. 4.14).

Histologic Features

Ischemia elicits a chain of interrelated events: necrosis, edema, inflammatory reaction, macrophage activation, and marginal astrocytic proliferation (Table 4.2).

Ischemic necrosis. During the first 24 to 48 hours, the ischemic tissue appears vacuolated, spongy, and stains faintly with eosin (Fig. 4.15). The distribution is patchy; faintly stained hypoperfused areas alternate with hyperemic areas (luxury perfusion) due to loss of autoregulation and early venous filling. The hypoperfused but potentially viable tissue around the ischemic core, the so-called *penumbra*, provides the rationale for instituting therapy to rescue it from being incorporated into the infarction.

The neurons, most vulnerable to ischemia, are first to succumb. Red neurons are the hallmark of ischemia; they shrink and show bright eosinophilia of the perikaryon, dissolution of the Nissl substance, and homogenization of the nucleus (see Fig. 4.15). Other neurons appear as dark neurons with shrunken peri-

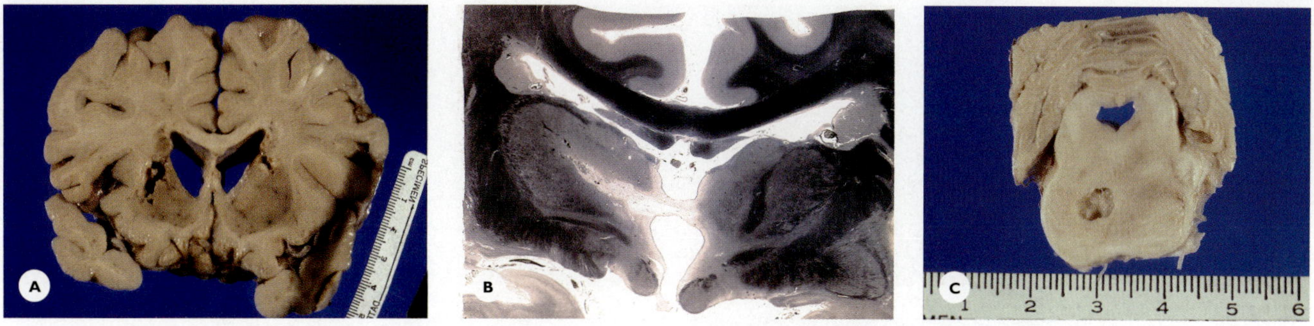

FIGURE 4.12
Lacunar infarcts. **A.** Basal ganglia (lenticulostriate artery). **B.** Thalamus (thalamoperforating artery). **C.** Pons (paramedian branches of BA).

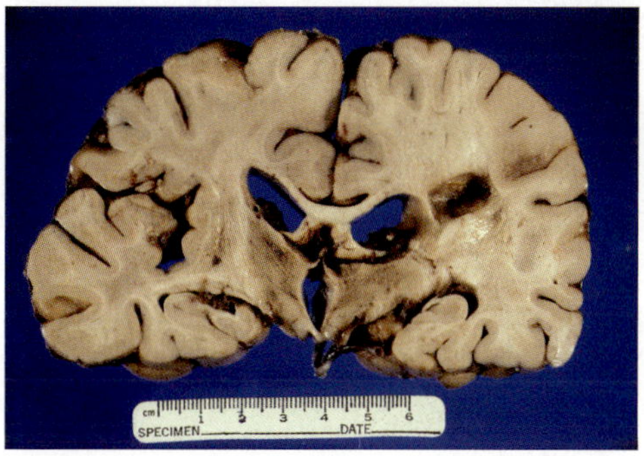

FIGURE 4.13
Giant white-matter lacunar infarct in the border zone between cortical and deep penetrating arteries.

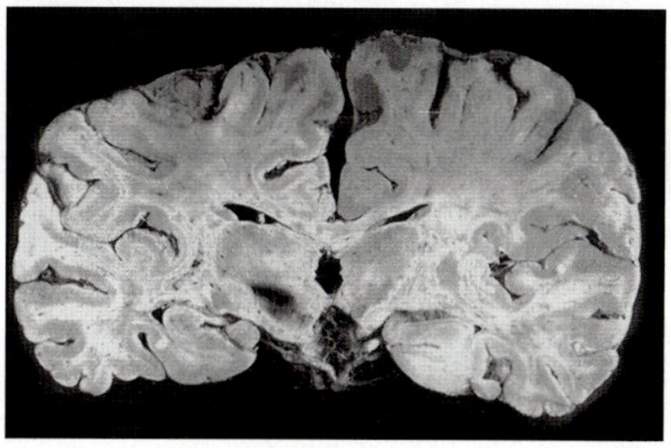

FIGURE 4.14
Concomitant hemorrhagic and ischemic strokes in a 75-year-old hypertensive woman. She developed ballistic movements in her right extremities, followed 4 days later by left hemiparesis. Gross section shows a fresh hemorrhage in the left subthalamic nucleus and a recent right MCA infarct.

TABLE 4.2.

Approximate Timetable of Histologic Events in Ischemic Necrosis

1. Tissue Necrosis Neurons Myelin Glial cells Axons 1 hr — 3–4 days	3. Inflammation; PNL 24–72 hrs
	4. Macrophage Activation 48–72 hrs
	5. Capillary Proliferation 48 hrs
2. Edema Cytotoxic Vasogenic 3 hrs 72 hrs	6. Marginal Astrocytosis 48 hrs–days

PNL, polymorphonuclear leukocytes.

karyon, or as ghost neurons with pale perikaryon and nucleus.

As the neurons undergo necrosis, changes also occur in the myelin, nerve fibers, and glial cells. The myelin first loses its affinity for Luxol fast blue. Then, by about the third day, the myelin gradually disintegrates into neutral lipid globules. Along with the myelin, the nerve fibers break into small fragments, and residual axonal retraction balls may remain at the margin of the infarct. Within the severely affected ischemic areas, the oligodendrocytes and astrocytes also disintegrate. The capillaries, least vulnerable to ischemia, show endothelial hypertrophy and hyperplasia (see Fig. 4.15).

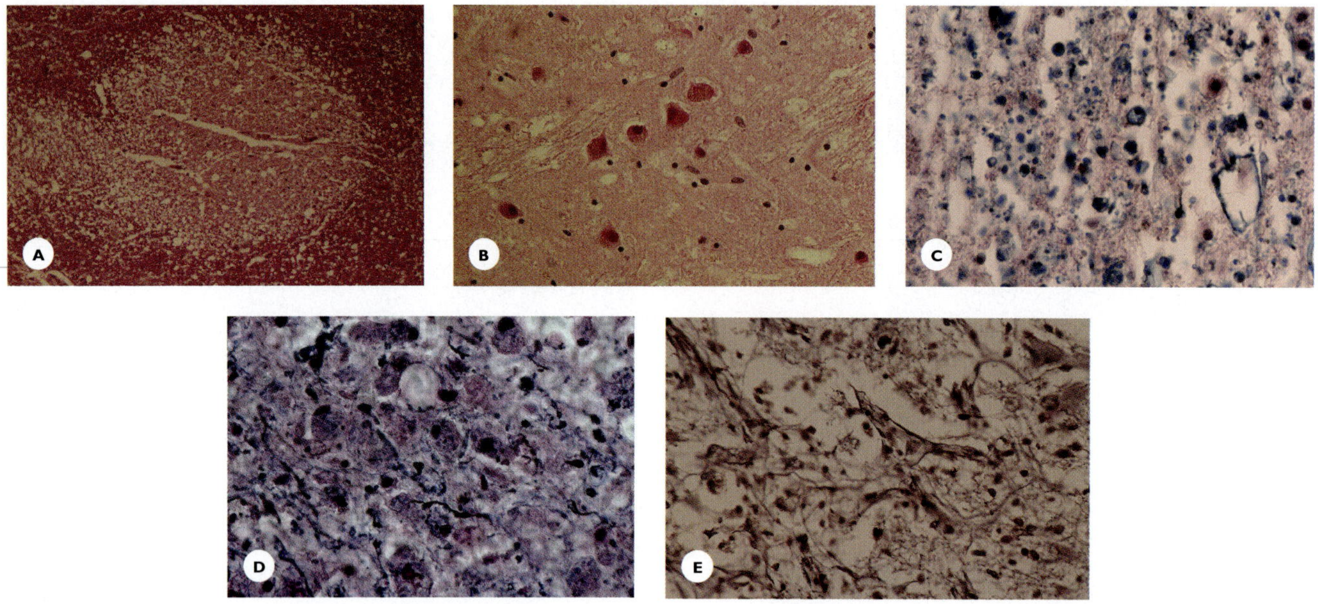

FIGURE 4.15
Histologic evolution of infarcts. Ischemic necrosis. **A.** Ischemic tissue stains faintly with eosin, is vacuolated and spongy. **B.** Ischemic (red) neurons display a strongly eosinophilic, shrunken perikaryon and a homogenous dark basophilic nucleus (HE). **C.** Myelin disintegrates into small lipid globules (LFB-CV) and (**D**) the axons into small fragments (Holmes stain). **E.** Capillaries are prominent (reticulin stain).

Edema. Two types of edema develop in ischemic tissue: cellular and vasogenic.

In *cellular (cytotoxic) edema*, swelling of the neurons and astrocytes develops within a few hours after the ischemic insult. This swelling results from the opening of the ion pump and the excessive inflow of sodium, chloride, and water into the intracellular compartment and outflow of potassium into the extracellular compartment.

Vasogenic edema develops 2 to 3 days after the ischemic insult and reaches its peak by the fifth or sixth day. It results from breakdown of the blood–brain barrier and the escape of fluid and protein into the extracellular space, chiefly into the white matter. The white matter swells and stains faintly with Luxol fast blue. The myelin sheaths are separated from each other, and the pericapillary spaces are filled with plasma fluid (Fig. 4.16).

Inflammatory reaction. During the first 24 to 38 hours, the ischemic tissue is invaded by polymorphonuclear leucocytes (Fig. 4.17). This inflammatory reaction, mediated by cytokines, aggravates the ischemic injury by producing toxic substances and obstructing the microcirculation.

Macrophage activation. By about the third day, the leucocytes are replaced by macrophages derived from blood monocytes and activated microglial cells. The macrophages phagocytose the tissue debris and remove it to the blood vessels and subarachnoid space (Fig. 4.18). So, gradually, the infarcted tissue is transformed into a cystic cavity, the lumen of which is traversed by a fine fibrous meshwork derived from surviving capillaries (Fig. 4.19).

Marginal astrocytic proliferation. At the margin of the ischemic tissue, the astrocytes proliferate into large gemistocytic astrocytes, forming a transition zone between the infarct and the healthy tissue (see Fig. 4.19).

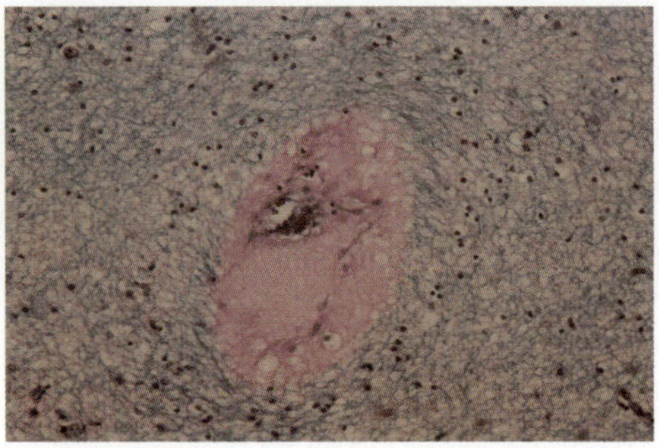

FIGURE 4.16
Histologic evolution of infarcts. Vasogenic edema. **A.** Plasma fluid fills the perivascular space (LFB-CrV-E).

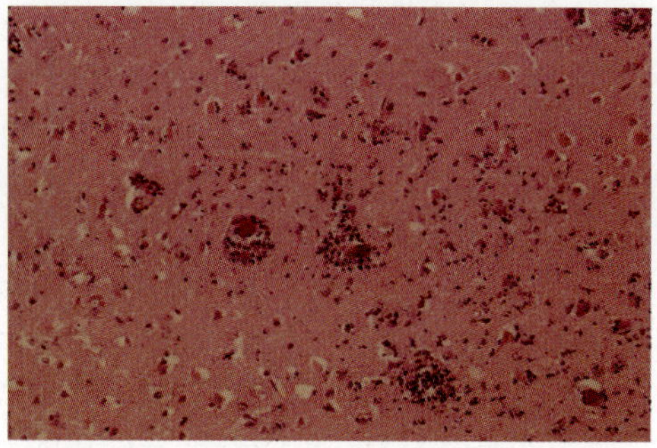

FIGURE 4.17
Histologic evolution of infarcts. Inflammatory reaction. Polymorphonuclear leukocytes invade the ischemic tissue during the first 24 hours (HE).

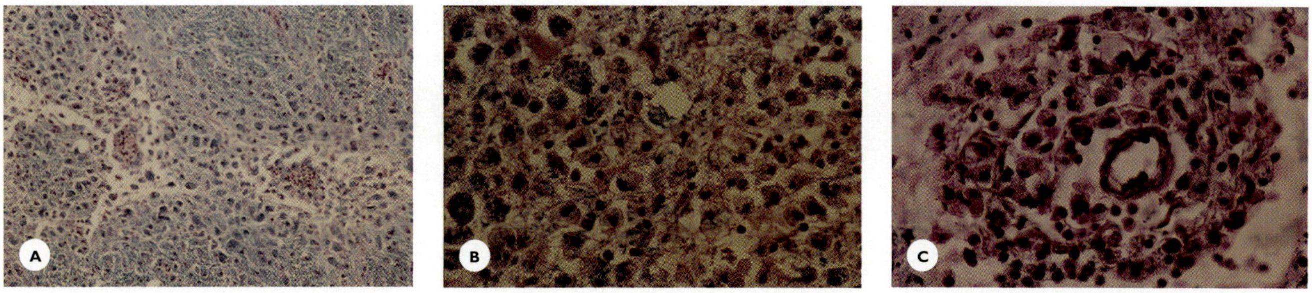

FIGURE 4.18
Histologic evolution of infarcts. Macrophage activation. **A.** By the second and third day, macrophages invade the necrotic tissue. **B.** Cytoplasms of macrophages are filled with tissue debris, which is then removed to the perivascular spaces. **C.** Collection of macrophages around a blood vessel (LFB-CV-E).

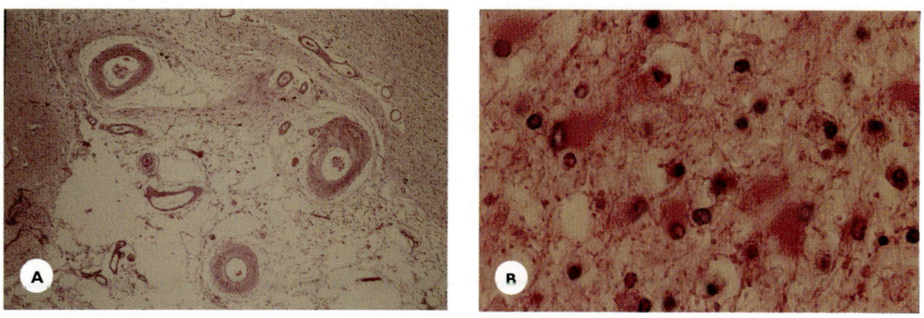

FIGURE 4.19
Histologic evolution of infarcts. Marginal astrocytic proliferation. **A.** Chronic cavitated infarct contains a few remaining capillaries and macrophages within the lumen. **B.** The margin consists of proliferated gemistocytic astrocytes (HE).

Pathomechanism

Reduction or cessation of rCBF, by disrupting the oxygen and glucose supply to the nervous tissue and by preventing elimination of harmful metabolites, induces a chain of deleterious processes leading first to neuronal death and ultimately destroying all tissue. Glutamate-mediated excitotoxicity and lactic acidosis play key roles in ischemic necrosis.

Excitotoxicity. Ischemia initiates the release and excessive accumulation of the excitatory neurotransmitters glutamate and aspartate and related amino acids in the extracellular space. By exciting the neuronal membrane receptors, these neurotransmitters depolarize the synaptic membranes, allowing ionic and water exchange; the inflow of sodium, chloride, and water into the neurons; and the outflow of potassium into the extracellular space. Most important, they promote the entry of calcium into the neurons. Intracellular overload of calcium interferes with mitochondrial and metabolic functions and eventually destroys the neurons.

Lactic acidosis. Ischemia leads to anaerobic glycolysis and the formation of lactic acid and free radicals. The harmful effects of lactacidosis and free radicals, along with some other toxic metabolites, culminate in the breakdown of all components of neural tissue.

Clinical Aspects

Presentation. Ischemic stroke accounts for about 80% of all strokes. The clinical presentation is determined by the severity of the ischemic attack and its cause, and also by the adequacy of the collateral circulation and the presence of any stroke risk factors (Table 4.3).

Transient ischemic attack (TIA). A mild and short ischemic attack produces transient impairment of neuronal function. Focal neurologic symptoms and signs develop suddenly, progress rapidly, and usually resolve within less than 24 hours. Clinical features of TIAs in the carotid and vertebrobasilar arterial territories are summarized in Table 4.4.

Completed stroke. A severe ischemic attack lasting approximately from thirty minutes to 1 hour produces an infarction: The neurologic deficits remain prolonged or permanent.

Classification. There are three subtypes of ischemic strokes based on their pathomechanism (Table 4.5):

- *Thrombotic stroke,* accounting for about 50% of ischemic strokes, is often preceded by TIAs. The symptoms worsen steadily or stepwise during the first 24 to 48 hours (evolving stroke).
- *Embolic stroke,* accounting for about 30% of ischemic strokes, has a very abrupt onset and rapid evolution of neurologic deficits that are maximal from the onset. The source of the embolus—heart, aorta, cervicocranial arteries—is usually evident, and the infarct is often hemorrhagic.
- *Hemodynamic stroke,* accounting for 10% to 30% of ischemic strokes, results from systemic hypoperfusion in the territory of a severely stenotic artery. Cardiovascular diseases that affect the systemic circulation are present, and the infarcts are preferentially located in watershed regions and terminal arterial fields.

TABLE 4.3.
Stroke Risk Factors

Stroke Risk Factors
Age, gender, race
Hypertension
Arteriosclerosis
Cardiac diseases
Hyperlipidemia
Diabetes mellitus
Oral contraceptive use
Illicit substance abuse
Cigarette smoking
Chronic alcohol abuse
Obesity
Migraine
Sedentary lifestyle

TABLE 4.4.
Transient Ischemic Attacks

Carotid Territory	
Transient monocular blindness	
*Hemiparesis	
*Hemisensory deficit	
Aphasia (D)	
Vertebrobasilar Territory	
Diplopia	Dysarthria
Binocular visual loss	Bilateral motor/ sensory deficits
Vertigo	Loss of consciousness
Ataxia	

*Contralateral. D, dominant hemisphere.

TABLE 4.5.
Ischemic Stroke

Causes and Presentation		
Thrombus	**Embolus**	**Hemodynamic failure**
	Cardiogenic / Arterial	
Stepwise Fluctuating Hx of TIA	Sudden Rapid progression Hemorrhagic infarct	Systemic hypoperfusion Local arterial stenosis Watershed infarct

Clinical Features

Clinical features of ischemic stroke greatly depend on the size and location of the infarcts. Large hemispheric and brainstem infarcts present with depression of alertness ranging from somnolence through lethargy to coma. During the acute stage, ischemic edema when severe, aggravates the clinical course and may endanger the patient's life. Seizures may occur during the acute stage or several weeks or months later. Mortality rate ranges from 10% to 20% during the first month. Cardiac and pulmonary complications account for about half the deaths. Neurologic deficits, particularly motor, remain in about 50% of survivors. Behavioral changes, depression, and cognitive decline add to the clinical picture. Multiple cortical or subcortical infarcts, depending on their locations, are the substrates of multiinfarct dementia.

Stroke Syndromes

Ischemic strokes produce distinct syndromes for each arterial territory. Table 4.6 summarizes the common clinical manifestations of carotid territory infarcts. The occlusion of the internal carotid artery presents chiefly with features of a middle cerebral artery (MCA) territory infarct; contralateral motor and sensory deficits, visual field defect, and aphasia when the lesion is in the dominant hemisphere. If the occlusion extends beyond the point of origin of the ophthalmic artery, ipsilateral blindness occurs. Anterior cerebral artery (ACA) territory infarct is distinguished by motor and sensory deficits, predominantly in the leg. Neuropsychological dysfunctions are associated with infarcts in the territories of cortical branches of the MCA and the ACA.

Infarcts in the territories of the vertebrobasilar arteries produce a great variety of syndromes (Table 4.7). Posterior cerebral artery syndromes generally present with various combinations of visual, sensory, and neuropsychological deficits. Large brainstem infarcts are the most detrimental, causing either a sudden loss of consciousness with extensive neurologic deficits or a "locked-in" syndrome with consciousness intact. It is important to differentiate between coma and conditions that superficially may be mistaken for coma (Table 4.8). Cross syndromes of unilateral brainstem infarcts manifest with ipsilateral cranial nerve deficits (3rd to 12th) and contralateral motor and sensory deficits.

Diagnostic Evaluation

Specific diagnostic tests are aimed at defining the cerebral lesion and identifying any vascular and cardiac pathology. Neuroimaging using structural and functional magnetic resonance imaging (MRI) and computed tomography (CT) scan are most valuable in eliminating diseases that can mimic a stroke, differentiating between an ischemic and a hemorrhagic stroke, and monitoring progression of edema and hemorrhagic complications (Table 4.9):

1. From about 8 to 24 hours after the onset of symptoms, CT scan shows the infarct as a low-density area within an arterial supply territory (Fig. 4.20). Earlier indirect signs, however, are present as loss of differentiation between the cortex and the white

TABLE 4.6(A).
Internal Carotid Territory Infarcts Syndromes of Middle Cerebral Artery (1)

Clinical Features	*Cortical and Deep Branches*	*Superior Division*	*Inferior Division*	*Lenticulostriate Artery*
Visual	*Homonymous hemianopia		Homonymous hemianopia/ upper quadrantanopia	
Conjugate horizontal gaze	Paresis to opposite side	Paresis to opposite side		
Motor	*Hemiplegia face, arm → leg	*Hemiplegia face, arm → leg	None/Minimal	*Hemiparesis
Sensory	*Hemisensory deficit	*Hemisensory deficit		*Hemisensory deficit
Language	Global aphasia (D)	Expressive aphasia (D)	Receptive aphasia (D)	
Neuropsychological dysfunction	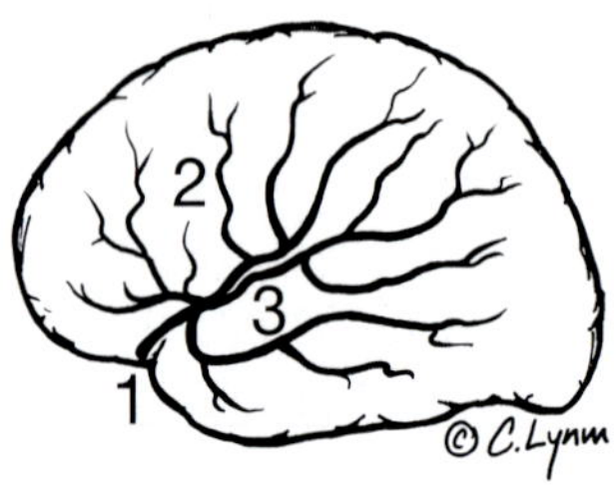	Agraphia (D), Alexia (D) Gerstmann syndrome; agraphia, acalculia, finger agnosia, right-left confusion	Constructional apraxia (nD) Dressing apraxia (nD) Agitated delirium	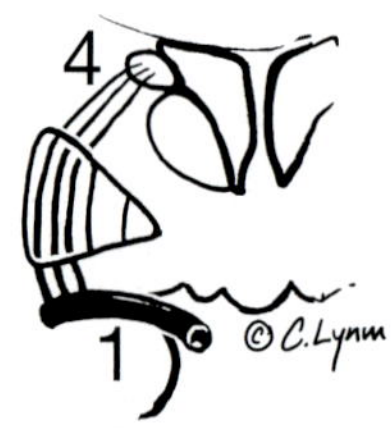

*Contralateral, (D) dominant hemisphere, (nD) nondominant hemisphere. KEY: 1, MCA; 2, superior division; 3, inferior division; 4, lenticulostriate artery.

TABLE 4.6(B).
Syndromes of Branches of Internal Carotid Artery (2)

Clinical Features	*Anterior Cerebral Artery*	*Anterior Choroidal Artery*	*Ophthalmic Artery*
Visual		*Homonymous hemianopia quadrantanopia	Amaurosis fugax Partial/total blindness
Motor	*Paresis of leg, minimal of arm bilateral: Central paraplegia	*Hemiparesis	
Sensory	*Deficit over leg	*Hemisensory deficit	
Language	Transcortical motor aphasia (D)		
Neuropsychological dysfunction	Frontal lobe: abulia Bilateral: akinetic mutism, Gait apraxia	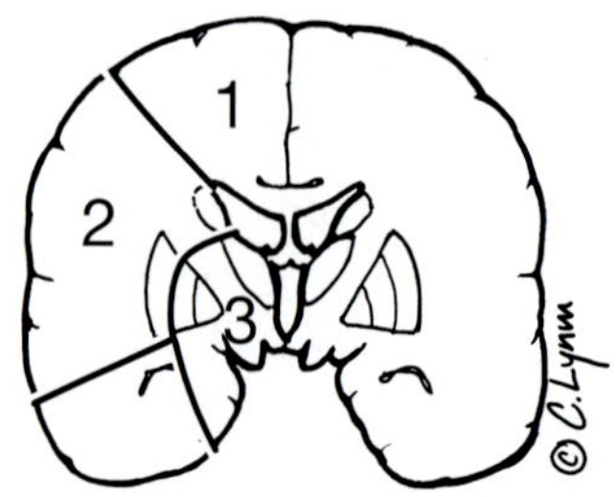	
Other	*Grasp reflex Sucking reflex Urinary incontinence		

*Contralateral; D, dominant hemisphere. KEY: 1, ACA; 2, MCA; 3, AchA.

TABLE 4.7(A).
Subclavian Steal Syndrome

An occluded or stenosed subclavian artery, proximal to the origin of the vertebral artery, steals the blood flow from the vertebral artery by reversing its direction.

Ipsilateral to stenosis

Delayed radial pulse
Reduced BP
Supraclavicular bruit
Exercise of the arm can induce TIAs in posterior circulation

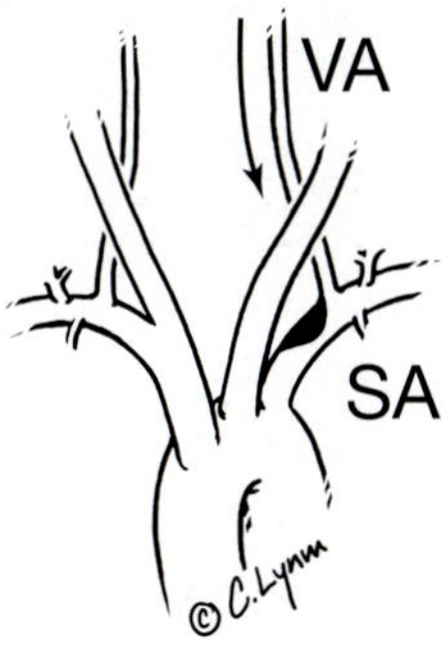

VA, vertebral artery; SA, subclavian artery.

matter, and effacement of sulci. A large infarct, by the second or third day, is surrounded by edema, which produces a mass effect with ventricular compression and midline shift (Fig. 4.21).

2. From about 1 to 3 weeks, a subacute infarct often shows peripheral enhancement due to neovascularity (luxury perfusion). Sometimes, by the second week, the infarct is poorly visualized, a phenomenon referred to as *fogging*.
3. From 3 to 4 weeks on, a chronic infarct appears as a well-delineated, low-density lesion with a dilated ipsilateral ventricle due to tissue loss.

MRI demonstrates the infarction earlier than does the CT scan, within a few hours after the ictus, and is particularly useful in diagnosing lacunar infarcts. An acute infarct appears as a hyperintense (bright) lesion with a

TABLE 4.7(B).
Posterior Cerebral Artery Infarcts

Occipitotemporobasal Syndromes

Occipitotemporal artery	Calcarine artery	
	Unilateral	***Bilateral*
*Homonymous hemianopia Visual agnosias; inability to recognize objects, colors, faces (prosopagnosia) (D) Alexia without agraphia (inability to read—ability to write) (D) Spatial disorientation (nD).	*Homonymous hemianopia	Cortical blindness (pupillary light reflex is present) Denial or unawareness of blindness

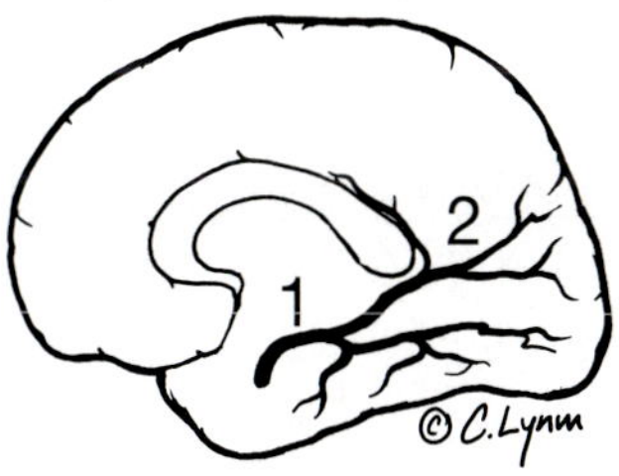

Thalamic Syndromes

Thalamogeniculate artery	Thalamoperforating artery	
	Unilateral	*Bilateral*
Sensory loss for all modalities Dysesthesias Spontaneous pain Athetotic hand posturing Intention tremor Choreoathetosis Homonymous hemianopia	Hemiataxia Tremor Choreoathetosis	Hypersomnia Korsakoff amnestic syndrome Subcortical dementia Vertical gaze abnormalities

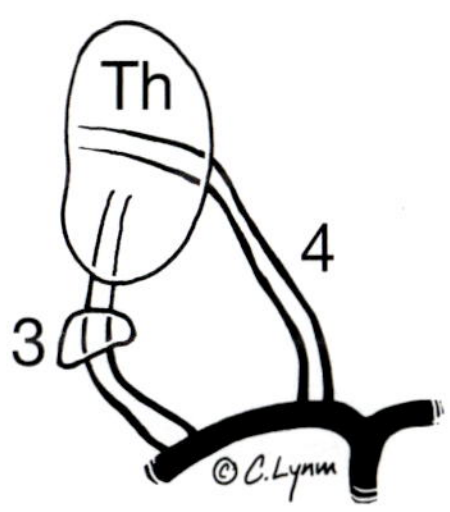

*Contralateral; D, dominant hemisphere; nD, nondominant hemisphere; **Anton syndrome. KEY: 1, occipitotemporal atery; 2, calcarine artery; 3, thalamogeniculate artery; 4, thalamoperforate artery.

TABLE 4.7(C).
Midbrain Syndromes

**Peduncular Arteries*			*Basilar Artery*
Weber Syndrome *Ipsilateral* 3rd nerve palsy *Contralateral* Hemiplegia	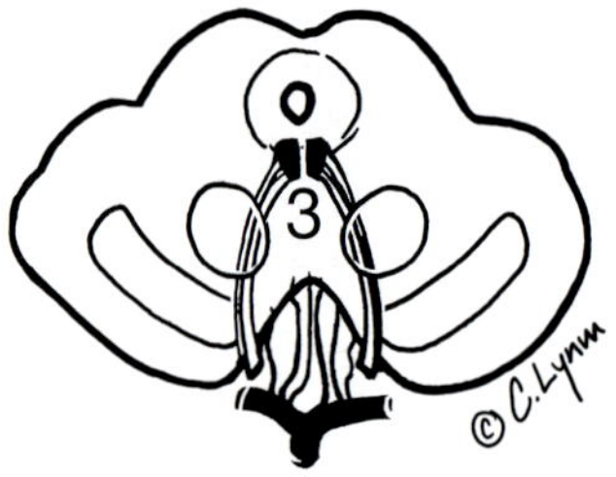	**Benedikt Syndrome** *Ipsilateral* 3rd nerve palsy *Contralateral* Intention tremor	**Top of the Basilar Syndrome** Vertical gaze palsy Skew deviation of eyes Pupillary changes Somnolence Hallucinosis Confusion Visual field defect

*Branches of PCA and BA. KEY: 3, oculomotor nerve.

TABLE 4.7(D).
Pontine Syndromes

Basilar Artery Infarcts

*Locked-in syndrome
- Quadriplegia
- Facial diplegia
- Anarthria, Dysphagia
- Consciousness; intact

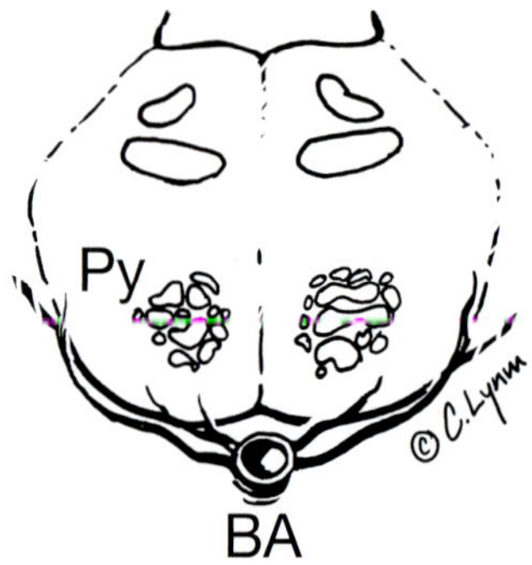

**Pontine tegmentum and basis syndrome

Unilateral	*Bilateral*
Ipsilateral	Coma
Cranial nerve 6th, 7th palsy	Quadriplegia
Gaze palsy	Bulbar paralysis
Contralateral	Facial diplegia
Hemiparesis	
Hemihypesthesia	

*Paramedian arteries.
**Circumferential branches of superior and anterior inferior cerebellar arteries.
KEY: BA, basilar artery; Py, pyramids.

TABLE 4.7(E).
Medullary Syndromes

Lateral Medullary Syndrome

Posterior inferior cerebellar artery (PICA)

Ipsilateral	*Contralateral*
Loss of pain and temperature sensations over the face	Loss of pain and temperature sensations over the body and extremities
Loss of cornea reflex	
Horner syndrome	
Ataxia	
Paralysis of soft palate, pharynx, larynx	

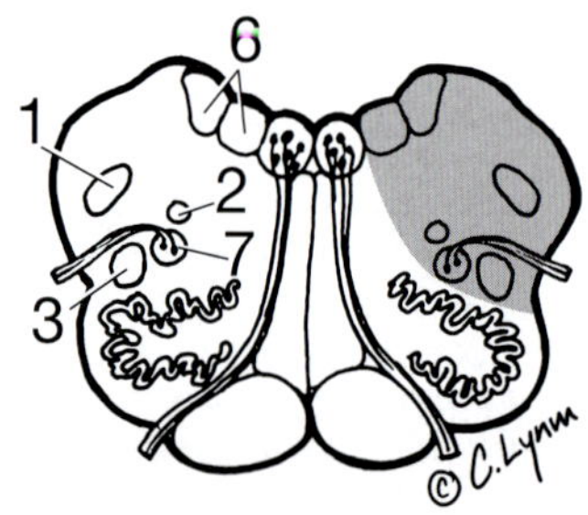

Medial Medullary Syndrome

Anterior spinal artery/Vertebral artery

Ipsilateral	*Contralateral*
12th nerve palsy	Hemiparesis Loss of position and vibration sensations

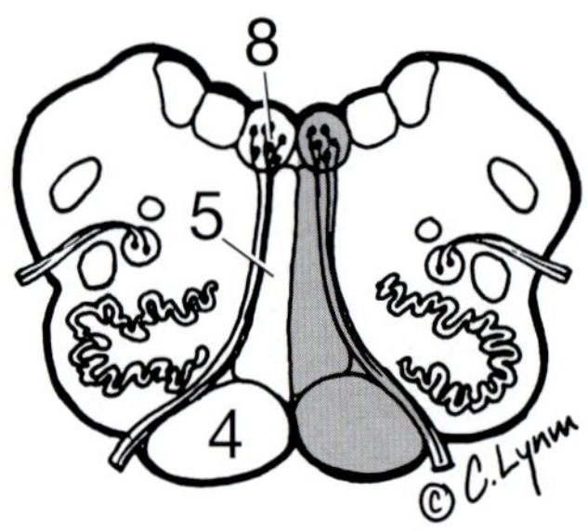

KEY: 1, Spinotrigeminal tract; 2, sympathetic tract; 3, spinothalamic tract; 4, pyramids; 5, medial lemniscus; 6, acoustic/vestibular nucleus; 7, vagus motor nucleus; 8, hypoglossus nucleus.

TABLE 4.7(F).
Cerebellar Syndromes

Ataxia of gait, trunk, and ipsilateral limbs
Variable midbrain, pontine, medullary deficits

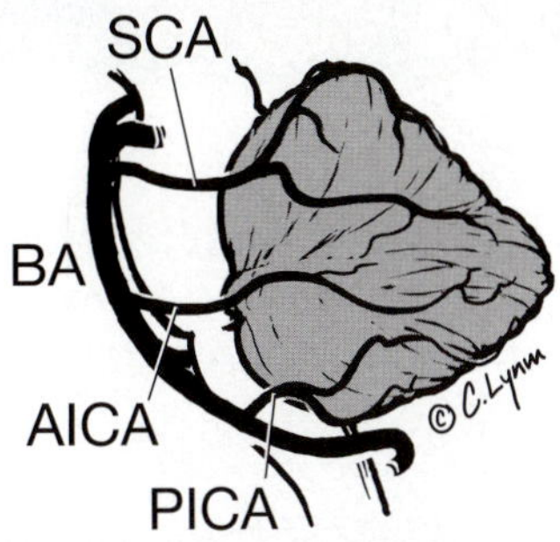

KEY: SCA, superior cerebellar artery, midbrain; AICA, anterior inferior cerebellar artery, pons; PICA, posterior inferior cerebellar artery, medulla; BA, basilar artery.

TABLE 4.8.
Comparison Between Coma, Locked-In Syndrome, and Akinetic Mutism

Clinical Features	*Coma*	*Locked-in Syndrome*	*Akinetic Mutism*
Consciousness	Lost	Intact	Intact
Motor activity	None	None; due to quadriplegia	None/severely reduced
Speech	None	None; due to anarthria	Mute/reduced to yes–no
Autonomic functions	Altered	Retained	Retained
Brain Stem reflexes	Altered	Retained	Retained
Anatomical sites	Brain stem Diencephalon Bihemispheric Cortex/white matter	Pontine basis	Fronto-orbital-cingular regions Diencephalon

TABLE 4.9 (A).
CT Appearance of Cerebral Infarct and Hemorrhage

Stage	*Infarct*	*Hemorrhage*
Hyperacute 1–24 h	Sulcal effacement	Hyperdense
Acute 24 h–3 days	Hypodense Edema	Hyperdense Edema
Subacute 4 days+	Hypodense Mass effect Ventricular compression Ring-enhancement	Hyperdense ↓ Isodense
Chronic 14 days+ weeks	Hypodense Ventricular dilatation	Hypodense Ring-enhancement

TABLE 4.9 (B).
MRI Appearance of Cerebral Infarct and Hemorrhage

Stage	*Infarct*	*Hemorrhage*
Hyperacute <12 hrs	T1-Hypointense T2-Hyperintense	T1-Isointense T2-Hyperintense
Acute 24 h–3 days	T1-Hypointense T2-Hyperintense	T1-Hypo-isointense T2-Hypointense
Subacute 4 days 7+ days	T1-Enhancing T2-Hyperintense	T1-Hyperintense T2-Hypointense T1-Hyperintense T2-Hyperintense
Chronic 14 days + weeks	T1-Hypointense T2-Hyperintense	T1-Hypo-isointense T2-Hypointense

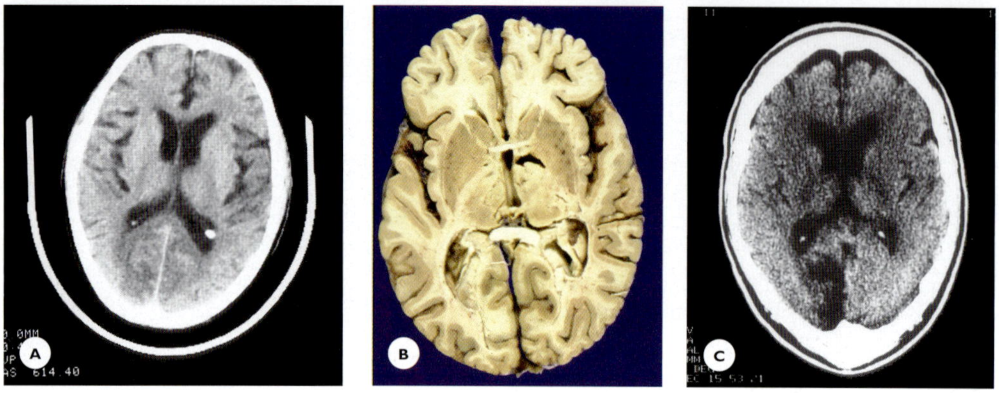

FIGURE 4.20

CT scan images of infarcts. PCA infarcts in a 65-year-old man who developed cortical blindness following a severe hypotensive episode and died 4 days later. **A.** Axial CT scan taken 1 day after the episode shows slightly hypodense lesions in medial aspects of occipital lobes. **B.** Horizontal section of the brain shows acute infarcts in supply territories of PCAs. **C.** Intensely hypodense appearance of an old PCA infarct.

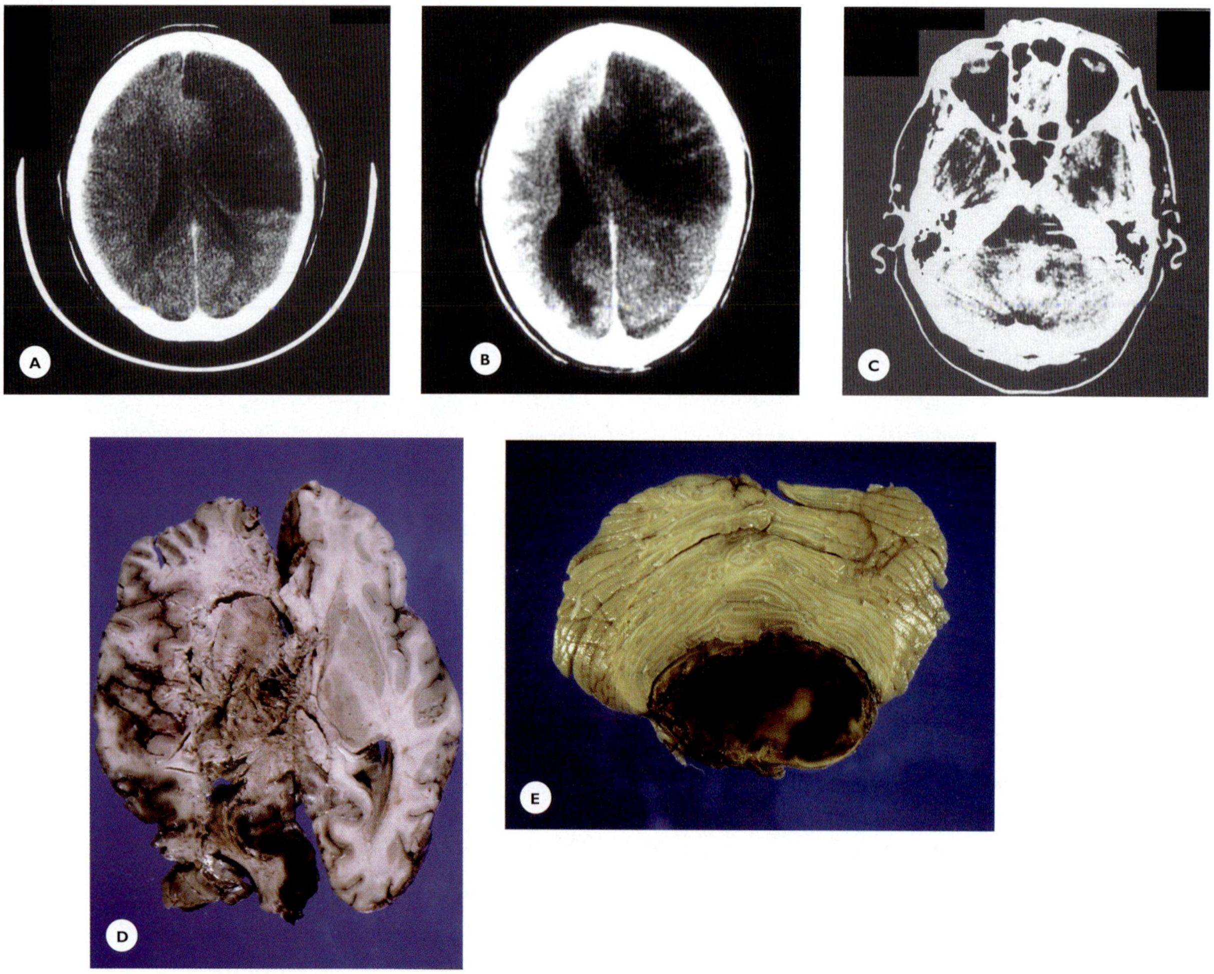

FIGURE 4.21

Sequential CT scan of an internal carotid artery (ICA) infarct, with progressive mass effect from edema. A 58-year-old hypertensive man, following a few short TIAs, developed right hemiparesis, sensory deficit, and expressive aphasia. Nine days later, he died. Initial CT scan showed only obliteration of sulci in the left cerebral hemisphere (**A**). Three days later, a left hemispheric, large, hypodense lesion in the territory of the MCA and ACA compressed the ipsilateral ventricle (demarcation between infarct and edema is poorly defined). **B.** Eight days later, an increase occurred in the size of the lesion and of the mass effect, with obliteration of the ventricle and midline shift. **C.** A pons hemorrhage was also present (hyperdense lesion). **D.** Horizontal section shows a markedly swollen left hemisphere. The infarct obliterates the lateral and third ventricles. A fresh hemorrhagic infarct is present in the occipital lobe and (**E**) a massive hemorrhage in the pons, both consequences of edema and increased brain volume.

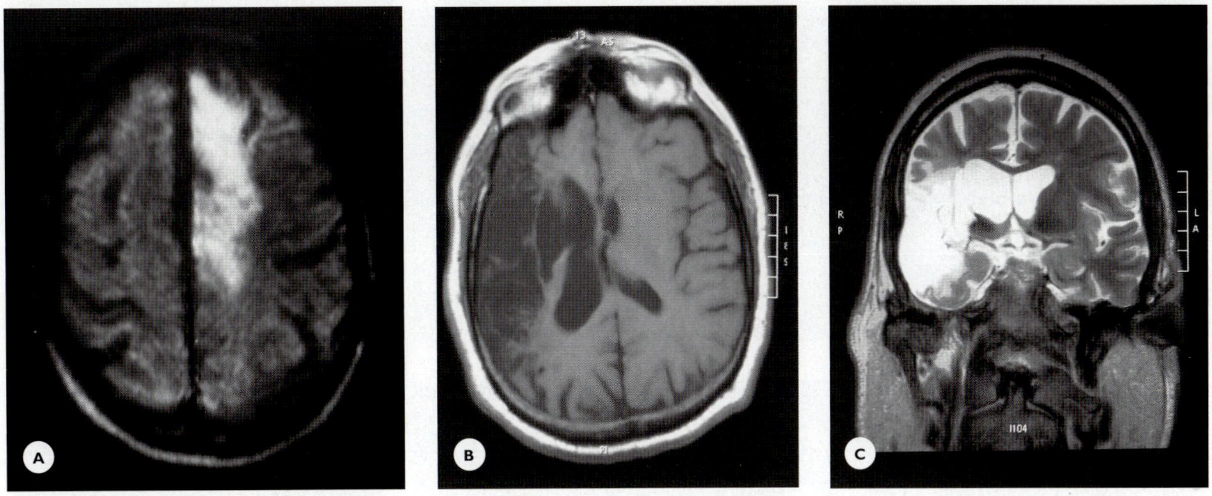

FIGURE 4.22
MR images of cerebral infarcts. **A.** Acute ACA infarct appears as a hyperintense lesion on axial T2-weighted image. **B.** Old MCA infarct is hypointense on T1-weighted image and hyperintense (**C**) on T2-weighted image. Note the enlargement of adjacent lateral ventricle indicating chronicity of the lesion.

mass effect on T2-weighted images. A chronic infarct is hypointense on T1 and hyperintense on T2-weighted images (see Table 4.9; Fig. 4.22).

Functional MRI with diffusion- and perfusion-weighted images is particularly valuable in identifying the ischemic territory within minutes postictally, thereby making early therapeutic intervention possible. Such images are also helpful in monitoring therapeutic efficacy.

The pathology of the cervical and cerebral arteries is conveniently demonstrated with magnetic resonance angiogram (MRA) (Fig. 4.23). Color-flow Doppler is a useful screening test to demonstrate severe arterial stenosis and occlusion of the cervical and intracranial arteries. An invasive four-vessel angiogram is performed in selected cases at the discretion of the vascular surgeon (see Fig. 4.23).

Hemorrhagic Stroke

The pathologic substrate of a hemorrhagic stroke is either an intracerebral hematoma or a subarachnoid hemorrhage (Table 4.10).

Spontaneous Intracerebral Hematoma

Etiology

The majority of intracerebral hemorrhages are associated with hypertension, which affects the small parenchymal arteries and arterioles and leads to fibrosis, hyalinosis, and fibrinoid necrosis. Such diseased arterioles easily rupture, causing the hemorrhage.

Less common causes of hemorrhages are vascular malformations, vasculopathies, hemorrhagic diseases, and hemorrhage within tumors (see Table 4.10; also see the section, Various Stroke Etiologies).

Pathology

Hypertensive hemorrhages have predilections for the basal ganglia (50%), the thalamus (10%), the pons and the cerebellum (5%–15%). Less common sites are the cerebral hemispheric white matter (lobar hemorrhage) and the ventricles (Fig. 4.24). Large basal ganglia and thalamus hemorrhages are accompanied by significant edema and may, during the first days, extend into the ventricles. A variant of basal ganglia hemorrhage occurs in the head of the caudate nucleus, which is supplied by the lateral striatal arteries. The pontine hemorrhage

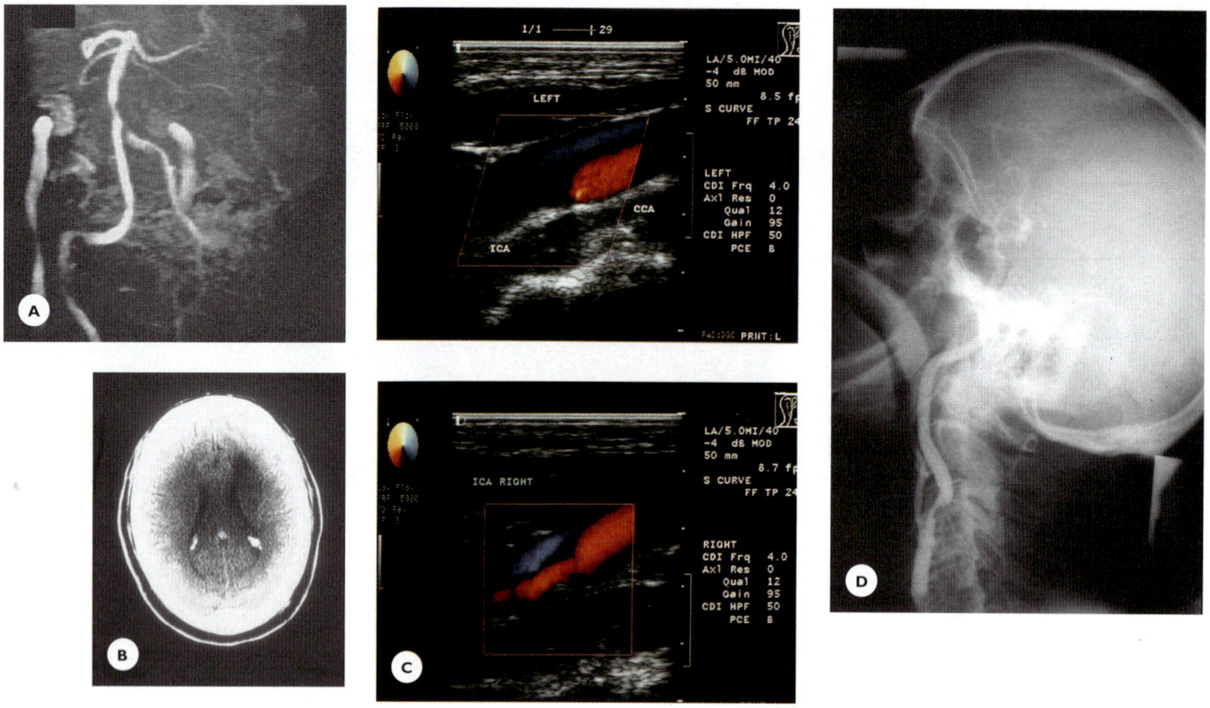

FIGURE 4.23
Vascular images. **A.** MRA of a 69-year-old man with history of TIAs in the vertebrobasilar circulation shows occlusion of the left vertebral artery and stenosis of the basilar artery. **B.** CT scan of a 62-year-old man shows a recent large left-MCA infarct. **C.** Color-flow Doppler shows sharp occlusion of the left ICA and severe stenosis of the right ICA. **D.** Conventional angiogram in a 70-year-old man with history of TIAs in carotid circulation shows severe stenosis of ICA above the bifurcation.

TABLE 4.10.
Cerebral Hemorrhage

Cerebral Hemorrhage

- **Parenchymal**
  - Hypertension
  - Arteriolosclerosis
  - Vascular malformation / Amyloid angiopathy / Vasculopathy/Vasculitis / Hemorrhagic diseases / Iatrogenic complications
- **Subarachnoid**
  - Vascular malformation
  - Rupture of berry aneurysm

may occupy the basis or may form confluent hemorrhages in the tegmentum and the basis. A large cerebellar hemorrhage carries the risk of tonsillar herniation, subsequent medullary compression, and acute respiratory failure. Early diagnosis and surgical evacuation of the clot is life saving.

The hematoma breaks down and liquefies after a few days. Its resorption may take several weeks or even months, depending on the size. Ultimately, a cystic cavity, with brown-stained walls from hemosiderin, replaces the hematoma (see Fig. 4.24).

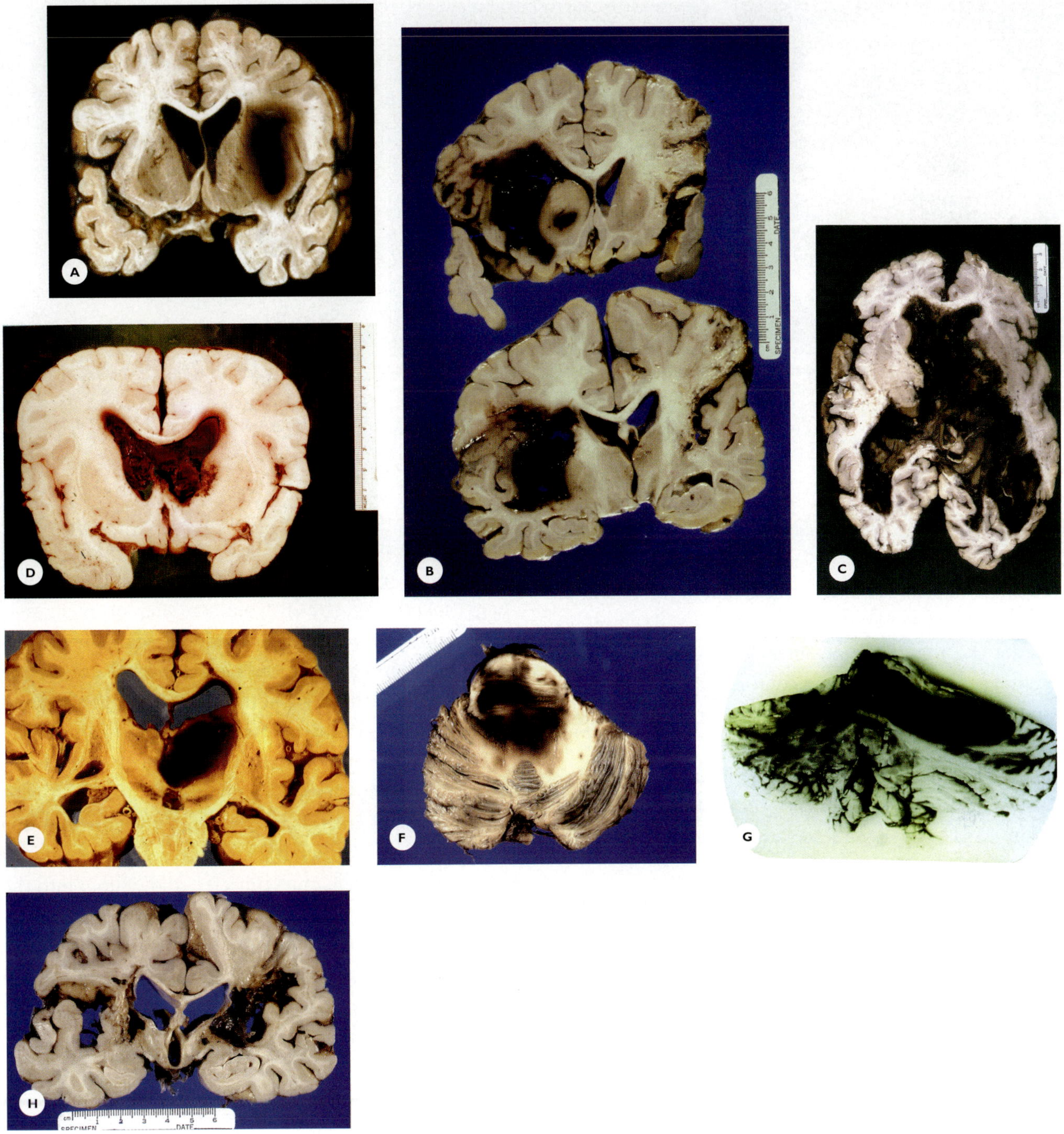

FIGURE 4.24

Topographic distribution of hypertensive intracerebral hemorrhages. **A.** Small putaminal hemorrhage. **B.** Massive basal ganglia hemorrhage extending into the ventricle. The parenchyma surrounding the hemorrhage is swollen, and the ventricle is compressed. **C.** Massive basal ganglia hemorrhage ruptured into the ventricle. **D.** Small caudate hemorrhage associated with massive ventricular hemorrhage. **E.** Thalamus hemorrhage. **F.** Pontine hemorrhage. **G.** Cerebellar hemorrhage. Note the herniation of the cerebellar tonsils. **H.** Cystic cavities with brown stained walls from hemosiderin at the site of resolved basal ganglia hemorrhage.

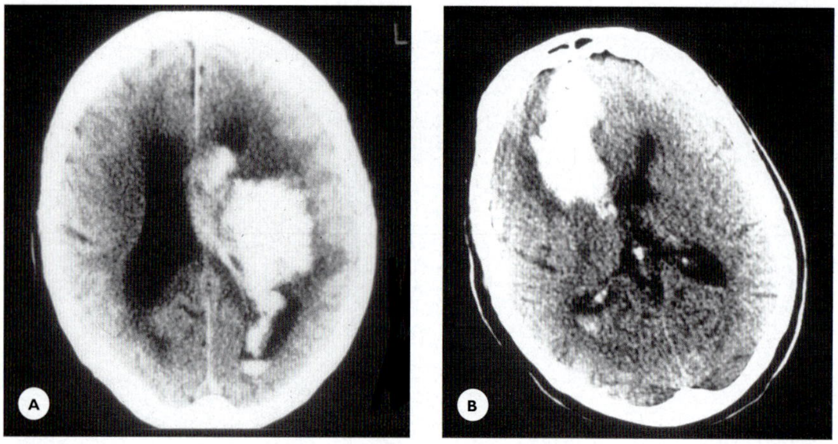

FIGURE 4.25
CT images of hypertensive cerebral hemorrhages. **A.** Nonenhanced axial CT scans show an acute hyperdense hemorrhage extending into the ventricle. **B.** Acute hyperdense lobar hemorrhage in the frontal lobe extends into the anterior horn.

Clinical Features

Hypertensive intracerebral hemorrhage accounts for about 10% to 12% of all strokes. The onset is abrupt. Generalized symptoms include headaches, vomiting, confusion, depressed consciousness ranging from stupor to coma and, in some patients, seizures. Focal symptoms indicate the site of the hemorrhage. Expansion of the hemorrhage and edema may continue, causing deterioration for about 24 hours. Early mortality remains high, at 30% to 40%.

CT scan readily demonstrates the acute parenchymal hematoma as a hyperdense (bright) lesion, usually surrounded by a hypodense area caused by edema (Fig. 4.25). Acute hemorrhage on MR T1-weighted images appears as a hypointense (dark) and on T2-weighted images as a hyperintense (bright) lesion. With time, as the oxyhemoglobin gradually disintegrates into methemoglobin and then into hemosiderin, the appearance of the hemorrhage changes. An old hemorrhage on the CT scan appears as a hypodense lesion indistinguishable from an old infarct and, on T1- and T2-weighted MR images, as a hypointense lesion (see Table 4.9).

Hypertensive Encephalopathy

Chronic and poorly controlled hypertension produces an encephalopathy with headaches, altered mentation, and occasionally seizures. Fibrinoid necrosis of the small arteries, edema, and petechiae are the cerebral findings.

Subarachnoid Hemorrhage

Etiology and Pathology

The rupture of a saccular (berry) aneurysm is the most common cause of a nontraumatic subarachnoid hemorrhage (SAH) (Fig. 4.26). Common sites of aneurysms are the circle of Willis at the junctions of major arteries and at their first bifurcation. Less common sites are the tip of the basilar artery and the junction of the vertebral arteries. Aneurysms vary in size from a few millimeters to 2 to 3 cm (giant aneurysms). They are often multiple, situated bilaterally as mirror images (Fig. 4.27). A ruptured saccular aneurysm commonly bleeds into the basal cisterns of the subarachnoid space, less often into the brain parenchyma or ventricles, and seldom into the subdural space.

Less common causes of SAH are mycotic (infectious) and fusiform (arteriosclerotic) aneurysms, vascular malformations, vasculopathies, and hematologic diseases (see Table 4.10).

Clinical Features

Subarachnoid hemorrhage accounts for approximately 8% of hemorrhagic strokes and is somewhat more common in younger patients and women.

Prodromal symptoms with localized, often pulsating headaches and third nerve palsy may precede the aneurysmal rupture. The highly characteristic presentation of SAH is abrupt, with severe, often excruciating headaches and meningeal signs. Altered mentation, extraocular muscle palsy, subhyaloid hemorrhage, and

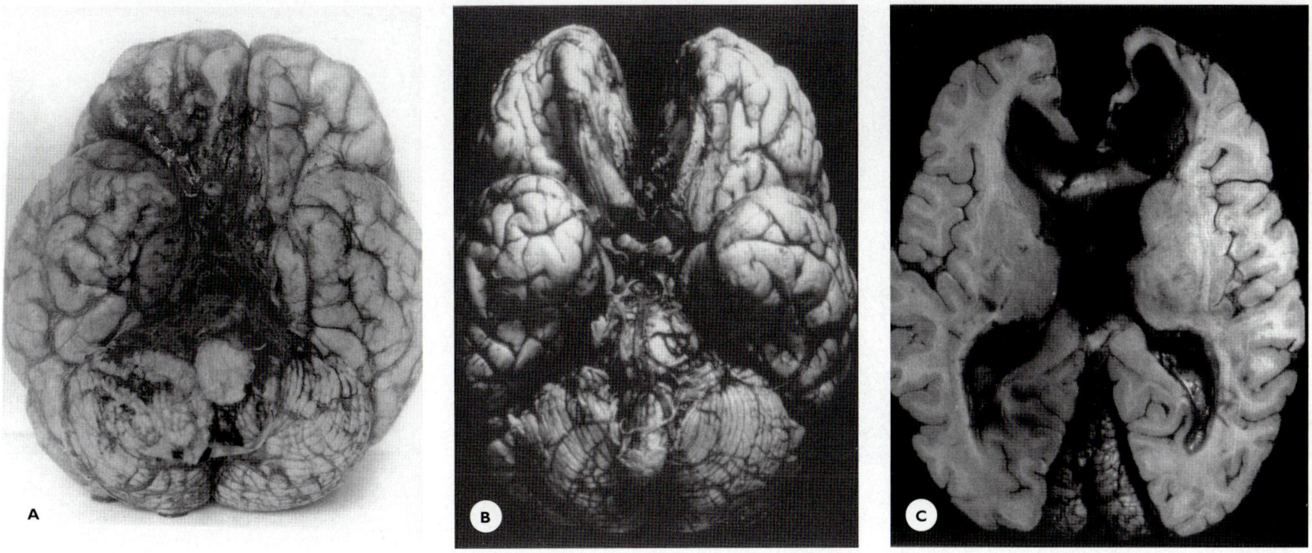

FIGURE 4.26
Subarachnoid hemorrhage. **A.** Massive fresh hemorrhage in basal subarachnoid space from rupture of an anterior communicating artery aneurysm. Note the hemorrhage in the optic nerve. **B** and **C.** An anterior communicating aneurysm ruptured into the corpus callosum and ventricles.

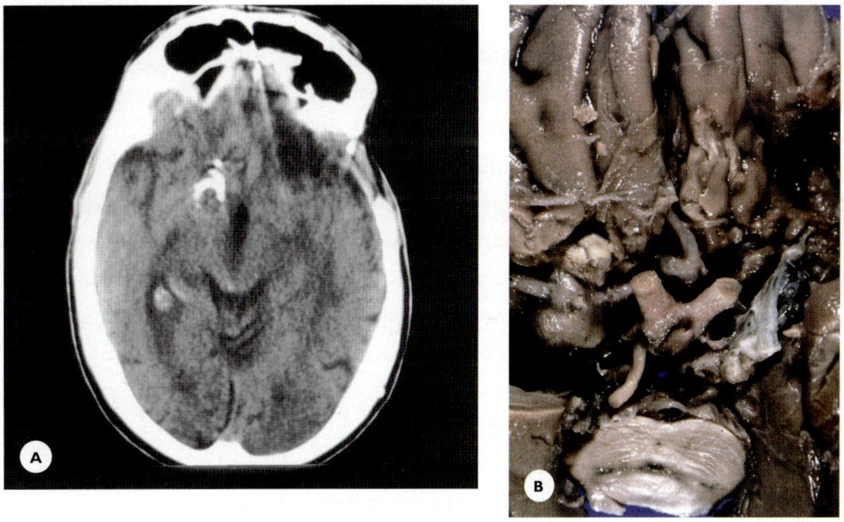

FIGURE 4.27
Mirror image aneurysms of MCAs. A 26-year-old man underwent clipping of a ruptured left MCA aneurysm. He died at age 73 of carcinoma of the lung. **A.** A nonenhanced CT scan of the head done a few weeks prior to his death shows a cherry-sized, low-density structure with a hyperdense rim in the right Sylvian fissure. **B.** Base of the brain shows surgical clips in the left Sylvian fissure and a large, partially calcified and thrombosed asymptomatic right MCA aneurysm, mirror image of the ruptured left MCA aneurysm.

occasionally, focal neurologic signs and seizures are present. CT scan identifies the SAH in the majority of cases, and MRA and conventional angiogram identify the aneurysm (Fig. 4.28). Mortality is high; approximately 20% of patients die within 24 hours. One-third die of the initial insult, and about one-fourth die of recurrent bleeding, frequently during the second and third weeks.

The SAH carries the risk of serious complications, notably:

- Ischemia and infarction due to vasospasm in the proximity of the bleeding aneurysm or embolization from intraluminal thrombus
- Syndrome of inappropriate antidiuretic hormone secretion (SIADH) and cardiac arrhythmias due to hypothalamic dysfunction

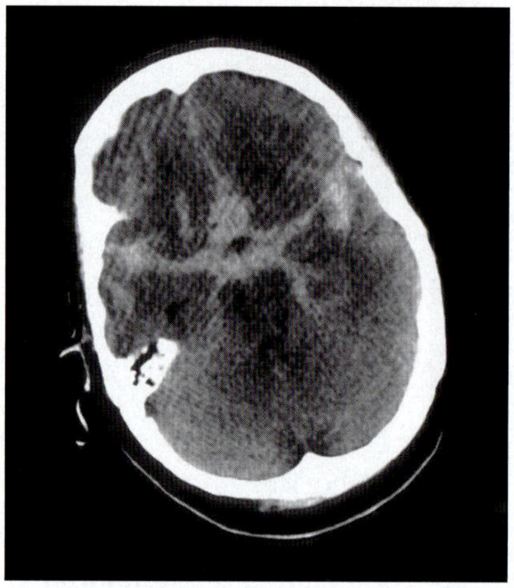

FIGURE 4.28
CT scan of subarachnoid hemorrhage. **A.** Axial nonenhanced CT scan shows acute hemorrhage in the basal cisterns and Sylvian fissures.

TABLE 4.11.
Stroke Predisposing Diseases in the Young

Cardiac Diseases	*Vascular Diseases*
Rheumatic valvular disease Mitral valve prolapse Prosthetic heart valve Congenital heart disease Myxoma Cardiomyopathy in neuro-degenerative diseases and myopathies	Fibromuscular dysplasia Arterial dissection Systemic lupus erythematosus Vascular malformation Takayasu's arteritis Moyamoya disease Vasculopathy secondary to illicit substances Inherited vascular diseases Early atherosclerosis
Hematologic Diseases	***Inherited Metabolic Diseases***
Sickle cell disease Thrombotic thrombocytopenia Hemophilia Leukemia Antiphospholipid antibody syndrome Venous thrombosis	Homocystinuria MELAS; Mitochondrial Encephalomyopathy, Lactic acidosis, Stroke-like Episodes Fabry's disease

- Hydrocephalus, which may develop during the acute stage or several months later

During the acute stage, the circulation and absorption of the cerebrospinal fluid (CSF) is obstructed by the hemorrhage and, during the chronic stage, by fibrotic adhesions between the arachnoid and pia.

Cerebral aneurysm often coexists with cerebral and visceral vascular malformations, moyamoya disease, polycystic kidneys, pancreatic cysts, fibromuscular dysplasia, coarctation of the aorta, and Ehlers-Danlos and Marfan syndromes (see next section, Various Stroke Etiologies).

VARIOUS STROKE ETIOLOGIES: STROKE IN THE YOUNG

In addition to arteriosclerosis of the cerebral arteries, diseases of the heart, and hypertension, a variety of conditions predispose to strokes;,vasculitis and vasculopathies, hematologic disorders, iatrogenic complications, and abuse of illicit substances being the most prevalent. These and several other conditions (see following sections) predispose to strokes at any age, but are particularly common and important causes of strokes that affect younger subjects, ranging in age from infancy through childhood and adolescence, to adulthood. Additional causes of strokes in the young are cardiac diseases particular to the young, early atherothrombosis of hereditary dyslipoproteinemia, and some inherited metabolic and neurodegenerative diseases (Table 4.11). In a significant number of patients, the etiology remains undetermined.

Stroke in the young population accounts for 5% of all strokes; the incidence of ischemic stroke is only slightly higher than that of hemorrhagic. Stroke in the pediatric age group usually presents with headaches and acute hemiplegia, often associated with seizures. Because of diverse etiologies, young stroke patients require a comprehensive cardiovascular, hematologic, and metabolic screening.

The prognosis of ischemic stroke among young subjects is favorable, and mortality is low. Recovery ranges from complete to partial, with variable motor deficits, movement disorder, seizures and, in children, learning difficulties and mental retardation. Prognosis of intracerebral hemorrhage is less favorable, and mortality in subarachnoid hemorrhage is high, possibly reaching 40%.

Nonarteriosclerotic Diseases of Cerebral Arteries

This group encompasses vascular diseases of varied etiologies, including inflammatory and. noninflammatory vasculopathies, hereditary arteriopathies, malformations, and mineralization related to aging.

The diagnosis of these diseases often presents difficulties; early diagnosis, however, is important because appropriate therapy may halt or even reverse the disease process. The clinical presentation varies across a broad spectrum. The disease may begin acutely as a TIA or a full blown stroke, or it may progress gradually with headaches, multifocal neurologic signs, seizures, behavioral changes, psychosis, and cognitive decline often progressing to dementia. Several diseases also affect the systemic blood vessels and produce visceral and cutaneous changes. Segmental constriction (beading) of the arterial wall, as seen on angiogram, is characteristic for some; for others, the definite diagnosis may require tissue biopsy. The cerebral pathology also ranges widely: Some angiopathies have a predilection for the large, and some for the small vessels; infarctions and hemorrhages may be solitary or multiple, small or large.

Inflammatory Vascular Diseases

Immune-Mediated Vasculitis

Giant cell temporal arteritis, a granulomatous inflammation of the temporal artery may also involve the ophthalmic artery, branches of the carotids, and the systemic blood vessels. Mononuclear cells and multinucleated giant cells infiltrate the vessel walls, thickening the intima and the media; thus, the lumen becomes significantly reduced, and the temporal arterial wall becomes tender and pulseless. The disease commonly affects individuals over 50 years of age. Headache in the temporal region and elevated sedimentation rate are diagnostic.

Polyarteritis nodosa usually occurs in middle-aged adults and involves the medium-sized and small leptomeningeal and parenchymal arteries and the nutrient arterioles of the peripheral nerves. In the acute stage, the vessel wall undergoes fibrinoid necrosis, with massive polymorphonuclear infiltration. In the chronic stage, dense fibrosis with residual inflammatory cells replaces the vessel wall (Fig. 4.29). The kidneys, liver, and gastrointestinal tract are commonly involved.

Systemic lupus erythematosus (SLE) affects individuals from adolescence to old age. The small cerebral arteries undergo fibrinoid necrosis, mononuclear infiltration, hyalinization, and fibrosis. The lumen is often occluded by a thromboembolus. Characteristic visceral manifestations are verrucous endocarditis, glomerulonephritis, and interstitial pneumonia. Patients may harbor lupus anticoagulant antibodies and present the antiphospholipid antibody syndrome.

Wegener's granulomatosis occurs in middle-age. It is characterized by granulomatous necrosis of the small- and medium-sized arteries, often in a segmental fashion. Frequently, the respiratory tract and kidneys are also affected.

Takayasu's arteritis (aortic arch syndrome, pulseless disease) is common in young women. A granulomatous

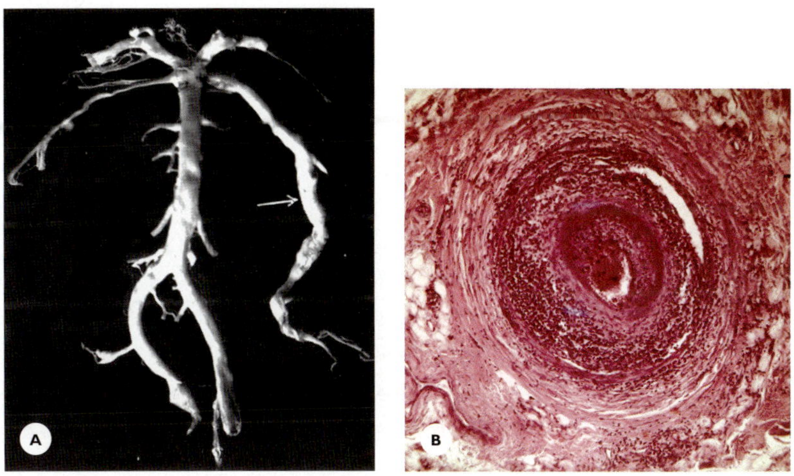

FIGURE 4.29
Polyarteritis nodosa in a 47-year-old man. **A.** The walls of cerebral arteries are grayish and show segmental constriction and distension (string sign). **B.** A nutrient artery of the sciatic nerve shows acute fibrinoid necrosis with polymorphonuclear and monocytic leukocytes (HE).

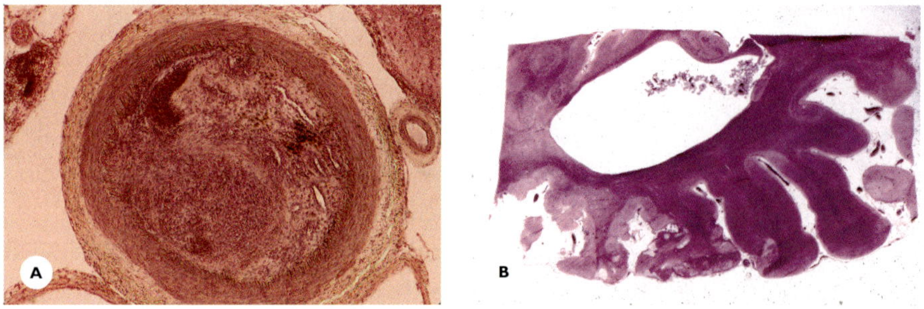

FIGURE 4.30
Thromboangiitis obliterans in a 50-year-old man. **A.** Leptomeningeal artery shows marked intimal proliferation and thrombotic occlusion. **B.** The cortex shows multiple small cystic infarctions (HE).

proliferative inflammatory process with giant cells involves the aorta and its branches, leading to severe luminal narrowing and occlusion.

Primary central nervous system angiitis is characterized by necrosis and infiltration of small- and medium-sized arteries with mononuclear cells and multinucleated epithelial cells. The inflammation may extend into the meninges.

Infectious Vasculitis

A number of bacteria and fungi that infect the nervous system often produce an acute inflammatory, necrotizing, or chronic granulomatous vasculitis of the cerebral blood vessels. Spirochetes may infect the blood vessels: *Treponema pallidum* in neurosyphilis and *Borrelia burgdorferi* in Lyme disease. HIV-associated vasculitis is prone to cause ischemic episodes in both adults and children. Vasculitis of the large cerebral arteries accounts for the hemiplegia that develops contralaterally to a facial or ocular herpes zoster infection. Post varicella vasculopathy is a potential risk for stroke in children.

Noninflammatory Vasculopathies

Thromboangiitis obliterans occurs chiefly in middle-aged men who smoke heavily. It commonly involves the peripheral arteries. The disease may also involve the medium-sized and small meningeal and cerebral arteries, producing intimal proliferation, luminal obliteration, and multiple small infarctions (Fig. 4.30).

Moyamoya disease affects young adults. The basal cerebral arteries undergo severe intimal thickening and luminal occlusion. Subsequently, an abnormal collateral vascular network develops at the base of the brain. This network appears on angiogram as a puff of smoke, hence the name moyamoya (Japanese; puff of smoke).

Fibromuscular dysplasia occurs among the middle-aged, mostly in women. The cervical carotids and the vertebrals show segmental muscular fibrous thickening and loss of the elastic layer, which appear on angiogram as string of beads. The disease presents with ischemic stroke and is an important cause of arterial dissection.

Amyloid angiopathy affects the leptomeningeal and the medium-sized and small cortical arteries. The amyloid deposited in the media and adventitia of arteries stains positively with Congo red and shows green birefringence under polarized light. It immunoreacts for β-amyloid peptide, a cleavage product of amyloid precursor protein. The disease affects the elderly and is associated with Alzheimer's disease. It causes small infarctions and intracerebral lobar hemorrhages (Fig. 4.31).

Hereditary Arteriopathies

Cerebral autosomal dominant arteriopathy with subcortical infarcts and leukoencephalopathy (CADASIL) affects young and middle-aged adults. It is associated with mutations of *Notch 3* gene on chromosome 19. The disease involves the leptomeningeal and small parenchymal arteries, and the small arteries of the peripheral nerves, muscles, and skin. The vessel walls are fibrotic and hyalinized, and basophilic and PAS-positive granules are deposited in the media. Skin biopsy and genetic studies confirm the diagnosis.

Familial cerebral amyloid angiopathy, a rare autosomal dominant disorder of the small arteries, predisposes to ischemic and hemorrhagic strokes. The *Dutch variety* affects elderly subjects, and the vascular deposits contain β-amyloid peptide. The *Icelandic variety* affects

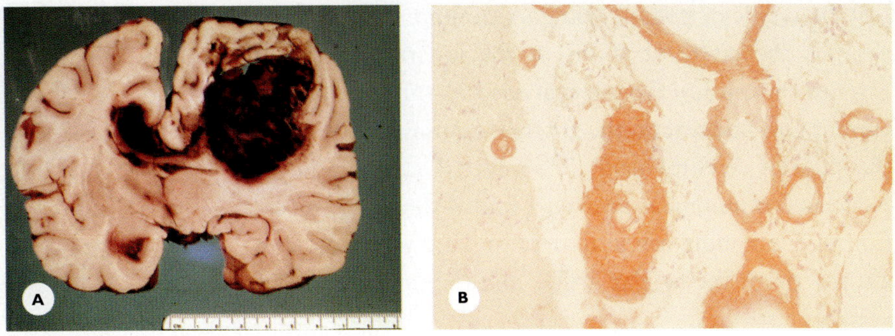

FIGURE 4.31
Amyloid angiopathy. **A.** Amyloid angiopathy associated with lobar centroparietal hemorrhage in a 72-year-old man. **B.** Amyloid deposits in walls of small blood vessels (Congo red).

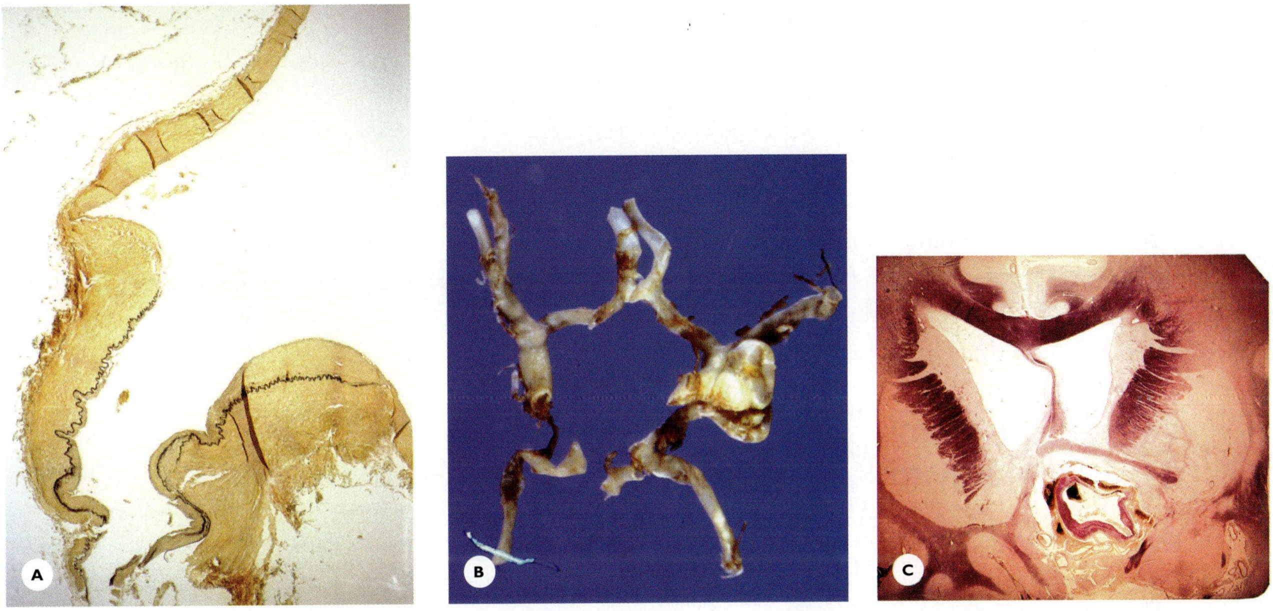

FIGURE 4.32
Aneurysms. **A.** Histologic section of a MCA aneurysm. The muscular and elastic layers of the artery end abruptly at the neck of the aneurysm. The aneurysmal wall consists of fibrous tissue (van Gieson-orcein). **B.** Circle of Willis dissected from the base of the brain shows a cherry-sized unruptured aneurysm at the point of junction of the MCA and posterior communicating artery **C.** Macrosection of an unruptured ACA aneurysm.

younger subjects, and the vascular deposits contain cystatin C, an abnormal microprotein (cystatin C amyloid angiopathy).

Ehlers-Danlos syndrome, an autosomal dominant or recessive disorder of collagen synthesis, predisposes to aneurysmal formation, carotid-cavernous fistula, and arterial dissection.

Marfan's syndrome, an autosomal dominant disorder of connective tissue, manifests with cardiovascular (aortic dissection, aneurysmal dilatation), ocular (lens dislocation), and skeletal (elongated habitus) anomalies.

Vascular Malformations

Malformations of the cerebral arteries may remain clinically silent, or may present with seizures and focal symptoms and signs, and may also produce ischemic or hemorrhagic events.

Saccular (Berry) Aneurysm

An aneurysm is a focal dilatation in the wall of an artery. The muscular and elastic layers taper off or end at the margin of the aneurysm. The aneurysmal wall consists of fibrous tissue only (Fig. 4.32). The aneurysm may be sessile or pedunculated. A common site of aneurysm is the circle of Willis at the junction of major arteries (Fig. 4.32); the internal carotid and the anterior communicating artery, the anterior communicating and the anterior cerebral artery, the internal carotid and the posterior communicating artery, and at the first bifurcation of the middle cerebral arteries. Less common sites are the tip of the basilar artery and the junction of the vertebral arteries.

Etiologic considerations include congenital weakness of the arterial wall, degeneration from hemodynamic stress, or vestigial remnant of embryonic arteries.

Clinical Features

Aneurysm has the highest incidence between the ages of 30 and 60 years, but it may occur in adolescence and old age. It is very rare in infants and children. It is slightly more common in women, and familial cases are known. Subarachnoid hemorrhage from the rupture of an aneurysm is the second major cause of hemorrhagic strokes.

An unruptured aneurysm may remain clinically silent or may cause pulsating headaches, TIAs, and focal symptoms and signs through local pressure (see Fig. 4.32). In carotid territories, aneurysms produce visual deficit, visual field defect, and an isolated third nerve palsy. An aneurysm within the cavernous sinus presents with frontal and orbital headache, oculomotor and abducens palsies, Horner syndrome, and sensory deficit over the forehead and maxilla (V/1 and V/2 divisions). When it ruptures, it produces a carotid-cavernous (arteriovenous) fistula with pulsating exophthalmos, bruit over the eye, hemorrhagic edema of the eyelid, and visual failure from retinal hemorrhage and occlusion of central retinal vein. In vertebrobasilar territories, aneurysms produce trigeminal, acoustic, or lower cranial nerve deficits and brainstem symptoms and signs.

Angiomas

Angiomas, congenital conglomerates of abnormal vascular channels, are classified as arteriovenous, cavernous, and venous angiomas and capillary telangiectasis (see Chapter 11). Seizures and headaches are characteristic clinical manifestations. Ischemic episodes result when the angioma steals (shunts) blood from the surrounding parenchymal arteries (sump effect). Subarachnoid and parenchymal hemorrhages are major complications (Fig. 4.33).

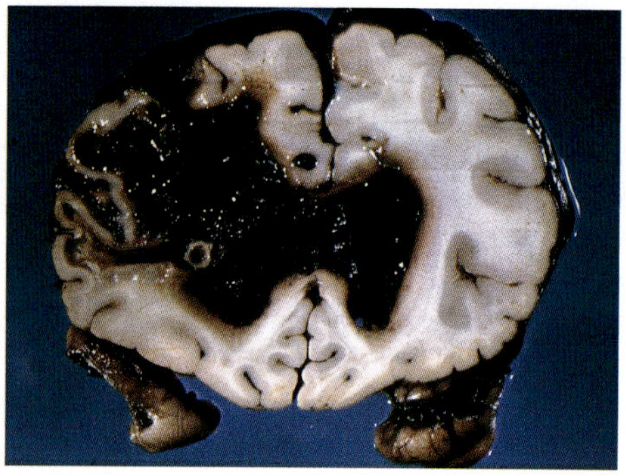

FIGURE 4.33
Angioma. Massive frontal lobe hemorrhage from rupture of an arteriovenous malformation.

Dolichoectasia

Dolichoectasia is the diffuse elongation, distention, and tortuosity of the extracranial and intracranial cerebral arteries; the vertebrobasilar and the posterior cerebral arteries are affected most often. Atherosclerosis accentuates the anomaly. Histologically, the arterial wall is thin and the elastica is disrupted or virtually absent (Fig. 4.34). Dolichoectasia is associated with ischemic stroke, subarachnoid hemorrhage, and various symptoms caused by the pressure exerted on adjacent structures: visual impairment, vertigo, tinnitus, facial spasm, trigeminal neuralgia, hydrocephalus, and cranial nerve deficits. It is identifiable on MRA and occasionally on CT scan.

Anomalies of Basal Cerebral Arteries

The *persistence of the embryonic origin of the posterior cerebral artery from the carotid artery* is a common incidental autopsy finding (Fig. 4.35). Subsequently, the supply territory of the posterior cerebral artery becomes liable to circulatory insufficiency in the carotid artery.

In hypoplasia of one vertebral artery, the basilar artery is the continuation of the normal vertebral artery.

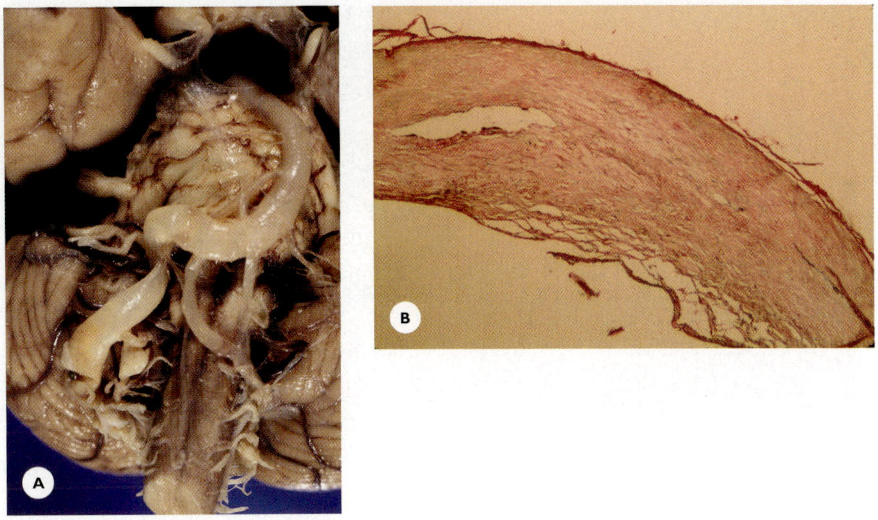

FIGURE 4.34
Dolichoectasia in an 83-year-old man. **A.** The basilar artery is tortuous, its wall is thin and soft, and the lumen distended. The artery is the continuation of the thin-walled right vertebral artery. **B.** The wall of the basilar artery is fibrotic, the elastic lamina is fragmented and partially missing (Verhoeff elastic stain).

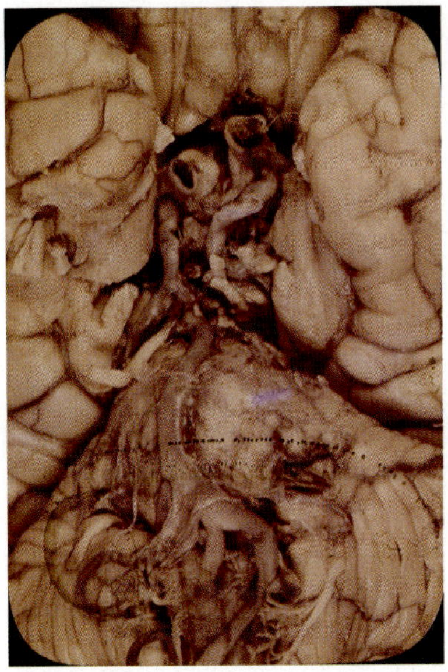

FIGURE 4.35
Anomalous origin of the PCAs from the respective carotid arteries.

Subsequently, the supply territory of the hypoplastic artery becomes vulnerable to falls in systemic blood pressure.

The *persistence of the trigeminal artery* between the cavernous section of the carotid artery and the basilar artery has been associated with trigeminal neuralgia.

Mineralization Related to Aging

Siderocalcinosis

Calcium and iron deposits in the walls of the small arteries and capillaries are common incidental autopsy findings in the brains of elderly population (Fig. 4.36). Usual sites are the basal ganglia, where they are detectable on CT scan, the white matter of the hippocampus, and the dentate nucleus of the cerebellum. They may cause rarefaction and spongiosis of the parenchyma.

Hematologic Diseases

Cerebral infarctions and hemorrhages are serious complications of a variety of blood disorders affecting the red and white cells, the platelets, and the coagulation mechanism. Some diseases are inherited, but the majority are acquired.

Disorders of Red and White Blood Cells

Sickle cell anemia, an inherited hemoglobin disorder, is characterized by the replacement of hemoglobin A (HbA) with hemoglobin S (HbS sickle hemoglobin). Homozygotes have all HbA replaced with HbS (HbSS) and carry the disease, whereas heterozygotes have less than 40% HbS (HbSA) and carry the sickle cell trait. HbSA occurs in about 8% to 10% of African

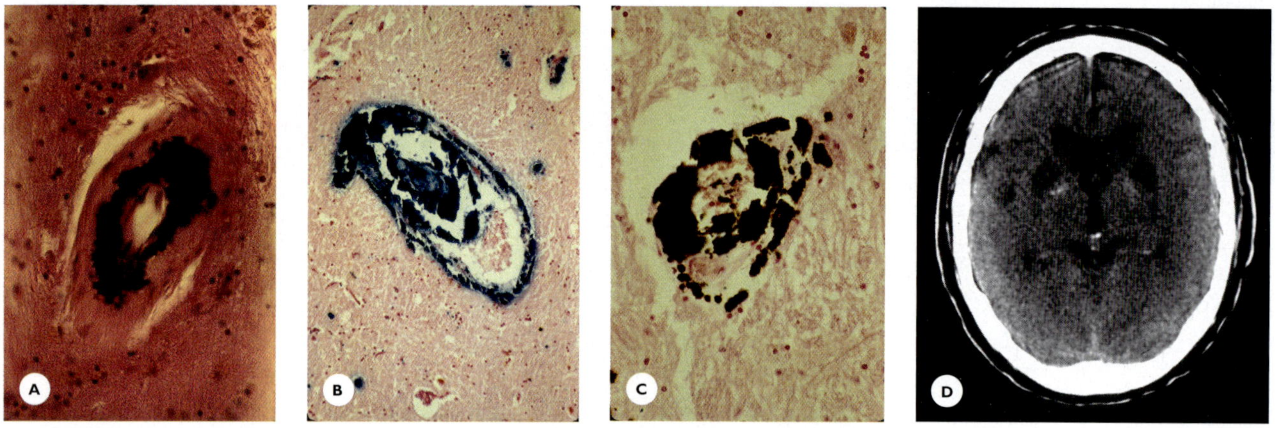

FIGURE 4.36
Siderocalcinosis of blood vessels in globus pallidus. Basophilic mineral deposits **A.** in the intima and media (HE), **B.** in full thickness of the wall, partially obliterating the lumen (Gomori iron stain) and, **C.** destroying the vessel's wall (Von Kossa calcium stain). **D.** CT scan showing mineralization in globus pallidus.

Americans. A number of situations associated with low arterial oxygen tension (chronic anemia, infection, heat stroke, physical overexertion) are apt to precipitate sickling of the erythrocytes.

Stroke, more often ischemic than hemorrhagic, occurs at any age from childhood to old age, and frequently is recurrent. The incidence is particularly high in children, and small infarctions may develop in the absence of clinical evidence of a stroke. The ischemic events result from occlusion of arterioles and capillaries by sludging of sickled erythrocytes, or from thrombotic occlusions of larger arteries. The cerebral pathology is characterized by small and large infarctions, often situated in the watershed region between arterial territories. Ischemic events may occur even in individuals with sickle cell trait (Fig. 4.37).

In *polycythemia vera*, hyperviscosity from an increased concentration of erythrocytes reduces the cerebral blood flow, leading to TIAs and eventually infarction (Fig. 4.38).

The *hyperleukocytosis* of leukemias is a serious risk for cerebral hemorrhage (see Fig. 4.38).

Disorders of Platelets

Thrombocythemia is associated with TIAs and infarctions.

Thrombocytopenia is associated with bleeding that ranges from petechiae to massive intracerebral hematoma (see Fig. 4.38).

Thrombotic thrombocytopenic purpura is characterized by hyalin platelet thrombi in the small cere-bral arteries and microinfarctions (see Fig. 4.38). Purpuric skin lesions, hemolytic anemia, focal neurologic symptoms, seizures, and mental changes are clinical manifestations.

Disorders of Coagulation

Hemophilia A and B (Christmas disease) are sex-linked recessive diseases caused by a deficiency of clotting factor VIII and IX, respectively. They are major causes of childhood intracerebral hemorrhages.

In *inherited hypercoagulability,* mutation of coagulation factor V gene (factor Leiden) has been associated with ischemic strokes in children. Diseases with protein-C, protein-S, and antithrombin-III deficiencies are inherited in an autosomal dominant pattern. They affect young adults and present with recurrent venous thrombosis.

Antiphospholipid antibody syndrome is an important acquired coagulation disorder in young individuals (Fig. 4.39). Antiphospholipid antibodies (aPL) are a group of circulating immunoglobulins (IgG, IgM, and

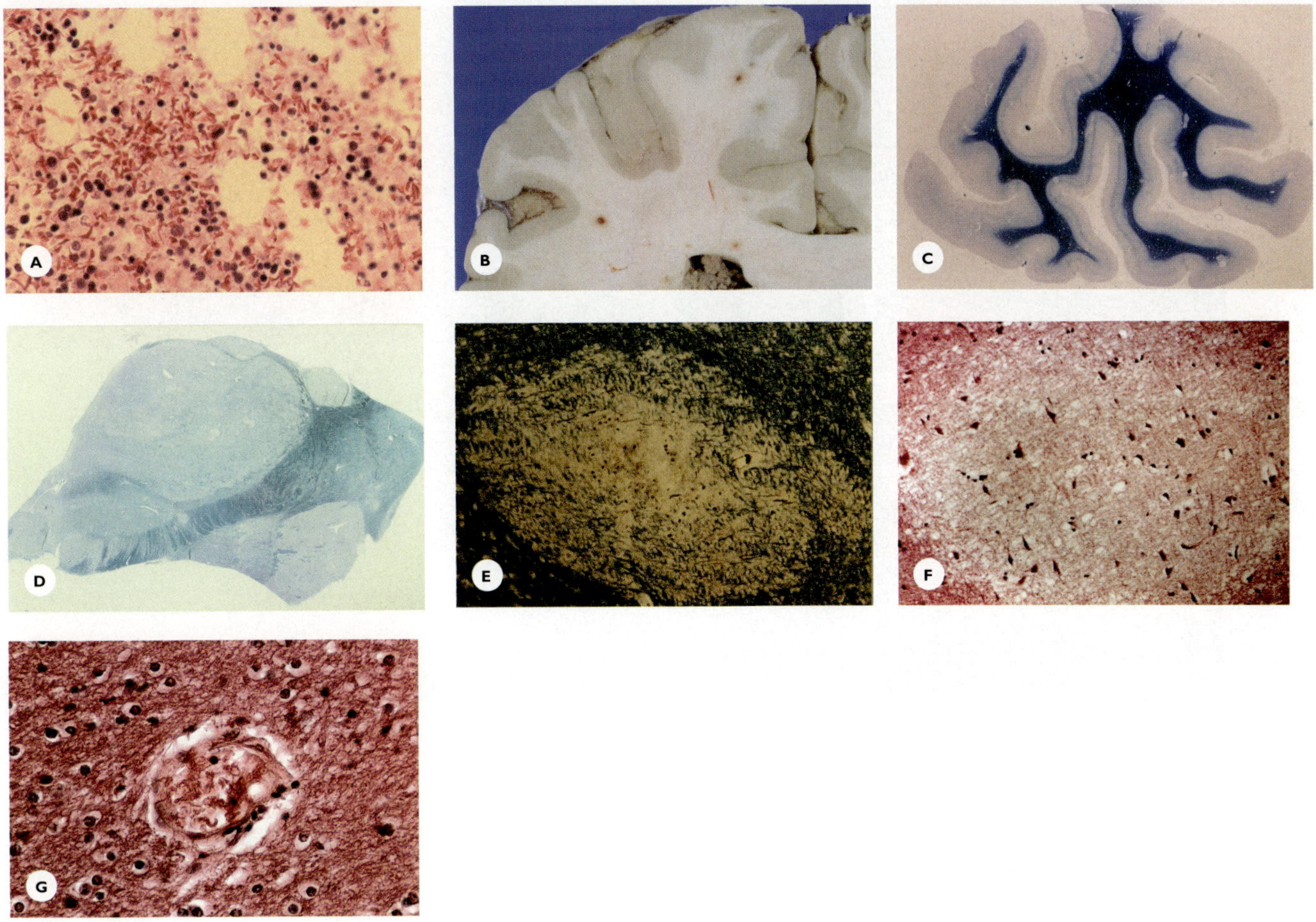

FIGURE 4.37
Sickle cell crisis with fulminant fatal hypoxic-ischemic encephalopathy in a 20-year-old African American woman with sickle cell trait. Following strenuous physical exercises, her illness began with abdominal and joint pain, and culminated 3 days after the onset in coma and death. **A.** Bone marrow shows closely packed sickled erythrocytes and hemorrhages (HE). **B.** Petechiae are scattered throughout the white and gray matter. **C.** Multiple discrete lesions are dispersed in the cortex and white matter of the occipital lobe and in (**D**) thalamus and basal ganglia (LFB-CV). **E.** Within the lesions, the myelin and nerve fibers are variably destroyed (Holmes stain). **F.** The cortex shows focal ischemic neuronal necrosis (HE). **G.** Sludging and sickling of erythrocytes are noticeable in the lumen of a small vessel (HE).

IgA). Among them, the anticardiolipin antibody and the lupus anticoagulant are the best characterized. Antiphospholipid antibodies are present in a high percentage of patients with lupus erythematosus. The aPL antibodies predispose to intravascular thrombotic events and infarctions through a complex immune-mediated mechanism.

The syndrome is associated with widespread recurrent arterial and venous thrombosis in the brain, retina, visceral organs, and peripheral blood vessels. Characteristic neurologic manifestations are TIAs, ischemic strokes, amaurosis fugax, migraine-like headaches, seizures, ischemic encephalopathy and, in severe cases, the disease progresses to dementia. Cardiac valvular diseases (verrucous endocarditis), cutaneous lesions (livedo reticularis), and recurrent abortions in women are common systemic manifestations. Thrombocytopenia, prolonged activated thromboplastin time and prothrombin time, and high titers of antiphospholipid antibodies are laboratory hallmarks of the syndrome.

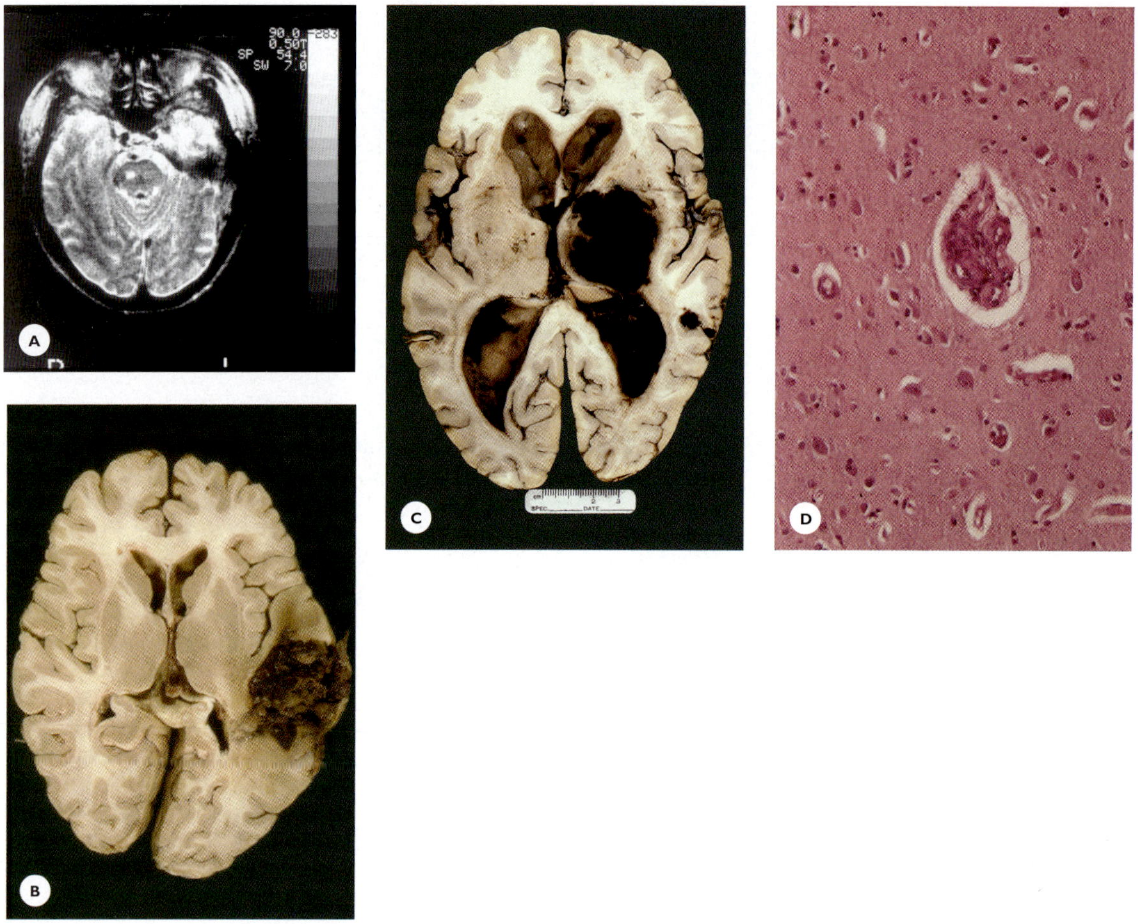

FIGURE 4.38
Complications of hematologic diseases. **A.** Polycythemia vera in a 67-year-old man. MRI shows a pontine lacunar infarct. **B.** Acute myelocytic leukemia in a 52-year-old man complicated by temporal lobe hemorrhage. **C.** Thrombocytopenia in a 67-year-old alcoholic patient associated with thalamic hemorrhage. **D.** Thrombotic thrombocytopenic purpura. Hyalin platelet thrombus occludes the lumen of a capillary (HE).

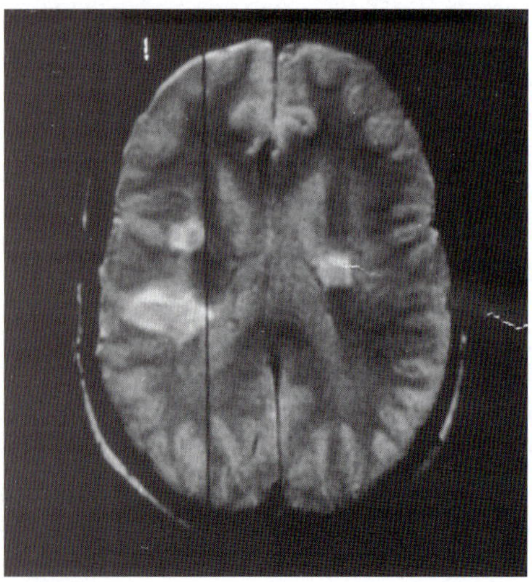

FIGURE 4.39
Antiphospholipid antibody syndrome in a 48-year-old man. He suffered his first stroke at age 31 years and the second at age 33. T2-weighted MRI shows multiple infarcts in territories of MCAs. Recurrent TIAs, slowly progressive neurologic deficits, dysarthria, and memory decline define his clinical course.

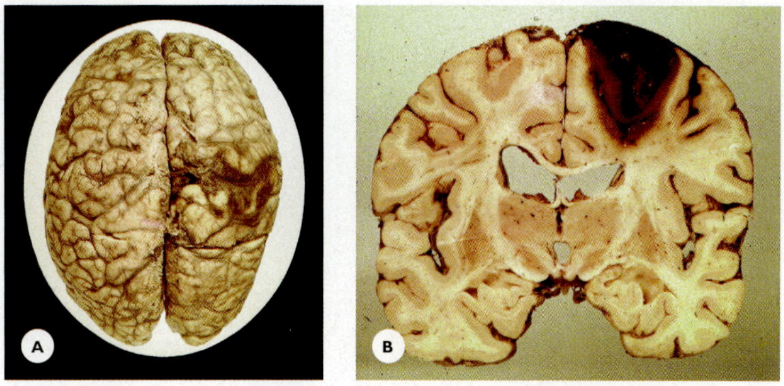

FIGURE 4.40
Venous thrombosis associated with a hemorrhagic infarct.

Antiphospholipid antibodies have been associated with malignancies, Lyme disease, HIV infection, and benign intracranial hypertension. They occasionally occur in patients treated with Dilantin, valproic acid, and phenothiazine drugs. In all these conditions, they seldom produce the syndrome.

Disseminated intravascular coagulation (DIC), a thrombohemorrhagic disorder, is associated with a variety of diseases, including infection, liver disease, neoplasm, trauma, burns, and obstetric complications. Fibrin thrombi in the small arteries and capillaries of the brain, viscera, and skin cause microinfarcts and microhemorrhages. Hemorrhages are more common in acute disease, whereas infarcts are more common in chronic disease.

Cerebral sinovenous thrombosis may develop in a variety of clinical settings, including liver disease, nephrotic syndrome, fracture, burns, malignancy, pregnancy, postpartum and postoperative states, the use of birth control pills, and dehydration. It can cause subarachnoid and intracerebral hemorrhages and bland or hemorrhagic infarcts. The lesions are commonly situated in the cortex and subcortical white matter (Fig. 4.40).

Other Conditions

Iatrogenic Complications

Diagnostic procedures and major surgeries for coronary artery and valvular diseases, heart transplant, and various organ and bone marrow transplants carry the highest risk for cerebral hemorrhage and infarction. Subdural and intracranial hemorrhages are rare complications of spinal anesthesia. Chiropractic manipulation of the neck poses a potential risk for the dissection of vertebral and carotid arteries.

Among prescription drugs, anticoagulants and fibrinolytic agents carry the risk of subdural, subarachnoid, and cerebral hemorrhages (Fig. 4.41). The use of oral contraceptives has been associated with thrombotic infarction, and the risk may increase in women over 35 years of age.

Vascular Complications of Illicit Substance Abuse

Stroke, more often hemorrhagic than ischemic, is a major complication of the abuse of illicit substances such as amphetamine, heroine, cocaine or crack, T's (Talwin), and blues (pyribenzamine). The pathogenesis is multifactorial, including drug-induced vasculitis, sympathomimetic effect with vasospasm or hypertensive crisis, and embolization from infective endocarditis or intravascular foreign material.

Cerebral Neoplasms

Highly vascular primary tumors (glioblastoma, oligodendroglioma) and metastatic tumors (melanoma, choriocarcinoma, renal and bronchogenic carcinomas) are prone to bleed, mimicking a hemorrhagic stroke (Fig. 4.42).

Hereditary Metabolic Diseases

Mitochondrial myopathy, encephalopathy, lactic acidosis, and stroke-like episodes (MELAS), a maternally

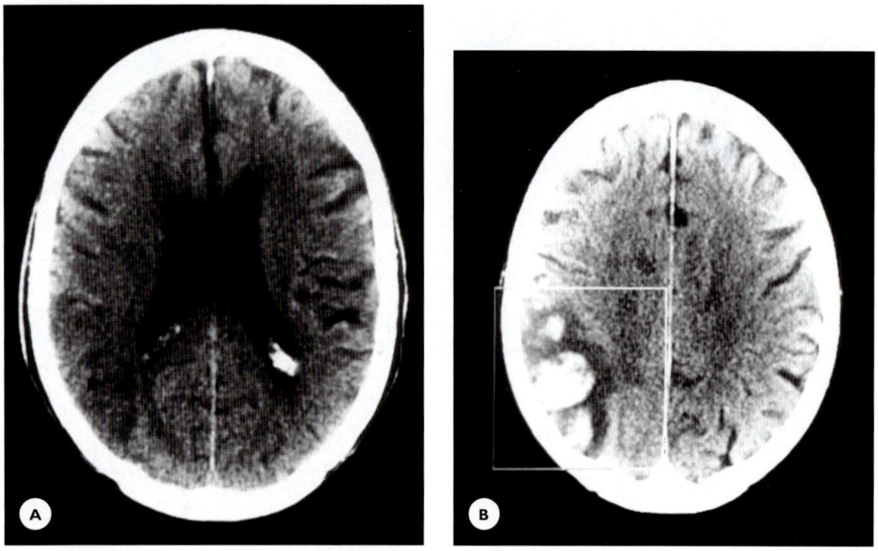

FIGURE 4.41
Complication of anticoagulation. **A.** CT scan of a 73-year-old man treated with Coumadin for chronic atrial fibrillation shows a recent left parietal infarct. **B.** CT scan repeated 3 days later because of mental changes shows an acute hemorrhage within the infarct.

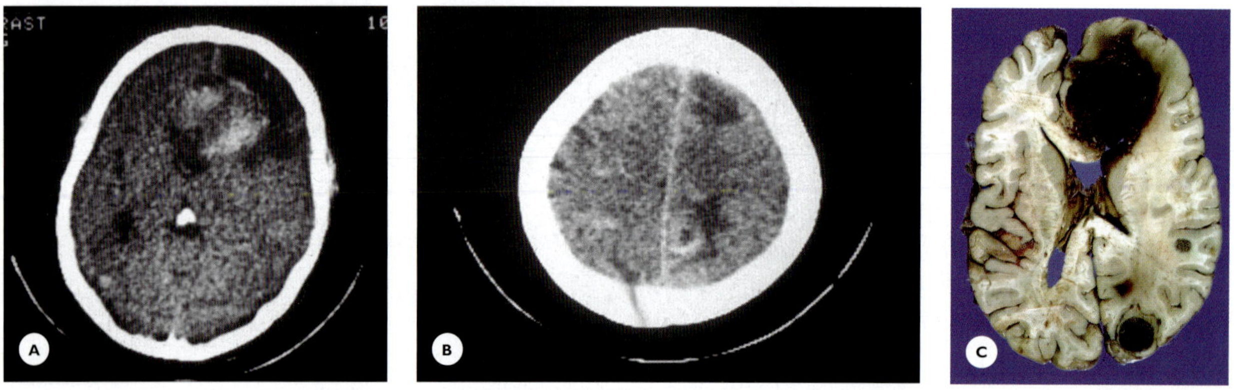

FIGURE 4.42
Bleeding within neoplasm mimicking a stroke. A 59-year-old man, in good health, suddenly collapsed. A few hours later, he was lethargic, his left side was paralyzed, a mild right ptosis was present, and the right pupil was slightly larger than the left, indicating incipient transtentorial uncal herniation. Three days later, he died. His medical history was significant for excision of a cutaneous melanoma 9 years earlier. A noncontrast CT scan of the head shows: (**A**) a large right frontal and (**B**) a small right occipital hyperdense lesion surrounded by hypodense edema with mass effect. The brain shows (**C**) circumscribed hemorrhagic lesions corresponding to the large frontal and the small occipital lesions shown on the CT scan, and also a third small parietal lesion—histologically, all melanomas.

transmitted mitochondrial disease of young individuals, presents with recurrent ischemic events leading eventually to multiple infarctions.

Homocystinuria, an autosomal recessive disorder of methionine metabolism, affects chiefly infants and children and is associated with multiple ischemic strokes. The blood vessels display fibrous thickening and luminal occlusion.

Fabry's disease, a sex-linked recessive lysosomal metabolic disease, is characterized by cutaneous angiokeratoma and deposits of glycosphingolipids in the neurons, visceral organs, and blood vessels. The disease predisposes to stroke in children and young adults.

Arterial Dissection

Dissection of the cervical carotid and vertebral arteries may occur spontaneously or due to trauma to the head or neck. It is an important cause of death in the young and middle-aged. Rupture of the arterial wall produces

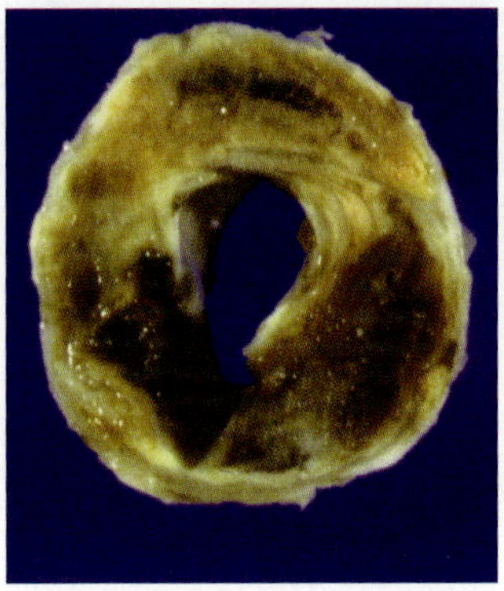

FIGURE 4.43
Arterial dissection. Nontraumatic massive mural hematoma in a carotid endarterectomy specimen.

an intramural hemorrhage and subsequent luminal reduction (Fig. 4.43). It carries the risk of local thrombosis and embolization. The pathogenesis is poorly understood: Weakness of the arterial wall and fibromuscular dysplasia predispose to dissection.

A dissection of the carotids and vertebrals presents with unilateral headaches, neck pain, Horner syndrome, ipsilateral cranial nerve deficits, and TIAs. It may culminate in a cerebral hemispheric or brainstem infarct. Angiogram confirms the diagnosis by demonstrating segmental luminal narrowing (string sign).

CEREBRAL PATHOLOGY IN ARTERIOLOSCLEROSIS: VASCULAR DEMENTIA

Arteriosclerosis of the small cerebral arteries produces distinct pathologic conditions:

- Subcortical arteriosclerotic encephalopathy
- Lacunar state
- Granular cortical atrophy
- Cribriform state

These conditions may occur alone, but more often they appear in various combinations and manifest with a variety of neurologic symptoms and signs. Most notably, they contribute to the pathology of vascular dementia. Typical neurologic manifestations are parkinsonian features, slow and small step-gait, postural instability, bradykinesia or akinesia, rigidity, pyramidal signs, spasticity, pseudobulbar palsy and dysarthric speech, seizures, and urinary incontinence.

The dementia associated with diseases of the small parenchymal arteries is classified as *subcortical dementia*, to distinguish it from cortical multiinfarct dementia, which is associated with diseases of the large arteries. Small-vessel dementia is characterized by slow psychomotility, apathy, poor judgment, lack of insight, moderate memory impairment, and emotional and behavioral changes.

Subcortical arteriosclerotic encephalopathy or *Binswanger's disease* presents clinically as a slowly progressive subcortical dementia, often complicated by minor strokes. The majority of patients are hypertensive and have several stroke risk factors. Neuroimaging, particularly MRI, is helpful to support the diagnosis, although the changes are not specific. MR images show large periventricular hyperintense lesions (caps and rims), and multiple small and large, often symmetrical lesions in the hemispheric white matter. They are referred to as *leukoaraiosis* (Greek; white, rarefaction) (Fig. 4.44).

Grossly, the hemispheric and the periventricular white matter is faintly discolored and slightly softened. The histology is characterized by arteriosclerotic changes of the small vessels, multifocal demyelinations in the hemispheric white matter and periventricular zones, and subependymal gliosis (Fig. 4.45).

The vascular changes consist of fibrotic and hyalin thickening of the arteriolar and capillary walls, enlargement of the perivascular spaces, and a dense periadventitial fibrosis. Some perivascular spaces are filled with plasma fluid.

The myelin changes vary from pale staining and rarefaction, through swelling and varicosities, to breakdown. The extent varies from patchy to diffuse, often extending from the ventricles to the cortex, sparing the subcortical U fibers. Within the demyelinated areas, the density of the nerve fibers is reduced, and the astrocytes are moderately proliferated. Macrophages are sparse. The ependymal lining of the ventricles is disrupted, and subependymal astrocytosis can be prominent. The periventricular veins show collagenosis and luminal stenosis.

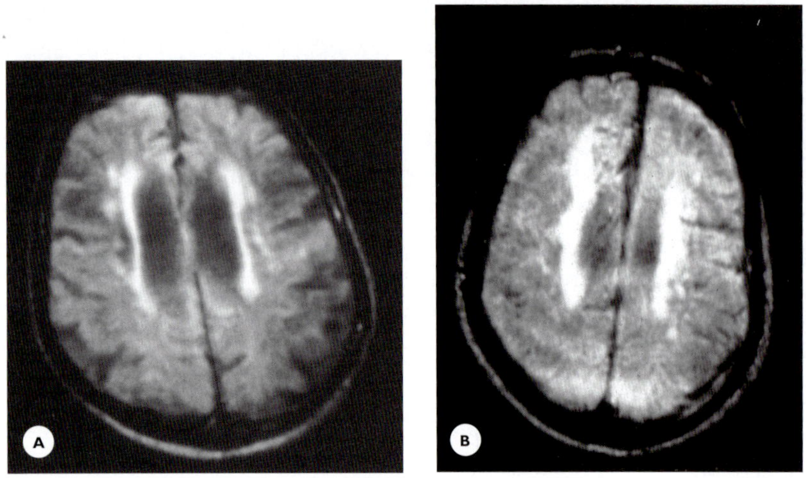

FIGURE 4.44
Subcortical arteriosclerotic encephalopathy, Binswanger's disease (BD). **A** and **B.** Horizontal T1-weighted MR images show periventricular and multiple small and large confluent hyperintense lesions in the hemispheric white matter. The ventricles are enlarged.

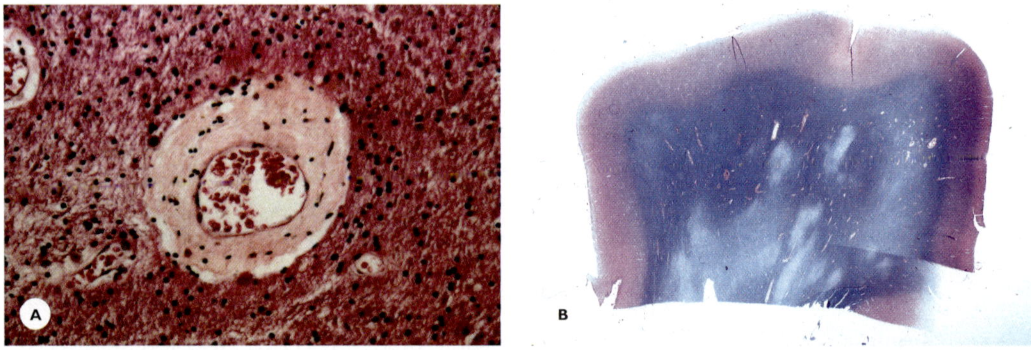

FIGURE 4.45
Binswanger's disease. **A.** Fibrohyalinosis and mural thickening of a small blood vessel in the white matter (HE). **B.** Diffuse and multifocal ischemic demyelination (LFB-CV).

The pathomechanism of the disease is not fully elucidated. The demyelination is attributed to chronic ischemia associated with systemic hypotension due to cardiac failure or impaired autoregulation. A suggested alternate mechanism is a late effect of vasogenic edema associated with hypertension.

Lacunar state refers to multiple small cystic cavities that result from the removal of ischemic debris. These lacunae are commonly situated in the subcortical gray structures, brainstem, and hemispheric white matter. Some produce distinct clinical syndromes (Fig. 4.46; Table 4.12).

In *granular cortical atrophy*, grossly, the cortical surface contains multiple small depressed soft and firm areas. Histologically, these are minute glial scars, small cystic cavities, and laminar cortical necrosis (Fig. 4.47).

Cribriform state refers to multiple miniature cavities, often visible grossly as round, oval, or slit-like smooth-walled cavities averaging 0.5 to 2 mm in size. Typically, they are situated in the basal ganglia and hemispheric white matter. Histologically, the cavities are dilated perivascular spaces that contain one or two thick-walled arterioles or capillaries surrounded by fine fibrous strands or dense collagenous fibers (Fig. 4.48). Corpora amylacea line some cavities. The perivascular myelin may be rarefied, but frank myelin breakdown and macrophage reaction are absent.

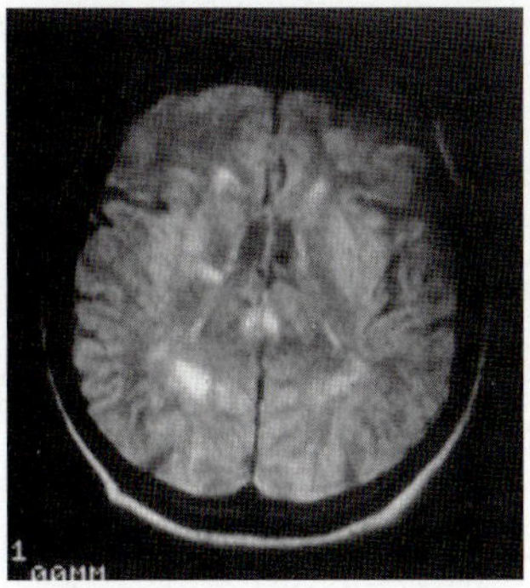

FIGURE 4.46
Lacunar infarct. MRI shows a lacunar infarct in the internal capsule, which manifested with pure hemiparesis in a 58-year-old hypertensive man.

TABLE 4.12.
Common Lacunar Syndromes

Syndrome	*Presentation*	*Localization*
Pure motor	Hemiparesis	Posterior limb of internal capsule Pontine basis
Pure sensory	Hemisensory deficit	Thalamus
Ataxic-hemiparesis	Hemiparesis ipsilateral ataxia	Posterior limb of internal capsule Thalamus Pontine basis
Dysarthria—clumsy hand syndrome	Dysarthria, clumsiness of a hand	Internal capsule pontine basis
Pseudobulbar palsy	Facial diplegia Dysarthria Dysphagia Compulsive laughing and crying	Bilateral corticobulbar tracts

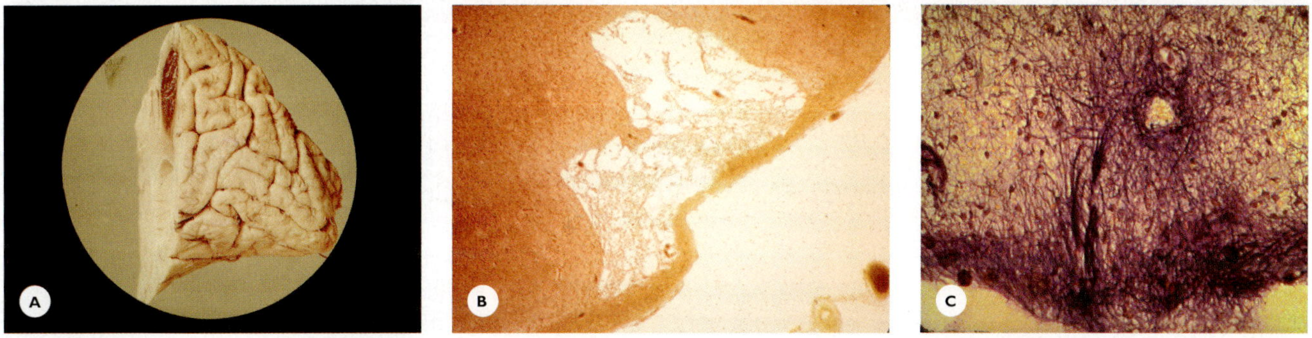

FIGURE 4.47
Granular cortical atrophy. **A.** Gross appearance in the occipital lobe. Cortex from different cases shows (**B**) small vascular cavity (HE) and (**C**) subpial and pericapillary glial scars (Holzer stain).

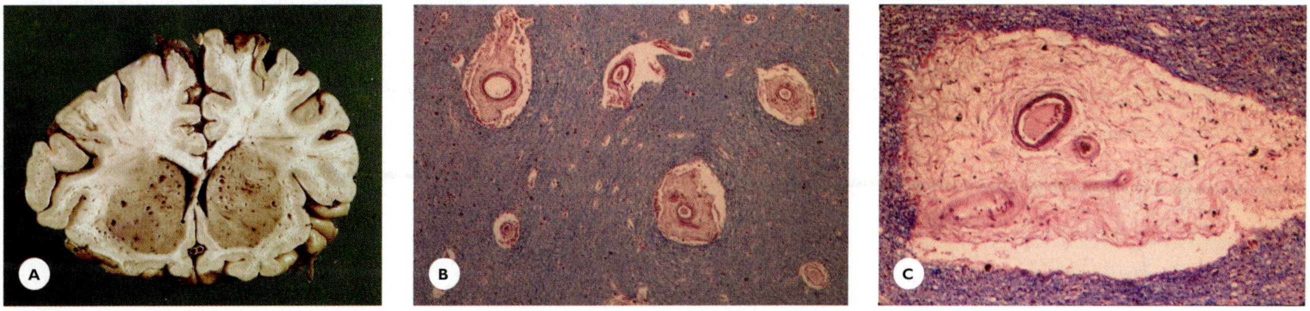

FIGURE 4.48
Cribriform state. **A.** Severely dilated, round perivascular spaces in the basal ganglia and slit-like cavities in the subinsular white matter. **B** and **C.** The dilated perivascular spaces are filled with fine collagenous fibrillary strands. Occasional hemosiderin pigments are noted (LFB-CV-E).

BIBLIOGRAPHY

Biller, J., Mathews, K. D., & Love, B. B. (Eds.). (1994). *Stroke in children and young adults.* Boston: Butterworth–Heinemann.

Bogousslavsky, J., & Caplan, L. R. (Eds.). (2001). *Stroke syndrome,* 2nd ed. Cambridge, U.K.: Cambridge University Press.

Caplan, L. R. (1993). *Stroke: a clinical approach,* 2nd ed. Boston: Butterworth–Heinemann.

Fisher, M. (Ed.) (1994). *Clinical atlas of cerebrovascular disorders.* London: Mosby.

Garcia, J. H. (1992). The evolution of brain infarcts: a review. *J Neuropathol Exp Neurol 51,* 387–393.

Kalimo, H. (2005). *Pathology & Genetics. Cerebrovascular Diseases.* ISN Neuropath Press. Basel, Switzerland.

Kark, J. A., Posey, D. M., Schumacher, H. R., & Ruehle, C. J. (1987). Sickle-cell trait as a risk factor for sudden death in physical training. *N Engl J Med 317,* 781–787.

Nencini, P., Barriffi, C. M., Abbate, R., et al. (1992). Lupus anticoagulant and anticardiolipin antibodies in young adults with cerebral ischemia. *Stroke 23,* 189–193.

Pullicino, P. M., Caplan, L. R., & Hommel, M. (Eds.). (1993). *Cerebral small artery disease,* Advances in Neurology, Vol. 62. New York: Raven Press.

Ruchoux, M. M., Maurage, C.A. (1997). CADASIL: Cerebral autosomal dominant arteriopathy with subcortical infarcts and leukoencephalopathy. *J Neuropathol Exp Neurol 56,* 947–964.

Welch, K. M. A., Caplan, L. R., Reis, D. J., et al. (Eds.) (1997). *Primer on cerebrovascular diseases.* San Diego: Academic Press.

REVIEW QUESTIONS

1. A cerebral infarct can be caused by:
   A. Thrombotic occlusion of extracranial cerebral arteries
   B. Thrombotic occlusion of intracranial arteries
   C. Atheromatous embolus
   D. Severe hypotensive episode
   E. Any of these

2. An infarct caused by an atheromatous embolus from the ICA is characterized by which of the following?
   A. It is a common occurrence in the caudate.
   B. It is bland.
   C. It is often hemorrhagic.
   D. It commonly occurs in the white matter.
   E. It is common in the thalamus.

3. An acute infarct shows all of the following histological changes *except*:
   A. Capillary hyperplasia
   B. Infiltration with neutrophils
   C. Red neurons
   D. Oligodendroglial proliferation
   E. Macrophage reaction

4. An infarct in the basis of the pons produces the "locked-in" syndrome, which is characterized by all of the following *except*:
   A. Quadriplegia
   B. Vertical gaze paralysis
   C. Dysarthria
   D. Dysphagia
   E. Has basilar artery thrombosis as its cause

5. A large, old, MCA infarct on the CT scan appears as:
   A. A hyperdense lesion
   B. A hypodense lesion with an indented adjacent ventricle
   C. A hypodense lesion with a dilated adjacent ventricle
   D. A hyperdense lesion in the thalamus
   E. A hypodense lesion in the thalamus

6. Concerning the clinical presentation of bilateral occipital infarcts, all of the following can apply *except*:
   A. Blindness
   B. Loss of pupillary light reflex
   C. Confusion
   D. Denial of blindness
   E. Agitation

7. The most common site of a hypertensive intracranial hemorrhage is the:
   A. Pons
   B. Thalamus
   C. Frontal lobe
   D. Basal ganglia
   E. Midbrain

8. Lateral medullary syndrome (Wallenberg syndrome) usually results from occlusion of the:
   A. Basilar artery
   B. Anterior superior cerebellar artery
   C. Anterior spinal artery
   D. Posterior inferior cerebellar artery
   E. Anterior inferior cerebellar artery

9. The brain requires an average constant blood flow of:
   A. 80 to 90 mL/100 g/min
   B. 90 to 100 mL/100 g/min
   C. 50 to 60 mL/100 g/min
   D. 40 to 50 mL/100 g/min
   E. 30 to 40 mL/100 g/min

10. Complications of subarachnoid hemorrhage include:
    A. Hydrocephalus
    B. Infarct
    C. Cardiac arrhythmias
    D. All of these
    E. None of these

11. Concerning fibromuscular dysplasia, all of the following statements are correct *except*:
    A. It affects small parenchymal arteries.
    B. It is more common in middle-aged women.
    C. It can cause arterial dissection.
    D. It can cause an ischemic stroke.
    E. It affects large arteries.

12. Hereditary arteriopathies include all of the following *except*:
    A. Familial cerebral amyloid angiopathy
    B. Thromboangiitis obliterans
    C. Cerebral autosomal dominant arteriopathy with subcortical infarcts and leukoencephalopathy (CADASIL)
    D. Marfan's syndrome
    E. Ehlers-Danlos syndrome

13. Concerning subcortical arteriosclerotic encephalopathy, all of the following statements are correct *except*:
    A. It presents with dementia.
    B. MRI shows periventricular lesions.
    C. MRI shows small and large white matter lesions.
    D. It is a disease of the extracranial carotid arteries.
    E. It is a disease of the small parenchymal arteries.

14. Stroke in the young can be caused by:
    A. Vascular malformation
    B. Homocystinuria
    C. Cardiac diseases
    D. All of these
    E. None of these

(Answers are provided in the Appendix.)

CHAPTER 5

Neurodegenerative Diseases

Dementias
Motor Neuron Diseases
Extrapyramidal Diseases
Cerebellar and Spinocerebellar Degenerations
Multiple System Atrophy

The progressive deterioration and ultimate death of the neurons within selective anatomic regions characterize the neurodegenerative diseases. Notably, the group encompasses common and less common but important dementing diseases and movement disorders. Some diseases present only with dementia, some only with motor disorder, and some with both.

Neurodegenerative diseases affect all ages from infancy on, but they occur chiefly during midlife or later. The clinical symptoms and signs indicate the anatomic regions involved in the disease process. The course is slowly progressive over several years, leading inevitably to severe mental and neurologic disabilities and, among long-time survivors, to a terminal vegetative state. As yet, no therapy is curative.

The etiology of neurodegenerative diseases remains elusive. Some diseases are sporadic, some inherited, and some both. A vast amount of information has accumulated on the genetic basis of several diseases. In an increasing number, the gene or its chromosomal locus has been identified. It is noteworthy that the genetic mechanism, in one group of inherited diseases, differs from that of classical Mendelian genetics. These diseases result from the expansion of trinucleotide repeats encoding for polyglutamine tracts and are referred to as polyglutamine diseases. Genetic testing is gaining wide use to confirm the diagnosis in symptomatic patients suspected of suffering from an inheritable neurodegenerative disease.

The degeneration of the neurons is confined to definite anatomic regions: in dementias, to the cerebral cortex; in movement disorders, to anatomically and functionally related structures within the motor, extrapyramidal, or cerebellar systems (multisystem degenerations).

The presence of inclusion bodies, derived from abnormal aggregations of proteins in the cytoplasms or nuclei of the neurons and glial cells (astrocytes, oligodendrocytes), characterizes the pathology of a number of dementias and movement disorders. Hence the concept that disturbances in protein metabolism play a fundamental role in the pathogenesis of neurodegenerative diseases. The molecular components of these inclusions have been identified using immunohistochemical technics. Two kinds of inclusions are those that stain positively for tau protein, a microtubule-associated protein involved in microtubule assembly, and those that stain positively for α-synuclein, a presynaptic protein involved in synaptic function. Diseases that display tau protein or α-synuclein–positive inclusions are classified as *tauopathies* or *synucleinopathies*, respectively. Furthermore, cytoplasmic and nuclear inclusions in several diseases display immunoreactivity for ubiquitin, a stress protein involved in protein degradation. An emerging trend is to link certain clinical phenotypes to particular protein abnormalities. Such correlations, based on neuropathologic studies, enhance diagnostic accuracy and may suggest therapeutic strategies.

The neurons in degenerative diseases die generally by apoptosis (programmed cell death). A failure of the neurons to cope with oxidative stress likely promotes apoptosis. A slow, chronic form of excitotoxic neurodegeneration is an alternative mechanism. Oxidative stress renders the neurons vulnerable to the slowly evolving effects of excitatory neurotransmitters. Persistent overexcitation of the neurons ultimately leads to their deaths.

For presentation, neurodegenerative diseases are classified into five categories based on their chief clinical features and the anatomic distribution of the lesions:

- Dementias
- Motor neuron diseases
- Extrapyramidal diseases
- Cerebellar and spinocerebellar degenerations
- Multiple system atrophy

DEMENTIAS

Dementia is defined as "impairment in short- and long-term memory, associated with impairment in abstract thinking and judgment, other disturbances of higher cortical function, and personality changes. The disturbance is severe enough to interfere significantly with work or usual social activities or relationships with others." The diagnosis of dementia is not made if these symptoms occur in patients with altered levels of consciousness (*Diagnostic and Statistical Manual of Mental Disorders, 4th edition, DSM-IV*). Dementia is a prominent feature of a number of neurologic, general medical, and psychiatric diseases. It is imperative to identify the treatable and reversible etiologies of dementia before considering a primary neurodegenerative process as the underlying cause (Table 5.1).

Degenerative dementias are a heterogeneous group. Two major forms are dementias caused by diffuse cortical degeneration and dementias caused by lobar (circumscribed) cortical degeneration. The former form encompasses Alzheimer's disease and dementia with Lewy bodies, and the latter form characterizes the frontotemporal lobar dementias. Diagnosing the various subforms of dementias can be challenging because definitive diagnosis requires neuropathologic verification. A demonstration of the presence of specific neuronal and glial inclusions is most valuable in confirming the diagnosis and in differentiating between various subforms and eliminating other degenerative diseases of cognitive decline.

TABLE 5.1.
Etiologies of Dementias

Etiologies of Dementias
Specific causes
Cerebrovascular diseases
Normal pressure hydrocephalus
Endocrine/metabolic diseases
Toxic disorders
Head injury
Infectious diseases
Mass lesion
Hereditary neurometabolic diseases
Prion diseases
Psychiatric disorders
Neurodegenerative diseases

Diffuse Cortical Dementias

Alzheimer's Disease

Clinical Features

Alzheimer's disease (AD), the most common cause of organic dementias, affects an estimated 4 million individuals in the United States, where it is the fourth major cause of death. Primarily a disease of the elderly, it affects more women than men. The onset is usually after the age of 50 to 55 years, and the incidence increases steadily with advancing age. It affects 10% of the population over age 65 years and 40% over 85 years. The disease has a worldwide distribution. It occurs sporadically or is inherited in an autosomal dominant pattern. About half of early-onset AD cases are familial.

AD begins insidiously, with a failing memory. This is followed by a progressive decline of cognitive functions such as language, writing, reading, calculation, motor skills, visuospatial orientation, and sensory gnostic functions. Along with the cognitive decline, psychiatric symptoms and changes in personality, mood, and affect emerge. Some patients become withdrawn or apathetic, others agitated. During the course of the disease, neurologic signs appear, such as snout, sucking, and grasp reflexes (primitive reflexes, frontal release signs); postural abnormalities; akinesia and rigidity; paratonia in the extremities; and loss of sphincter control. Seizures and myoclonic jerks develop in a small number of patients. The course is slowly progressive. The patients gradually become mute, bedridden, and unaware of their environment. The usual course ranges from 6 to 12 years, seldom longer.

The diagnostic evaluation of patients with suspected AD requires a multidisciplinary approach and close monitoring of the progression of cognitive decline. Structural imaging using computed tomography (CT) scan and magnetic resonance imaging (MRI) is standard procedure. These imaging procedures are important in eliminating diseases that are not degenerative. Their usefulness in the decisive diagnosis of AD is limited. Cerebral atrophy, evidenced by dilatation of the subarachnoid space, and enlargement of the lateral and third ventricles, commonly occurs in dementias. However, atrophy may occur in normal elderly individuals and, conversely, demented patients may display normal or mildly abnormal imaging. Enlargement of the rhinal sulcus and temporal horn, indicating atrophy of the entorhinal cortex and hippocampus, occurs in AD and also in lobar dementias. White matter changes such as hyperintense periventricular caps and rims and scattered small foci (*leukoaraiosis*; Greek, white rarefaction) often are seen on the MR images of AD patients. They represent periventricular edema or ischemic demyelination associated with small-vessel disease. Functional imaging using single photon emission computed tomography (SPECT) shows perfusion deficits and, using positron emission tomography (PET), hypometabolism in the frontal, temporal, and parietal regions.

Specific laboratory tests are used to eliminate endocrine dysfunction and vitamin deficiency. Cerebrospinal fluid (CSF) examination is indicated when an infectious etiology of dementia is suspected. Commercially available biomarkers for AD are not used routinely in the evaluation of patients. A definite diagnosis is based on the clinical criteria of probable AD (Clinical diagnosis of Alzheimer's disease: report of the NINCDS, ADRDA Work Group, 1984) along with histologic verification by autopsy, rarely by biopsy.

Pathology

Grossly, the brain volume is diminished, with brain weight ranging between 1,250 and 1,000 g or less. The exterior shows an atrophy of the convolutions and widening of the sulci. The atrophy is generalized, although the most severely affected regions are the frontal and temporomesial lobes. On sections, the cortical ribbon is thin, particularly the frontal cortex, the entorhinal cortex, and the hippocampus. The amount of the white matter is diffusely reduced and the lateral ventricles, including the temporal horns, are enlarged (hydrocephalus ex-vacuo) (Figs. 5.1 and 5.2).

A number of histologic changes occur in AD, but the diagnostic hallmarks are the neuritic plaques (NP) and the neurofibrillary tangles (NFT) (Table 5.2). Both are demonstrated in sections stained with silver. Immunohistologic stains identify their molecular components. These features are not altogether specific for AD, because both are found in normal aging, and the neurofibrillary

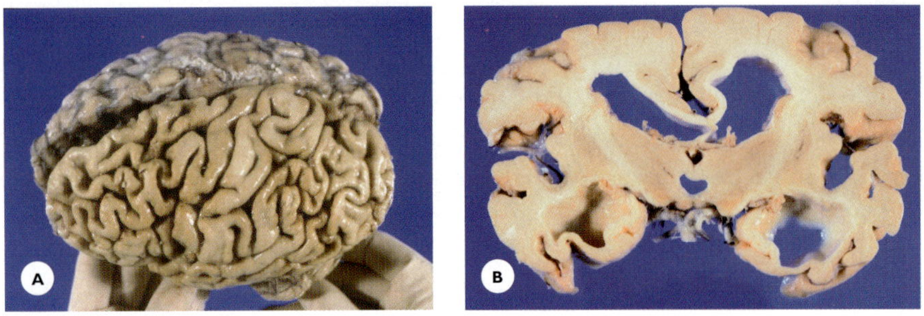

FIGURE 5.1
Alzheimer's disease. Onset of intellectual decline at 69 years of age, clinical course 6 years. **A.** The 1,090-g brain shows prominent atrophy of the frontal lobes. **B.** Transverse slice shows severe atrophy of the hippocampal convolutions and enlargement of the temporal horns.

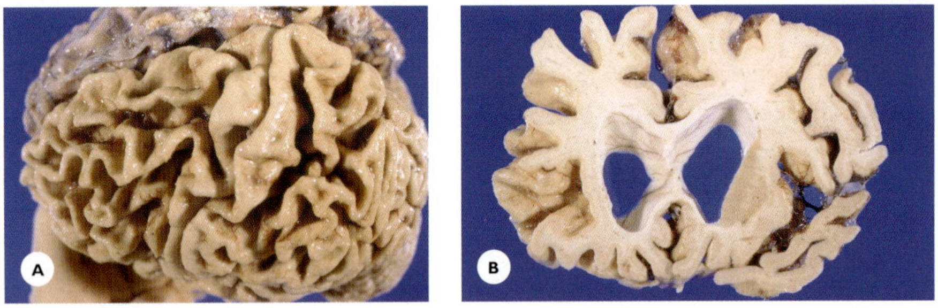

FIGURE 5.2
Alzheimer's disease. Onset of memory decline at 52 years, course 17 years. **A.** The 800-g brain shows extremely severe generalized convolutional atrophy. **B.** The width of the cortex is reduced to 1.5 to 2 mm. The white matter is atrophic, and the ventricles are dilated.

TABLE 5.2.
Histology of Alzheimer's Disease

Neuritic plaques
Neuronal changes
- Neurofibrillary tangles
- Granulovacuolar degeneration
- Hirano bodies
- Synaptic losses

Neuronal losses
Amyloid angiopathy

tangles are also found in a variety of diseases (see Chapter 2). However, their number and distribution in AD are highly characteristic. They typically appear first in the entorhinal cortex, then in the hippocampus, amygdala, neocortical areas, and the basal nucleus of Meynert. They are infrequent in the basal ganglia, hypothalamic region, rostral brainstem, and cerebellar cortex. Several guidelines have been established for the pathologic diagnosis of AD. According to guidelines of the Consortium to Establish a Registry of Alzheimer's Disease (CERAD), the density of the neuritic plaques is assessed in several neocortical and limbic areas as sparse, moderate, or frequent and is compared with the age of the patient. Then, this age-related score, along with the clinical history, is used to formulate a diagnosis of definite, probable, possible, or normal.

Neuritic (senile) plaques. These extracellular round or spherical argyrophilic structures, measuring 150 to 200 microns, are dispersed in the neuropil. Some may appear in hematoxylin-eosin (HE)-stained sections as acellular eosinophilic homogenous or fibrillary aggregations (Fig. 5.3).

Three morphologic forms of the neuritic plaques, corresponding to stages of their evolution, are distinguished: diffuse, classic, and burnt-out.

A *diffuse* or primitive plaque consists of fibrils of preamyloid that immunoreact for amyloid β-amyloid peptide (Aβ) and some for β-amyloid precursor protein (βAPP) (Fig. 5.4).

A classic or mature plaque has three components: a dense central core of amyloid, dystrophic neurites, and periplaque glial cells.

The central core stains positively with Congo-red and, when viewed in polarized light, it shows the characteristic Maltese cross pattern of amyloid. It fluoresces in thioflavin-S–stained sections viewed in ultraviolet light. Its major component is Aβ, the cleavage product of βAPP (Fig. 5.5). In addition to β-APP and Aβ-peptide, the plaques contain α-synuclein and other amyloid-

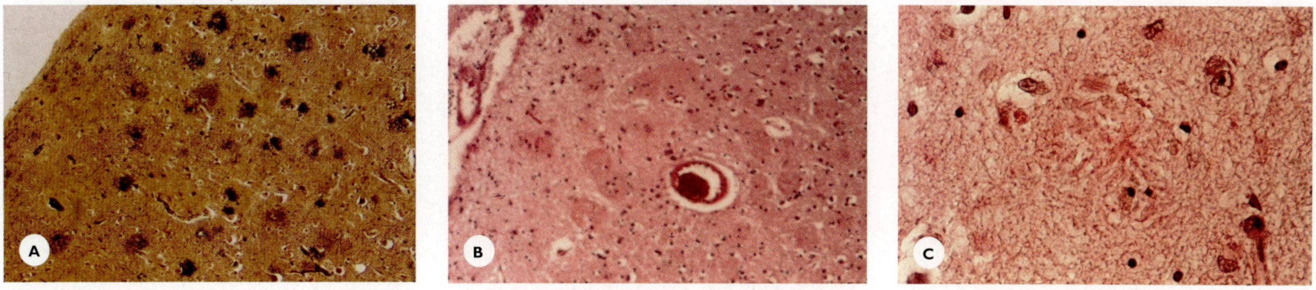

FIGURE 5.3
Alzheimer's disease. **A.** Neuritic plaques in the frontal cortex are demonstrated in silver-stained section (Bodian stain). **B.** Some are noticeable in hematoxylin-eosin (HE)-stained section. **C.** Higher-magnification view shows a fibrillary pattern (HE).

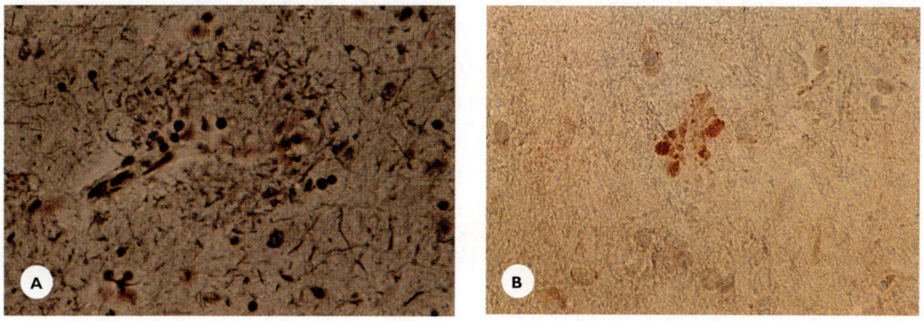

FIGURE 5.4
Alzheimer's disease. **A.** Diffuse (primitive) neuritic plaque (Bodian stain) (**B**) contains amyloid precursor protein (APP) (immunostain).

associated proteins. The amyloid core is surrounded by argyrophilic filamentous, rod-shaped, and granular structures derived from dystrophic neuronal processes and presynaptic terminals. They immunoreact for tau protein (see Fig. 5.5). A variable number of reactive astrocytes and activated microglial cells surround the dystrophic neurites (see Fig. 5.5).

A *burnt-out* or compact plaque contains only an amyloid core (Fig. 5.6).

Neurofibrillary tangles. These argyrophilic structures within the cytoplasm of the pyramidal neurons have a basket-shaped, flame-shaped, or globose form. Some can be detected as bluish fibrillary structures in HE-stained sections. At the electron microscope level, the tangles appear as paired helical and straight filaments. Their major molecular component is abnormally phosphorylated tau, a microtubule-associated protein. The diseased neurons eventually die, leaving the tangles as the only remnants (ghost neurons). Neuropil threads of degenerating neuronal processes are dispersed throughout the cortex (Fig. 5.7).

Granulovacuolar degeneration and *Hirano bodies* are found in the pyramidal neurons of the hippocampus. The granulovacuolar degeneration appears as small basophilic cytoplasmic granules within vacuoles. The Hirano bodies are eosinophilic, rod-shaped structures within or adjacent to the cell body (Fig. 5.8).

Loss of synapses. A progressive loss of synaptic connections between neurons is an essential feature of AD pathology.

Loss of neurons in the neocortical areas and hippocampus ranges from moderate to severe and, in some cases, is total. The cortex, depleted of neurons, shows spongiform changes and replacement astrocytosis (Fig. 5.9).

Amyloid angiopathy. Amyloid is deposited in the walls of the small leptomeningeal and cortical arteries and capillaries. Its composition is similar to that of the amyloid in the neuritic plaques (Fig. 5.10).

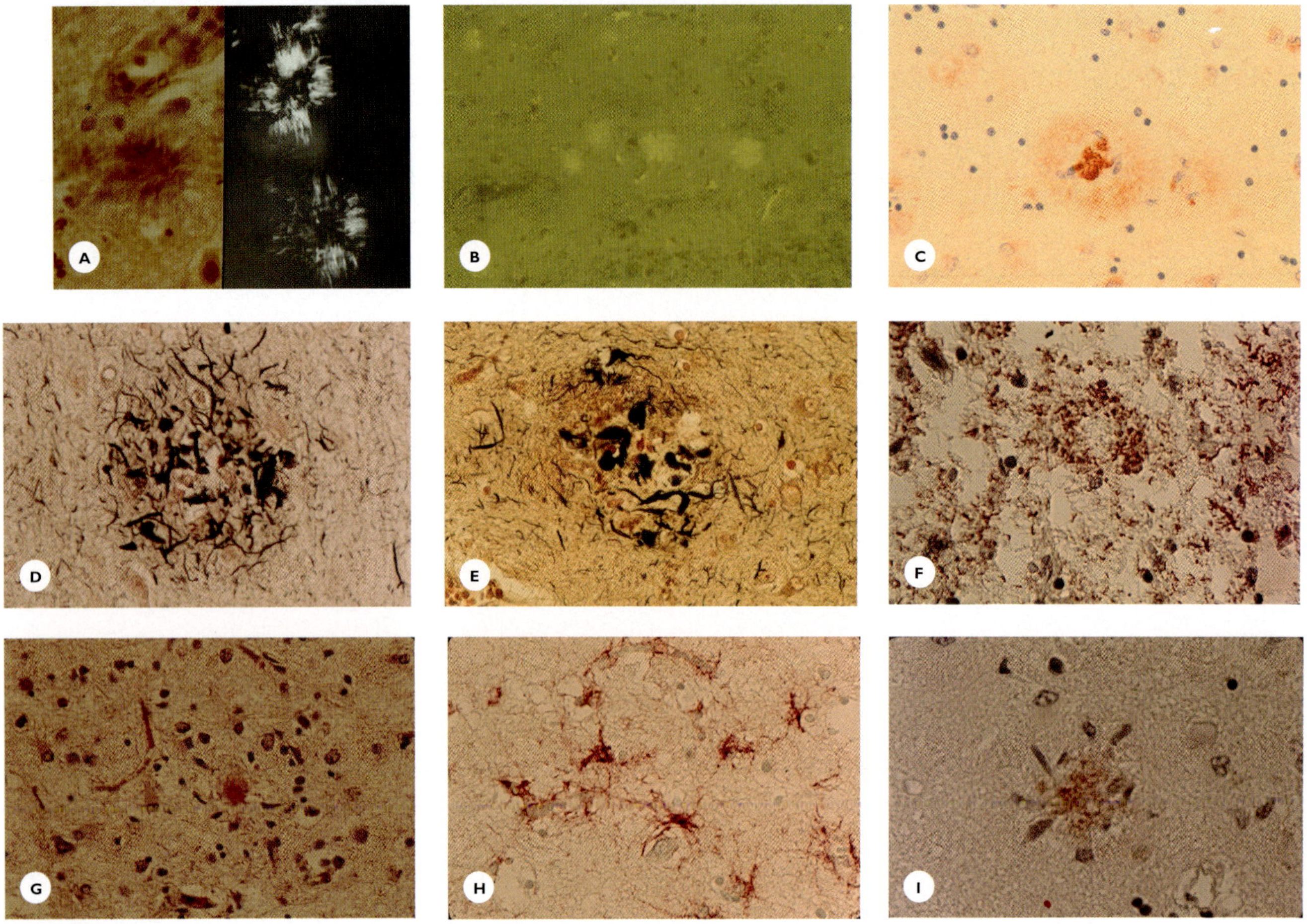

FIGURE 5.5
Alzheimer's disease. Classic (mature) neuritic plaque. **A.** The central amyloid core stains positively with Congo red and gives the characteristic Maltese-cross pattern in polarized light, (**B**) fluoresces in thioflavin S-stained sections in ultraviolet light, and (**C**) contains β-amyloid peptide (immunostain). **D** and **E.** The central core is surrounded by argyrophilic dystrophic neuronal processes (Gallyas silver stain), which (**F**) immunoreact for tau protein (immunostain). **G.** Periplaque glial reaction (HE), consists of (**H**) astrocytes (GFAP–immunostain), and (**I**) rod-shaped microglial cells (HE–Congo red).

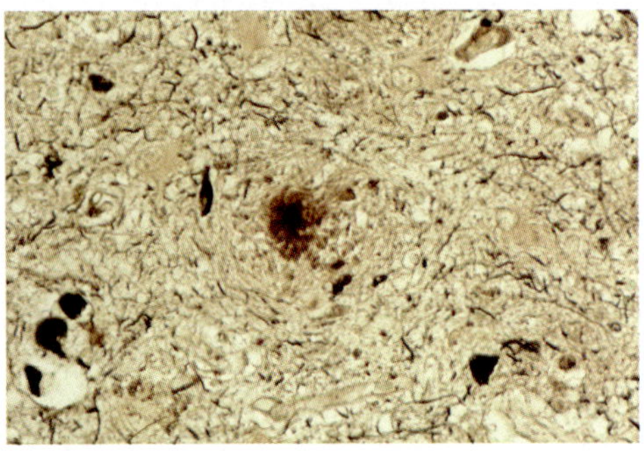

FIGURE 5.6
Alzheimer's disease. Burnt-out neuritic plaque consists of amyloid core only, lacking dystrophic neurites (Bodian stain).

Neurochemical Pathology

Neuronal degeneration results in deficiencies of the major neurotransmitters. Neuronal losses in the basal nucleus of Meynert are responsible for deficiencies of acetylcholine and its enzyme, choline acetyltransferase in limbic and neocortical areas. Cholinergic deficiency is strongly implicated in the memory deficit of AD. Neuronal losses in the locus ceruleus account for norepinephrine deficiency in the cortex; and losses in the pontine raphe nuclei account for serotonin deficiency in the cortex and subcortical structures.

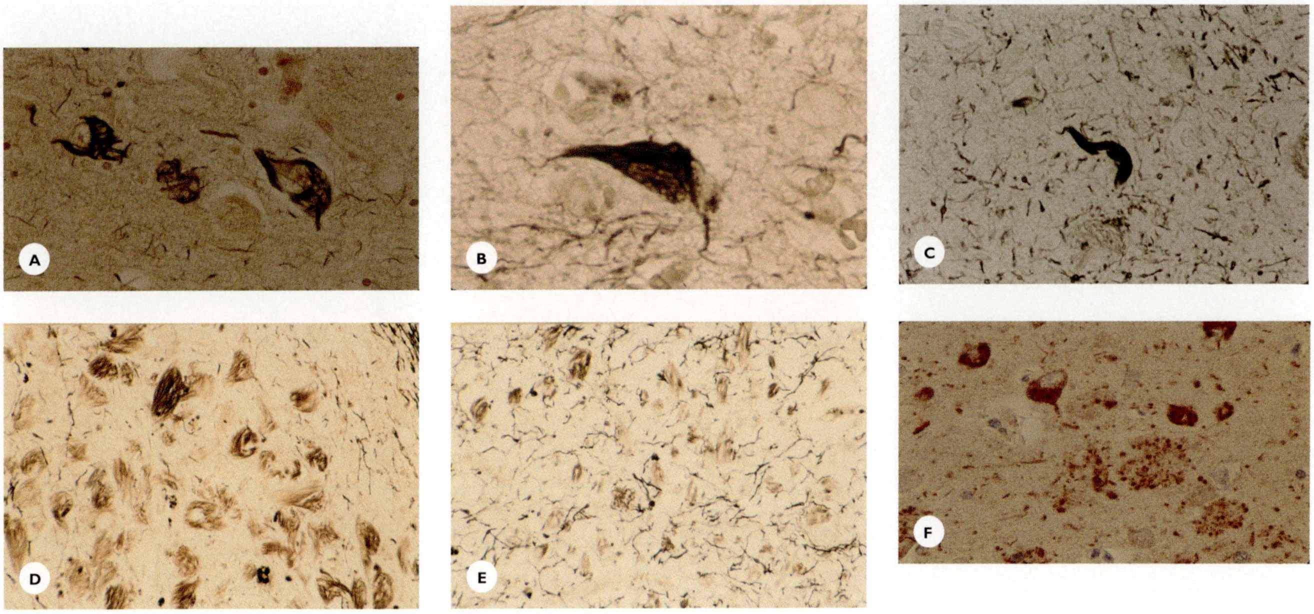

FIGURE 5.7
Alzheimer's disease. Neurofibrillary tangles (NF). **A.** Argyrophilic cytoplasmic tangles showing torch- and basket-shaped configurations. **B.** Twisted bundles. **C, D,** and **E.** Residual ghost tangles and neuropil threads (Gallyas silver stain). **F.** Tau-immunoreactivity of tangles (immunostain).

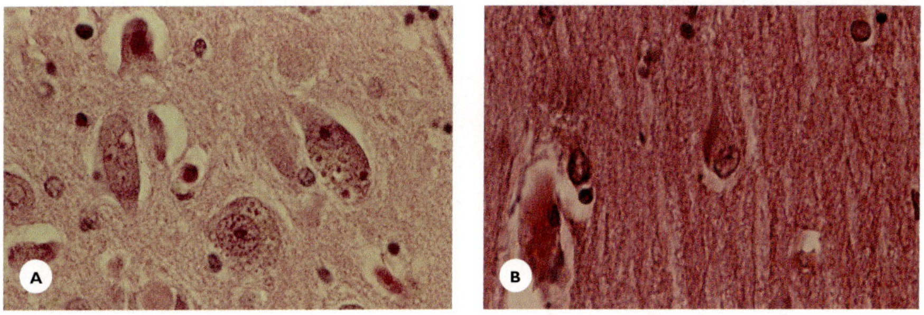

FIGURE 5.8
Alzheimer's disease. Neuronal changes. Hippocampal pyramidal neurons showing (**A**) granulovacuolar degeneration and (**B**) Hirano body (HE).

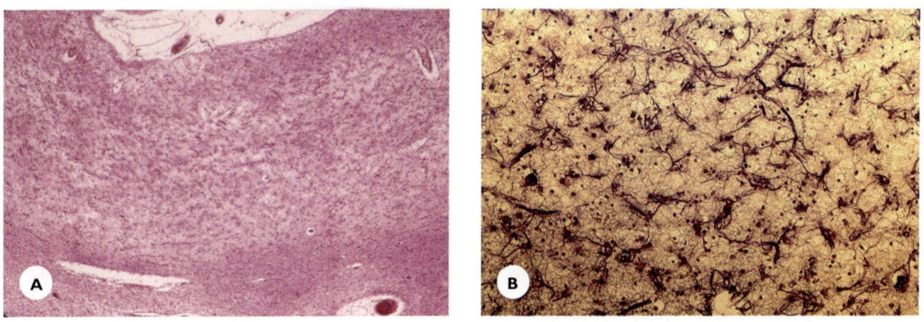

FIGURE 5.9
Alzheimer's disease. Cortical neuronal losses. **A.** Severe cortical neuronal degeneration and status spongiosus (HE). **B.** Prominent replacement astrocytic gliosis (Holzer stain).

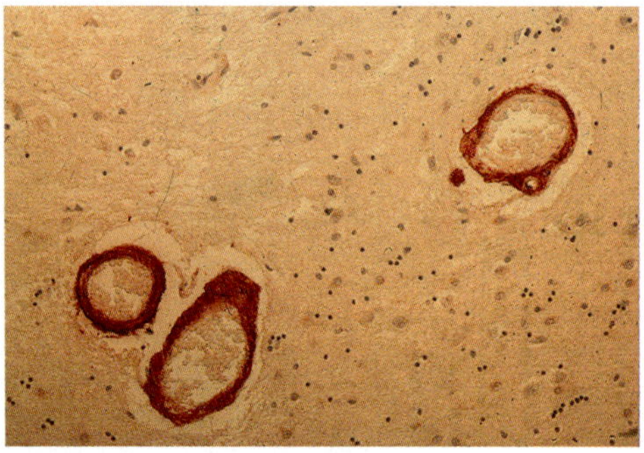

FIGURE 5.10
Alzheimer's disease. Amyloid angiopathy. Congo red–positive amyloid deposits around and within the walls of small cortical blood vessels (Congo-red stain).

TABLE 5.4.
Alzheimer's Disease

Molecular Pathology

Neuritic Plaques	Neurofibrillary Tangles
↓	↓
Amyloid β peptide	Abnormal Tau-protein

↘ Neuronal Death ↙

TABLE 5.3.
Genetics of Alzheimer's Disease

APP: Chromosome 21
Early onset
Autosomal dominant
Presenilin 1: Chromosome 14
Early onset
Autosomal dominant
Presenilin 2: Chromosome 1
Early onset
Autosomal dominant

APOE4: Chromosome 19
Susceptibility gene
Late onset
Familial and sporadic

APP, amyloid precursor protein; APOE4, apolipoprotein E4.

Etiology

The etiology of AD remains elusive. Aging, familial occurrence, Down's syndrome, elevated blood levels of apolipoprotein 4 (APOE4) and homocysteine, and head injury are risk factors. Among environmental factors, aluminum, zinc, and silicon toxicities have been associated with the disease, but none has been confirmed.

Genetic factors have a key role in the pathogenesis of AD (Table 5.3). Mutations in the *APP* gene on chromosome 21 and mutations in presenilin 1 and presenilin 2 genes on chromosomes 14 and 1, respectively, are implicated in early-onset autosomal dominant AD. A susceptibility gene—the gene of APOE4 on chromosome 19—is linked to late-onset sporadic and familial AD. APOE4, a blood lipoprotein, is elevated in about 45% to 60% of AD patients. Carriers of the gene are at risk for the disease.

Pathogenesis

AD is viewed as a protein metabolic disorder (Table 5.4). Several major steps in the formation of the neuritic plaques and neurofibrillary tangles have been identified, although others remain to be discovered.

Neuritic plaques. Amyloid precursor protein (APP), the generator of the neuritic plaques, is a neuronal membrane glycoprotein with an extracellular component. The overexpression of APP leads to its cleavage by the enzymes γ- and β-secretase into Aβ-peptides 40 and 42, respectively. It is postulated that an extracellular accumulation of Aβ-peptides results from the secretion of Aβ-40 by the neurons and from the release of excessively accumulated Aβ-42 by the dying neurons. Aβ-peptides are apt to aggregate into fibrillary structures that result in primitive (diffuse) plaques. Adding to the Aβ-plaques are α-synuclein, a synaptic protein, and other nonamyloid components (proteoglycans, APOE, cholesterol). Aβ-peptide is toxic to the neurons. Dystrophic neurites derived from dendrites, axons, and synaptic terminals of degenerating neurons congregate around the primitive plaques, converting them into classic, mature plaques. The appearance of activated microglia and astrocytes outside the dystrophic neurites completes the process of plaque formation.

Neurofibrillary Tangles

Tau protein, a microtubule-associated cytoskeletal protein, is normally present in a phosphorylated state. Abnormally phosphorylated tau protein aggregates into cytoplasmic filamentous structures—neurofibrillary tangles—that interfere with neuronal metabolism and eventually lead to neuronal death.

Clinical–Pathologic Correlates

Failing memory, the presenting cognitive deficit, correlates well with the early and severe involvement of the entorhinal–hippocampal structures of the limbic lobe, which is essential for memory and learning. As the neuronal degeneration gradually extends to the frontal, temporal, parietal, and occipital neocortex, the dementia evolves; more and more cognitive deficits appear, in conjunction with psychiatric symptoms and neurologic signs. Ultimately, the cerebral cortex becomes diffusely involved, and the dementia becomes global and profound.

Researchers dispute which of the basic pathologic lesions—neuritic plaques, neurofibrillary tangles, or synaptic losses—best correlates with the cognitive decline. Both the neurofibrillary tangles and the synaptic losses are thought to be crucial for the development of dementia.

Clinical Application of Neuropathologic Features

The discoveries of molecular pathology and neurochemical abnormalities in AD initiated vigorous clinical investigations in two major areas: diagnostic and therapeutic.

The neuropathologic features of AD also provide the basis for finding reliable biomarkers to make early and accurate diagnoses. β-Amyloid, a component of neuritic plaques, and tau protein, a component of neurofibrillary tangles, are commercially available CSF markers. β-Amyloid levels were found to be low and tau protein levels high in the CSF of a number of patients with suspected AD when compared with normal age-matched controls. Presently, the assays make the diagnosis more likely but *not definite* in subjects aged 70 or over with a clinical history of dementia.

The basic pathologic features of AD became targets for therapeutic strategies aiming to prevent or delay the progression of the disease, slow its course, and improve cognitive deficits. Several features already have been targeted for therapeutic application: (a) the cholinergic deficiency state in the limbic and neocortical regions initiated therapy with cholinesterase inhibitors; (b) the activation of microglia around neuritic plaques, implying an inflammatory element in the disease process, prompted therapy with nonsteroidal anti-inflammatory agents; (c) elevated blood levels of APOE4 in a number of AD patients became the rationale for using cholesterol-lowering drugs; and (d) immunization with β-amyloid peptide was intended to reduce the amyloid burden in the neuritic plaques. The treatment, however, was discontinued because a minority of patients developed neurologic complications consistent with meningoencephalitis from which two patients died.

Dementia with Lewy Bodies

Clinical Features

Dementia with Lewy bodies (DLB), also called diffuse Lewy body dementia (DLBD), is the second most common degenerative dementia in the elderly, after AD. It is somewhat more common in men. It may coexist with AD and Parkinson's disease. Cognitive decline, visual hallucinations, parkinsonian features, syncope, sensitivity to neuroleptics, sleep abnormalities, and a slowly progressive and fluctuating course are characteristic.

Pathology

Generalized cortical atrophy with frontal-temporal predominance and discoloration of the substantia nigra are distinctive gross features (Fig. 5.11).

Histologically, the presence of Lewy bodies in cortical neurons is the hallmark of the disease (see Fig. 5.11). These bodies are eosinophilic cytoplasmic inclusions, similar structurally to the Lewy bodies found in the substantia nigra of patients with idiopathic Parkinson's disease. They typically immunoreact with α-synuclein and ubiquitin (Table 5.5). Lewy bodies and Lewy

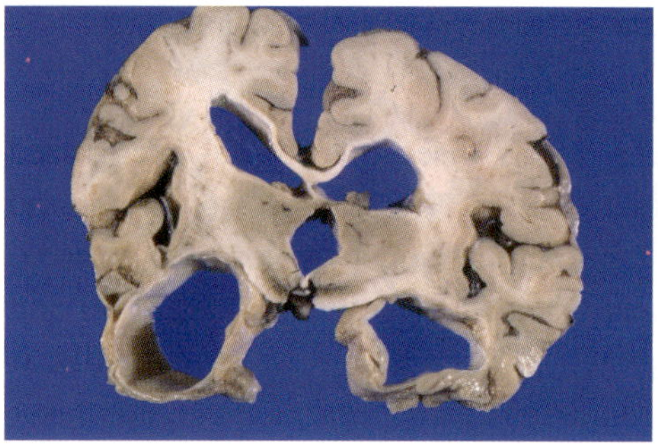

FIGURE 5.13

Pick's disease. A 60-year-old man became irritable and his memory began to decline. His cognitive skills slowly deteriorated and, by age 66, his short- and long-term memory, object naming, counting, and simple motor activities were greatly impaired. During the following years, he gradually became mute, physically abusive, and wheelchair bound. Following a 16-year clinical course, he died at age 76. Transverse section of the 1,100-g brain shows severe circumscribed symmetrical atrophy of the temporal lobes (knife-blade atrophy), sparing the posterior superior temporal convolutions. The temporal horns are markedly enlarged.

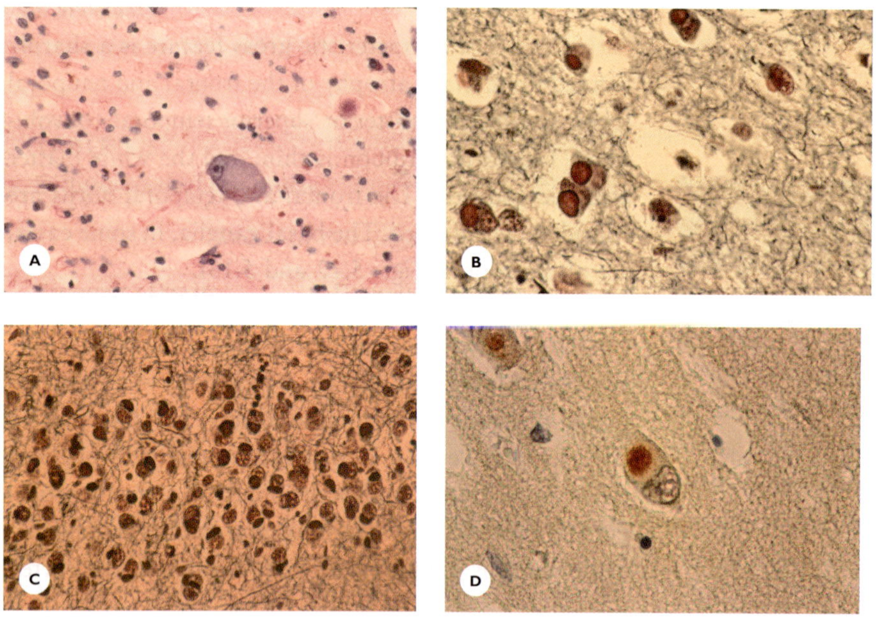

FIGURE 5.14

Pick's disease. **A.** A Pick cell in temporal cortex displays swollen perikaryon and peripherally displaced nucleus (HE). **B.** Pick bodies appear as argyrophilic globular cytoplasmic inclusions, and (**C**) are particularly numerous in the dentate gyrus (Bodian stain). **D.** The Pick body immunoreacts for tau protein (immunostain).

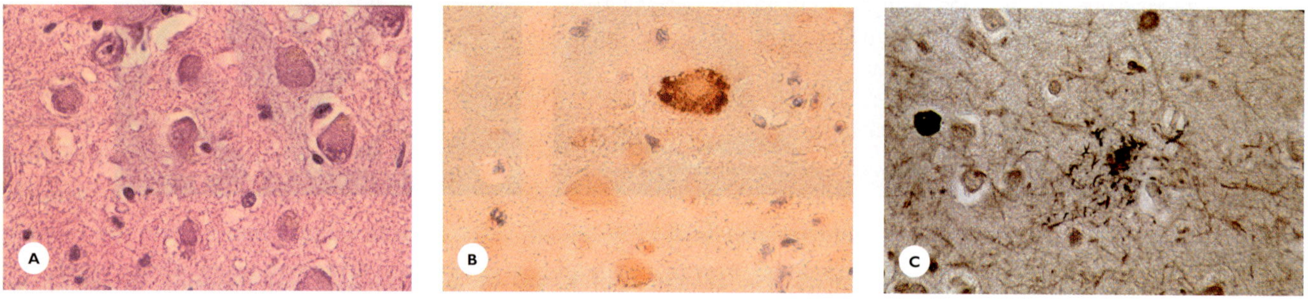

FIGURE 5.15

Corticobasal degeneration. **A.** Ballooned, achromatic neurons in the hippocampus are devoid of Nissl substance (HE) and (**B**) stain positively for tau protein (immunostain). **C.** Astrocytic plaque in cerebral cortex (Gallyas stain).

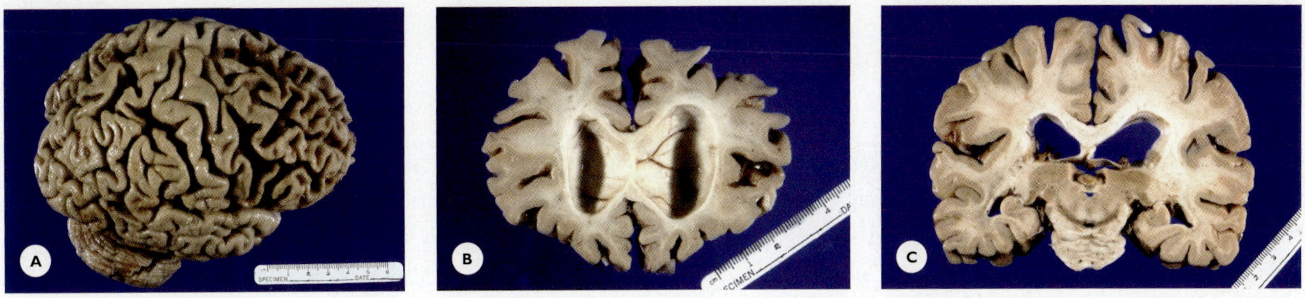

FIGURE 5.16

Tau-immunopositive fronto-temporal dementia. A 73-year-old man developed partial complex seizures with automatism at age 48 years. Memory decline became evident at age 53 years and steadily progressed. Gradually, he became confused, disoriented, very slow and withdrawn, needing assistance in all his daily activities. A few years prior to his death, he became mute, bedridden, and incontinent. He died 20 years following the onset of memory decline. Family history was not contributory. **A.** Lateral aspect of the brain shows severe frontal lobe atrophy. **B.** The cortical ribbon in the frontal lobe is reduced in width, the white matter is severely atrophic, and the anterior horns are enlarged. **C.** Atrophy of the temporal lobe is moderate.

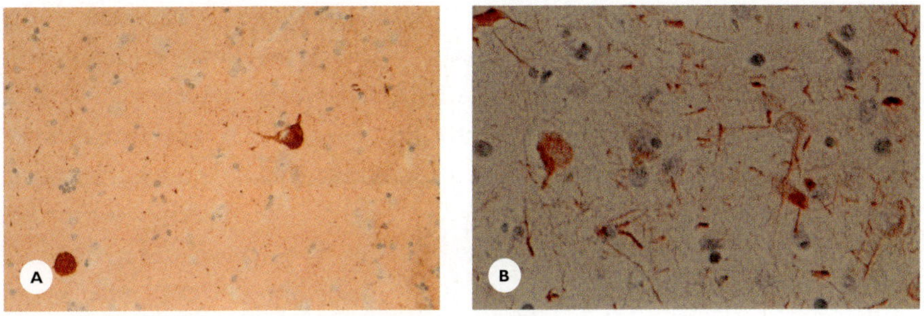

FIGURE 5.17

Amygdala shows (**A**) tau-immunopositive neurons and (**B**) neuritic threads (immunostain).

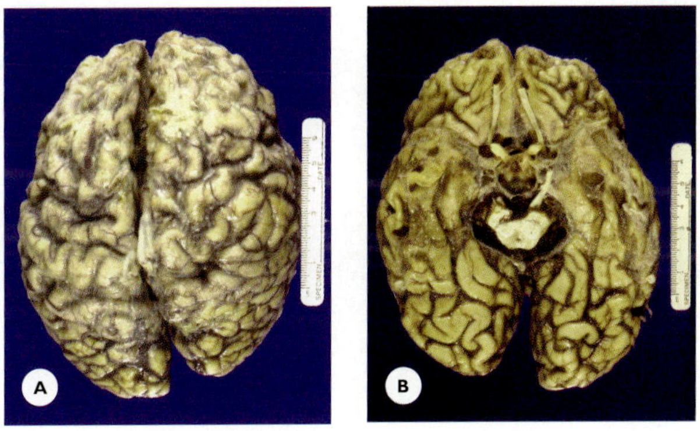

FIGURE 5.18

Fronto-temporal dementia with ubiquitin-only immunopositive neuronal inclusions. The illness of this 67-year-old man began with memory impairment at age 47. This was followed by progressive deterioration of language and other cognitive functions. He became violent, physically abusive, and exhibited oral tendencies, placing inedible objects in his mouth, drinking detergent, and urine. By the age of 60, he was mute, incontinent, and wheelchair bound. He had positive snout, sucking, and grasp reflexes and cogwheel rigidity in all extremities. He died of an acute cardiorespiratory arrest following a 20-year clinical course. His family history was noncontributory. The brain shows (**A**) severe circumscribed atrophy of the frontal and (**B**) anterior temporal and mesio-temporal convolutions.

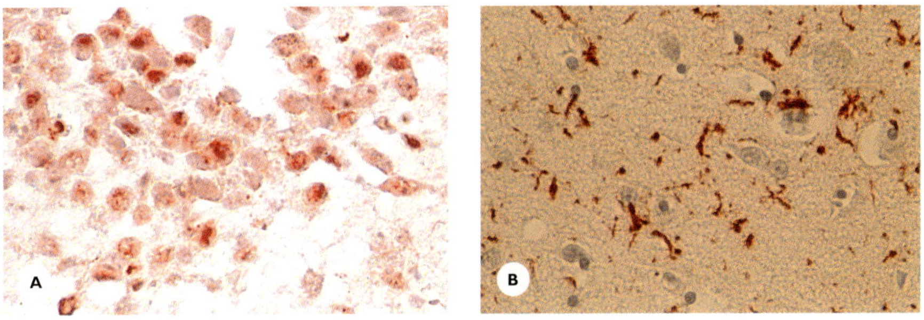

FIGURE 5.19

A. Dentate gyrus displays neurons with ubiquitin-immunoreactive inclusions. **B.** Cortex shows ubiquitin-positive threads (immunostain).

is depleted of neurons, becomes spongy, and displays a dense astrofibrosis. The white matter is variably devoid of myelin, which is replaced by astrogliosis. Astrocytes in the cerebral cortex and oligodendrocytes in the white matter may display argyrophilic and tau-immunoreactive cytoplasmic inclusions.

Dementia with Parkinsonism Linked to Chromosome 17

Clinical features. This is a familial dementia inherited in an autosomal dominant pattern: The interest of the disease lies in its association with mutations in the *Tau* gene on chromosome 17. The disease begins between the ages of 30 and 50 years and manifests with behavioral changes, features of Klüver-Bucy syndrome, cognitive decline, frontal lobe dementia, and akinetic rigidity that is unresponsive to dopamine therapy.

Pathology. Frontotemporal atrophy and discoloration of the substantia nigra and locus ceruleus are distinct gross findings. Major histologic changes are neuronal losses and the presence of argyrophilic tau-immunopositive cytoplasmic inclusions in the neurons, astrocytes, and oligodendrocytes. Common sites of neuronal losses and replacement gliosis are the frontal and limbic cortex, substantia nigra, basal ganglia, and amygdala. The neuronal inclusions are round, oval, or ring-shaped, and are found in the cerebral cortex and affected subcortical gray structures. Astrocytes with tau deposits appear as tufted astrocytes and astrocytic plaques. Oligodendrocytes in the cerebral, cerebellar, and brainstem white matter display coil-shaped inclusions.

Dementia with Corticobasal Degeneration

Clinical features. Corticobasal degeneration (CBD) is a slowly progressive neurodegenerative disease of mid to late life. It occurs sporadically; few familial cases have been recorded. Prominent clinical features include combinations of:

- Limb dystonia and apraxia, often unilateral or asymmetrical
- Akinetic-rigidity
- Postural instability
- Postural and action tremor and
- Cortical sensory impairment
- Eye-movement abnormalities
- Focal myoclonus
- Alien limb phenomenon (the extremity feels foreign)
- Frontal lobe behavioral changes
- Aphasia
- Cognitive decline

Pathology. Grossly, the atrophy is confined to the superior frontoparietal convolutions, including the pre- and postcentral convolutions; to the basal ganglia; and to the midbrain tegmentum. The substantia nigra is depigmented, and the globus pallidus may have a rustye color. The temporal lobe is usually spared, except in cases presenting with aphasia and severe dementia. The histology is characterized by (a) the presence of achromatic neurons, (b) tau-immunoreactive neuronal inclusions, (c) glial inclusions, (d) neuropil threads, and (e) neuronal losses and gliosis.

The achromatic or ballooned neurons are devoid of Nissl substance, stain faintly with eosin, are weakly argyrophilic, and immunoreact for phosphorylated neurofilaments, α-B-crystalline, and tau protein. They are found chiefly in the affected frontal cortex, limbic areas, and amygdala (Fig. 5.15).

The tau-positive, argyrophilic neuronal inclusions, called *corticobasal* bodies, are widely distributed in the cortex, subcortical gray structures, and brainstem.

The glial inclusions are argyrophilic, tau-positive astrocytic plaques, thorn-shaped and tufted astrocytes in the cerebral cortex; and oligodendrocytic coiled bodies in the white matter. The tau-positive neuropil threads of glial and neuronal origin are abundant in the gray and white matter. Neuronal losses and astrogliosis, usually moderate, occur in the cerebral cortex, substantia nigra, striatum, thalamus, midbrain, medullary olives, and cerebellar dentate nuclei.

FTLDs with Ubiquitin-Only Pathology

Dementia with Motor Neuron Disease

In this rare condition, the patient presents with behavioral changes, frontal lobe dementia, and an amyotrophic picture showing weakness, muscle wasting, fasciculation and, ultimately, dysarthria and dysphagia.

Grossly, the frontotemporal lobes are atrophic, and the substantia nigra is discolored. Histologically, the spinal cord and brainstem show degeneration of the motor neurons. Neuronal losses are present in the atrophic cortex, striatum, thalamus, and substantia nigra. Ubiquitinated neuronal cytoplasmic inclusions are characteristic, and occur in the granule cells of the dentate fascia of the hippocampus, frontal and temporal cortex, brainstem, and spinal motor neurons.

Dementia with Ubiquitin-Only-Positive Neuronal Inclusions

Clinically, this group of dementias is often referred to as *dementias with motor neuron disease-inclusions*, although features of amyotrophic lateral sclerosis (ALS) are not present. Grossly, the brain shows a circumscribed atrophy of the frontal and/or temporal lobes (Fig. 5.18). The histology is distinguished by the presence of ubiquitin-only immunoreactive neuronal inclusions. They are neither argyrophilic nor eosinophilic, and they do not immunoreact for tau protein. The inclusions are commonly found in the granule cells of the dentate fascia of the hippocampus. Ubiquitin-positive neurites and occasional neuronal inclusions occur in the superficial cortical layers (Fig. 5.19). The limbic and neocortical areas show neuronal losses and microvacuolation, chiefly in the external layers. Astrogliosis is moderate to severe in the affected areas.

Dementias Lacking Distinctive Histologic Features

This is a heterogenous group of sporadic and familial dementias affecting individuals in their fifth and sixth decades. Primary progressive aphasia, cognitive decline, and behavioral changes occur in various combinations. The pathology, confined to the frontotemporal lobes, consists of neuronal losses, spongiosis, and astrogliosis, particularly in the outer cortical layers. Conventional and sensitive silver stains and currently applied immunohistologic stains fail to reveal neuronal or glial inclusions.

MOTOR NEURON DISEASES

Motor neuron diseases (MNDs) are characterized clinically by a progressive loss of muscle power brought about by the primary degeneration of lower or upper motor neurons or both. In lower MNDs, the weakness is associated with muscle wasting, fasciculation, hypotonia, and a decrease or loss of tendon reflexes. In upper MNDs, the weakness is associated with spasticity, hyperactive reflexes, and Babinski sign. Some diseases are sporadic, and some inherited. Individuals of all ages from birth to late midlife can be affected. The diagnosis depends primarily on the symptoms and signs. An electromyogram (EMG) showing a denervation pattern confirms degeneration of the lower motor neurons.

The three groups of MNDs are: (Table 5.7): (a) ALS, entailing concurrent degeneration of upper and lower motor neurons; (b) spinal muscular atrophies, entailing degeneration of lower motor neurons only; and (c) primary lateral sclerosis and hereditary spastic paraparesis, entailing degeneration of upper motor neurons only.

Amyotrophic Lateral Sclerosis

Clinical Features

ALS, the most common MND, begins during the fifth or sixth decade of life. The incidence is estimated to be 1 to 2 per 100,000 per year. The disease is usually sporadic, although familial incidences with autosomal dominant inheritance occur in about 5% to 10% of

TABLE 5.7.
Motor Neuron Diseases

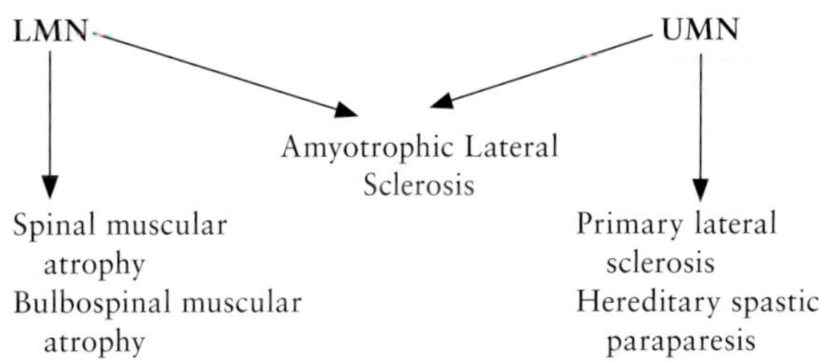

LMN, lower motor neuron; UMN, upper motor neuron.

cases. Some familial cases are associated with mutations in a gene on chromosome 21 that encodes the free radical–scavenging enzyme copper/zinc superoxide dismutase–1 (SOD1). SOD1 converts cytotoxic oxygen radicals to hydrogen superoxide. A rare juvenile variant with autosomal recessive or x-linked inheritance is associated with mutation in a gene (*alsin*) on chromosome 2. In the etiology of sporadic cases, oxidative stress and the excitotoxic effect of the neurotransmitter glutamate are considered.

The clinical presentation is characterized by a concurrence of symptoms and signs involving both the lower and upper motor neurons. The disease usually begins in the spinal cord, with weakness in extremities, increased or diminished to absent tendon reflexes, Babinski sign, increased or diminished muscle tone, muscle wasting, and fasciculations. Bulbar symptoms usually develop late in the course of the disease but, in a small number of cases, introduce the disease. The bulbar palsy combines the features of brainstem motor neurons (bulbar palsy) with those of corticobulbar tracts (pseudobulbar palsy). It presents with facial weakness, nasal or dysarthric speech, brisk or absent gag and jaw reflexes, dysphagia, atrophy and fasciculation of the tongue, and emotional lability with spontaneous laughing or crying. The course averages from 2 to 10 years.

Pathology

Grossly, the spinal cord and motor nerve roots and, less often, the motor cortex are atrophic. The histology is characterized by a degeneration of the motor neurons in the spinal cord, brainstem (nuclei of the 3rd, 4th, and 6th cranial nerves are spared), and motor cortex along with a degeneration of the corticospinal and corticobulbar tracts (Fig. 5.20). The degeneration of the cortico-

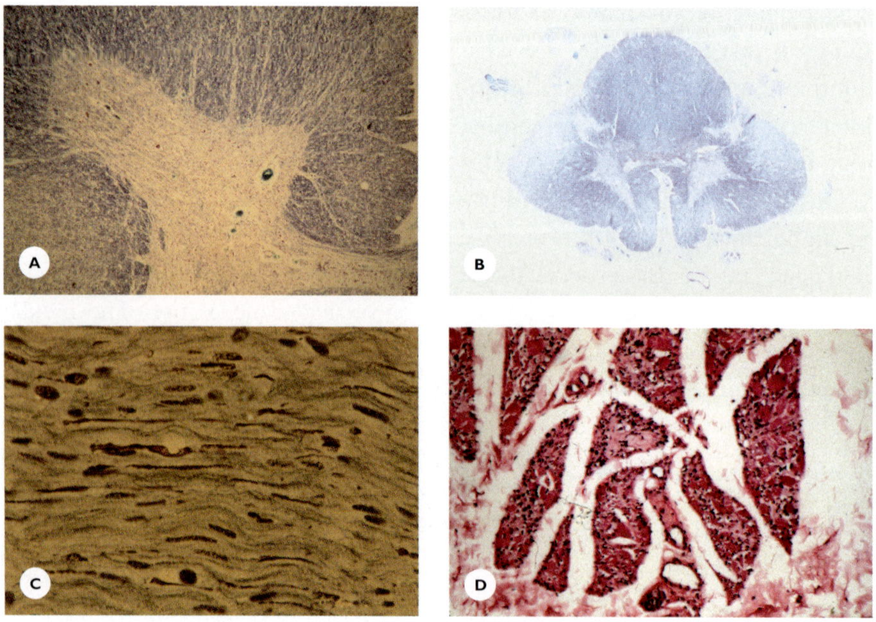

FIGURE 5.20
Amyotrophic lateral sclerosis (ALS). A 68-year-old man had been diagnosed with ALS at age 58 years when he noticed weakness, some wasting, and twitching in muscles of his arm. The weakness gradually progressed, involved his legs and, by the age 66, he was bedridden. On examination, he was quadriplegic with generalized muscle wasting and fasciculations. Reflexes were hypoactive in the arms, and hyperactive with clonus and Babinski sign in the legs. Sensation was normal. Facial muscles were slightly weak, and fasciculation was present in the tongue. Speech was dysarthric. Following a 13-year clinical course, he died at age 71. **A.** The anterior horn of the cervical cord is depleted of motor neurons. **B.** The thoracic cord shows degeneration of the lateral and anterior corticospinal tracts (LFB-CV). **C.** The spinal motor nerve root shows axonal and myelin degeneration (Holmes stain). **D.** The skeletal muscle shows denervation with severely atrophic muscle fibers arranged in groups (HE).

spinal tracts is most prominent in the lower spinal cord segments, and it can be traced up through the brainstem to the internal capsule (dying-back axonal degeneration). Surviving spinal motor neurons display small eosinophilic inclusions (Bunina bodies), larger hyalin bodies, and ubiquitin-positive, filamentous, skein-like inclusions (Table 5.8). The motor nerve roots show axonal and myelin degeneration; the skeletal muscles exhibit denervation (group) atrophy (see Fig. 5.20).

Neuronal losses outside the motor system may occur in the thalamus, basal ganglia, dentate gyrus, and cerebellum. ALS may occur in association with frontotemporal dementia and the parkinsonism–dementia complex of Guam. (See the section Extrapyramidal Diseases.)

Spinal Muscular Atrophy

A degeneration of the motor neurons in the spinal cord and brainstem characterize the spinal muscular atrophies (SMAs). These diseases, accounting for 10% of MNDs, are inherited and chiefly affect children of various ages. Based on age of onset, several types are distinguished (Table 5.9). Neonatal and early infantile, infantile, and juvenile types are transmitted as an autosomal recessive trait. They are associated with mutations in the survival motor neuron gene (*SMN1*) on chromosome 5. Adult-onset SMA, has an autosomal recessive or dominant mode of inheritance and a slowly progressive course. Clinical findings are weakness, muscle wasting, fasciculations, hypotonia, absent tendon reflexes and, late in the course, dysphagia and dysarthria. The clinical course is the shortest in neonates, ranging from a few weeks to 2 months; it is longer in infants—2 to 3 years—and juveniles may reach adulthood. Early death is from respiratory failure and bulbar involvement.

Pathology

Grossly, the spinal cord and motor nerve roots are atrophic. The histology is characterized by a loss of spinal and bulbar motor neurons (Figs. 5.21 and 5.22). Microglial nodules indicate the sites of neuronal losses. Acute cases show ballooned chromatolytic neurons and neuronophagia. Outside the motor system, chromatolytic neurons occur in the thalamus, and neuronal losses occur in the Clarke's columns of the spinal cord and sensory root ganglia. Skeletal muscles show denervation atrophy, mostly of type 2 fibers.

TABLE 5.8.
Amyotrophic Lateral Sclerosis

Molecular Pathology	
Neuronal Inclusions	
Bunina bodies	Eosinophilic
Hyalin bodies	Eosinophilic
Skeins of threads	Ubiquitin-positive
Spherical bodies	Ubiquitin-positive

TABLE 5.9.
Spinal Muscular Atrophies

Diseases	*Age of Onset*	*Clinical Course*	*Inheritance*
SMA 1 Werdnig-Hoffmann Disease	Early infantile	Acute	Autosomal recessive
SMA 2	Infantile	Chronic	Autosomal recessive
SMA 3 Kugelberg-Welander disease	Juvenile	Chronic	Autosomal recessive
SMA 4	Adult	Chronic	Autosomal recessive/ Autosomal dominant
Bulbospinal muscular atrophy (Kennedy's disease)	Adult	Chronic	X-linked recessive Triplet repeat disorder

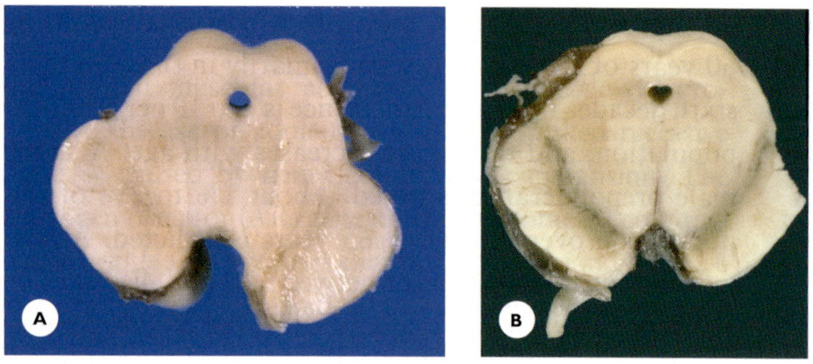

FIGURE 5.23
Idiopathic Parkinson's disease (iPD). A 66-year-old man suffered from Parkinson's disease from the age of 50 years. The brain shows (**A**) discoloration of the substantia nigra compared to (**B**) normal control.

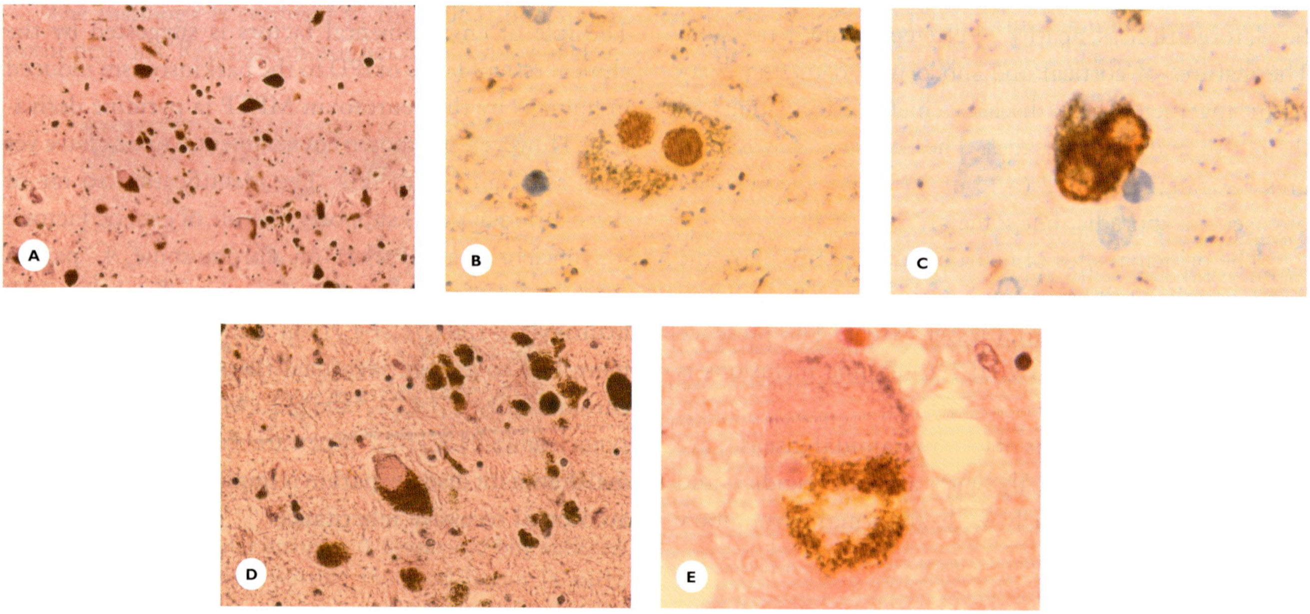

FIGURE 5.24
Idiopathic Parkinson's disease. Substantia nigra shows (**A**) severe neuronal losses and melanin pigments freely dispersed in the parenchyma. Lewy bodies immunoreact for (**B**) α-synuclein and (**C**) ubiquitin (immunostains). **D.** Hyalin body is present in a pigmented neuron (HE). **E.** Locus ceruleus shows a Lewy body (HE).

Pathology

The pathology of iPD encompasses nigral and widespread extranigral neuronal degenerations. A discoloration of the substantia nigra and locus ceruleus is a distinctive gross feature (Fig. 5.23). The essential histology is a degeneration of the melanin-containing neurons in the compact zone of the substantia nigra and the presence of Lewy bodies in remaining neurons (Fig. 5.24). As the neurons degenerate, melanin pigments are found within macrophages or dispersed freely in the neuropil. An astrocytic gliosis eventually forms at the site of neuronal losses. Surviving neurons display *Lewy bodies* and pale hyaline bodies. The Lewy bodies, histological hallmarks of iPD, are intracytoplasmic, eosinophilic, laminated inclusions often surrounded by a halo. Their molecular components are α-synuclein, a synaptic protein, and ubiquitin, a cellular stress protein (Table 5.11). α-Synuclein–positive dystrophic Lewy neurites are also present. The hyaline bodies are pale, eosinophilic, granular structures that displace the melanin and the nucleus (Fig. 5.24).

Common sites of neuronal degenerations and of Lewy bodies and Lewy neurites outside the substantia nigra are the locus ceruleus, dorsal nucleus of vagus, hypothalamus, midbrain raphe nuclei, pedunculopontine and ventral tegmental nuclei, basal nucleus of Meynert,

TABLE 5.11.
Idiopathic Parkinson's Disease

Molecular Pathology
Lewy bodies: Eosinophilic α-Synuclein–positive Ubiquitin-positive

amygdala, hippocampus, intermediolateral column of the spinal cord, and autonomic ganglia. Recent reports indicate astrocytic and oligodendrocytic involvement with argyrophilic and α-synculein–positive cytoplasmic inclusions in areas of neuronal degeneration.

Several factors are considered in the pathomechanism of neuronal degeneration, including apoptosis, excitotoxic neurodegeneration, mitochondrial dysfunction, and the formation of free radicals derived from the auto-oxidation of dopamine into neuromelanin.

Neurochemical Pathology and Clinical Correlates

The pigmented nigral neurons synthesize the neurotransmitter dopamine and transport it to the striatum along the nigrostriatal pathway. In the striatum, the dopamine acts on the neurons possessing D_1 and D_2 receptors. The striatum also contains GABAergic spiny neurons and cholinergic interneurons. The inhibitory neurotransmitter γ-aminobutyric acid (GABA) and the excitatory neurotransmitters acetylcholine (ACh) and glutamate are involved in complex neural circuits subserving motor activities. Depletion of the mostly inhibitory dopamine in the striatum upsets the balance between the excitatory and the inhibitory neurotransmitters, resulting in the motor manifestations of iPD. The akinetic rigidity is attributed directly to dopamine deficiency in the striatum, whereas the tremor at rest is related to neuronal activity in the globus pallidus. It is estimated that a greater than 50% loss of nigral neurons and a 50% to 80% reduction in striatal dopamine results in clinical symptoms.

Neurons in several extranigral sites synthesize specific neurotransmitters and transmit them to the mesolimbic cortex, neocortex, and deep gray structures. Deficiencies of these neurotransmitters are implicated in some of the neuropsychiatric and autonomic features of iPD. Degeneration of dopaminergic neurons in the ventral tegmental nuclei is associated with cognitive decline. The degeneration of noradrenergic neurons in the locus ceruleus is associated with affective changes and autonomic symptoms, and the degeneration of serotonergic neurons in the brainstem correlates with depression and sleep disorder. Neuronal degeneration in the noradrenergic dorsal vagus nucleus accounts for autonomic dysfunction, and degeneration of cholinergic forebrain basal nucleus adds to cognitive decline.

Parkinson's Disease Plus Dementia

Severe dementia occurs in about 10% to 20% of patients with Parkinson's disease. Likely causes are concomitant AD, dementia with Lewy bodies, and vascular pathology.

Parkinsonism or Parkinsonian Syndrome

Parkinsonism or *parkinsonian syndrome* refers primarily to the motor features of iPD that occur in a number of neurodegenerative diseases, in diseases with specific etiologies, and in some inherited metabolic diseases (Table 5.12). Clinical and pathologic overlaps between iPD and degenerative diseases with parkinsonism often pose diagnostic difficulties. Table 5.13 presents differentiating clinical and pathologic features of major diseases with parkinsonism.

Progressive Supranuclear Palsy, Steele-Richardson-Olszewski Disease

Clinical Features

Progressive supranuclear palsy (PSP) affects middle-aged and elderly individuals. The disease is sporadic, but a few familial occurrences have been reported, some associated with mutations in the tau gene. The annual incidence rate is 5 per 100,000 population; this figure increases with advancing age.

The disease presents a broad spectrum of symptoms and signs including (a) supranuclear vertical and horizontal gaze palsy; (b) motor disturbances, such as bradykinesia-akinesia, rigidity of the neck, axial, and

TABLE 5.12.
Diseases with Parkinsonism

Degenerative	*Acquired*		*Hereditary*
Progressive supranuclear palsy	Infection	Toxin	Wilson's disease
Striatonigral degeneration	Trauma	MPTP	Neuroacanthocytosis
Corticobasal dementia	Dementia pugilistica	Carbon monoxide	Hallervorden-Spatz disease
Chromosome 17-linked dementia	Vascular diseases	Manganese	
Parkinsonism-dementia complex of Guam	Hypoxic-ischemic insult	Neuroleptics	
Postencephalitic parkinsonism	Mass lesion		
Multiple system atrophy			

TABLE 5.13(A).
Neurodegenerative Diseases with *Parkinsonism

***Diseases*	*Differentiating Clinical Features*
PSP	Gaze palsy, Axial dystonia, Pseudobulbar palsy
CBD	Limb apraxia, Alien-limb phenomenon, Cortical sensory deficit, Aphasia
FTDP-17	Autosomal dominant inheritance. Mutation in tau gene on chromosome 17
MSA	Cerebellar ataxia, Dysautonomia of Shy-Drager syndrome

*Parkinsonism refers principally to motor disturbances of idiopathic Parkinson's disease (iPD).
PSP, progressive supranuclear palsy; **CBD, corticobasal degeneration; FTDP-17, frontotemporal dementia parkinsonism linked to chromosome 17; MSA, multiple system atrophy.

limb muscles, neck dystonia, impaired gait, postural instability with frequent falls, and pseudobulbar palsy; and (c) behavioral changes and cognitive decline. The clinical course averages from 5 to 10 years.

Pathology

Grossly, the substantia nigra and locus ceruleus are discolored. The basal ganglia, brainstem tegmentum, and cerebral cortex are variably atrophic.

The histology is characterized by neuronal degeneration in distinct anatomic regions and the presence of neuronal and glial cytoplasmic inclusions (Table 5.14).

Neuronal Degeneration

The principal sites of neuronal degeneration are (a) the substantia nigra and the pallidostriatal structures, (b) the mesencephalic and pontine tegmentum, and (c) the cerebral cortex, chiefly the frontal and limbic areas. The thalamus, subthalamic nucleus, pontine nuclei, medullary tegmentum, inferior olives, and cerebellum are variably affected. The fiber tracts of the degenerated neurons are severely or completely demyelinated. Astrocytic fibrosis in the affected regions is moderate to severe (Figs. 5.25 through 5.27).

Neuronal and Glial Cytoplasmic Inclusions

Neuronal and glial cytoplasmic inclusions are argyrophilic and immunoreact for tau protein. The neuronal inclusions are fibrillary tangles, mostly in globose form. Tau-positive neurons and threads and curly fibers of dystrophic neurites are dispersed throughout the neuropil (Fig. 5.28). Glial inclusions occur in both astrocytes and oligodendrocytes. The astrocytic inclusions are thorn-shaped or tufted astrocytes and astrocytic plaques. The oligodendrocytic inclusions are coiled bodies of filaments around the nuclei (Fig. 5.29).

TABLE 5.13(B).
Neurodegenerative Diseases with Parkinsonism: Differentiating Pathologic Features

		Cytoplasmic Inclusions				
Diseases	*Neuronal Degeneration*	*Neurons*	*Astrocytes*	*Oligodendrocytes*	*Molecular Component*	*Staining Characteristic*
PSP	Midbrain and brainstem, limbic cortex	Neurofibrillary tangles	Tufted Thorn-shaped	Coiled bodies	Tau protein	Argyrophilic
CBD	Frontoparietal cortex, basal ganglia, substantia nigra	Corticobasal bodies	Plaques Tufted Thorn-shaped	Coiled bodies	Tau protein	Argyrophilic
FTDP-17	Frontotemporal cortex, substantia nigra, basal ganglia	Round/oval tangle-like	Plaques Tufted Thorn-shaped	Coiled bodies	Tau protein	Argyrophilic
MSA	Cerebellum, striatum Substantia nigra Autonomic neurons	Oval, round		Oval, round triangular (Papp-Lantos inclusions)	α-synuclein	Argyrophilic

TABLE 5.14.
Progressive Supranuclear Palsy

Molecular Pathology
Tau-positive inclusions → Neurons; Glial cells
Glial cells → Astrocytes; Oligodendrocytes

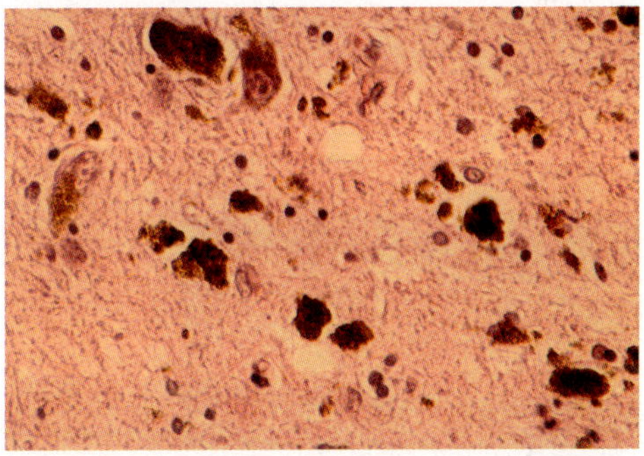

FIGURE 5.25
Progressive supranuclear palsy (PSP). A 65-year-old man presented with a 6-year history of difficulty walking and frequent falls, inability to look up or down, difficulty speaking and swallowing, and declining memory. Family history was not contributory. On examination, he was not able to articulate words, but was able to follow simple commands. The vertical and horizontal eye movements were severely restricted. The muscle tone was increased in the neck, trunk, and extremities, but strength was good. No tremor was noted. He needed assistance to rise from a chair and ambulate. The gait was slow and shuffling. Tendon reflexes were brisk, plantar reflexes were flexor, and the vestibulo-ocular reflex was present. He died at age 66 following a 7-year clinical course. Midbrain shows degeneration of the substantia nigra (HE).

Clinical–Pathologic Correlates

The degeneration of the mesencephalic and pontine tegmental neurons accounts for the supranuclear gaze palsy. The degeneration of the nigropallidostriatal system accounts for the parkinsonian features, and the degeneration of the neurons in the mesolimbic and frontal cortex accounts for the behavioral changes and cognitive decline.

Striatonigral Degeneration

Striatonigral degeneration is a slowly progressive degenerative disease of middle age that greatly resembles Parkinson's disease. Rigidity, akinesia, and postural

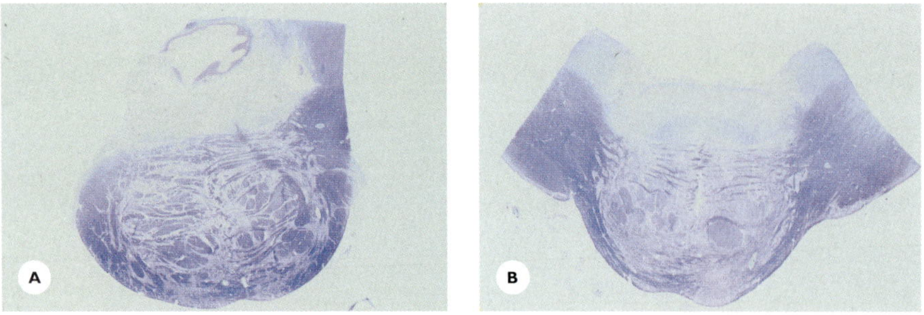

FIGURE 5.26
Progressive supranuclear palsy. Pons. **A** and **B.** The tegmental fiber tracts are demyelinated due to extensive and severe neuronal degenerations (LFB-CV).

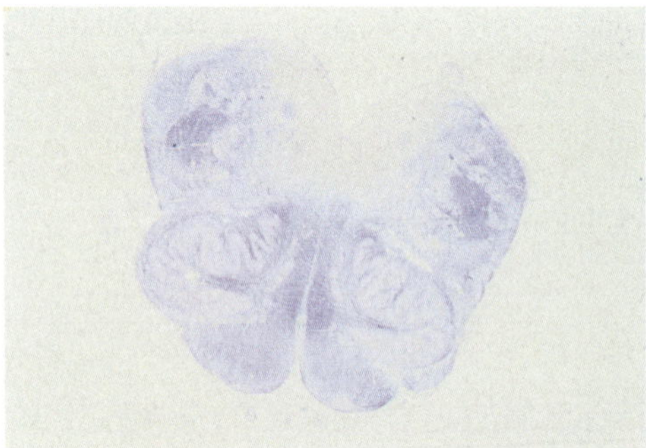

FIGURE 5.27
Progressive supranuclear palsy. Medulla. The tegmentum stains faintly due to severe neuronal and myelin losses (LFB-CV).

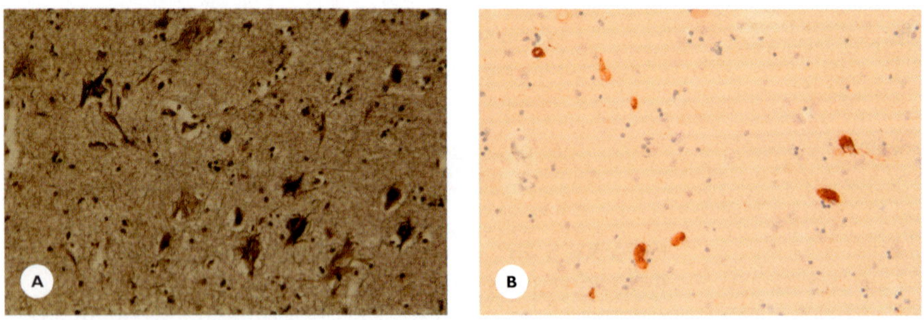

FIGURE 5.28
Progressive supranuclear palsy. Neuronal inclusions. **A.** Neurofibrillary tangles are present in the entorhinal cortex (Bodian stain). **B.** Tau-positive neurons are present in the thalamus (immunostain).

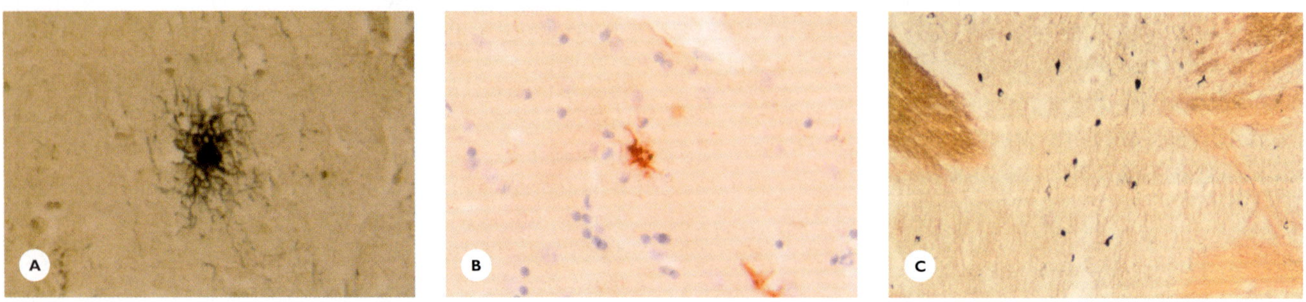

FIGURE 5.29
Progressive supranuclear palsy. Glial inclusions. **A.** Astrocytes display argyrophilic (Gallyas stain) and (**B**) tau-immunoreactive inclusions (astrocytic plaque; immunostain). **C.** Oligodendrocytes display argyrophilic coiled bodies (Gallyas stain).

instability are major clinical features. But, unlike Parkinson's disease, it is unresponsive to dopamine therapy. The pathology is characterized by neuronal losses, particularly severe in the striatum and variable in the substantia nigra, which displays no Lewy bodies. Striatonigral degeneration is a component of multiple system atrophy.

Corticobasal Degeneration

This disease is presented under the section on neurodegenerative dementias. A summary of pertinent features is given in Table 5.13.

Postencephalitic Parkinsonism

This disease has been reported among survivors of the epidemic of von Economo encephalitis lethargica that occurred in Europe in 1915 and in the United States in 1918. The parkinsonism developed many years following the encephalitis and afflicted young adults and children. It presented with parkinsonian features, extraocular muscle palsy, and oculogyric spasm, which is a tonic conjugate deviation of the eyes lasting minutes or hours.

Grossly, the substantia nigra and locus ceruleus are depigmented. The histology is characterized by (a) lympho-plasmacytic perivascular infiltrations, particularly severe in the brainstem; (b) neuronal losses and gliosis in the substantia nigra, locus ceruleus, and brainstem; (c) the presence of argyrophilic, tau-positive neurofibrillary tangles in neurons of the brainstem, hippocampus, frontal, temporal, and insular cortex; and (d) the presence of tau-positive cytoplasmic inclusions in astrocytes.

Parkinsonism-Dementia Complex of Guam

This disease occurs among the Chamorro tribe of Guam. It presents with parkinsonian features and progressive dementia, and it may be associated with ALS (see the section, Motor Neuron Diseases). Grossly, the brain is atrophic, and the substantia nigra and locus ceruleus are discolored. The histology is characterized by neuronal losses that are particularly severe in the hippocampus, temporal and frontal cortex, hypothalamus, substantia nigra, and locus ceruleus. Variable neuronal losses are present in the thalamus and basal ganglia. Tau-immunopositive neurofibrillary tangles are evident in the remaining neurons of affected areas. Neuritic plaques and neuropil threads are inconspicuous.

Diseases with Abnormal Involuntary Movements

Huntington's Disease

Huntington's disease (HD), a disorder of trinucleotide repeat expansion, is inherited in an autosomal dominant trait. The HD gene on chromosome 4 encodes the protein huntingtin, which is widely expressed in the central nervous system. The gene contains a CAG-trinucleotide repeat that normally expands up to 26. In HD patients, the repeat length expands to over 36. A repeat length of over 100 is associated with juvenile-onset disease and is usually transmitted by the father.

Clinical Features

The disease presents in the third and fourth decades of life; successive generations have an earlier onset (anticipation phenomenon). The prevalence is 5 to 10 per 100,000 population. Choreic movements, psychiatric features, and dementia characterize the clinical picture. The choreic movements—abrupt, brief, asymmetric, and jerky—involve the face, tongue, and extremities. They occur spontaneously and during voluntary activities, eventually leading to severe impairment of gait, speech, and swallowing. The juvenile variant presents with akinetic rigidity, dystonia, and seizures, and has a shorter clinical course.

The psychiatric symptoms are manifold, including behavioral and personality changes, distractibility, mood and affective disorders, mainly depression, and psychosis often resembling schizophrenia. These symptoms are combined with a cognitive decline that slowly progresses to dementia. Alcoholism and suicide have a high incidence among HD patients. The clinical course averages from 10 to 15 years.

CT scan and MRI show variable cortical atrophy, mostly of the frontal lobes; enlargement of the anterior horns; and atrophy of the caudates. Subsequently, the

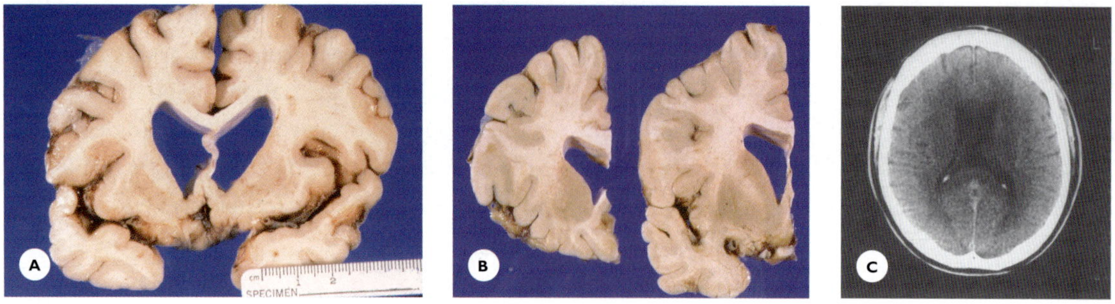

FIGURE 5.30
Huntington's disease. This 50-year-old man had a family history of Huntington's disease. He was diagnosed with the disease at age 37 years and died 13 years later. Transverse section shows (**A.**) moderate convolutional atrophy, severe atrophy of the caudates and putamens, and flattening of the walls of the enlarged anterior horns as compared with (**B.**) normal control. **C.** CT scan of the head from a different patient with Huntington's disease shows flattening of the lateral ventricular walls.

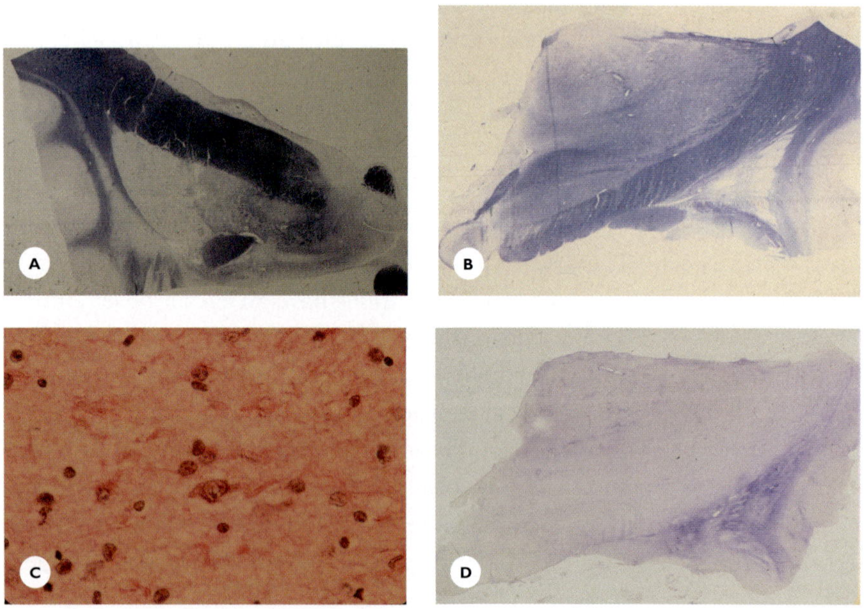

FIGURE 5.31
A and **B.** The putamen and the caudate show marked atrophy and myelin losses (LFB-CV), (**C**) neuronal losses (HE), and (**D**) dense astrogliosis (Holzer stain).

lateral walls of the anterior horns lose their normal curvature and become straight or concave (Fig. 5.30).

Pathology

Grossly, the cerebral cortex is atrophic, the white matter is diminished in volume, and the lateral ventricles are enlarged. The distinctive pathology is confined to the striatum; the caudate and putamen are severely atrophic (see Fig. 5.30).

The histology is characterized by severe neuronal degeneration in the striatum, particularly of the medium-sized GABAergic spiny neuron. The neuronal losses are accompanied by a reduction of myelinated fibers and astrogliosis (Fig. 5.31). The cerebral cortex shows variable neuronal losses. The presence of ubiquitin-immunoreactive nuclear inclusions in remnant spiny neurons and ubiquitinated neurites in the affected regions is characteristic.

The chemical pathology is characterized by a deficiency of the inhibitory neurotransmitter γ-aminobutyric acid (GABA) and of the enzyme glutamate decarboxylase.

Dystonias

Primary torsion dystonia, characterized by twisting movements of extremities with sustained muscle contractions and abnormal posturing, generally affects children and young adults. It occurs either sporadically or is inherited as an autosomal dominant condition. Limited pathologic studies describe neuronal degenerations and astrocytosis in the caudate and putamen.

Neuroacanthocytosis

This disease is characterized by choreiform movements, dystonia, orofacial dyskinesia, cognitive deficit, peripheral neuropathy, seizures, and acanthocytosis (thorny erythrocytes) in the peripheral blood, and a normal lipoprotein concentration. It is inherited in an autosomal recessive or dominant fashion and affects individuals in the third and fourth decades. Neuronal losses in the striatum and, to a lesser degree, in the pallidum characterize the pathology.

TABLE 5.15.

Cerebellar and Spinocerebellar Degenerations

Hereditary
Autosomal recessive
Friedreich's ataxia
Ataxia telangiectasia
Cerebellar ataxia with isolated vitamin E deficiency
Autosomal dominant
Spinocerebellar ataxias
Dentatorubro-pallidoluysial atrophy
Episodic ataxias
Sporadic
Olivopontocerebellar atrophy
Idiopathic cerebellar ataxia

TABLE 5.16.

Trinucleotide Repeat Diseases

Huntington's disease
Bulbospinal muscular atrophy (Kennedy's disease)
Friedreich's ataxia
Dentatorubropallido-luysial atrophy
Adult-onset spinocerebellar ataxias

CEREBELLAR AND SPINOCEREBELLAR DEGENERATIONS

Ataxia, or disturbance of coordination of movements and of gait and balance, tremor of the extremities and head, dysarthric speech, and disorders of eye movement, are distinctive clinical features of cerebellar and spinocerebellar degenerations. This group encompasses inherited and sporadic diseases (Table 5.15).

Sporadic cerebellar ataxias are the olivopontocerebellar atrophy (see the section Multiple System Atrophy) and the idiopathic cerebellar ataxias of midlife.

Inherited cerebellar and spinocerebellar ataxias (ICSCA) occur from infancy to adulthood. The clinical presentation is manifold. The ataxia is associated with combinations of various symptoms and signs relating to the cranial nerves and to the pyramidal, extrapyramidal, and sensory systems. Systemic manifestations are characteristic for some. The pattern of inheritance is autosomal recessive or autosomal dominant (see Table 5.15). Notably, several diseases are trinucleotide repeat disorders caused by expanding cytosine-adenine-guanine (CAG) repeats that code for polyglutamine tracts, hence the name *polyglutamine diseases* (Table 5.16). An expansion of the repeats from the normal range of 10 to 30 to over 40 to 90 results in diseases (Table 5.17). Longer repeats cause an earlier age of onset and greater severity of the disease in offspring, a feature referred to as *genetic anticipation.*

Diagnostic evaluation is aimed first at eliminating sporadic degenerative ataxias and cerebellar diseases with specific causes, and second, at differentiating between various forms of inherited cerebellar ataxias (Table 5.18). Molecular genetic tests are available to detect and measure triplet expansion.

The pathology is widespread. The cerebellum, brainstem, and spinal cord are usually affected. Additional lesions occur in various subcortical gray structures and peripheral nerves. The presence of neuronal nuclear inclusions that derive from aggregations of expanded polyglutamine-containing proteins are characteristic of triplet-repeat diseases.

TABLE 5.17.
Genetic Features of Trinucleotide Repeat Diseases

Disease	*Gene Product*	*Chromosome*	*Repeats*	*Abnormal Length*	*Normal Length*
FA	Frataxin	9	GAA	66–1700	9–55
DRPLA	Atrophin 1	12	CAG	34–79	7–23
SCA 1	Ataxin 1	6	CAG	42–81	16–36
SCA 2	Ataxin 2	12	CAG	35–64	15–34
SCA 3/MJD	Ataxin 3	14	CAG	68–79	13–36
SCA 6	CACNA1A	19	CAG	20–33	4–181
HD	Huntingtin	4	CAG	36–121	6–34
BSMA	Androgen receptor	X	CAG	38–62	9–34

FA, Friedreich's ataxia; DRPLA, dentatorubro-pallidoluysial atrophy; SCA, spinocerebellar ataxia; MJD, Machado-Joseph disease; GAA, guanine-adenine-adenine; CAG, cytosine-adenine-guanine; HD, Huntington's disease; BSMA, bulbospinal muscular atrophy (Kennedy's disease)

TABLE 5.18.
Etiologies of Cerebellar Diseases

Primary Degenerative

Acquired
- Vascular
- Infection
- Toxin
  - Alcohol, phenytoin,
  - Barbiturate, lithium,
  - Mercury, lead,
  - Thallium, solvents
- Myelin diseases
- Paraneoplastic
- Heat stroke, hypoxia,
- Metabolic
  - Hypothyroidism
- Neoplasm

Inherited Metabolic
- Lysosomal diseases
- Mitochondrial diseases
- Hartnup disease
- Aminoacidurias
- Acanthocytosis (Abetalipoproteinemia)

Prion Diseases
- Sporadic Creutzfeldt-Jakob disease
- Gerstmann-Sträussler-Scheinker disease

Friedreich's Ataxia

Clinical Features

Friedreich's ataxia (FA) presents during childhood or adolescence with gait and limb ataxia, loss of sense of joint position and vibration, and loss of tendon reflexes. During the course of the disease, which averages from 20 to 25 years, optic atrophy, sensorineural hearing impairment, weakness and spasticity in lower extremities, Babinski sign, and dysarthria develop. Characteristic systemic manifestations include skeletal anomalies with scoliosis and pes cavus, hypertrophic cardiomyopathy, and occasional diabetes mellitus. FA, an autosomal recessive disease, is caused by an expansion of guanine-adenine-adenine (GAA) repeats in the frataxin gene on chromosome 9. Expansion of the repeats is from 90 to more than 100. The normal number of repeats is 6 to 27.

Pathology

The brunt of pathology falls on the cerebellum, peripheral nerves, and spinal cord. The cerebellar pathology is confined to the dentate nuclei, which show extensive neuronal losses. Purkinje cell degeneration is usually mild. The peripheral nerves and sensory nerve roots show axonal and myelin degeneration, and the sensory spinal ganglia show neuronal losses. In the spinal cord, the posterior columns, the dorsal and ventral spinocerebellar tracts, the neurons in the Clarke's columns, and the pyramidal tracts are degenerated (Fig. 5.32). Neuronal losses are present in the cuneate and gracile nuclei, and in the cochlear and vestibular nuclei. Degeneration of the optic nerves adds to the pathology.

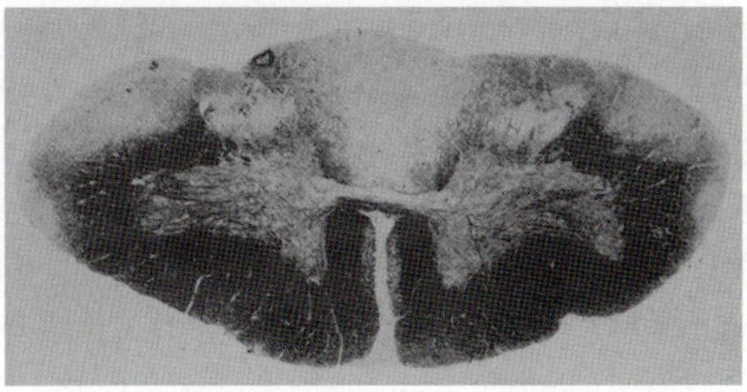

FIGURE 5.32
Friedreich's ataxia in a 5-year-old boy whose older brother, aged 15 years, suffered from a similar illness. Spinal cord shows degeneration of the posterior columns, pyramidal tracts, and spinocerebellar tracts (Weil stain).

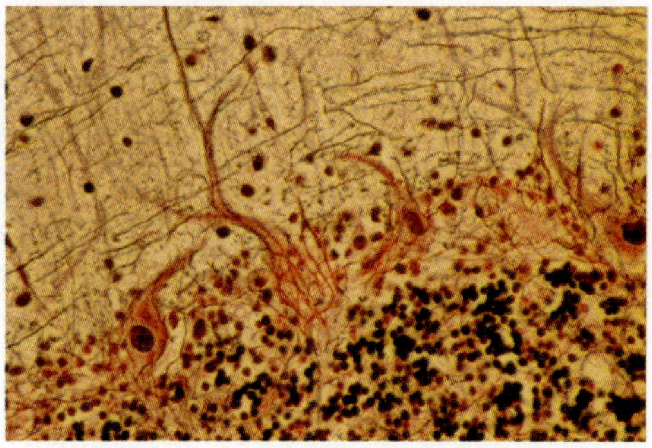

FIGURE 5.33
Ataxia telangiectasia. A 22-year-old man, diagnosed with AT before the age of 2 years, had bilateral conjunctival telangiectasia and nystagmus. From the age of 9 years, he was confined to a wheelchair because of progressing gait ataxia. His medical history was remarkable for multiple episodes of infection. He died of pneumonia following resection of a pulmonary abscess. The cerebellar cortex shows Purkinje cell losses, empty basket cells and replacement Bergmann astrocytosis (Bodian stain).

Ataxia Telangiectasia, Louis-Bar Syndrome

Clinical Features

Ataxia telangiectasia (AT) is a complex syndrome with nervous system, ocular, cutaneous, and visceral manifestations. It is an autosomal recessive disorder associated with mutations in the ataxia telangiectasia mutated (ATM) gene on chromosome 11. Its prevalence is estimated at 1 per 80,000 live births.

The disease begins during infancy or early childhood with slowly progressive cerebellar ataxia. Nystagmus and gaze apraxia are characteristic ocular signs. Patients who survive beyond adolescence develop dysarthric speech, choreoathetosis, weakness, muscle wasting, and an impaired vibratory sense. Characteristic somatic features include conjunctival and cutaneous telangiectasia, retarded growth or dwarfism, progenic changes of the hair and skin (premature aging), and delayed development of sex characteristics. Defective immune mechanism, sinopulmonary infection, and a tendency to malignancy, mostly lymphomas or leukemias, complete the syndrome. Serum levels of α-fetoprotein and carcinoembryonic antigen are increased, and levels of immunoglobulin A (IgA) and E (IgE) are decreased.

Pathology

Extensive Purkinje cell degeneration characterizes the cerebellar pathology (Fig. 5.33). Residual cells may contain eosinophilic cytoplasmic inclusions. Cerebral lesions include cortical neuronal atrophy, neuronal losses in the basal ganglia, and gliosis in the hemispheric white matter. The spinal cord, in advanced cases, shows degeneration of the posterior columns and atrophy of the motor neurons. Pathologic changes outside the nervous system include hypoplasia of the thymus and lymphoid tissues, ovarian or testicular dysgenesis, and large bizarre cells in the anterior pituitary gland.

Cerebellar Ataxia with Isolated Vitamin E Deficiency

Cerebellar ataxia with isolated vitamin E deficiency, an autosomal recessive disorder, is associated with mutations of the α-tocopherol transfer protein gene. Clinically, the disease resembles FA. Progression is preventable with vitamin E supplement.

Dentatorubro-Pallidoluysial Atrophy

Dentatorubro-pallidoluysial atrophy (DRPLA) occurs from infancy to adult life. It is relatively common among the Japanese. It is inherited as an autosomal dominant trait and is associated with an expanded CAG repeat in the DRPLA gene on chromosome 12. The CAG repeats expand to 54 to 79; the normal number of repeats is from 6 to 35. Progressive cerebellar ataxia is associated with combinations of choreoathetosis, myoclonus, seizures, and mental retardation in children, and with dementia in adults. On radiograph, a thick skull is noted. On MRI T2-weighted images, cerebellar and brainstem atrophy and hyperintense lesions in the hemispheric white matter, pallidum, and thalamus are characteristic.

Grossly, the brainstem and the cerebellum are atrophic, and the globus pallidus has a brown-tan discoloration. Histology:, the disease is confined to the cerebellum and its efferent connection —, the red nucleus, and to the globus pallidus and its efferent connection, the subthalamic nucleus. A loss of neurons occurs in the dentate nucleus, and myelin pallor and gliosis is noted in the dentate hilus and the superior cerebellar brachia. The remaining dentate neurons display grumose degeneration with eosinophilic and argyrophilic granular materials around the perikaryon and dendrites. They derive from axonal terminals of the Purkinje cells. The red nuclei show gliosis and some neuronal losses. The globus pallidus and the subthalamic nucleus show neuronal losses and gliosis, and a loss of myelin occurs in the pallidosubthalamic tracts. Variable neuronal losses occur in the cerebral cortex, and myelin losses and gliosis are present in the hemispheric white matter.

The presence of neuronal inclusions is characteristic. The dentate neurons display round, eosinophilic, nuclear and filamentous cytoplasmic inclusions. Both immunoreact for ubiquitin and expanded polyglutamine tracts. Neurons with intranuclear inclusions, which represent aggregates of expanded polyglutamine tracts, are widely distributed.

Episodic Cerebellar Ataxias

Episodic ataxias (EA), rare autosomal dominant conditions, are characterized by ataxic episodes lasting from seconds to minutes (type EA1) or from hours to days (type EA2). The diseases map to loci on chromosomes 12 and 19, respectively.

Adult-Onset Inherited Spinocerebellar Ataxias

This group of spinocerebellar ataxias (SCA) comprises autosomal dominant diseases, the majority are caused by triplet (CAG) repeat expansions. To date, 17 genetic types (SCA 1 through 17) have been identified with their chromosomal loci. The genes of SCA-1, -2, -3, -7, -8, -10, and -11 encode for the protein ataxin. Mutations of the *SCA-6* gene affect calcium-channel function (Table 5.17). The prevalence of SCAs is estimated at 5 per 100,000 persons. The age of onset is between 40 and 50 years. It is earlier in successive generations (anticipation); occasional infantile and childhood cases occur, depending on the repeat length.

Clinical Features

The cerebellar symptoms and signs are associated with a wide range of neurologic disorders in various combinations, such as visual deficit, extraocular muscle palsy, spasticity, akinetic-rigidity, choreoathetosis, dystonia, bulbar symptoms, amyotrophy, sensory deficit, and cognitive decline.

Pathology

Cerebellar and brainstem atrophy are usual gross findings. Histologically, the cerebellar degeneration involves the cortex or the dentate neurons (Fig. 5.34). In the spinal cord, the motor neurons and the posterior columns are commonly involved. Neuronal losses occur in the basal ganglia, substantia nigra, thalamus, and brainstem. The neurons display intranuclear inclusions that immunoreact for ubiquitin and polyglutamine tracts.

MULTIPLE SYSTEM ATROPHY

Multiple system atrophy (MSA), a sporadic neurodegenerative disease of adults, combines the clinical and pathologic features of three conditions, namely, olivopontocerebellar atrophy (OPCA), striatonigral degeneration (SND), and dysautonomia of the Shy-Drager syndrome (SDS). Occurring together, they form a clinicopathologic entity that is defined by the presence of distinct oligodendrocytic and neuronal cytoplasmic inclusions.

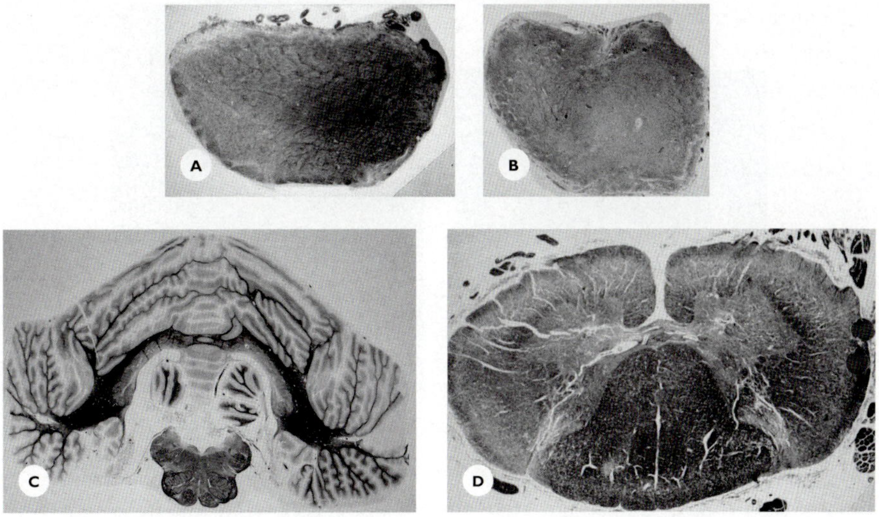

FIGURE 5.34

Adult-onset hereditary spastic spinocerebellar ataxia. A 43-year-old man developed rapidly progressing visual impairment, cerebellar ataxia, and weakness in all extremities. By age 44, he was blind and had pale, sharply outlined discs. Deep tendon reflexes were brisk, and Hoffmann and Babinski signs were present on both sides. All extremities were weak and spastic. Cerebellar ataxia and intention tremor were present in the upper extremities. Sensation was normal. His condition steadily deteriorated and, at age 49, he died. His mother and two sisters, aged 51 and 37 years, respectively, suffered from a similar illness. **A** and **B.** The optic nerves are partially demyelinated (Weil stain). **C.** The cerebellar cortex and white matter are diffusely atrophic. **D.** The corticospinal tracts and the spinocerebellar tracts are degenerated in the spinal cord (Weil stain).

Clinical Features

A combination of cerebellar dysfunction, parkinsonian features, and autonomic failure characterize the clinical picture. In some patients, cerebellar, and in others, parkinsonian symptoms predominate. The Shy-Drager syndrome may occur with either one.

Ataxia of gait is usually the presenting cerebellar symptom, followed by ataxia of limbs, dysarthria, and ocular signs such as nystagmus, ocular dysmetria, fixation instability, and jerky pursuit movements. The parkinsonian features include rigidity, bradykinesia-akinesia, postural instability, hypokinetic dysarthria, and tremor. The autonomic failure consists of orthostatic hypotension, bladder dysfunction (urinary frequency, urgency, retention), bowel dysfunction (constipation), and sexual (male erectile) dysfunction. Spasticity, hyperreflexia, sleep disorder, respiratory stridor, and hypoventilation add to the syndrome. The course averages from 6 to 10 years. MRI demonstrates cerebellar atrophy and enlargement of the fourth ventricle, indicating pontine atrophy (Fig. 5.35).

Pathology

Grossly, the cerebellar cortex is atrophic, the basis of the pons and middle cerebellar peduncles are shrunken, and the inferior olives are flattened (see Fig. 5.35). The substantia nigra and locus ceruleus are discolored, and the putamen is atrophic with grayish discoloration. Histologically, widespread degeneration of the neurons in three anatomic systems and the presence of distinct glial and neuronal cytoplasmic inclusions are the defining features.

Neuronal degeneration occurs in the olivopontocerebellar system, the striatonigral system, and the autonomic nervous system. Extensive degeneration of the Purkinje cells characterizes the cerebellar pathology. The basket cells are empty, and axonal spheroids (torpedoes) of the degenerated Purkinje cells are commonly found in the granular layer. A prominent Berg-

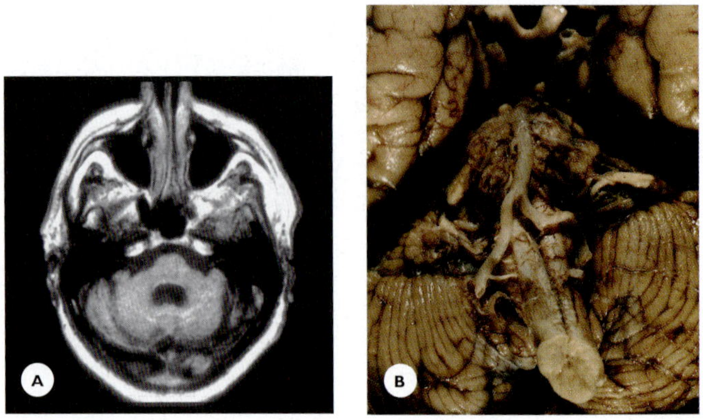

FIGURE 5.35
Multiple system atrophy. A 62-year-old man presented with a history of gait imbalance that began at age 58. At 60 years of age, he had lost sensation of the urinary bladder and gradually became incontinent. Impotence and constipation had begun a few years earlier. The incoordination gradually involved first the lower, then the upper extremities. His speech became slurred. The unsteadiness of gait progressed and, by 62 years of age, he was confined to a wheelchair. No similar disease had occurred in his family. On examination, his mentation appeared normal. His speech was severely dysarthric. He had severe cerebellar ataxia in all extremities and nystagmus on lateral gaze. Reflexes were symmetric, with plantar flexor reflexes. Muscle strength and sensation were normal. He was unable to walk and could stand only a few minutes with bilateral assistance. On changing from a supine to a sitting position, his blood pressure consistently dropped by 20 mm Hg while his pulse remained unchanged. **A.** MRI shows atrophy of the cerebellum and enlargement of the fourth ventricle. **B.** The cerebellar cortex is severely atrophic, the pontine basis is reduced in volume, and the inferior olives are flattened.

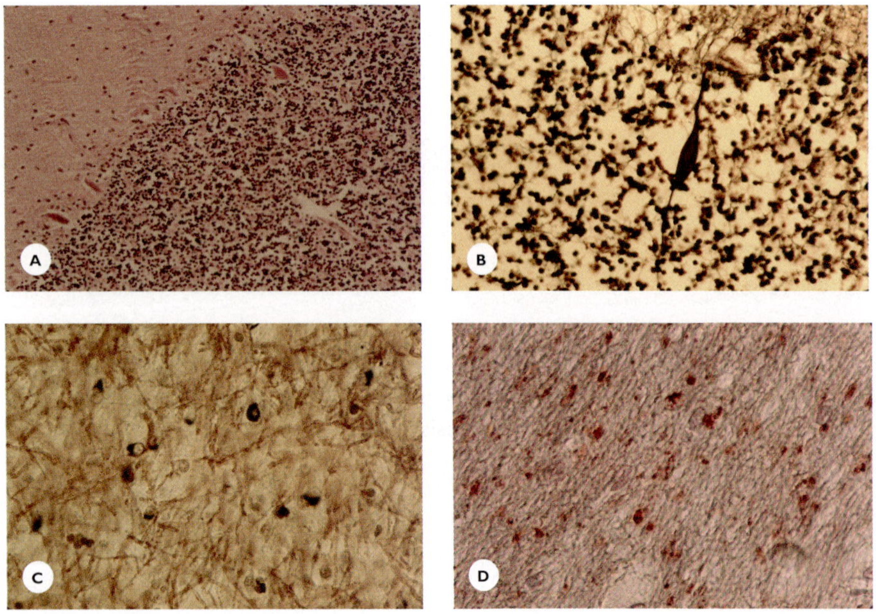

FIGURE 5.36
Multiple system atrophy. Cerebellum shows **A.** severe Purkinje cell losses and prominent Bergmann astrocytosis (HE), **B.** Axonal spheroid (torpedo) of the degenerated Purkinje cells (Bodian stain). **C.** Argyrophilic (Gallyas stain). **D.** Ubiquitin-positive cytoplasmic inclusions in oligodendrocytes of the white matter (immunostain).

mann astrocytic layer marks the site of Purkinje cell losses (Fig. 5.36). The neurons in the griseum pontis degenerate, and their cerebellar projections—the transverse pontine fibers and middle cerebellar peduncles—are demyelinated (Fig. 5.37). The medulla shows degeneration of the neurons in the inferior olives and variable myelin losses in the inferior cerebellar peduncles (Fig. 5.38).

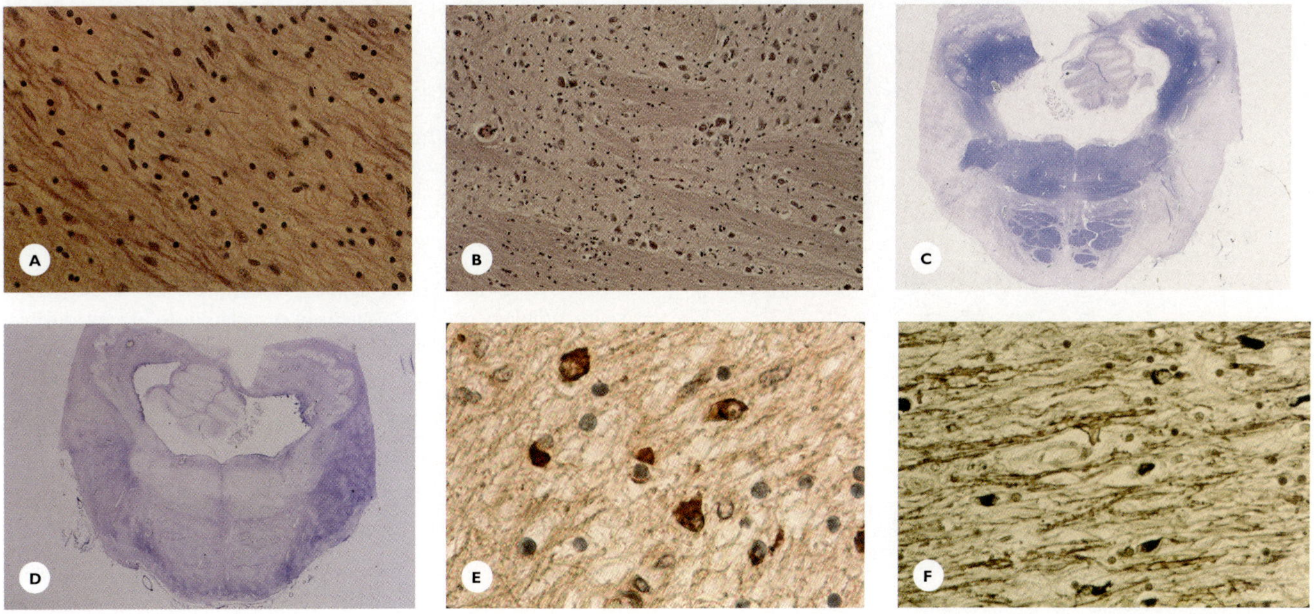

FIGURE 5.37
Multiple system atrophy. **A.** Pons shows extensive neuronal losses in griseum pontis compared with (**B**) normal control (HE), (**C**) demyelination of transverse pontine fibers and middle cerebellar brachia (LFB-CV); (**D**) astrofibrosis at the site of transverse pontine fibers and middle cerebellar brachia (Holzer stain); (**E**) argyrophilic conical cytoplasmic inclusions in oligodendrocytes (Gallyas stain); and (**F**) α-Synuclein–immunoreactivity of inclusions (immunostain).

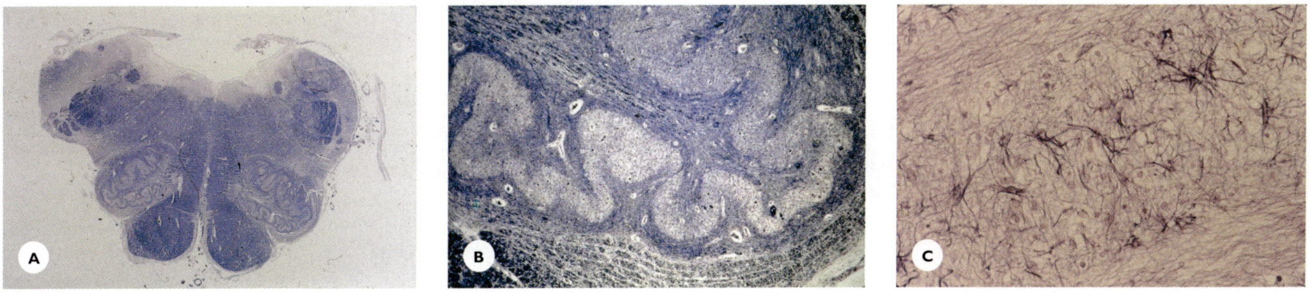

FIGURE 5.38
Multiple system atrophy. Medulla shows (**A**) loss of myelin in olivocerebellar fibers and inferior cerebellar brachia (LFB-CV), (**B**) neuronal losses in the inferior olivary nuclei (LFB-CV), and (**C**) dense astrogliosis (Holzer stain).

Neuronal losses and gliosis are prominent in the putamen and variably severe in the substantia nigra (Fig. 5.39). Changes in the autonomic nervous system consist of losses of sympathetic neurons in the intermediolateral columns of the thoracic and lumbar spinal cord and losses of parasympathetic neurons in the sacral cord (Fig. 5.40).

Cytoplasmic inclusions in the oligodendrocytes and neurons (Papp-Lantos inclusions), are the hallmark lesions of MSA (Table 5.19). They are argyrophilic, best demonstrated using sensitive silver stain (Gallyas method) and appear as round, oval, conical, flame- or crescent-shaped structures. The inclusions are distinguished by immunoreactivity for α-synuclein and ubiquitin (see Figs. 5.36 and 5.37). They commonly occur in the frontal motor cortex and adjacent white matter, basal ganglia, brainstem reticular formation, pontine basis, cerebellar white matter, and middle cerebellar brachia.

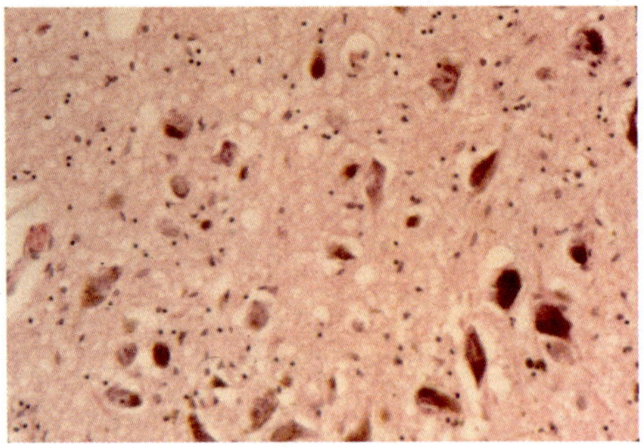

FIGURE 5.39
Multiple system atrophy. Midbrain shows moderate losses of pigmented neurons of the substantia nigra (HE).

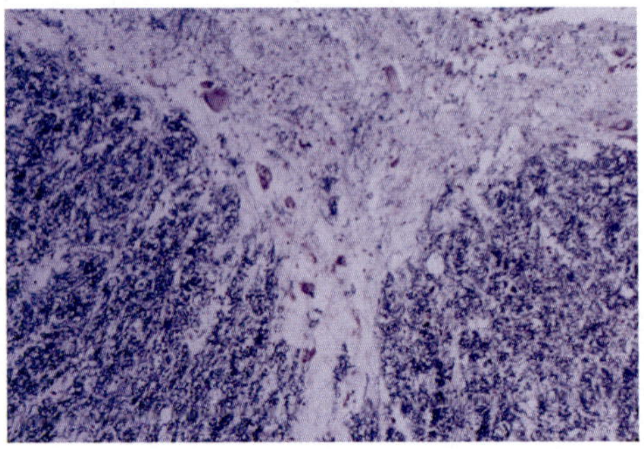

FIGURE 5.40
Multiple system atrophy. Thoracic spinal cord shows loss of sympathetic neurons in the intermediolateral column (LFB-CV).

TABLE 5.19.
Multiple System Atrophy

Molecular Pathology

Cytoplasmic Inclusions

Oligodendrocytes → α-Synuclein-positive, Ubiquitin-positive, Argyrophilic ← **Neurons**

α-Synuclein-positive
Ubiquitin-positive
Argyrophilic

BIBLIOGRAPHY

Cummings, J. L., ed. (1990). *Subcortical dementia.* New York: Oxford University Press.

Cummings, J. L. (2003). Toward a molecular neuropsychiatry of neurodegenerative diseases. *Ann Neurol 54*, 147–154.

Dickson, D. W. (2003). *Neurodegeneration: the molecular pathology of dementia and movement disorders ISN.* Basel: Neuropath Press.

Forrer, T., Rovira, M. B., Sanchez Guerra, M. L., et al. (2004). Neuropathology and pathogenesis of encephalitis following amyloid-β immunization in Alzheimer's disease. *Brain Pathol 14,* 11–20.

Hodges, J. R., Davies, R. R., Xuereb, J. H., et al. (2004). Clinicopathological correlates in frontotemporal dementias. *Ann Neurol 56*, 399–406.

Kolozin, B. & Behl, C. (2000). Mechanisms of neurodegenerative disorders Part 1: Protein aggregates. *Arch Neurol 57*, 793–804.

Markesbery, W. R. (Ed.). (1998). *Neuropathology of dementing disorders.* London: Arnold.

McKhann, G., Drachman, D., Folstein, M., et al. (1984). Clinical diagnosis of Alzheimer's disease: Report of the NINCDS–ADRDA Work Group under the auspices of Department of Health and Human Services Task Force on Alzheimer's Disease. *Neurology 34,* 939–944.

McKhann, G. M., Alberts, M. S., Grossman, M., et al. (2001). Clinical and pathological diagnosis of frontotemporal dementia: Report of Work Group on Frontotemporal Dementia and Pick's Disease. *Arch Neurol 58*, 1803–1809.

Mirra, S. S., Heyman, A., McKeel, D. et al. (1991). The consortium to establish a registry for Alzheimer's disease (CERAD) Part II Standardization of the neuropathological assessment of Alzheimer's disease. *Neurology 41*, 479–486.

Trojanowski, J. Q. & Growdon, J. H. (1998). A new consensus report on bio-markers for the early antemortem diagnosis of Alzheimer's disease; current status, relevance to drug discovery and recommendations for future research. *J Neuropath Exp Neurol 57,* 643–644.

Trojanowski, J. Q. & Dickson, D. (2001). Update on the neuropathological diagnosis of frontotemporal dementias. *J Neuropath Exp Neurol 60,* 1123–1126.

Whetsell, W. O., Jr. (1996). Current concepts of excitotoxicity. *J Neuropath Exp Neurol 55*, 1–13.

REVIEW QUESTIONS

1. Histopathologic changes characteristic of Alzheimer's disease (AD) are:
   A. Lewy bodies
   B. Neurofibrillary tangles
   C. Amyloid angiopathy
   D. Neuritic plaques
   E. Neuronal losses

2. Neurofibrillary tangles are:
   A. Best revealed with phosphotungstic acid hematoxylin (PTAH)
   B. Argyrophilic
   C. Composed of fibrillary acidic protein
   D. Composed of hyperphosphorylated tau protein
   E. Common in the hippocampus

3. A neuritic plaque is composed of:
   A. An amyloid core
   B. Rod-shaped eosinophilic structures
   C. Dystrophic neurites
   D. Activated microglial cells
   E. Reactive astrocytes

4. Neuritic plaques:
   A. Are common in the white matter
   B. Are argyrophilic
   C. Contain amyloid precursor protein (APP)
   D. Contain Aβ-peptide
   E. Are revealed with thioflavin-S in polarized light

5. Genes associated with early-onset, dominantly inherited AD are:
   A. Presenilin 1 on chromosome 14
   B. APP gene on chromosome 21
   C. Gene of apolipoprotein (APOE)4 on chromosome 4
   D. All of these
   E. None of these

6. Pathologic features of Pick's disease include:
   A. Knife-edge atrophy of the parieto-occipital lobes
   B. Argyrophilic cytoplasmic inclusions
   C. Knife-edge atrophy of the frontotemporal lobes
   D. Eosinophilic cytoplasmic inclusions
   E. Tau-positive cytoplasmic inclusions

7. Dementia with parkinsonism linked to chromosome 17 is characterized by:
   A. Mutations in α-synuclein gene
   B. Depigmentation of the substantia nigra
   C. Argyrophilic inclusions in the neurons
   D. Mutations in tau-gene on chromosome 17
   E. Astrocytic plaques in the cortex

8. Clinical features of dementia with corticobasal degeneration include:
   A. Limb dystonia
   B. Akinetic rigidity
   C. Alien limb phenomenon
   D. All of these
   E. None of these

9. The pathology of dementia with corticobasal degeneration includes:
   A. Tau-positive neuronal inclusions
   B. Argyrophilic astrocytic inclusions
   C. Achromatic neurons
   D. Lewy bodies in the substantia nigra
   E. Hirano bodies in the hippocampus

10. Histopathologic features of amyotrophic lateral sclerosis (ALS) are:
    A. Degeneration of corticospinal tracts
    B. Degeneration of spinothalamic tracts
    C. Degeneration of spinal motor neurons
    D. Eosinophilic inclusions in the motor neurons
    E. Neurogenic muscle atrophy

11. Characteristics of spinal muscular atrophies are:
    A. They are common in children.
    B. They present with weakness, atrophy, fasciculation and loss of vibration sensation.
    C. They are caused by trinucleotide repeat expansion.
    D. All of these.
    E. None of these.

12. All of the following characterize idiopathic Parkinson's disease (iPD) *except*:
    A. Akinetic rigidity
    B. Dopamine deficiency
    C. Depigmentation of substantia nigra
    D. Tau-positive argyrophilic inclusions in the neurons of the substantia nigra
    E. In dominantly inherited PD mutation in α-synuclein gene (Park 1) on chromosome 4

13. Clinical findings characteristic of progressive supranuclear palsy (PSP) include:
    A. Neck dystonia
    B. Vertical gaze palsy
    C. Bilateral Babinski signs
    D. All of these
    E. None of these

14. Pathologic findings characteristic of PSP are:
    A. Degeneration of corticospinal tracts
    B. Degeneration of substantia nigra
    C. Neurofibrillary tangles in the hippocampus
    D. Lewy bodies in the neocortex
    E. Tau-positive inclusions in the astrocytes

15. Lewy body dementia is clinically distinguished by:
    A. Parkinsonian features
    B. Visual hallucinations
    C. Syncope
    D. All of these
    E. None of these

16. Characteristics of Huntington's disease (HD) are:
    A. It is dominantly inherited.
    B. The huntingtin gene maps to chromosome 4.
    C. It is a disorder of CAG trinucleotide repeat expansion.
    D. Juvenile cases are associated with short repeats.
    E. Juvenile cases are associated with long repeats.

17. Somatic features of ataxia telangiectasia include:
    A. Retarded growth
    B. Progenic changes (early aging) of skin
    C. Delayed sexual development
    D. All of these
    E. None of these

18. Histopathologic characteristics of olivopontocerebellar atrophy (OPCA) are:
    A. Degeneration of Purkinje cells
    B. Degeneration of brachium conjunctivum
    C. Tau-positive inclusions in the oligodendrocytes
    D. α-Synuclein–positive inclusions in oligo-dendrocytes
    E. Loss of sympathetic neurons in the spinal cord

19. Clinically, OPCA may present with:
    A. Cerebellar ataxia
    B. Autonomic dysfunctions
    C. Parkinsonian features
    D. All of these
    E. None of these

20. All of the following characterize Friedreich's ataxia *except*:
    A. It is an autosomal dominant disorder
    B. It is associated with expansion of GAA repeats
    C. Skeletal anomalies are present
    D. The cerebellar dentate neurons are degenerated
    E. The sensory nerve roots are degenerated

(Answers are provided in the Appendix.)

CHAPTER 6

Infectious Diseases

Bacterial Infections
Viral Infections
Mycotic Infections
Syphilitic Infections
Parasitic Infections
Miscellaneous Infections

Infectious diseases of the central nervous system (CNS) are particularly important because of their increasing incidence and high fatality. Major predisposing factors to infections are diseases and therapies associated with immunosuppression: notably, AIDS, malignancies, poorly controlled diabetes, long-term antibiotic therapy, high doses of corticosteroids, cytotoxic and immunosuppressive drugs, and organ and bone marrow transplants. Blood transfusions and the intravenous use of illicit substances are important sources of infections (Table 6.1). Some diseases occur sporadically; others occur in epidemics. A great variety of pathogens can infect the nervous system.

The assessment of an infectious disease should include the following points: (a) the portal of entry of the pathogen; (b) the route to the neural tissue; and (c) the characteristic inflammatory response of the neural tissue to a particular pathogen.

Some microorganisms are detected in histologic sections stained with hematoxylin-eosin (HE), but most are only visualized using special stains. Other microorganisms are identified only in tissue cultures or by techniques based on polymerase chain reaction (PCR) or using immunologic stains.

Some pathogens evoke an acute inflammation, presenting with a sudden onset and rapid progression of clinical symptoms. Others evoke a slowly evolving inflammation over several weeks, months, or even years, presenting a protracted clinical course. Still other pathogens are opportunistic—they remain dormant in the nervous tissue and only become pathogenic under an altered immune state in the host.

The inflammation may resolve with no residual tissue damage, resulting in complete recovery. But, in severe cases, residual necrosis or scarring leave the patient with neurologic and psychiatric deficits.

TABLE 6.1.
Risk Factors for CNS Infections

Immunosuppression by:	
Diseases	Acquired immunodeficiency syndrome (AIDS)
	Malignancies
	Primary immunodeficiency states
Therapies	Chemotherapies,
	Corticosteroid therapy
	Solid organ and bone marrow transplantations
	Radiation therapy
	Antiviral, antibacterial therapies
Blood transfusion	
Intravenous abuse of illicit substances	

TABLE 6.2.
Age Prevalence of Major Pyogenic Infections

Age	*Microorganisms*
Neonates	*Escherichia coli*
	B. streptococcus
	Listeria monocytogenes
	Staphylococcus aureus
6 mos.–2 yrs.	*Haemophilus influenzae*
Children–young adults	*Neisseria meningitidis*
Adults	*Streptococcus pneumoniae*

BACTERIAL INFECTIONS

Acute Purulent Inflammatory Diseases

Pyogenic bacterial diseases are among the most common infections of the CNS. The nervous system may be infected in any of the following ways:

- By hematogenous spread during septicemia from a distant infection; common sources are lung abscesses, bronchiectasis, subacute bacterial endocarditis, osteomyelitis, and pelvic infections
- By direct spread from sinusitis, mastoiditis, otitis media, and dental abscesses
- By penetrating traumatic skull injuries
- By diagnostic (lumbar and ventricular puncture) and neurosurgical procedures (ventriculoperitoneal shunt)
- In neonates, by amniotic fluid or from the maternal genital tract during parturition
- In fetuses, by transplacental transmission.

Two major purulent inflammations are leptomeningitis and cerebral abscess.

Purulent Leptomeningitis

Purulent leptomeningitis refers to an inflammation of the pia and arachnoid with a purulent exudate in the subarachnoid space. *Streptococcus pneumoniae*, *Neisseria meningitidis*, and *Haemophilus influenzae* are responsible for about 75% of these infections.

Clinical Features

Purulent leptomeningitis occurs at all ages from birth through old age. The age-related preferences of common bacteria are listed in Table 6.2. The onset is sudden, with fever, headaches, photophobia, and nuchal rigidity. Severe cases are complicated by an altered state of consciousness, seizures, cranial nerve deficits, and focal neurologic symptoms and signs. The cerebrospinal fluid (CSF) shows elevated cell count, chiefly with polymorphonuclear leukocytes (PNLs), increased protein levels, and decreased glucose levels. The causative microorganisms are identified in the sediment of the CSF using Gram stain and by culturing the CSF and blood. Polymerase chain reaction (PCR) and immunologic techniques identify the bacteria within hours of onset.

Once the bacteria have reached the subarachnoid space, they evoke an acute inflammatory reaction that produces a purulent exudate, vascular-circulatory changes, and edema. The exudate is composed of PNLs, plasma fluid, protein, and a few erythrocytes. The cerebral blood flow increases, and the blood vessels dilate and become engorged. The release of toxic substances from bacteria and disintegrating leukocytes produces cytotoxic edema. The breakdown of the blood–brain barrier allows an escape of fluid and protein into the extracellular compartment and produces vasogenic edema. Subsequently, the brain volume increases, and the intracranial pressure rises. When it becomes severe, herniations develop, carrying the risk of sudden death.

Pathology

Grossly, the brain is swollen, the blood vessels are congested, and a purulent greenish yellow exudate fills the subarachnoid space and the basal cisterns, obscuring the cortical surface (Fig. 6.1).

Histologically, the subarachnoid space is filled with PNLs, phagocytic cells, fibrin, and a few erythrocytes. The inflammation may involve the arterial and venous walls, and the exudate may extend into the parenchyma along the perivascular spaces (see Fig. 6.1).

With time, the vascular congestion and exudate gradually resolve, usually without sequelae. In some severe cases, late complications may develop, such as (a) internal hydrocephalus due to leptomeningeal fibrosis and obstruction to CSF circulation in the subarachnoid space; (b) infarction due to vasculitis and arterial and venous thrombosis; or (c) subdural effusion, a common complication of *Haemophilus influenzae* meningitis.

Meningococcus Meningitis

Infection with gram-negative *Neisseria meningitidis* has a virulent and fulminant variant with a high mortality (Fig. 6.2). The disease occurs sporadically or in epidemics. The primary infection, a nasopharyngitis, spreads to the brain via the bloodstream. The meningitis is associated with the Waterhouse-Friderichsen syndrome, which is characterized by petechiae and ecchymotic purpuric lesions in the skin and hemorrhages in the visceral organs, chiefly the adrenals. Disseminated intravascular coagulopathy often complicates the clinical picture.

Anthrax Meningoencephalitis

Infection with *Bacillus anthracis* is acquired through cutaneous contact, inhalation, or ingestion. The bacilli

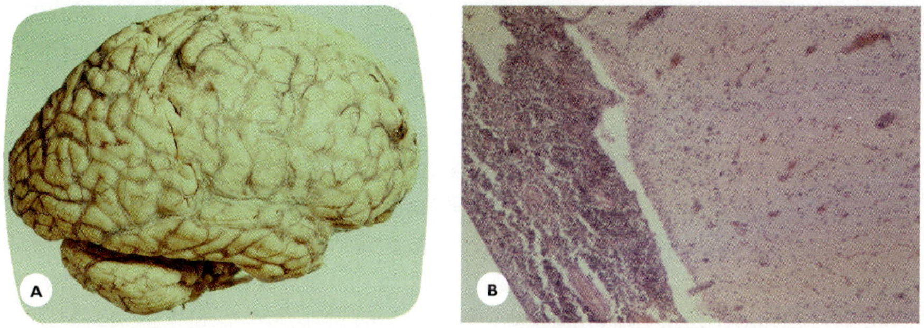

FIGURE 6.1
Acute purulent leptomeningitis caused by β-hemolytic streptococci in a 71-year-old man. **A.** Thick yellow exudate fills the subarachnoid space over the lateral aspects of the cerebral hemispheres. **B.** Dense exudate of PNLs, a few lymphocytes and erythrocytes, and some fibrin fills the subarachnoid space (HE).

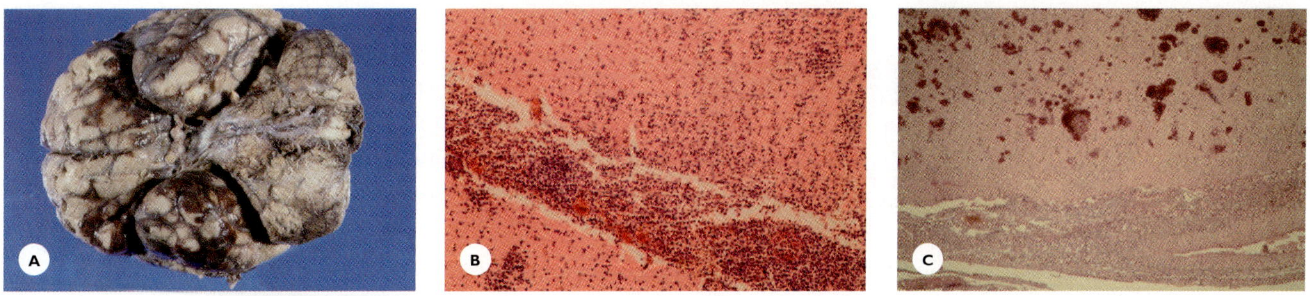

FIGURE 6.2
Fulminant meningococcus meningitis. An 18-year-old male presented in the emergency room with a sudden onset of headaches, fever, and generalized malaise. Examination of the CSF revealed an increased cell count with PNLs, increased protein levels, and the presence of gram-negative meningococci. On the second day, he developed purpuric skin rashes and required assisted ventilation. Soon he went into septic shock, eventually became comatose and, on the fourth day of his illness, he died. At autopsy, both adrenal glands were hemorrhagic. **A.** The brain is markedly swollen, the leptomeninges clouded, and the blood vessels congested. Patchy and confluent hemorrhages fill the basal subarachnoid space. **B.** The subarachnoid space is filled with PNLs, red blood cells, macrophages, and fibroblasts. The exudate extends into the superficial cortical layers. **C.** The cerebral cortex is hemorrhagic and necrotic (HE).

produce an acute, fulminant meningitis or meningoencephalitis with a high mortality rate. Examination of the CSF, which is usually bloody, yields an elevated white cell count, a high protein level, a low glucose level, and the presence of gram-positive bacilli. Computed tomography (CT) scan and magnetic resonance imaging (MRI) reveal subarachnoid and parenchymal hemorrhages and, with the use of contrast material, enhance the leptomeninges.

The cerebral pathology is characterized by a purulent, hemorrhagic exudate in the subarachnoid space. Necrotizing vasculitis, inflammatory infiltrates, and multiple hemorrhages and infarcts characterize the parenchymal changes. The bacilli are readily demonstrated using Gram stain.

Abscesses

Brain abscess is the second major bacterial infection. Lung abscess, bronchiectasis, bacterial endocarditis and, particularly in children, congenital heart disease with right-to-left shift, are common sources of the infection. Blood-borne abscesses are usually multiple in the distribution of the terminal branches of major arteries. The infection may reach the brain from the paranasal sinuses, mastoid, or teeth. These abscesses are usually solitary in the frontal or temporal lobes or cerebellum. Penetrating skull injuries are also important causes of cerebral abscesses.

Pathology

Grossly, an abscess begins as a circumscribed purulent encephalitis (Fig. 6.3). Within a few days, the center of the inflammation liquefies. This acute stage of abscess formation is associated with a vasogenic edema that produces increased intracranial pressure and herniation of the hippocampus and cerebellar tonsils. During this stage, the abscess may rupture into the ventricles, producing a pyocephalus, and it may extend into the subarachnoid space, producing a purulent leptomeningitis.

Histologically, the purulent necrotic tissue is gradually surrounded by highly vascular granulation tissue (see Fig. 6.3). This, in 2 to 3 weeks, forms a thick collagenous capsule around the purulent center. Meanwhile, outside the capsule, astrocytes proliferate, separating the abscess from the healthy tissue.

Multiple disseminated embolic microabscesses are usually encountered in chronically ill, debilitated elderly individuals. Acute bacterial endocarditis caused by staphylococcus is a major source of infection. Clinically, the disease presents as a septic encephalopathy. The abscesses, a few millimeters in size, are usually situated at the cortical–white matter junction.

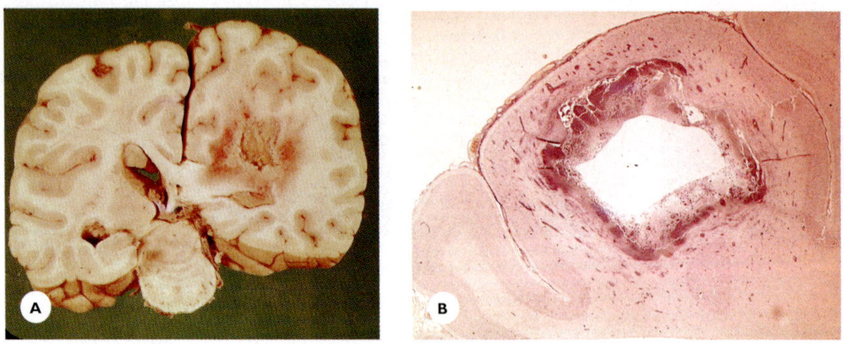

FIGURE 6.3
Metastatic cerebral abscesses from the lung, caused by *Streptococcus pneumoniae* in a 38-year-old man, a chronic alcoholic. **A.** A subacute abscess is situated deep in the parietal white matter. Its center contains liquefied pus, and the wall contains purulent hemorrhagic necrotic tissue surrounded by massive edema. Pus from the ruptured abscess covers the ependyma of lateral ventricles. **B.** Macrosection of a second abscess, situated in the frontal lobe at the junction of cortex and white matter; it is surrounded by a thin capsule of granulation tissue (cresyl violet).

Subdural abscess (empyema), a collection of pus on the undersurface of the dura, is usually associated with infections of the ear, facial sinuses, and with thrombophlebitis of the dural sinuses.

Epidural abscess, a collection of pus on the outer surface of the dura, is associated with osteomyelitis of the skull and infection of adjacent structures.

Spinal epidural abscess, a complication of back injury, skin infection, or osteomyelitis of the vertebrae, is a surgical emergency. Dural abscesses may be difficult to diagnose. MRI and CT scan are most useful in confirming the diagnosis.

Other Purulent Inflammations

Purulent encephalitis is caused by septic emboli from the lung, heart, bone, or other distant septic foci. PNLs diffusely infiltrate the cerebral cortex and the deep gray structures (Fig. 6.4).

Thrombophlebitis of the major cranial sinuses is commonly associated with infections of the brain, ear, facial and nasal sinuses, and skin.

Mycotic aneurysm, an inflammatory necrosis of the vascular wall caused by septic emboli, carries a potential risk for rupture, with subsequent infection and intracerebral and subarachnoid hemorrhages.

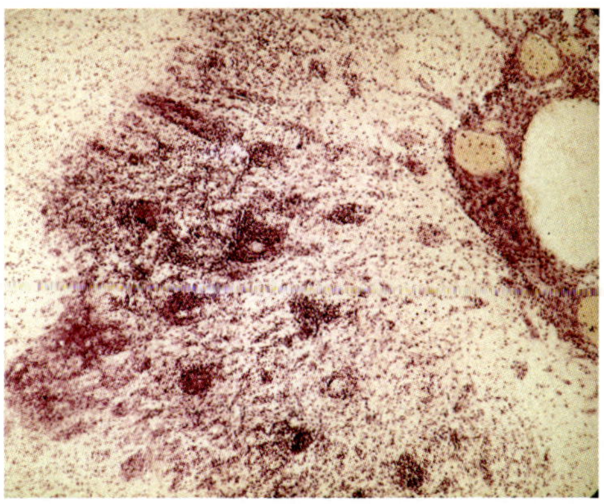

FIGURE 6.4
Purulent encephalitis in a young woman with bacterial endocarditis. Dense perivascular and diffuse parenchymal polymorphonuclear infiltrations are present in the cerebral cortex (cresyl violet).

Subacute and Chronic Granulomatous Inflammatory Diseases

Mycobacterium tuberculosis of human type, an acid-fast bacillus, is the major pathogen of tuberculous infections of the nervous system. The incidence of tuberculosis is increasing, particularly in HIV-infected individuals and abusers of illicit substances.

Tuberculous Granulomatous Meningitis

Clinical Features

Tuberculous meningitis may occur at any age. In children, it is often part of a disseminated miliary tuberculosis. Unlike purulent meningitis, the symptoms evolve over several weeks. Cranial nerve signs, often ocular nerve palsies, are common. Increased intracranial pressure develops after a few weeks due to obstructive hydrocephalus.

The CSF shows pleocytosis with PNLs and lymphocytes; this changes after a few days to predominantly lymphocytes, high protein levels, and low glucose and chloride levels. The demonstration of the bacilli in CSF sediment is often difficult, and their growth in culture requires several weeks. Contrast-enhanced CT scan and MRI demonstrate the basal exudate, hydrocephalus, tuberculomas, and infarcts.

Pathology

The primary infection, commonly in the lungs or lymph nodes, may be active or latent, although, in some cases, no clinical evidence of an extraneural infectious focus is found. The microorganisms reach the meninges or the vessel wall via the bloodstream and produce a small tubercle. From here, the microorganisms invade the subarachnoid space and evoke a granulomatous meningeal reaction. Grossly, this reaction is characterized by multiple small meningeal tubercles and a thick gelatinous exudate. The exudate is typically confined to the basal cisterns and subarachnoid space, extending into the spinal subarachnoid space (Fig. 6.5).

The histology is characterized by: (a) meningeal tubercles composed of lymphocytes, plasma cells, epithelioid cells, Langhan's-type multinucleated giant cells, and areas of caseation necrosis; and (b) subarachnoid exudate containing fibrin and massive perivascular and diffuse infiltrations with mononuclear cells and caseations (Fig. 6.5). The inflammation usually involves the vascular walls and the cranial nerve roots. It may extend into the parenchyma, where it produces a granulomatous meningoencephalitis.

Late complications of tuberculous meningitis are infarction due to thrombotic occlusion of inflamed vascular walls and hydrocephalus due to fibrotic obliteration of the subarachnoid space and obstruction to CSF circulation.

Tuberculoma. Microtubercles may develop into large granulomas, which produce mass effect and raised intracranial pressure (Fig. 6.6).

VIRAL INFECTIONS

A great number of viruses have affinity for the neural tissue and account for a significant number of serious neurologic diseases, especially in patients who are immunosuppressed.

Viral infections of the CNS occur sporadically or in epidemics, either worldwide or in particular geographic areas. Viruses can infect individuals of all ages from infancy to old age, but some favor particular age groups. Viruses enter the host via respiratory or oral routes, sexual contact, or cutaneous inoculation. Mothers can infect fetuses transplacentally and neonates during parturition from a genital infection or from breast milk.

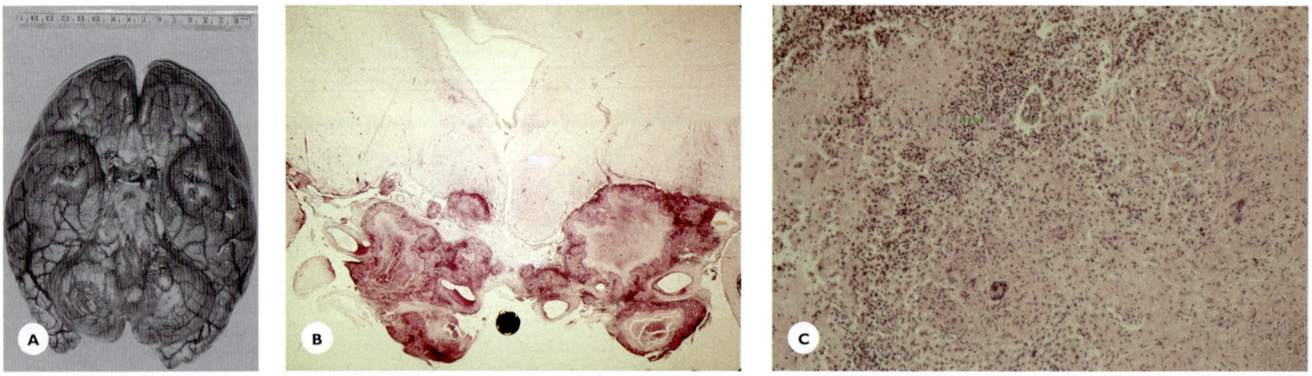

FIGURE 6.5
Tuberculous meningitis/encephalitis. **A.** Thick gelatinous exudate fills the basal cisterns **B.** Macrosection of the infundibulum shows massive granulomatous exudate in the subarachnoid space (Cresyl violet). **C.** Subarachnoid exudate shows lymphoplasmacytic infiltrations, Langhans'-type multinucleated giant cells, and epithelioid cells, and areas of caseous necrosis (HE).

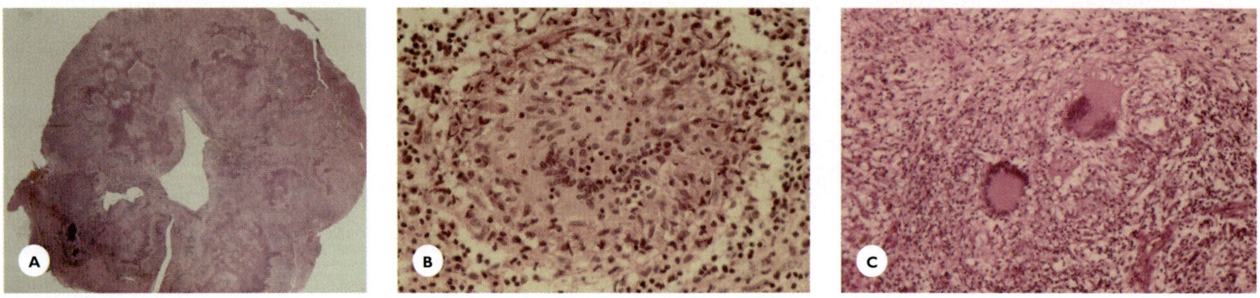

FIGURE 6.6
Tuberculoma. **A.** Macrosection of a cherry-sized tuberculoma surgically excised from the cerebellum of a 32-year-old man. **B.** Multiple microtubercles with (**C**) Langhans'-type multinucleated giant cells (HE).

Most viruses, after replication in distant organs, reach the nervous system via the bloodstream during a temporary phase of viremia. A few viruses reach the neural tissue along peripheral nerves, through retrograde axonal transport.

Once the viruses reach the neural tissue, they can afflict it in several ways. Most viruses evoke an acute aseptic inflammation of the leptomeninges, brain, and/or spinal cord. Some latent viruses, when reactivated, produce either an acute inflammatory or a slowly progressive inflammatory/demyelinating disease. Other viruses (teratogenic) produce malformations in the fetuses of infected pregnant women, and a few viruses (oncogenic) are apt to produce neoplasms.

Acute Aseptic Meningitis, Encephalitis, and Myelitis

Clinical Features

Meningitis presents with fever, general malaise, headaches, photophobia, nuchal rigidity, nausea, vomiting, and muscle aches. Altered states of consciousness, focal neurologic deficits, and seizures are common in encephalitis. Flaccid mono- or paraparesis suggests myelitis. The CSF yields a mild to moderate pleocytosis, typically with lymphocytes; however, during the initial stage, PNLs may also be present. Protein is moderately elevated and glucose is normal. Viral-specific DNA and RNA are identified in the CSF and blood using PCR assay and *in-situ* hybridization.

Pathology

Grossly, the brain and spinal cord are swollen with congested blood vessels. The histology of acute infections by different viruses is basically similar—variations occur mainly in the severity and distribution of lesions. General features are perivascular and diffuse mononuclear cell infiltrations, neuronal or glial destruction, and the presence of intranuclear or intracytoplasmic viral inclusions. In meningitis, the subarachnoid space is filled typically with lymphocytes—mostly T-helper cells, fewer T-suppressor/cytotoxic cells, and B cells. In encephalitis and myelitis, the severity of perivascular cuffings varies: The parenchyma, in severe cases, may undergo necrosis (Fig. 6.7). Most viruses have an affinity for the neurons, or for both the neurons and the glial cells. The infected neurons are surrounded by clusters of polymorphonuclear cells, lymphocytes, activated microglial cells, and macrophages. The diseased neurons gradually disintegrate (lysis) and are phagocytosed by macrophages (neuronophagia). Eventually, residual microglial nodules (stars) replace the destroyed neurons (see Fig. 6.7).

Aggregates of viral particles may form inclusion bodies in the nucleus or cytoplasm of surviving neurons and glial cells. *Cowdry type A inclusions* are large, dense intranuclear eosinophilic bodies surrounded by a clear halo. *Cowdry type B inclusions* are small, often multiple, and lack a halo. Viral antigens are demonstrated using immunohistologic technique.

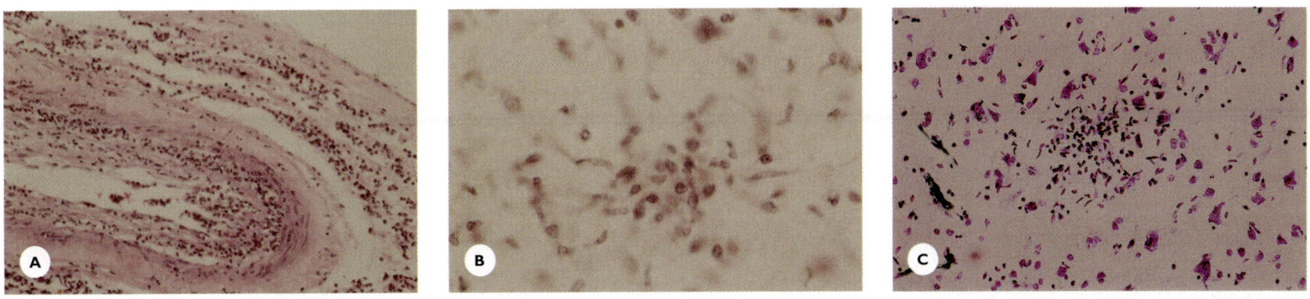

FIGURE 6.7
Histologic features of viral meningoencephalitides. **A.** Mononuclear cell infiltrations in the subarachnoid space and vascular wall. **B.** Mononuclear cells and activated microglia invade the neurons (neuronophagia). **C.** Residual glial nodule takes the place of destroyed neurons (Cresyl violet).

Classification

For presentation, viral infections of the CNS are grouped into the following classifications:

- RNA virus infections
- Herpesvirus infections
- Human immunodeficiency virus-1 (HIV-1) infections
- Chronic viral infections

Acute RNA Viral Infections

Infections caused by RNA viruses of various families occur among both children and adults. Some are important sources of epidemics (Table 6.3). Clinically, the diseases vary greatly, from a benign aseptic meningitis to an encephalitis or a myelitis, and the outcome ranges from full recovery to severe residual neurologic disabilities and even death. Distinct features of major acute RNA virus infections are briefly presented.

TABLE 6.3
RNA Viruses That Cause Acute Aseptic
Meningitis, Encephalitis, Myelitis

Enteroviruses	**Arboviruses**
Poliovirus	St. Louis encephalitis virus
Coxsackie virus	Eastern encephalitis virus
Echovirus	Western encephalitis virus
Paramyxoviruses	Venezuelan encephalitis virus
Mumps virus	California encephalitis virus
Measles virus	Japanese encephalitis virus
Parainfluenza virus	West Nile virus
Nipah virus	**Rhabdovirus**
Toga virus	Rabies virus
Rubella virus	

Enteroviruses

Enteroviruses are spread through the respiratory route or through fecal contamination (hand-to-mouth).

Poliovirus causes poliomyelitis, chiefly a childhood disease, which, before the introduction of the Salk vaccine, had a high mortality rate. The virus spreads from the oropharynx to the gastrointestinal tract and from there to the lymphoid tissue. Here, it replicates and disseminates to the nervous tissue via the bloodstream. Within the nervous tissue, the virus selectively affects the motor neurons of the spinal cord and brainstem and, variably, the cortical motor neurons.

Clinically, a few days following a nonspecific infection, the patient develops meningeal signs and flaccid paresis or paralysis of the extremities, which may extend to the bulbar muscles. Survivors of the acute illness are left with a residual weakness that gradually resolves, either partially or fully. Several years after a paralytic poliomyelitis, a *post polio syndrome* may develop, characterized by progressive weakness and atrophy of the affected muscles.

The pathology of poliomyelitis is characterized by perivascular lymphocytic infiltrations in the leptomeninges, spinal cord, and brainstem, and by neuronophagia and microglial nodules in the anterior horns of the spinal cord and brainstem gray matter (Fig. 6.8). The cortical motor, thalamic, hypothalamic, and cerebellar neurons are less affected. Residual neurons may show small intranuclear inclusions and, in chronic cases, the anterior horns are depleted of neurons and are gliotic (Fig. 6.9).

Coxsackie and *echovirus* infections in children and adults are major causes of aseptic meningitis and encephalitis. Cutaneous rashes, herpangina, carditis, and pleurodynia are systemic manifestations.

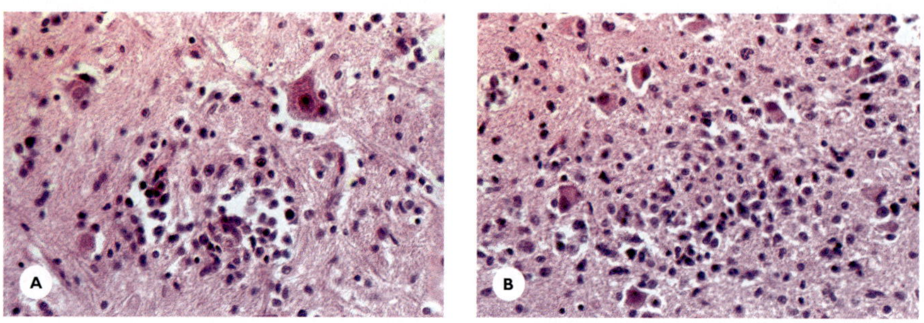

FIGURE 6.8
Acute poliomyelitis. **A.** Motor neurons in the medulla are invaded by activated microglia and mononuclear cells. **B.** Loose glial nodule at the site of disintegrated neurons (HE).

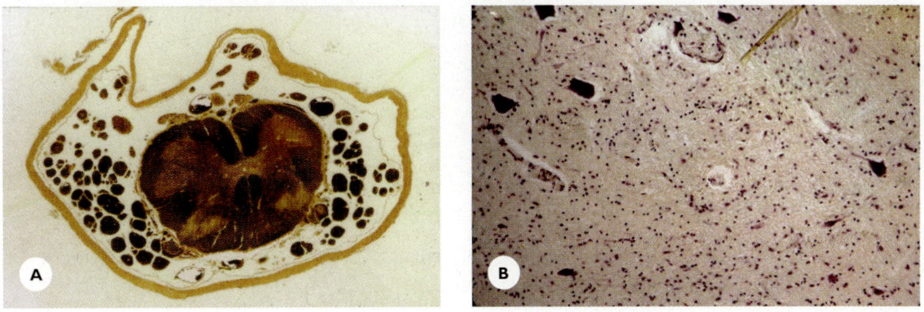

FIGURE 6.9
Chronic poliomyelitis. **A.** Lumbar spinal cord shows atrophy of one anterior horn (iron hematoxylin-picrofuchsin stain). **B.** Depletion of motor neurons (cresyl violet).

Paramyxoviruses

Paramyxoviruses are spread by contamination with infected saliva or respiratory droplets.

Mumps virus, the pathogen of parotitis and orchitis, causes an aseptic meningitis, less often an encephalitis.

Measles virus infections may present in various forms: (a) Aseptic meningitis complicates acute infections. (b) Postinfectious perivenous demyelinating encephalomyelitis, probably immune-mediated, develops 1 to 2 weeks following an acute infection. (c) Subacute measles inclusion body encephalitis is a rare but serious complication of the immunosuppressed state. (d) Subacute sclerosing panencephalitis develops in children and adolescents several years after an early childhood infection.

Parainfluenza virus rarely evokes an encephalitis.

Nipah virus, a newly identified paramyxovirus, is associated with an epidemic of encephalitis with high mortality in southeast Asia. The pathology is characterized by systemic vasculitis of the small vessels, thrombosis, and parenchymal necrosis.

Arboviruses

Arboviruses (arthropod-borne) belong to various families but share common features: (a) they are major causes of epidemics in particular geographic areas; (b) the diseases are acquired by mosquito and tick bites, commonly in late summer or early fall; and (c) from the site of inoculation, the viruses reach the nervous tissue through the bloodstream, evoking an aseptic meningitis or meningoencephalitis. The prognosis varies; it is less favorable among children and elderly individuals.

St. Louis encephalitis, the most common viral encephalitis, occurs throughout the United States. It has a relatively low mortality (5%–10%) and good recovery.

Eastern encephalitis has a high mortality (35%), and residual disabilities are severe, particularly in children.

Western encephalitis has low mortality, but sequelae are common in children.

Venezuelan and *California encephalitides* occur frequently in children. Mortality is high in cases of Venezuelan encephalitis and low in cases of California encephalitis.

Japanese encephalitis, the most common epidemic encephalitis, primarily affects children. The mortality is high (20%–35%) and, in survivors, the sequelae are serious.

West Nile virus infection occurs in several regions of the United States. The infection produces a meningoencephalitis or a myelitis with flaccid paraparesis mimicking poliomyelitis. Immunosuppressed and elderly individuals are at particular risk for the infection.

Rhabdovirus Family

The *rhabdovirus* family is represented by the *rabies virus*. The disease—rabies—is acquired by contamination with saliva from the bites of infected animals, commonly dogs, cats, raccoons, or bats. The viruses reach the nervous tissue along the axons of the peripheral nerves. A few cases of infection through the respiratory route and corneal transplant have been recorded. Following an incubation period ranging from several days to several months, the viruses evoke an acute, rapidly progressing fatal encephalomyelitis and radiculoganglionitis. Eosinophilic viral inclusions (Negri bodies) in the cytoplasm of the pyramidal neurons of the hippocampus and Purkinje cells of the cerebellum are characteristic.

Toga Virus Family

The *Toga virus* family is represented by the *rubella* virus, the pathogen of German measles, an acute benign exanthematous disease of children. It is noteworthy that the rubella virus is teratogenic: It is apt to induce malformations in the fetus of an acutely infected pregnant woman, mainly during the first trimester.

Herpesvirus Infections

The family of human herpesviruses encompasses the following important DNA viruses with strong affinity for the nervous tissue:

- Herpes simplex type 1 virus (HSV-1)
- Herpes simplex type-2 virus (HSV-2)
- Varicella zoster virus (VZV)
- Cytomegalovirus (CMV)
- Epstein-Barr virus (EBV)
- Human herpes viruses 6 and 7 (HHV 6 and 7)

They are all major causes of sporadic infections.

Herpesviruses, distributed worldwide, may infect the fetus in utero, neonates, and individuals of all ages. The initial infection may be inapparent or mild, producing fever, adenopathy, and nonspecific respiratory symptoms. Characteristically, following an initial infection, HSV-1, HSV-2, and VZV latently reside in the neurons, and CMV and EBV in the hematopoietic cells. Malignancies, febrile illnesses, diabetes, age-related decline of the immune system, and even emotional stress are potential risks for the reactivation of a latent infection. Among immunosuppressed individuals, those with HIV infection are most vulnerable. Once the viruses are reactivated, a variety of neurologic diseases arise in both immunocompetent and immunocompromised individuals.

Herpes Simplex Virus-1 Infection

Herpes simplex virus-1 infection is the major cause of sporadic and malignant encephalitis, chiefly in adults and young subjects. The infection is acquired by exposure to contaminated saliva or respiratory secretion. The virus initially causes a nasopharyngitis. By retrograde axonal transport, it reaches the trigeminal ganglia, where it becomes latent. Reactivation of the virus produces herpes vesicles on the lips (cold sore) or oral mucosa. The brain is infected by spread of the virus along the trigeminal nerve roots or dural nerves to the meninges and then to the frontal and basal temporal regions. Alternatively, it is suggested that a nasopharyngeal infection spreads along the olfactory nerves to the frontobasal and temporal regions, evoking an acute encephalitis.

Clinical Features

The onset is acute, presenting with meningeal symptoms and signs combined with behavioral changes, hallucinations, altered states of consciousness, and focal neurologic deficits. The course is fulminant, and the mortality is high, about 50% to 70%. Early diagnosis and the initiation of antiviral therapy are imperative, but even treated cases are often left with neurologic and psychiatric sequelae varying from personality changes, Korsakoff syndrome, and language and cognitive deficits, to a persistent vegetative state.

Herpes simplex virus–specific DNA is identified in the CSF using PCR. Neuroimaging adds to the diagnosis. CT scan during the early course of the disease shows bilateral, often asymmetrical, low densities in the orbital and temporomesial areas, mixed with hyperdense hemorrhages. On MRI, the lesions are hypointense on T1- and hyperintense on T2-weighted images. Electroencephalogram (EEG) may show periodic sharp and slow wave discharges at 2- to 3-seconds intervals. In a few cases, brain biopsy is performed to establish the diagnosis; immunofluorescent stain is a quick diagnostic tool to identify the viral antigen.

Pathology

The pathology is characterized by a hemorrhagic necrotizing encephalitis, typically confined to the frontoorbital cingular and temporomesial regions (Fig. 6.10). Grossly, the brain is swollen and the blood vessels congested. Petechial hemorrhages are scattered throughout the leptomeninges and cerebral cortex of the affected regions.

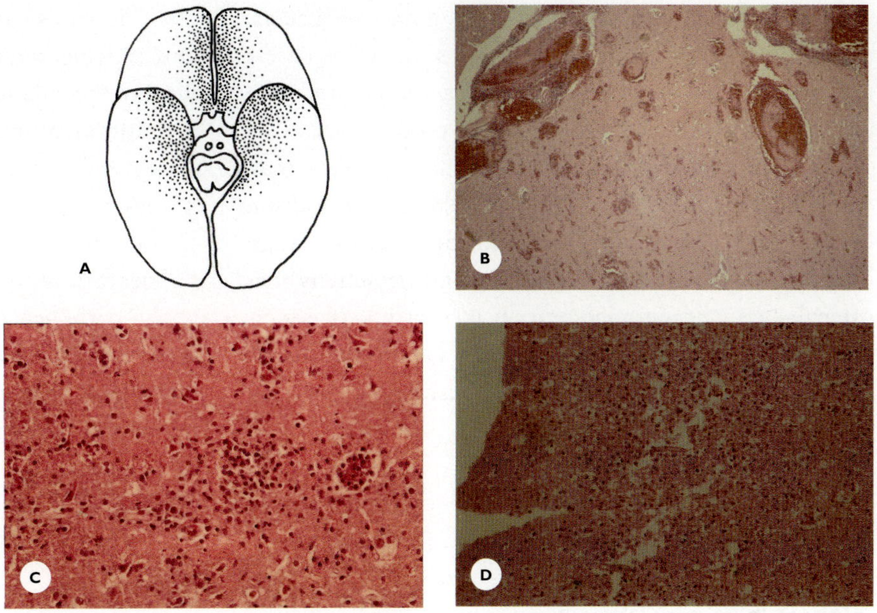

FIGURE 6.10
Herpes simplex-1 encephalitis (HSE). **A.** Schematic drawing shows the distribution of the lesions in the fronto-orbital and temporal regions. **B.** Perivascular hemorrhages in the subarachnoid space and cerebral cortex. **C.** Neuronophagia. **D.** Cortical necrosis (HE).

The histology is characterized by (a) perivascular and diffuse infiltrations with lymphocytes, some neutrophils, and macrophages in the leptomeninges and cerebral cortex; (b) pericapillary hemorrhages; (c) parenchymal necrosis; (d) neuronophagia and neuronal destruction; and (e) eosinophilic intranuclear inclusions in residual neurons and glial cells (see Fig. 6.10). In chronic cases, the brain shows atrophy, cystic necrosis, and gliosis in the frontotemporal regions.

Herpes Simplex Virus-2 Infection

Herpes simplex virus-2 infection is acquired through sexual contact. The virus resides in the sacral spinal ganglia. Reactivation causes genital herpes and, rarely, aseptic meningitis, myelitis, and radiculitis. Cerebral involvement is more common in neonates, and it results from a spread of infection either to the fetus or to the newborn during parturition through an infected birth canal. The viruses evoke a severe disseminated visceral inflammation and a necrotizing encephalitis.

Varicella-Zoster Virus Infection

Varicella-zoster virus (VZV) infection, acquired through the respiratory route, causes varicella in children and zoster in adults. *Varicella* (chickenpox) is a benign exanthematous disease of young children; the clinical course may be more serious in adults. Rarely, varicella is complicated by cerebellitis, postinfectious encephalomyelitis, and the encephalopathy of Reye's disease.

Varicella-zoster virus persists in the neurons of the spinal ganglia, less often in the ganglia of the trigeminal or the facial cranial nerves. Reactivated viruses may afflict the peripheral and the CNS, the skin and the blood vessels, in both immunocompetent and immunosuppressed individuals.

Herpes Zoster

Herpes zoster (shingles) results when the viruses pass from the ganglia to the skin along the sensory nerves. It commonly occurs in adults, and the incidence increases in the elderly. Clinically, herpes zoster manifests with erythematous vesicles in the skin, associated with pain and sensory deficits in the dermatomes that correspond to the involved ganglia. Common sites are the thoracic dermatomes, the ophthalmic division of the trigeminal nerve (ophthalmic zoster), and the somatosensory branch of the facial nerve (otic zoster). Notably, painful radicular neuropathy may occur in the absence of cutaneous changes. Postherpetic neuralgia is often a protracted disabling complication with severe pain and paresthesias.

The pathology of herpes zoster is a *radiculoganglionitis* with mononuclear cell infiltrates. In severe cases, the ganglia are hemorrhagic and necrotic, and the inflammation extends into the spinal cord.

Granulomatous angiitis of the large arteries may complicate an ipsilateral ophthalmic zoster. Infarction in the territory of the artery accounts for a contralateral hemiplegia. *Vasculopathy* of the small vessels, which often occurs in immunocompromised patients, is associated with multiple infarcts and foci of demyelination.

Cytomegalovirus Infection

Neurologic diseases associated with cytomegalovirus infection are more often encountered in immunocompromised—particularly HIV-infected—patients. The infection is acquired by exposure to infected saliva or respiratory secretion, transfusion, and possibly by sexual contact. Fetuses are infected by transplacental transmission and, neonates are infected by feeding with infected breast milk.

Acute infections have a broad spectrum of clinical–pathological presentations: aseptic meningitis; encephalitis characterized by presence of microglial nodules; ventriculitis, often necrotizing with calcifications; radiculomyelitis and radiculoneuropathy (Guillain-Barré syndrome); and retinitis. The virus may infect the glial cells, ependymal cells, neurons, and vascular endothelial cells. The infected cells enlarge and contain intranuclear (owl's-eye) and, less often, intracytoplasmic inclusions (Fig. 6.11).

Congenital and neonatal CMV infections cause microcephaly, mental retardation, seizures, hearing impairment, chorioretinitis, and cerebral malformations (see Chapter 13).

CT scan of the head displays punctate subependymal calcifications. Contrast-enhanced CT and MRI display the subependymal lining of the ventricles. MRI is useful in demonstrating associated malformations.

Epstein-Barr Virus Infection

EBV infection, acquired by exposure to infected saliva, is the pathogen of infectious mononucleosis. Nervous system complications are diverse and include aseptic meningitis, encephalitis, cerebellitis, myelitis, and peripheral neuropathies. EBV has oncogenic potential and is causally linked to the primary B-cell lymphoma of the brain, a complication of immunosuppression, chiefly in HIV-infected patients.

Human Herpesvirus-6 Infection

Human herpesvirus-6 causes exanthem subitum (roseola) and febrile seizures. Aseptic meningitis or meningoencephalitis may complicate an acute infection. Necrotizing encephalitis and inflammatory demyelination occur in immunocompromised adults.

Human Immunodeficiency Virus Infection

The human immunodeficiency virus-1 (HIV-1), a RNA-retrovirus, infects the immune system and the neural tissue, leading to a slowly progressive, multifaceted disease with a fatal outcome. Since the isolation of the virus in 1983, HIV infections have become epidemic worldwide; an estimated 60 million individuals have been infected. The incidence is still rising, particularly in Africa and Asia. HIV-associated diseases are a leading cause of death among men aged 25 to 45 years.

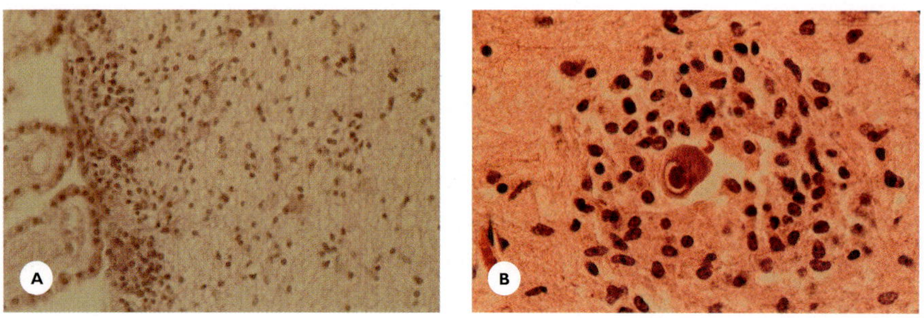

FIGURE 6.11
Cytomegalovirus encephalitis. **A.** Periventricular mononuclear cell infiltration. **B.** Intranuclear inclusion in a cytomegalic cell (HE).

HIV infection is transmitted by several routes: (a) sexual contact, among both homosexual men and heterosexual men and women; (b) blood transfusion; (c) intravenous illicit substance abuse; (d) transmission from mother to infant via placenta, during delivery, or via breast milk; and (e) via infected blood or needlestick injury among health care workers (this risk is considered minimal).

The virus infects the $CD4^+$ T lymphocytes and the macrophages. Infection of $CD4^+$ T cells results in a slowly progressive decline and ultimate loss of these cells, along with a decline of all cellular components of the immune system. The infection of the macrophages is significant, because they carry the viruses to the nervous system. When the viruses reach the neural tissue, they infect the cells of macrophage/microglial lineage and usually remain clinically asymptomatic for months to years. Occasionally, 3 to 6 weeks after infection, the viruses may produce a transient encephalopathy, myelopathy, or aseptic meningitis, all attributed to HIV-induced immunologic processes. The infection becomes clinically symptomatic when immunosuppression is severe; that is, when the $CD4^+$ cell count drops below 200 microliters (guidelines of the Center for Disease Control). This final stage of the disease, known as acquired immunodeficiency syndrome (AIDS) is associated with a variety of neurologic complications, some directly related to the virus and some related to the immunosuppressed state of the host.

HIV-Related Nervous System Diseases

The viruses may infect the brain, spinal cord, and peripheral nerves.

Cerebral Diseases

Involvement of the brain may present in three forms, often in combination: HIV encephalitis, HIV leukoencephalopathy, and diffuse poliodystrophy. The clinical manifestations are collectively referred to as *AIDS-dementia complex*, *HIV-associated dementia*, or *HIV-associated cognitive motor complex*. These disorders develop in about 15% to 20 % of HIV patients and are major causes of disabilities and death.

Clinical features. The disease begins with a slowing of mental activities, difficulty with concentration, apathy, social withdrawal, and personality changes, followed by progressive memory impairment and loss of verbal skills, leading to a profound dementia and, ultimately, to a vegetative state. During the course of the disease, seizures, gait difficulty, weakness, ataxia, and tremor develop, and frontal release signs appear. Strokes—hemorrhagic or ischemic—due to hematologic and cardiovascular changes, may complicate the clinical course.

Diagnostic evaluation. Proton magnetic resonance spectroscopy (MRS) is valuable in detecting metabolic abnormalities during early stages of the disease and in monitoring therapeutic efficacy. A decrease in N-acetyl-transferase (NAA), a neuronal marker, suggests neuronal and axonal damage, whereas an elevation in choline, a cellular membrane marker, suggests myelin breakdown. In more advanced stages of infection, neuroimaging demonstrates atrophy of the gray and white matter. The leukoencephalopathy appears on CT scan as hypodense, and on MRI T2-weighted images it appears as hyperintense, ill-defined white matter lesions. They produce no mass effect and do not enhance with contrast material. Examination of the CSF is useful in eliminating opportunistic infections.

Clinical course. After the onset of dementia, the course averages from a few to several months. Treatment with highly active antiretroviral therapy (HAART) apparently slows the progression of dementia, prolongs survival time, and decreases the incidence of some opportunistic infections. However, drug-resistant viral strains have caused a rise in the incidence of HIV encephalitis and the appearance of a malignant HIV leukoencephalopathy.

Encephalitis. Grossly, the brain volume is diminished, the convolutions are moderately atrophic, and the ventricles are dilated (Fig. 6.12).

The histology is characterized by a microglial nodular encephalitis (Fig. 6.13). Multiple discrete nodules composed of microglial cells and macrophages and multinucleated giant cells are dispersed throughout the cerebral cortex, white matter, deep gray structures, brainstem, and cerebellum. The multinucleated giant cells, derived from a fusion of macrophages, are the diagnostic hallmark of HIV infection. The microglia and macrophages and the multinucleated cells immunoreact for HIV p24 antigen. Perivascular lymphocytic cuffings are variable.

Leukoencephalopathy. Focal and diffuse myelin changes range from pallor and rarefaction to breakdown and phagocytosis of myelin debris. Axonal degeneration and axonal spheroids are detected in severely affected areas. Astrocytic proliferation accompanies the myelin changes (Fig. 6.14).

A severe leukoencephalopathy has been recognized in patients treated with HAART. It is characterized by extensive demyelination, axonal injury, and intense perivascular lymphocyte and macrophage infiltrations.

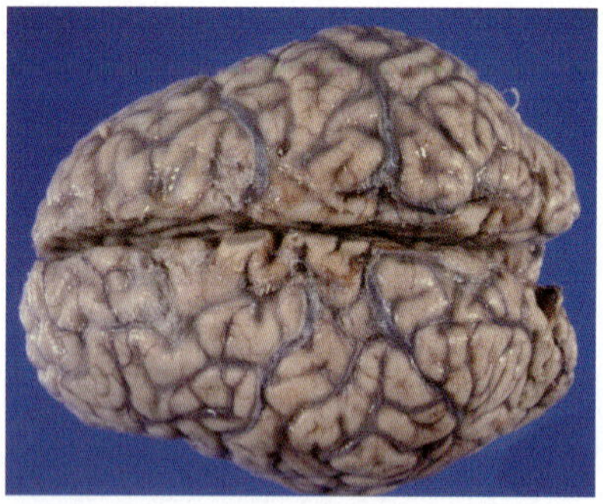

FIGURE 6.12
HIV encephalitis in a 44-year-old demented man. The brain shows a moderate convolutional atrophy.

Diffuse Poliodystrophy. The term refers to loss of dendritic processes and loss of neurons in the cerebral cortex and deep gray structures.

HIV Vacuolar Myelopathy

This distinct spinal cord complication of HIV infection is characterized by spongy degeneration of myelin in \the lateral and posterior columns. Clinically, it presents with slowly progressive spastic paraparesis, loss of position and vibratory senses, and incontinence (Fig. 6.15).

HIV Neuropathy

Involvement of the peripheral nerves manifests as bilateral distal symmetric neuropathies and, less often, as sensory or autonomic neuropathies, polyradiculopathies, and mononeuropathy multiplex. Segmental demyelination, axonal degeneration, perivascular lymphocytic infiltrations, and vasculitis are common (Fig. 6.16). Several etiologies include direct infection by HIV or cytomegalovirus, an immunologic mechanism, and nutritional, metabolic, and toxic factors.

HIV-Immunosuppression–Related Nervous System Diseases

This group of diseases comprises numerous opportunistic infections and the primary CNS lymphoma.

Opportunistic Infections

A great number of pathogens, dormant in the neural tissue, become reactivated by the immunosuppressed

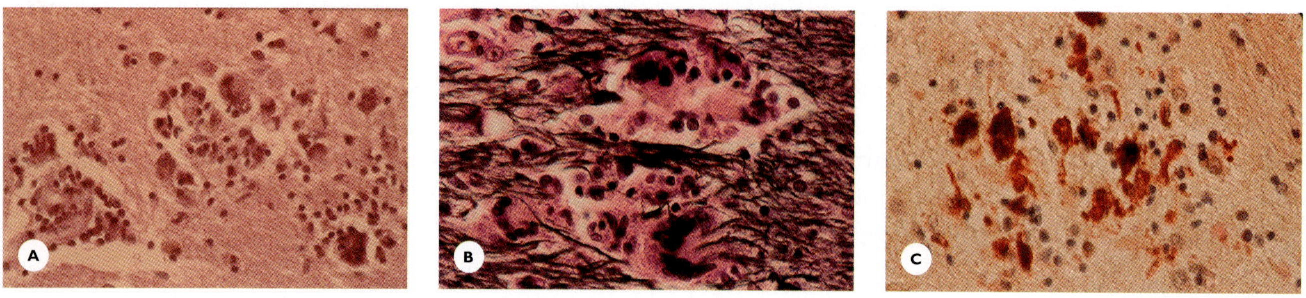

FIGURE 6.13
HIV-encephalitis. Microglial nodules with multinucleated giant cells (**A**) in the white matter (HE) and (**B**) brainstem (Holmes—H-E). **C.** Expression of HIV p24 antigen in cells of microglial nodule (immunostain).

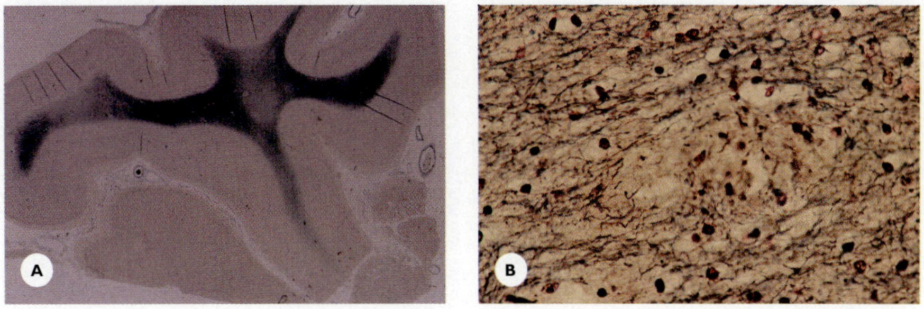

FIGURE 6.14
HIV leukoencephalopathy. **A.** Macrosection from the cerebral hemisphere shows multiple focal losses of myelin (LFB-CV-stain). **B.** Microscopic picture shows focal disintegration of myelin and axons (Holmes stain).

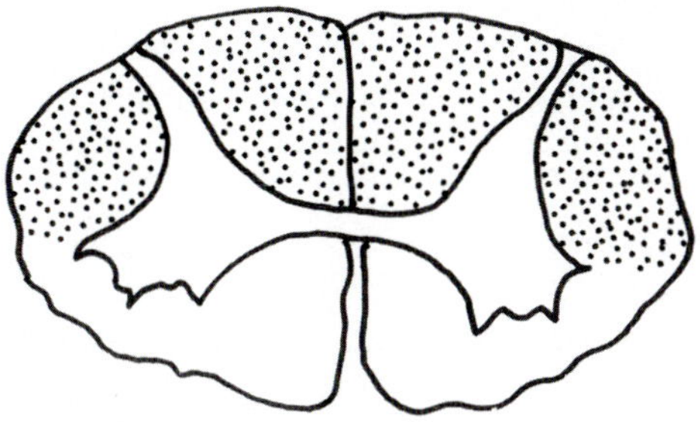

FIGURE 6.15
HIV myelopathy. Drawing of distribution of lesions in posterior and lateral columns.

TABLE 6.4.
Major Opportunistic Pathogens in AIDS

Viruses	**Fungi**
Cytomegalovirus	*Cryptococcus neoformans*
JC, SV40 viruses	*Candida*
Varicella-zoster	*Aspergillus fumigatus*
Herpes simplex 1 and 2	*Histoplasma capsulatum*
Epstein-Barr virus	*Coccidioides immitis*
Human herpes virus 6	**Protozoa**
Bacteria	*Toxoplasma gondii*
Mycobacterium tuberculosis	*Acanthamoeba*
Streptococcus pneumoniae	*Strongyloides stercoralis*
	Spirochaeta
	Treponema pallidum

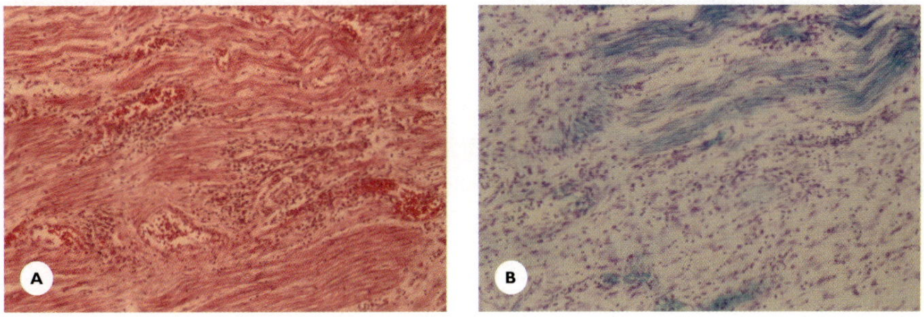

FIGURE 6.16
HIV polyneuropathy. A 40-year-old man presented with progressive flaccid paraparesis and loss of deep tendon reflexes. After a 6-month clinical course, he died. Peripheral nerve from the lumbosacral plexus shows (**A**) focal lymphocytic infiltrations and fibrosis (HE) and (**B**) myelin degeneration (LFB-CV).

state of the host and produce a broad spectrum of diseases (Table 6.4). Toxoplasmosis, CMV infection, and cerebral mycoses are the most common. Since the introduction of HAART, the incidence of these treatable infections has apparently declined. But, the incidence of *Mycobacterium tuberculosis* infection is rising. *Treponema pallidum*, in addition to causing meningitis and meningovascular syphilis, may evoke a severe necrotizing encephalitis (quaternary neurosyphilis).

Pathology. The pathologic features of opportunistic infections are generally similar to those that would occur in immunocompetent patients, but the inflammatory reaction may be less, the necrotic process more destructive, and the clinical course more malignant.

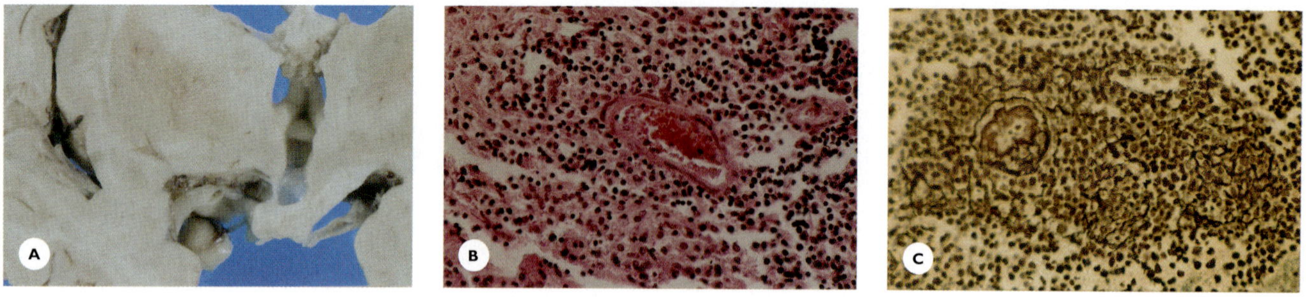

FIGURE 6.17
HIV-associated primary B-cell cerebral lymphoma in a 42-year-old man who died of *Pneumocystis carnii* pneumonia. **A.** Coronal section shows a poorly demarcated, grayish tan mass lesion with irregular margins in the basal ganglia. **B.** It consists of small- and medium-sized lymphocytes arranged around blood vessels (HE) and (**B**) surrounded by a rich reticulin network (Gömöri stain).

These patterns may change, however, in patients who have received HAART. The pathologic process may "burn-out"—lacking inflammation and detectable pathogens—probably due to patients' longer survival.

Primary Cerebral Lymphomas

These lymphomas occur in about 20% of AIDS patients. They are often multicentric and situated in the deep gray structures, corpus callosum, brainstem, and cerebellum. Grossly, they are poorly demarcated from the surrounding parenchyma, firm or friable, grayish or tan, and often necrotic. Histologically, they are pleomorphic, composed of small noncleaved cells and large immunoblastic cells of B-cell origin (Fig. 6.17). Some malignant B-cell lymphomas are causally associated with the Epstein-Barr virus.

Clinically, lymphomas present with focal neurologic symptoms and signs and altered mentation. On CT scan, they may appear as hypo-, iso-, or hyperdense lesions. With contrast material, they display ring or homogenous enhancement on CT and T1-weighted MRI.

HIV Infection in Children

An estimated 3 million children are infected with HIV, and an estimated 13% to 23% of these children develop an encephalitis characterized by nodules of microglial cells and multinucleated giant cells similar to those in infected adults. Perivascular lymphocytic infiltrations are prominent. In addition, vascular and parenchymal mineralization occurs in the basal ganglia and white matter (Fig. 6.18).

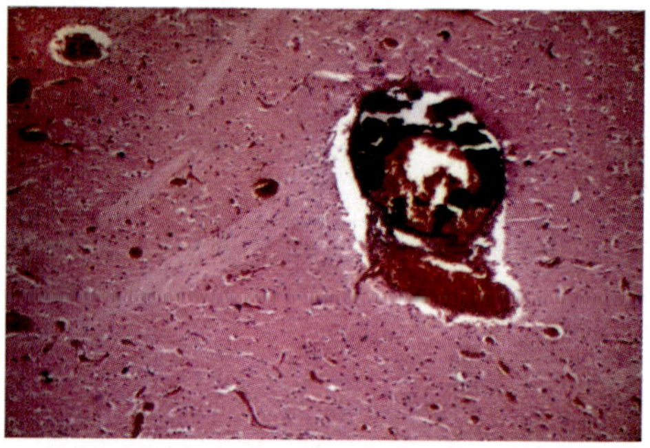

FIGURE 6.18
Vascular mineralization in childhood HIV infection (HE).

Clinically, the encephalitis presents as a progressive encephalopathy manifested by delayed brain growth, microcephaly, motor deficits, language and learning disorders, seizures, and behavioral changes.

Congenital opportunistic infections are rare in infants, but acquired infections and primary CNS lymphoma may occur in severely immunosuppressed older children. Cerebrovascular complications, such as hemorrhages and infarcts, also may occur.

Human T-Cell Leukemia/Lymphotropic Virus-1 Infection

Human T cell leukemia/lymphotropic virus-1 in the group of retroviruses is widely distributed in Africa,

South America and parts of Asia. The sexually transmitted infection presents as a slowly progressive myelopathy (tropical spastic paraparesis). The pathology is characterized by symmetrical degeneration of the long tracts, chiefly in the thoracic region, mononuclear cell infiltrations and hyalinosis of blood vessels.

Chronic Viral Infections

Chronic viral diseases develop when a virus that is dormant in the nervous tissue is reactivated. Several months or years after the initial infection, the disease unfolds, progressing slowly and leading to severe neurologic and mental disabilities and eventually to coma and death.

Progressive Multifocal Leukoencephalopathy (PML)

The disease is associated with the JC virus (named after the initials of the patient in whose brain the virus was first detected) and the SV40 virus, both papovaviruses. The disease commonly develops in immunocompromised adults and in patients with leukemias, lymphomas, and transplanted organs. Patients with AIDS are at high risk.

The onset of PML is insidious. The patient presents with behavioral changes, progressive cognitive decline and a variety of neurologic symptoms and signs. The clinical course is usually several months. CT scan demonstrates hypodense and MRI T2-weighted images hyperintense, usually nonenhancing multiple lesions, predominantly in the subcortical white matter, brainstem and cerebellum.

Grossly, multiple, ill-defined, soft, slightly granular areas are dispersed in the white matter of the cerebral hemispheres, brainstem, and cerebellum.

Histological features include (a) multiple confluent demyelinations with relative sparing of the axons (Fig. 6.19); (b) the presence of giant, bizarrely shaped, often multinucleated astrocytes and swollen oligodendrocytes in the demyelinated areas; (c) eosinophilic intranuclear viral inclusions in oligodendrocytes and astrocytes; and (d) perivascular lymphocytic infiltrations.

FIGURE 6.19
Progressive multifocal leukoencephalopathy. Multifocal myelin losses in subcortical white matter (myelin stain).

Measles Virus-Associated Diseases

Subacute Sclerosing Panencephalitis (SSPE)

The disease develops several years after an acute systemic measles infection. It is suggested that the risk is higher for those who had measles or measles immunization at a very early age. SSPE affects primarily children and adolescents. Behavioral changes, slowly progressive mental regression, seizures, myoclonus, and focal neurologic deficits characterize the clinical picture. In the acute stage, EEG often shows a burst-suppression pattern of high-amplitude slow-wave or spike and slow-wave complexes occurring at a rate of 4 to 20 seconds (Fig. 6.20). The CSF has high IgG levels with oligoclonal bands. Measles antibody titers in the CSF and serum rise during the course of the disease. Death occurs within several months or years after the initial symptoms.

Pathology: Grossly, the cerebral cortex is atrophic, and the hemispheric white matter is grayish and firm. The histology is characterized by (a) widespread perivascular lymphocyte and plasma-cell infiltrations in the cerebral hemispheres and brainstem; (b) variable neuronal losses in the cerebral cortex; (c) eosinophilic intranuclear inclusions in the neurons and oligodendrocytes; (d) diffuse myelin degeneration in the hemispheric white matter, accompanied by dense astrocytic gliosis; and (e) in some neurons, neurofibrillary tangles that may contain measles genomes (see Fig. 6.20).

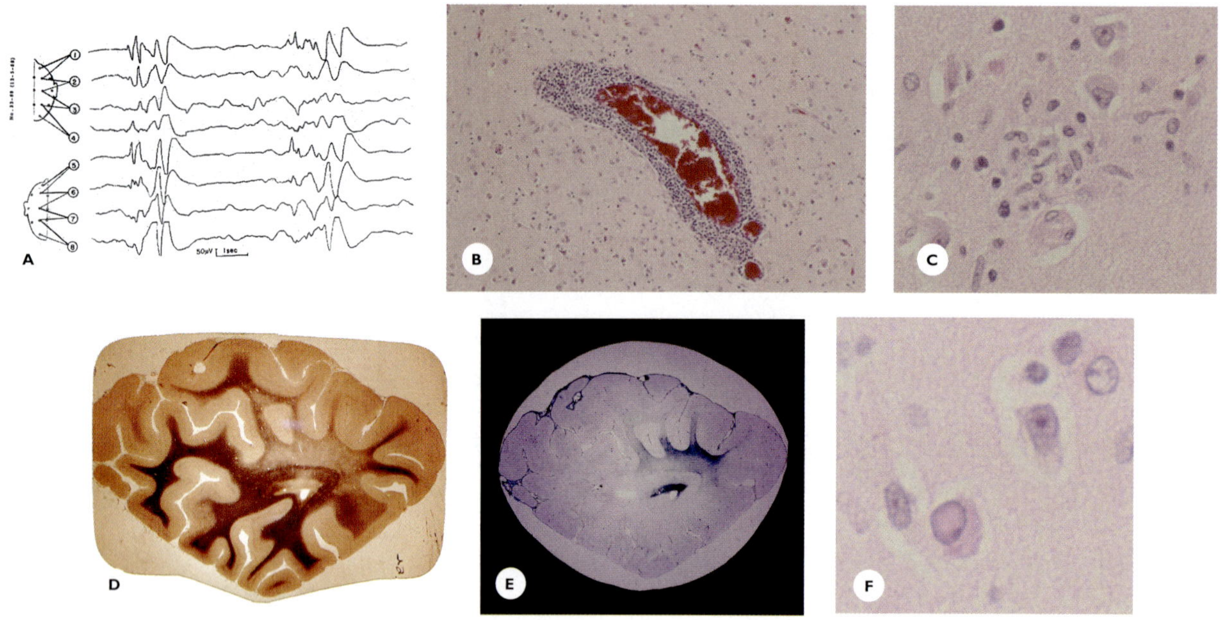

FIGURE 6.20

Subacute sclerosing panencephalitis (SSPE). A baby boy had measles at 11 months of age. He developed normally until 8 years of age, when his gait deteriorated and his behavior changed—he became hyperactive, distractible, and untidy. Seizures began around the same time. He continued to deteriorate, lost his motor skills and speech, became bedridden and incontinent, and displayed myoclonic jerks. At 10 years of age, he died. **A.** EEG shows periodic bursts of high-voltage slow complexes. **B.** Cerebral cortex shows perivascular cuffings with lymphocytes and plasma cells and **(C)** glial nodules (HE). White matter shows **(D)** myelin loss (Weil stain), **(E)** diffuse astrogliosis (Holzer stain), and **(F)** intranuclear inclusion in oligodendroglia (Lendrum stain).

Measles Inclusion Body Encephalitis

This is a rare condition which may develop several months after an acute measles infection. Immunocompromised subjects are particularly susceptible to the disease, which is fatal within a few weeks. The pathology, as the name implies, is characterized by the presence of intranuclear eosinophilic inclusions in the neurons and the glial cells. The inclusions contain viral antigen, demonstrable with immunohistochemical stain.

Progressive Rubella Panencephalitis

This disease develops years after a neonatal or childhood rubella infection. The pathology is characterized by a slowly progressive encephalitis and diffuse neuronal and myelin degenerations.

MYCOTIC INFECTIONS

Mycoses of the CNS commonly occur in patients with malignancies, lymphoproliferative and hematopoietic diseases, poorly controlled diabetes, infected prosthetic heart valves, and organ transplants, and also in patients receiving long-term antibiotics, chemotherapy, high-dose corticosteroids, and hyperalimentation. Patients with AIDS are particularly susceptible to fungal infections. Endemic infections are confined to the southeastern and southwestern United States.

The primary infection, usually in a distant organ, spreads hematogenously to the neural tissue. Less often, it extends directly to the brain from adjacent infectious foci. Cerebral involvement is often one manifestation of systemic mycosis. Once the fungi have reached the brain and/or spinal cord, a broad spectrum of inflammatory responses may occur, including granulomatous meningitis, meningoencephalitis, solitary or multiple granulomas, abscesses, and necrotizing vasculitis with septic hemorrhagic necrosis. The fungi are demonstrated readily in histologic sections using periodic acid-Schiff (PAS) and methenamine silver stains.

Mycotic infections may present acutely or may progress insidiously and slowly over weeks or months. Headaches, visual symptoms, nuchal rigidity, cranial nerve deficits, and low-grade fever are common presenting symptoms. Depending on the location of the pathologic lesions, focal symptoms and signs develop. Confusion, disorientation, psychiatric symptoms, and cognitive impairment evolve in chronic cases and may present diagnostic difficulties. A high suspicion for fungal infection and the use of appropriate tests secures the correct diagnosis.

An examination of the CSF reveals a moderate pleocytosis with lymphocytes and high protein and low sugar levels. Specific diagnostic tests include India ink preparation of the CSF sediment and blood smear, culture of CSF and blood, and immunologic tests for fungal antigen using enzyme linked immunosorbent assay (ELISA) and latex agglutination (LA) tests. Immunohistochemical-fluorescent antibody stain allows the rapid identification of fungi. Contrast-enhanced CT scan and MRI demonstrate meningeal involvement and parenchymal lesions.

Major mycotic infections of the nervous system are summarized in Table 6.5. Three of the most common are presented here.

Cryptococcosis

Cryptococcosis (torulosis) is the most prevalent cerebral mycosis. *Cryptococcus neoformans*, in yeast form, measures 5 to 12 microns. It is surrounded by a polysaccharide capsule that stains with Alcian blue and mucicarmine; it appears as a halo in sections stained with silver (Fig. 6.21).

The primary infection is commonly a granulomatous inflammation in the lungs. The fungi reach the brain by hematogenous dissemination and produce a granulomatous meningoencephalitis with thick, gelatinous exudate, minimal inflammatory reaction, and a few microgranulomas. These are composed of infiltrates of lymphocytes and plasma cells, epithelioid cells, fibroblasts, and multinucleated giant cells. The yeasts invade the brain along the perivascular spaces, expanding and

TABLE 6.5
Major CNS Mycotic Infections

Fungus	*Primary Site*	*Pathology*
Cryptococcus neoformans	Lung	Meningoencephalitis Abscess, granuloma
Aspergillus fumigatus	Lung Paranasal sinuses Orbit	Septic necrosis, Granuloma, abscess Meningitis Mycotic aneurysm, arterial thrombosis
Candida species	Skin, Oral cavity Gastrointestinal tract, Genitourinary tract	Meningitis Microabcesses Microgranulomas
Coccidioides immitis	Skin Lung	Acute/chronic granulomatous meningitis
Histoplasma capsulatum	Lung	Meningitis, granulomas
Blastomyces dermatitidis	Skin	Abcess Epidural abscess
Mucoraceae species	Nasal and oral cavities, nasopharynx	Hemorrhagic necrosis Cavernous sinus thrombosis Carotid artery thrombosis

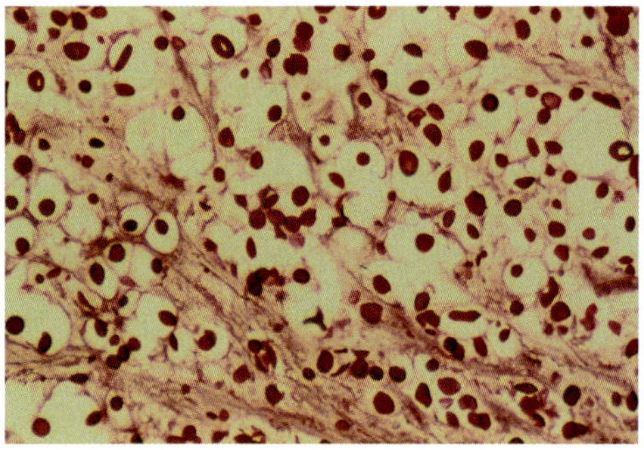

FIGURE 6.21
Cryptococcus meningoencephalitis. The subarachnoid space is densely packed with cryptococcus yeasts (silver stain).

gradually transforming them into multiloculated gelatinous cysts. Solitary abscesses are rare.

Aspergillosis

Aspergillus fumigatus, in the form of branching septate hyphae, measures 4 to 7 microns. The primary infection is usually a necrotizing hemorrhagic pneumonitis. From the lungs, the fungi reach the cerebral blood vessels, where they produce a necrotizing vasculitis and, subsequently, a septic hemorrhagic necrosis (Fig. 6.22).

Aspergillus may also invade the brain from infected paranasal sinuses, orbits, or ears to cause a meningitis. Abscesses and granulomas are common in disseminated aspergillosis. They may reach large sizes and cause increased intracranial pressure and mass effects (Fig. 6.23).

Candidiasis

Candida species grow as yeast and pseudohyphae. They are commonly found on the skin, mucous membranes of the oral cavity (thrush) and vagina, and in the gastrointestinal and genitourinary tracts. The fungi reach the brain via the bloodstream and produce multiple disseminated microabscesses and granulomas (Fig. 6.24). The clinical presentation is a septic encephalopathy. Candidiasis preferentially affects chronically ill elderly patients and poorly controlled diabetic patients.

SYPHILITIC INFECTIONS

The incidence of infection with the spirochete *Treponema pallidum* is rising among individuals infected with HIV and in those who abuse illicit substances.

The disease is acquired by venereal contact. In about 40% of cases, the spirochetes infect the nervous system via the bloodstream within several weeks to several months after the initial infection and produce a meningeal reaction. This may remain clinically asymptomatic and is diagnosed only by a positive serology test of the CSF.

Neurosyphilis may manifest clinically from 1 year to as long as 15 to 20 years after the initial infection. It presents under several forms, depending on the site of involvement: meninges, blood vessels, or parenchyma of the brain and spinal cord. The diagnosis is confirmed by examination of the CSF, which shows mild to moderate pleocytosis with lymphocytes and plasma cells, moderately increased protein and IgG immunoglobulin, and a positive serology for syphilis.

Chronic Basal Meningitis

Chronic basal meningitis presents 1 to 2 years after the initial infection, usually with meningeal and cranial nerve signs and occasionally with an acute hydrocephalus. Grossly, the leptomeninges are thickened and cloudy. Histologically, the subarachnoid space is filled with lymphocytes and plasma cells.

Meningovascular Syphilis

Meningovascular syphilis manifests 5 to 7 years after the initial infection and presents with meningeal and multifocal cerebral and/or spinal cord symptoms and signs.

The pathology is characterized by a proliferative endarteritis of the small, medium, and large arteries (Heubner endarteritis). A prominent endothelial proliferation along with mononuclear cell infiltrates in the media and adventitia lead to severe luminal narrowing and, eventually, occlusion and subsequent infarctions (Fig. 6.25).

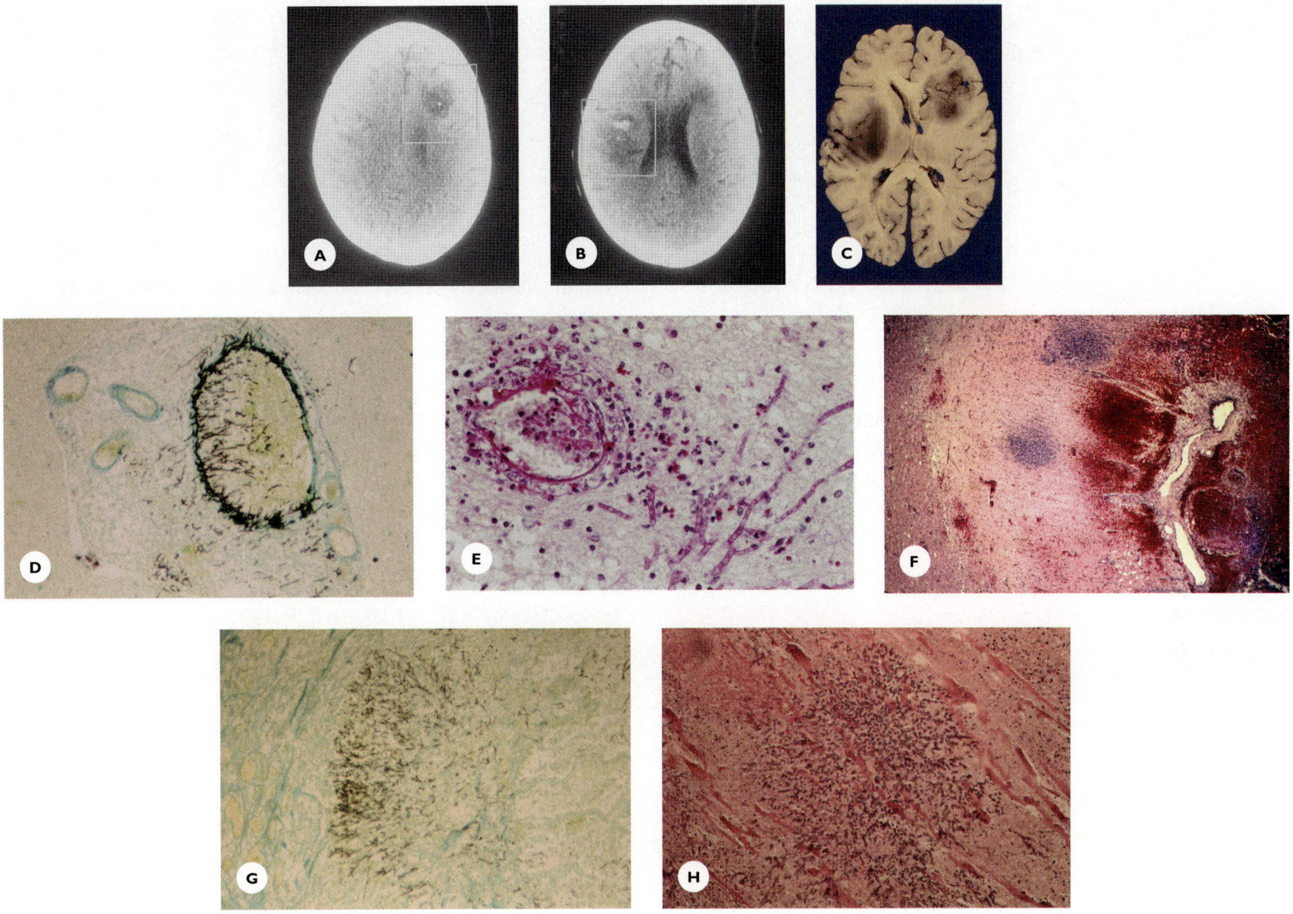

FIGURE 6.22
Cerebral and visceral aspergillosis. A 51-year-old man underwent nephrectomy for carcinoma that had already spread to the vertebrae and pelvis. Postoperatively, he received radiation, chemotherapy, and corticosteroids. Three years following surgery, he developed an acute pneumonitis that did not improve on broad-spectrum antibiotics. Three weeks later, he died. An unenhanced CT scan of the head shows two hypodense lesions: (**A**) one in the left frontal lobe and (**B**) the other with a hyperdense component in the right central region. **C.** Horizontal slice of the brain shows poorly defined hemorrhagic necrotic lesions in the left frontal and right central regions. **D.** Aspergillus hyphae fill the lumen and penetrate the wall of a small leptomeningeal artery (Grocott stain). **E.** Cerebral cortex showing freely dispersed aspergillus hyphae and necrotic blood vessel (PAS) and (**F**) hemorrhages and microabscesses (HE). Colonies of aspergillus hyphae in (**G**) the lung (Grocott stain) and (**H**) heart (HE).

Parenchymal Neurosyphilis

Parenchymal neurosyphilis presents 10 to 20 years after the initial infection under several forms.

The characteristic clinical features of *tabes dorsalis* are summarized in Table 6.6. Grossly, the posterior nerve roots of the spinal cord are thin and grayish, and the posterior columns are translucent and atrophic, chiefly in the lumbosacral segments.

Histologically, the spinal ganglia and the posterior nerve roots show lymphocytic infiltrations, fibrosis, and demyelination. The demyelination proceeds into the posterior columns, which eventually become demyelinated throughout the entire length of the spinal cord (Fig. 6.26).

General paresis (dementia paralytica, general paresis of the insane) presents with intellectual decline progressing to severe dementia, mood and personality

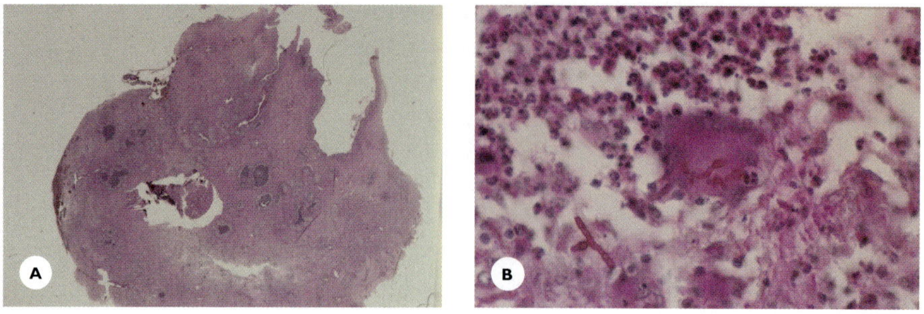

FIGURE 6.23
Aspergilloma. A 20-year-old man had a 1-week history of headaches, nausea, somnolence, and left-sided motor and sensory deficits. **A.** Surgical specimen of an egg-sized aspergilloma resected from the right centroparietal region contains multiple tiny abscesses. **B.** The microabscesses are separated by granulation tissue composed of fibroblasts, lymphocytes, plasma cells, and multinucleated giant cells. Aspergillus hyphae are apparent at the margin of the abscesses and inside a multinucleated giant cell (PAS stain).

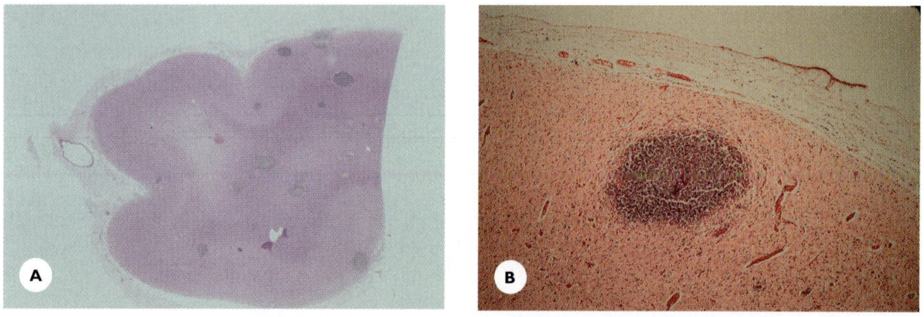

FIGURE 6.24
Cerebral candidiasis. **A** and **B.** Multiple microabscesses in the cortex and white matter (HE).

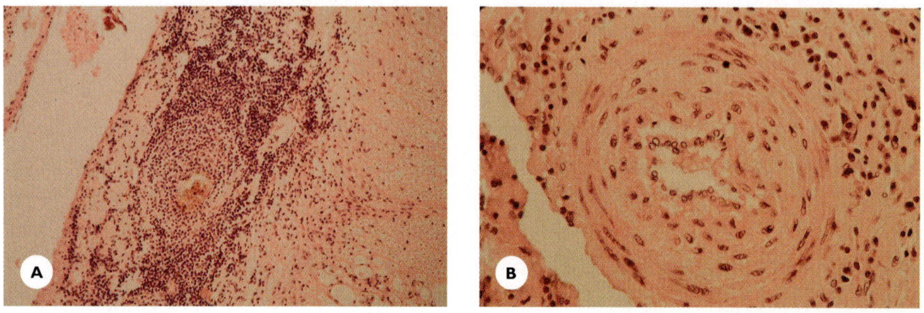

FIGURE 6.25
Meningovascular syphilis. **A.** Massive subarachnoid exudate with lymphocytes and plasma cells. **B.** Mural thickening and luminal reduction of a parenchymal artery (HE).

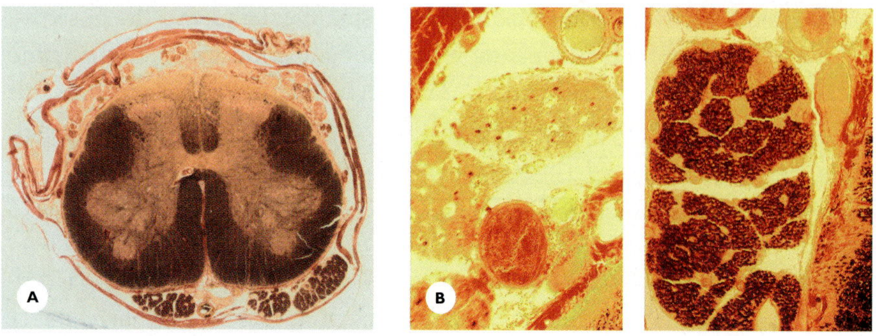

FIGURE 6.26
Tabes dorsalis. **A.** Macrosection of lumbar spinal cord section showing demyelination of the posterior nerve roots and posterior columns. **B.** Higher-power view of the demyelinated posterior nerve roots and the normal anterior nerve roots (iron hematoxylin-picrofuchsin stain).

changes, grandiose delusions, inappropriate joking, and disregard for social standards. Dysarthric speech, impaired visual acuity, pupillary changes, tremor, ataxia, myoclonic jerks, and seizures may develop any time during the course of the disease.

TABLE 6.6

Clinical Presentations of Tabes Dorsalis

Symptoms
- Lightning-lancinating pain in legs
- Paresthesias in extremities
- Visceral crisis; sharp pain of sudden onset, variable duration. and abrupt end

Signs
- Argyll-Robertson pupils: small, irregular unequal pupils, do not constrict to light, constrict on accommodation
- Optic atrophy
- Absent knee and ankle reflexes
- Loss of vibratory and position sensations
- Variable loss of touch, pain, and thermal sensations
- Romberg sign: positive
- Gait: sensory ataxic
- Autonomic dysfunction: urinary overflow, incontinence (insensitive atonic bladder), constipation, impotence
- Trophic changes: perforating ulcers in feet
- Charcot joints: insensitive arthropathy

Grossly, the brain volume is reduced. The leptomeninges are thick, mostly over the frontal lobes, which are severely atrophic. On sections, the ventricles are dilated and the ependyma is finely granular (granular ependymitis).

Histologically, general paresis is a syphilitic meningoencephalitis. Lymphocytic and plasma cell perivascular infiltrations are prominent in the leptomeninges, cerebral cortex, white matter, and deep gray structures. Hypertrophied, rod-shaped activated microglial cells diffusely infiltrate the cerebral cortex. Neuronal losses are widespread and particularly severe in the frontal lobes. Astrocytosis is usually proportional to the neuronal losses. In untreated cases, the spirochetes are demonstrable with silver stain (Fig. 6.27).

In *syphilitic optic atrophy*, a progressive loss of visual acuity may occur alone or may complicate tabes dorsalis and general paresis. The nerves show lymphocytic infiltrations, fibrosis, and degeneration of myelin.

Gumma or *syphilitic granuloma*, a very rare form of infection, presents as a firm mass in the meninges or brain parenchyma. Histologically, it contains areas of coagulation necrosis surrounded by epithelioid cells,

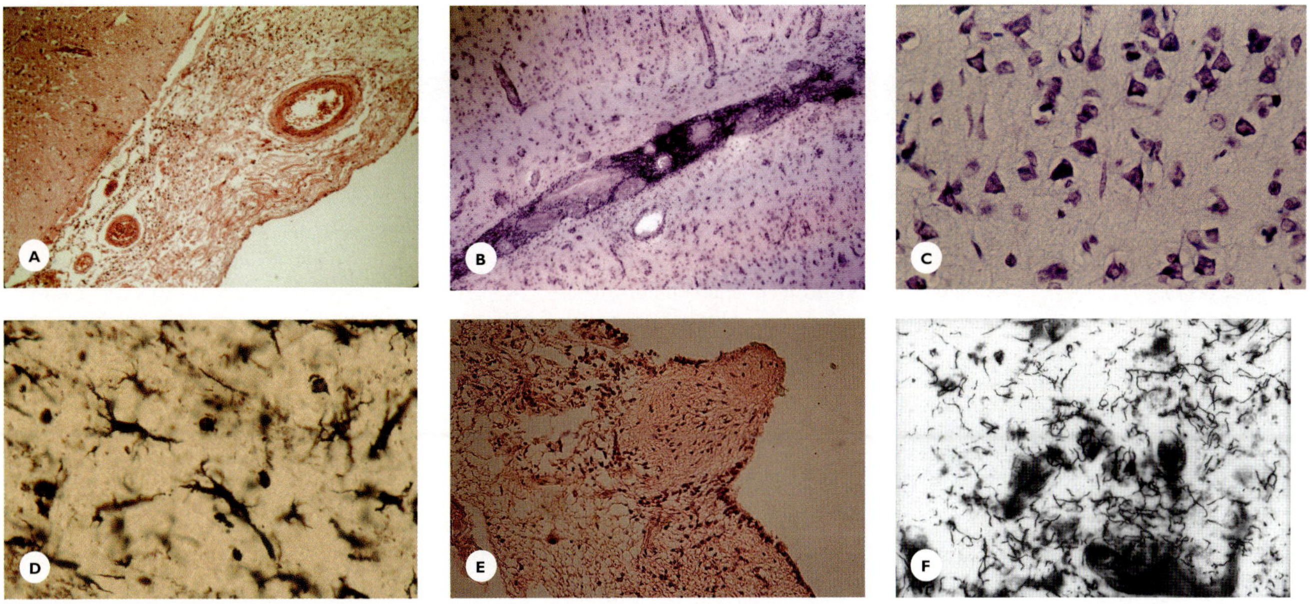

FIGURE 6.27
General paresis **A.** Chronic fibrotic leptomeningitis over the frontal lobe (HE). **B.** Perivascular infiltration with lymphocytes and plasma cells in the subarachnoid space and parenchyma (Cresyl-violet). **C** and **D.** Hypertrophied, rod-shaped microglia in the cerebral cortex (Cresyl-violet and Hortega silver stain). **E.** Ependymitis granulosa in the ventricular wall (HE). **F.** Colonies of spirochetes in an untreated case (silver stain).

lymphoplasmacytic infiltrations, fibroblasts, and occasional giant cells.

Congenital Neurosyphilis

A syphilitic infection of the mother can be transmitted across the placenta to the fetus at any time during pregnancy. The disease presents in childhood or early adolescence as a basal meningitis, hydrocephalus, or general paresis.

PARASITIC INFECTIONS

Parasitic infections by protozoa and helminths present with a broad spectrum of clinical features and pathologic lesions. Most have a worldwide distribution, but some are endemic and confined to certain countries and continents. The majority of infections are acquired orally, but a few are acquired through mosquito bites or cutaneous contact.

Some infections present acutely, whereas others remain dormant for months or years, until the host becomes immunocompromised. Seizures, headache, fever, altered mentation, focal neurologic deficits, and signs of increased intracranial pressure occur in various combinations. Early diagnosis is important, because most infections respond to therapy. The diagnosis is based on serologic tests, along with MRI and CT scan.

The pathology encompasses a great variety of lesions (Tables 6.7 and 6.8). In surgical and autopsy specimens, the parasites are identified using immunohistologic stains.

Protozoal Infections

Toxoplasmosis

Toxoplasmosis is one of the commonest opportunistic infections in immunocompromised individuals, mainly in patients with AIDS (Fig. 6.28). The infection by *Toxoplasma gondii* is acquired through the ingestion of undercooked meat infected with parasitic cysts. In a healthy host, the infection usually remains asymptomatic and seldom presents with meningeal or encephalo-

TABLE 6.7.
Protozoal Diseases

Diseases	*Protozoa*	*Mode of Infection*	*Neuropathology*
Toxoplasmosis	*Toxoplasma gondii*	Ingestion of meat contaminated with T cysts	Multifocal necrotizing encephalitis, granulomas, abscesses, microglial nodular encephalitis
Amoebiasis	*Entamoeba histolytica* *Naegleria fowleri* *Acanthamoeba*	Ingestion of E cysts Olfactory mucosa Respiratory tract	Abscess Meningoencephalitis Granulomatous encephalitis
Malaria	*Plasmodium falciparum*	Mosquito bite	Vascular necrosis Petechial hemorrhages Dürck (microglial) nodule
American trypanosomiasis Chagas disease	*Trypanosoma crusii*	Insect bite Transfusion Organ transplant Transplacental Breast feeding	Acute: microglial nodular encephalitis Chronic: autonomic nervous system involvement Cerebral infarct Reactivated: hemorrhagic meningoencephalitis
African trypanosomiasis Sleeping sickness	*Trypanosoma brucili*	Insect bite	Meningoencephalitis

TABLE 6.8
Helminthic Infections of the CNS

Diseases	*Helminths*	*Mode of Infection*	*Pathology*
Cysticercosis	*Taenia solium*	Ingestion of contaminated food with T solium eggs (fecal-oral route)	Cysticercus cysts, granulomas, calcifications, meningoencephalitis, granular ependymitis, vasculitis, obstructive hydrocephalus
Echinococcosis	*Taenia echinococcus*	Ingestion of contaminated food with T eggs (fecal-oral route)	Hydatid cysts; solitary or multiple
Trichinosis	*Trichinella spiralis*	Ingestion of undercooked pork meat contaminated with T larvae	Eosinophilic meningoencephalitis, vascular necrosis, thrombosis, ischemic/hemorrhagic lesions, granulomas
Schistosomiasis	*Schistosoma* species	Cutaneous infection	Clusters of ova, multiple granulomas, necrotizing vasculitis
Strongyloidiasis	*Strongyloides Stercoralis*	Cutaneous infection	Granulomas, abscesses, microinfarcts

pathic symptoms. A high percentage of population (20% to 70%) are seropositive for toxoplasmosis. In immunocompromised individuals, toxoplasmosis presents with meningeal and encephalitic symptoms or with signs of solitary or multiple mass lesions. The diagnosis is confirmed with serial serologic tests on serum and CSF. CT scan and MRI localize the lesions, which may display ring or homogeneous enhancement. Calcifications are found in the parenchyma and beneath the ventricles. The diagnostic value of brain biopsy is questionable. Because untreated cases have a fatal outcome, empirical therapy is justified.

The pathology may present as solitary or multiple necrotizing abscesses, coagulative necrotic granulomas, and microglial nodular encephalitis (Fig. 6.28). Toxoplasma organisms within cysts or freely dispersed in the parenchyma are demonstrated in sections stained with HE or by the Wright-Giemsa stain, but most reliably using immunohistologic methods.

Congenital toxoplasmosis is acquired transplacentally, either from an acute or reactivated infection of the mother. Characteristic clinical features are microcephaly, mental retardation, seizures, variable neurologic deficits, and chorioretinitis. Pathologic features are micrencephaly, extensive coagulative necrosis with calcifications, and hydrocephalus (see Chapter 14).

Amebiasis

Infections by one of the three species of amebae—*Naegleria fowleri*, *Acanthamoeba* sp., and *Entamoeba histolytica*—are rare but detrimental. Immunocompromised individuals are at risk for the infection.

Naegleria fowleri is found in freshwater and soil. It infects the nasal cavity and reaches the brain along the olfactory nerves to produce a fulminant hemorrhagic meningoencephalitis with PNLs.

Acanthamoeba sp. are found in fresh- and seawater. They reach the brain via the bloodstream, producing a subacute or chronic multifocal necrotizing granulomatous encephalitis.

Infection by *Entamoeba histolytica* is acquired by fecal–oral contamination. The organisms spread hematogenously from an intestinal infection or a liver abscess to the brain, producing single or multiple abscesses (Fig. 6.29).

Malaria

Malaria is endemic in tropical and subtropical regions, but may occur worldwide. Cerebral malaria develops several weeks after mosquito bites infect the host with *Plasmodium falciparum*. The encephalopathy is often

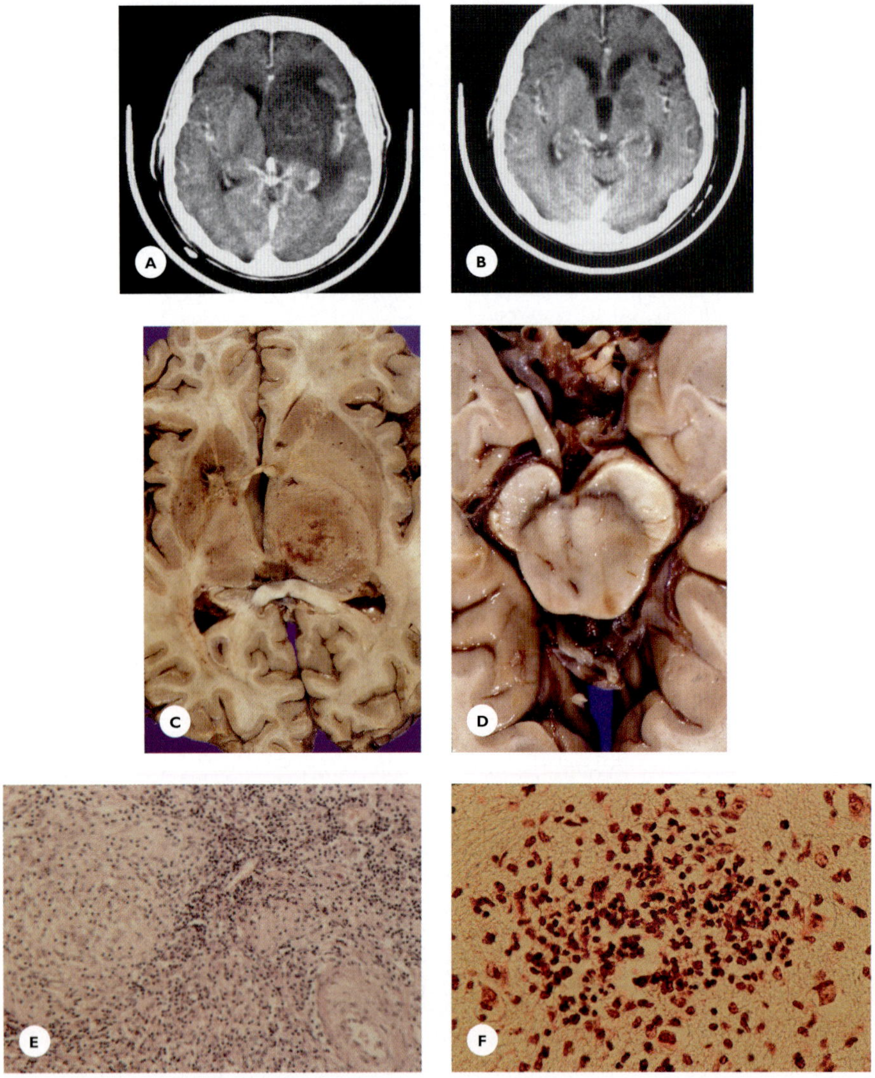

FIGURE 6.28
Cerebral toxoplasma granulomas. A 62-year-old HIV-positive man presented with a several-week history of generalized weakness, headaches, vomiting, confusion, and disorientation. **A.** CT scan of the head shows a large left frontal hypodense, nonenhancing lesion with mass effect. Despite a negative biopsy, the patient was treated for toxoplasmosis. **B.** CT scan 1 month later shows resolution of the lesion. After a 6-month clinical course, he died of numerous medical complications. **C.** Horizontal section of the brain shows the biopsy scar in the left caudate and a recent large toxoplasma granuloma in the right thalamus (**D**) extending into the brainstem. **E.** The granuloma shows coagulative necrosis, diffuse lymphocytic infiltrations, and (**F**) loose nodules of microglial cells and lymphocytes (HE).

fulminant; it results from obstruction of microcirculation by infected and sequestrated red blood cells, subsequent endothelial damage, and pericapillary ring hemorrhages and small infarcts. Malaria granulomas (Dürck nodules) are clusters of microglial cells scattered in the parenchyma.

Trypanosomiasis

Trypanosomiasis presents under two forms.

American trypanosomiasis or Chagas' disease has a high incidence in South and Central America. *Trypanosoma cruzi*, the causative protozoa, is carried in the feces of insects. Humans are infected with the excreted protozoa through an insect bite. The disease mainly afflicts children.

An acute infection presents as a microglial nodular encephalitis. Parasites are found within the cytoplasm of glial cells. Chronic infection presents with disorders of the autonomic nerves, cardiomyopathy, and changes of the digestive tract (mega-viscera). Cerebral infarcts are complications of the cardiac pathology.

A reactivated form of the disease is associated with immunosuppression, chiefly AIDS. The pathology is a multifocal necrotizing, hemorrhagic meningoencephalitis.

African trypanosomiasis or *sleeping sickness* is caused by *Trepanosoma brucei*. The pathology is a

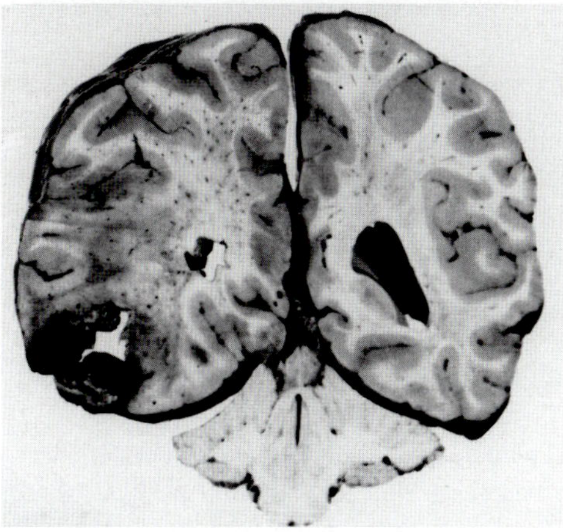

FIGURE 6.29
Entameba histolytica abscess. A 7-year-old girl with Down syndrome died 2 weeks following an acute *Entameba histolytica* enterocolitis. The brain shows a poorly demarcated abscess in the temporal lobe with purulent necrotic walls.

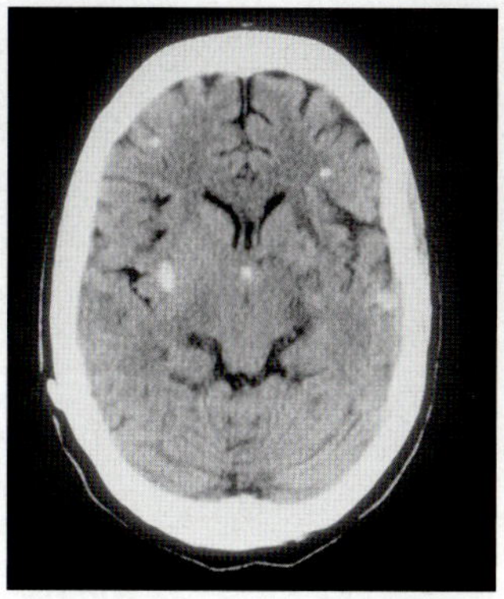

FIGURE 6.30
Cerebral cysticercosis. CT scan of the head shows multiple calcified cysticercus cysts in a 24-year-old woman who developed an acute hydrocephalus necessitating placement of a ventriculoperitoneal shunt. Note the presence of a calcified cyst at the foramen Monro. A cavum septum pellucidum is also present.

meningoencephalitis with perivascular mononuclear cell infiltrations.

Helminthic Infections

Neurocysticercosis

Neurocysticercosis caused by the tapeworm, *Taenia solium*, has a high incidence in Mexico, Africa, South and Central America, and India. In the United States, it is common in California.

Cysticercosis is acquired by the fecal–oral route through the ingestion of food contaminated by ova excreted in the feces of *Taenia* carriers. From the gastrointestinal tract, the ova are carried via bloodstream to the visceral organs, the muscles, and the brain, where they mature and become encysted. The cysts—single, multiple or racemose—measure 0.5 to 2 cm and vary greatly in location. Common sites are the cerebral and spinal subarachnoid space, the brain parenchyma, and the ventricles.

Clinically, the cysts manifest in a number of ways: Focal cerebral deficits, signs of spinal cord compression, psychiatric symptoms, and cognitive decline occur in various combinations. Seizures are common. Raised intracranial pressure due to obstructive hydrocephalus, and circulatory insufficiency due to arteritis may develop during the course of the disease. On CT scan, the cysts appear as hypodense, ring-enhancing lesions or calcified nodules (Fig. 6.30). MRI demonstrates the nonenhancing viable cysts and also the disintegrated cysts, which display ring or nodular enhancement with contrast material. The diagnosis is confirmed using ELISA or enzyme-limited immunoelectrotransfer blot (EITB).

Pathologically, the cyst wall consists of a hyaline–cuticular layer. Within the cyst, the larvae may remain viable for months or years and may provoke a leptomeningitis or encephalitis with plasma cells and eosinophils, and an ependymitis and arteritis. Dead larvae are embedded in granulation tissue or calcify (Fig. 6.31).

Echinococcosis

Echinococcosis (hydatoid disease) is acquired by the ingestion of food contaminated by eggs of *Taenia echinococcus*, a common intestinal parasite of dogs. The disease has a worldwide distribution and is prevalent in sheep- and cattle-breeding countries.

The embryos reach the liver through the portal system; through the systemic circulation, they reach the visceral organs, the brain and spinal cord, the skull, and vertebrae. Here they develop into cysts that contain

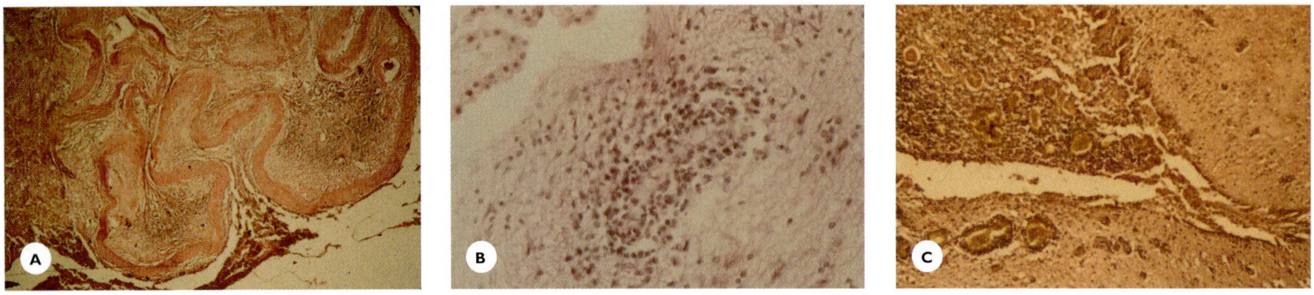

FIGURE 6.31
Cerebral cysticercosis, granular ependymitis, and acute obstructive hydrocephalus. A 44-year-old woman experienced episodic fever and two episodes of lymphocytic meningitis within 1 year prior to her death. Six days before she died, she developed acutely severe headache, confusion, constantly falling backwards, and urinary incontinence due to an acute hydrocephalus from occlusion of the third ventricle. **A.** A collapsed, dead cystocercous cyst in the dorsomedial aspect of the thalamus displays a structureless wavy collagenous wall (van Gieson). **B.** Wall of the third ventricle shows perivascular lymphocytic cuffing (HE). **C.** Granulation tissue infiltrates the floor of the third ventricle (von Gieson).

clear fluid and scoleces. The nervous system may also be secondarily involved from a ruptured hepatic or cardiac hydatid cyst. Spilling of the cyst contents may evoke an anaphylactic reaction and dissemination of infection.

Central nervous system echinococcosis is more common in children than in adults. The cysts are usually solitary and large, some reaching several centimeters. Clinically, they present as expanding mass lesions. On CT scan, they are round or oval, well-defined, hypodense cystic lesions with minimal or no ring enhancement.

Pathologically, the hydatid cyst can be granulosus or multiloculous (Fig. 6.32). The cyst wall consists of an inner germinal layer and an outer laminated layer. Mild mononuclear cell infiltrates and occasional foreign body giant cells surround the cysts.

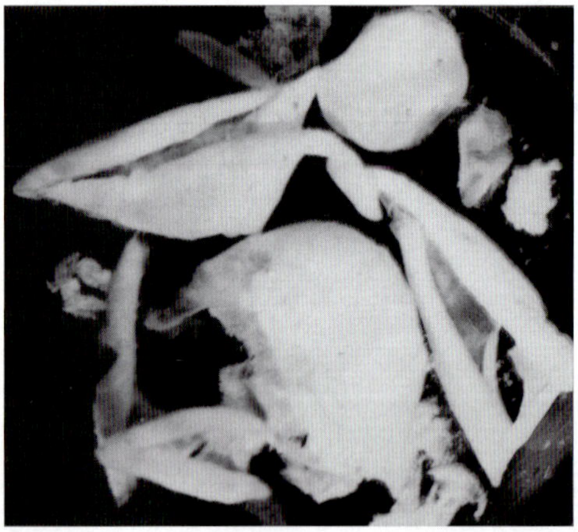

FIGURE 6.32
Cerebral echinococcosis. Hydatid cysts surgically excised from the left frontal lobe of a 32-year-old woman with a 9-month history of seizures, motor and sensory deficits, and aphasia.

Trichinosis

Trichinosis, caused by *Trichinella spiralis*, is acquired through the ingestion of meat contaminated with encysted trichinella larvae. From the intestinal tract, the larvae reach the skeletal muscles, visceral organs, and brain via the bloodstream.

Systemic manifestations include fever, eosinophilia, myalgia, facial edema, and cardiovascular and pulmonary symptoms. Common nervous system manifestations are headaches, seizures, altered mentation, focal neurologic signs, cranial nerve deficits, and psychiatric symptoms. Multiple small lesions with ring-like enhancement are evident on CT scan, and small hyperintense white-matter lesions are apparent on MRI. The diagnosis is confirmed using serology tests and muscle biopsy.

The cerebral pathology varies: It can be an eosinophilic meningoencephalitis, or multiple small hemorrhages, infarcts, and granulomas in the gray and white matter.

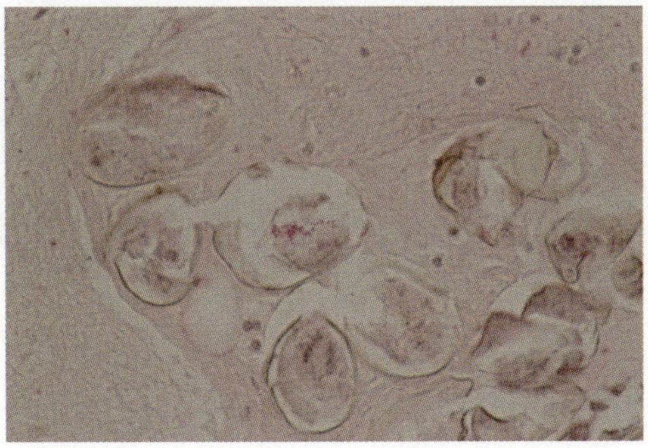

FIGURE 6.33
Cerebral schistosomiasis. *Schistosoma* ova in the subarachnoid space (HE).

Schistosomiasis

Schistosomiasis is acquired through cutaneous inoculation of the ova of one of the *Schistosoma* species. The ova invade the vascular walls and, via the bloodstream, reach the viscera and nervous tissue where they evoke a granulomatous inflammation with solitary or multiple granulomas (Fig. 6.33).

Strongyloidiasis

Strongyloidiasis is acquired through cutaneous infection with the larvae of *Strongyloides stercoralis*, an intestinal helminth. Neurologic complications develop during dissemination of the larvae to the visceral organs, skin, muscles, and brain. Immunosuppressed states, malignancies, and malnutrition promote the proliferation and dissemination of the larvae. Cerebral infection manifests as small granulomas, abscesses and, due to obstruction of capillaries by the larvae, microinfarcts.

MISCELLANEOUS INFECTIONS

Rickettsial Infections

Human infections by *Rickettsiae*, gram-negative cocobacilli are rare. The diseases (Rocky Mountain spotted fever, typhus, and scrub typhus) are acquired through tick, mice, or lice bites; the organisms spread hematogenously to the skin, muscles, visceral organs, and the brain. The pathology is characterized by perivascular lymphocytic infiltrations, vasculitis, microinfarcts, and petechial hemorrhages.

Lyme Disease

Lyme disease, a chronic systemic disease caused by the spirochete *Borrelia burgdorferi*, is acquired through a tick bite. Systemic manifestations include erythematous skin lesions, arthralgia, and cardiac and neurologic manifestations. Meningoencephalitic and myelitic syndromes and cranial and peripheral neuropathies are common features. A few pathologic studies report mononuclear cell infiltrations of the cranial and peripheral nerves and meningoencephalitis with microglial nodules.

Neurosarcoidosis

Sarcoidosis, a subacute or chronic inflammatory disease of undetermined etiology, affects the skin, visceral organs, eyes, parotid glands, and lymph nodes. In about 5% of cases, the brain and spinal cord are involved. Clinical features include cranial and peripheral nerve deficits and hypothalamic and pituitary symptoms and signs. The pathology is characterized by a noncaseating granulomatous meningoencephalitis. Grossly, the leptomeninges are thickened, and the subarachnoid space, mostly at the base of the brain, is filled with a gelatinous exudate. Histologically, noncaseating microgranulomas composed of epithelioid cells, mononuclear cells, and giant cells infiltrate the leptomeninges and underlying parenchyma, the ventricular walls, and the choroid plexus. The brunt of the inflammatory process is at the base, extending into the cranial and peripheral nerve roots.

Rasmussen's Encephalitis

A rare inflammatory disease of unknown etiology, it affects young individuals. Seizures and slowly progressive neurologic deterioration are major clinical features. The pathology is distinguished by a well-demarcated inflammatory process, localized to one cerebral hemisphere. It consists of perivascular mononuclear cell infiltrations, chiefly with T cells, focal and diffuse microglial reactions, and astrocytic gliosis. Neuronal losses, spongy degeneration, and even cavitations may add to the picture.

Whipple's Disease

Whipple's disease is caused by gram-positive bacilli. It presents with symptoms of malabsorption and variable central and peripheral nervous system symptoms. The pathology is characterized by multiple clusters of macrophages that contain PAS-positive bacilli. Such clusters are scattered throughout the brain and occasionally the peripheral nerves.

BIBLIOGRAPHY

Achim, C. L., & Wiley, C. (1998). Virus-mediated dementias. In W. R. Markesbery (Ed.). *Neuropathology of dementing disorders* (pp. 312–339). New York: Arnold.

Amlie-Lefond, C., Kleinschmidt-DeMasters, B. K., Mahalingam, R., et al. (1995). The vasculopathy of varicella–zoster virus encephalitis. *Ann Neurol 37*, 784–790.

Capello, M., & Hotez, P. J. (1993). Disseminated strongyloidiasis. *Semin Neurol 13*, 169–174.

Chimelli, L., & Scaravilli, F. (1997). Trypanosomiasis. *Brain Pathol 7*, 599–611.

Gottfredsson, M., & Perfect, J. R. (2000). Fungal meningitis. *Semin Neurol 20*, 307–322.

Gray, F., Chretien, F., Vallat-Decouvelaere, A. V., & Scaravilli, F. (2003). The changing patterns of HIV neuropathology in the HAART era. *J Neuropath Exp Neurol 62*, 429–440.

Johnson, R. T. (1998). *Viral infections of the nervous system*, 2nd ed. Philadelphia: Lippincott–Raven.

Kleinschmidt-DeMasters, B. K., & Gilden, D. H. (2001). The expanding spectrum of herpes virus infections of the nervous system. *Brain Pathol 11*, 440–451.

Meyer, M. A. (2003). Neurologic complications of anthrax. *Arch Neurol 60*, 483–488.

Mrak, R. E., & Young, L. (1994). Rabies encephalitis in humans—pathology, pathogenesis and pathophysiology. *J Neuropath Exp Neurol 53*, 1–10.

Roos, K. L. (2000). Acute bacterial meningitis. *Semin Neurol 20*, 293–306.

Sacktor, N., Lyles, R. H., Skolasky, R., et al. (2001). HIV-associated neurologic disease incidence changes: Multicenter AIDS Cohort Study, 1990–1998. *Neurology 56*, 257–260.

REVIEW QUESTIONS

1. The bacteria that most commonly cause acute purulent meningitis in neonates are:
   A. *Haemophilus influenzae*
   B. *Escherichia coli*
   C. *Neisseria meningitides*
   D. All of these
   E. None of these

2. *Haemophilus influenzae* meningitis is often complicated by:
   A. Epidural abscess
   B. Subdural empyema
   C. Subdural hygroma
   D. Myocarditis
   E. Multiple granulomas

3. Meningococcus meningitis can be complicated by:
   A. Skin petechiae
   B. Adrenal hemorrhage
   C. Disseminated intravascular coagulopathy
   D. All of these
   E. None of these

4. All of the following concerning tuberculous meningitis are correct *except*:
   A. The exudate is confined to the basal subarachnoid space.
   B. Tuberculous granulomas contain coagulative necrosis.
   C. The granulomas contain epithelioid cells and lymphocytes.
   D. The granulomas contain Langhans giant cells.
   E. The glucose level in CSF is low.

5. All of the following concerning general paresis are incorrect *except*:

   A. It is caused by gram positive bacilli.
   B. It presents with weakness of extremities.
   C. It is caused by Treponema pallidum.
   D. It complicates head trauma.
   E. Neurons display cytoplasmic inclusions.

6. Fungi are best revealed in paraffin sections using:

   A. Masson trichrome stain
   B. Grocott methenamine silver stain
   C. Phosphotungstic acid hematoxylin (PTAH)
   D. Von Kossa stain
   E. Congo red stain

7. All of the following concerning cerebral cryptococcosis are correct *except*:

   A. It can occur in HIV-infected individuals.
   B. The fungi invade small blood vessels.
   C. The infection spreads via the bloodstream from a pulmonary infection.
   D. The fungi are surrounded by a mucopolysaccharide capsule.
   E. The infection manifests as a meningitis.

8. Aspergillosis is characterized by all of the following *except*:

   A. The heart often is involved.
   B. The blood vessels show necrotizing vasculitis.
   C. The fungi appear as yeasts measuring 2 to 8 microns.
   D. Cerebral aspergillosis manifests as granulomas.
   E. Cerebral aspergillosis manifests as septic hemorrhagic necroses.

9. Histopathologic changes characteristic of herpes simplex type 1 encephalitis include all of the following *except*:

   A. Hemorrhages in the cerebral cortex
   B. Multifocal demyelinations in the white matter
   C. Necrosis in the cerebral cortex
   D. Eosinophilic cytoplasmic inclusions in the neurons
   E. Pathology in the basal-mesial aspects of the frontotemporal lobes

10. Cytomegalovirus encephalitis is characterized by all of the following *except*:

    A. It has a predilection for the walls of the ventricles.
    B. The glial cells display cytoplasmic inclusions.
    C. The glial cells display nuclear inclusions.
    D. It is prevalent among immunosuppressed individuals.
    E. CT scan displays massive calcifications in the cerebral and cerebellar cortex.

11. The histology of HIV-encephalitis is characterized by:

    A. Microglial nodules containing multinucleated giant cells
    B. Cytoplasmic eosinophilic inclusions
    C. Periventricular demyelination
    D. All of these
    E. None of these

12. Neurologic complications of AIDS in children are:

    A. Microcephaly
    B. Seizures
    C. Mineral deposits in the basal ganglia on CT scan
    D. All of these
    E. None of these

13. A fulminant parasitic hemorrhagic encephalitis acquired by swimming in fresh water is caused by:

    A. Entamoeba histolytica
    B. Schistosoma species
    C. Naegleria fowleri
    D. Taenia solium
    E. Trichinella spiralis

14. The following apply to neurocysticercosis:

    A. It often manifests with seizures.
    B. It may cause obstructive hydrocephalus.
    C. It is caused by infection with Taenia solium.
    D. It is caused by ingesting tapeworm eggs.
    E. All of these.

(Answers are provided in the Appendix.)

CHAPTER 7

Prion Diseases: Transmissible Spongiform Encephalopathies

Animal Prion Diseases
Human Prion Diseases

Prion diseases, a group of fatal neurodegenerative diseases affecting both humans and animals, are unique in that they can be both infectious (transmissible) and heritable. The causative pathogen is a proteinaceous infectious agent termed *prion protein* (PrPsc) (sc refers to scrapie). PrPsc is a protease-resistant isoform of a cellular prion protein (PrPc) (c refers to cellular) that is normally folded in the membranes of the neurons and glial cells of the central nervous system (CNS). PrPsc also is present in the lymphoreticular system, heart, and skeletal muscles. The gene of the human prion protein (*PRNP*) is located on the short arm of chromosome 20. *PRNP* is polymorphic at codon 129, encoding either for valine or methionine. The nonpathogenic PrPc, by changing the folding pattern, can convert to a pathogenic PrPsc spontaneously or by pathogenic mutations in *PRNP*. The PrPsc is unique in several respects: It consists solely of protein and lacks nucleic acid, it resists conventional sterilizing agents, it evokes neither inflammatory nor immune reaction, and it does not form neuronal inclusions. Due to its high infectivity, guidelines have been established for the handling of specimens from patients suspected of having a prion disease. By inoculation or ingestion, PrPsc is transmissible from animal to animal, from human to experimental animals, from human to human, and evidence exists for transmission from animal to human.

The characteristic pathologic feature shared by both human and animal diseases is a spongiform degeneration of the cerebral and cerebellar cortex and deep gray structures. Hence the name, transmissible spongiform encephalopathy.

Recent experimental studies raised the possibility of a role for Spiroplasma infection in the development of transmissible spongiform encephalopathies. Spiroplasma, an intracellular, highly infective, neurotropic bacteria spread by the oral route, reaches the neural tissue from the lymphatics. A possible interaction with prion proteins and a possible role in causing spongiform encephalopathies awaits elucidation.

ANIMAL PRION DISEASES

A number of prion diseases have been recognized in animals. Two of them—scrapie in sheep and bovine spongiform encephalopathy in cattle—are particularly important because of their relevance to human diseases.

Scrapie in Sheep

Investigations of scrapie contributed important information on the nature of prion diseases:

- These studies demonstrated the transmissibility of the disease to experimental animals with inoculation of scrapie-infected material.
- They established pathologic similarities between animal and human diseases
- They led to the discovery of the *prion protein* as the infectious agent responsible for both the animal and the human diseases.

Bovine Spongiform Encephalopathy in Cattle

Bovine spongiform encephalopathy (BSE or mad cow disease) was recognized in the United Kingdom in 1986, during the course of routine examinations of cattle fed with scrapie-infected food products.

Chronic Wasting Disease (CWD) of Deer and Elk

Outbreaks of CWD disease have been reported in several areas of the United States. Presently, a possible transmission to humans is unsupported.

HUMAN PRION DISEASES

Human prion diseases are rare. The yearly incidence is estimated to be 1 to 2 cases per million population. Point mutations, deletions, and insertions in the PrP gene produce a broad spectrum of diseases. The clinical and pathologic phenotypes are determined by homozygosity or heterozygosity for methionine or valine at codon 129. The diseases can be sporadic, familial, or acquired (Table 7.1). Sporadic occurrences account for about 85% of cases. About 10% to 15% are familial, with autosomal dominant inheritance. Acquired instances are rare, but the number may increase with the passage of time because incubation takes several years. The disease is acquired iatrogenically or by consumption of infected food products.

The group of human prion diseases encompasses kuru, a now-extinct disease, and four current conditions (see Table 7.1): Creutzfeldt-Jakob disease (CJD), Gerstmann-Sträussler-Scheinker disease (GSS), fatal familial insomnia (FFI), and new-variant CJD (nv CJD). The first three afflict mostly middle-aged and elderly individuals, and the fourth one affects younger subjects. The clinical presentation varies among the diseases, but all share progressing cognitive decline and neurologic deterioration, inevitably leading to death within several months or a year, seldom more. At present, no curative therapy is available. Genetic counseling is important in familial cases.

The diagnosis may be difficult in early stage of the disease. The differential diagnosis includes degenerative dementias, particularly of frontotemporal type. Electroencephalogram (EEG), magnetic resonance imaging (MRI), and cerebrospinal fluid (CSF) abnormalities, along with proper clinical features, support the diagnosis. EEG during the early stage of the disease shows synchronous periodic sharp wave complexes (PSWC) occurring at a rate of 1 to 2 per second. MRI abnormality is characterized by a hyperintensity of the basal ganglia and pulvinar on T2-weighted images. CSF fluid examination often shows elevated 14–3–3 protein and

TABLE 7.1.
Human Prion Diseases

Sporadic	*Inherited*	*Acquired*	
CJD FFI	CJD GSS FFI	Iatrogenic CJD	Oral route nvCJD Kuru

CJD, Creutzfeldt-Jakob disease; FFI, fatal familial insomnia; GSS, Gerstmann-Sträussler-Scheinker disease; nv, new-variant CJD.

elevated tau protein, but false positives and negatives may occur. Genetic studies reveal mutations in *PRNP* and identify homozygotes for methionine on codon 129; these homozygotes are at risk for developing the disease. Definite diagnosis rests on pathologic confirmation in autopsy or biopsy specimen.

Pathologically, the diseases share common features and also have distinguishing characteristics. Common features are (a) spongiform degeneration of the gray matter, (b) neuronal losses, (c) astrocytosis, and (d) deposits of prion protein (PrP) as amyloid precipitates. Identifying deposits of prion protein by using antibodies against them confirms the diagnosis.

Kuru

Kuru, the first recognized and now-extinct prion disease among the Forbe tribe in New Guinea, was transmitted by ritualistic cannibalism of the brain of affected dead persons. After a long incubation of several years, the disease presented with ataxia, tremor, and dementia. The pathology consisted of severe cerebellar cortical degeneration and the presence of Kuru (PrP amyloid) plaques.

Creutzfeldt-Jakob Disease

CJD, the most common prion disease, has worldwide distribution. It affects both genders equally. Most cases are sporadic, some are dominantly inherited, and some acquired. Iatrogenically acquired cases occurred through contaminated corneal transplant or cadaveric dura mater graft, use of inadequately sterilized surgical instruments, and the administration of extract of cadaveric pituitary hormone from patients dying of CJD.

Clinical Features

The average age of onset is 45 to 75 years, but it may occur earlier or later. Rapidly progressing dementia; myoclonus; combinations of cerebellar, pyramidal, extrapyramidal, and sensory symptoms and signs; and seizures characterize the clinical picture. The course is short; the patient is eventually in a vegetative state. Death usually occurs in less than 1 year. The EEG shows periodic sharp wave complexes. T2-weighted MR images may show hyperintensity in the basal ganglia, and the 14–3–3 protein level is often elevated in the CSF.

Rapidly progressing sporadic CJD may show homozygosity for methionine on codon 129, whereas a more slowly progressing disease often shows homozygosity for valine. Common genetic alterations in familial CJD are D178N and E200K. Mutation of the PrP gene at codon 178 causes aspartic acid (D) to be replaced by asparagine (N), and mutation at codon 200 causes glutamate (E) to be replaced by lysine (K). Insertion mutations have also been identified in familial cases.

Pathologic Features

Grossly, the brain shows variable atrophy of the convolutions, subcortical gray structures, and hemispheric white matter (Fig. 7.1). The histologic hallmark of the disease is microvacuolation and spongiform degenera-

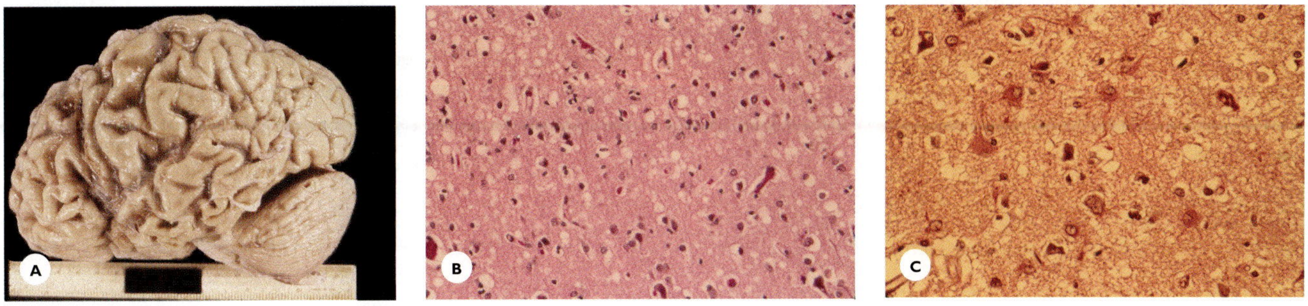

FIGURE 7.1
Creutzfeldt-Jakob disease. **A.** Severe diffuse cerebral atrophy. **B.** Cerebral cortex showing microvacuolation and neuronal losses and (**C**) prominent astrocytic proliferation (HE).

tion of the cerebral and cerebellar cortex and, variably, of the subcortical gray structures. The vacuoles are small, round or oval, often coalescing, and occurring in all cortical layers. Neuronal losses and astrocytosis are prominent (see Fig. 7.1). PrP precipitates as amyloid plaques in the cerebral and cerebellar cortex and, variably, in the deep gray structures. Immunohistologic stain identifies various forms of PrP deposits, including dense plaques (Kuru plaque); multicentric plaques; and granular deposits around neurons, synapses, and blood vessels and in vascular walls. In hematoxylin-eosin (HE)-stained sections, the plaques appear as homogenous eosinophilic structures.

Variants of CJD are (a) *Heidenhain disease* is distinguished clinically by cortical blindness and histologically by spongiosis and neuronal losses, predominantly in the occipital cortex (Fig. 7.2); (b) the *ataxic form* shows prominent cerebellar cortical degeneration (Fig. 7.3); (c) the *panencephalopathic form* entails additional degeneration of the white matter; and (d) the *amyotrophic and polyneuropathic forms* may introduce the disease or develop during its course. PrP deposits are found in the spinal cord gray matter and peripheral nerves.

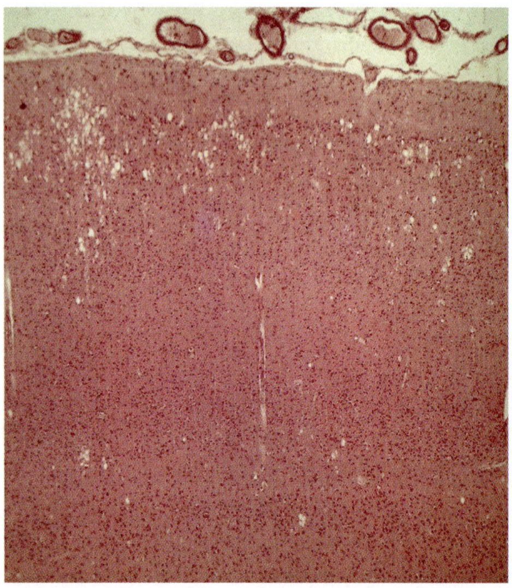

FIGURE 7.2
Heidenhain variant of CJD. A 56-year-old woman presented with progressive visual loss, myoclonic jerks, and dementia. She died 5 months after onset of symptoms. Microvacuolation in the occipital cortex (HE).

Gerstmann-Sträussler-Scheinker Disease

GSS disease, dominantly inherited, has a wide range of onset (20 to 60 years) and a more prolonged clinical course, with cerebellar ataxia in the foreground of clinical picture. Large PrP- and amyloid-containing plaques in the cerebellar cortex characterize the histology. Tau-immunoreactive neurofibrillary tangles occur in the cerebral cortex.

P102 L is a common genetic alteration. Mutations of the PrP gene at codon 102 result in the substitution of proline (P) with leucin (L).

Fatal Familial Insomnia

FFI, dominantly inherited or sporadic, is characterized by intractable insomnia, autonomic dysfunction (changes in blood pressure, heart rate, temperature, and respiratory rate), myoclonus, cerebellar ataxia, and pyramidal and extrapyramidal signs. Atrophy, neuronal losses, and severe gliosis of the thalamus are distinctive features. Spongiform changes and prion amyloid plaques are not conspicuous.

Mutation in the *PRNP* gene is the same as in familial CJD—D178N—but, in FFI, the gene encodes methionine at codon 178, whereas in familial CJD it encodes valine.

New-Variant CJD

In 1994 and1995, a little less than 10 years after the outbreak of BSE in Europe, a new variant of CJD (nvCJD) was recognized in the United Kingdom and France. The disease is distinguished by an earlier onset of behavioral changes and psychiatric symptoms, followed by cerebellar dysfunction and myoclonus. Later in the course, dementia develops. The course is protracted. Bilateral pulvinar hyperintensities on MRI are held to be characteristic. Because PrPsc is detectable in lymphoid tissue, immunohistochemical demonstration of PrP in tonsillar biopsy supports the diagnosis. Widespread spongy degeneration and an abundance of florid

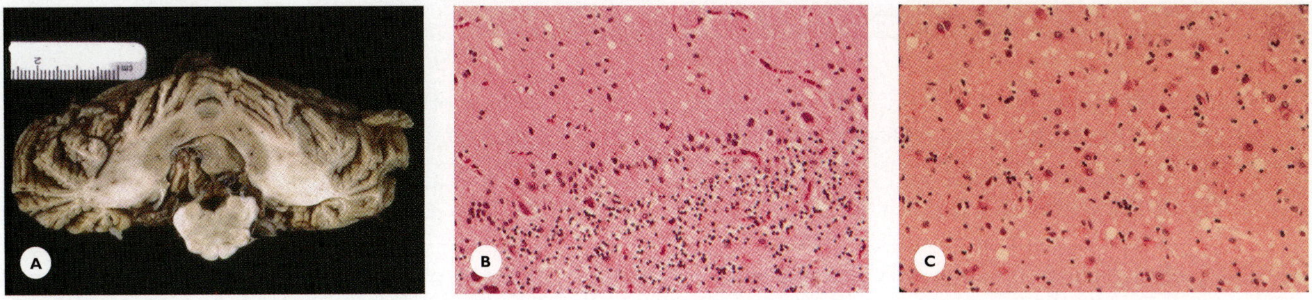

FIGURE 7.3
Ataxic-cerebellar variant of CJD. A 65-year-old woman presented with headaches, speech difficulty, gait impairment, and forgetfulness. Her symptoms steadily progressed. Her gait became severely ataxic, she displayed dysmetria in all extremities, and myoclonic jerks. Six months after the initial symptoms, she died. The cerebellum shows (**A**) severe diffuse cortical and white matter atrophy; (**B**) diffuse loss of Purkinje cells, rarefaction of granular cells layer, and microvacuolation in the molecular layer (HE); and (**C**) microvacuolation, neuronal loss and astrocytosis in basal ganglia (HE).

prion plaques (dense central cores surrounded by amyloid fibrils and outer spongiform halos) in the cerebral and cerebellar cortex characterize the histology. A causal association between this nvCJD and the consumption of meat products contaminated with BSE agent is gaining support. It has been shown that the PrPsc type in nvCJD is identical to that found in cattle infected with BSE.

BIBLIOGRAPHY

Bastian, F. O. (2005). Spiroplasma as a candidate agent for the transmissible spongiform encephalopathies. *J Neuropath Exp Neurol 64*, 833–838.

Dickson, D. (Ed.). (2003). *Neurodegeneration: the molecular pathology of dementia and movement disorders* (pp. 282–338). Basel: ISN Neuropath Press.

Epstein, L. G., & Brown, P. (1997). Bovine spongiform encephalopathy and a new variant of Creutzfeldt-Jakob disease. *Neurology 48*, 569–571.

Glatzel, M., Stoeck, K., Seeger, H., et al. (2005). Human prion diseases. *Arch Neurol 62*, 545–552.

Kovacs, T., Aranyi, Z., Szirmai, I., & Lantos, P. L. (2002). Creutzfeldt-Jakob disease with amyotrophy and demyelinating polyneuropathy. *Arch Neurol 59*, 1811–1814.

Kropp, S., Shultz-Schaeffer, W. Y., Finkenstaedt, M., et al. (1999). The Heidenhain variant of Creutzfeldt-Jakob disease. *Arch Neurol 56*, 55–61.

Prusiner, S. B. (1993). Genetic and infectious prion diseases. *Arch Neurol 50*, 1129–1153.

Schonberger, L. B. (1998). New variant Creutzfeldt-Jakob disease and bovine spongiform encephalopathy. *Infect Dis Clin North Am 12*, 111–121.

Will, R. G., Zeidler, M., Stewart, G. E., et al. (2000). Diagnosis of new variant Creutzfeldt-Jakob disease. *Ann Neurol 47*, 575–582.

REVIEW QUESTIONS

1. The infectious prion protein (PrPsc) is characterized by the following statement(s):
   A. It consists of protein and nucleic acid.
   B. It is a pathogenic isoform of a nonpathogenic prion protein (PrPc).
   C. It evokes an inflammatory reaction with lymphocytes.
   D. All of these.
   E. None of these.

2. The prion protein gene (PRNP):
   A. Is located on chromosome 20
   B. Is located on chromosome 26
   C. At codon 130, it codes for methionine
   D. At codon 129, it codes for either methionine or valine
   E. None of these

3. Diagnostic abnormalities encountered in Creutzfeldt-Jakob disease are:
   A. Vacuolated lymphocytes in circulating blood
   B. Elevated 14-3-3 protein in CSF
   C. Periodic sharp-wave complexes in EEG
   D. Abnormal auditory evoked potentials
   E. Hyperintensity of basal ganglia in T2-weighted MRI

4. Which of the following histologic changes characterize Creutzfeldt-Jakob disease?
   A. Spongiform degeneration of the cerebral cortex
   B. Neuronal losses
   C. Eosinophilic cytoplasmic inclusions in the remaining neurons
   D. Astrocytic proliferation
   E. Amyloid/prion plaques in the cerebral cortex

5. Which of the following statements characterize fatal familial insomnia?
   A. It is an autosomal recessive disorder.
   B. The pathology is confined to the basal ganglia.
   C. The pathology is confined to the thalamus.
   D. The disease is associated with point mutation of PRNP at codon 178.
   E. Autonomic dysfunctions are common.

6. The new variant of Creutzfeldt-Jakob disease is characterized by:
   A. Behavioral changes and psychiatric symptoms usually introduce the disease
   B. Cortical blindness is common in affected patients
   C. T2-weighted MRI may show hyperintensity of pulvinars
   D. Amyloid/prion plaques are abundant in the cerebral cortex
   E. Perivascular lymphocytic infiltrations are prominent

(Answers are provided in the Appendix.)

CHAPTER 8

Demyelinating Diseases

Diseases with Autoimmune Pathogenesis
Diseases with Probable Autoimmune Pathogenesis

The primary degeneration of central nervous system (CNS) myelin characterizes a heterogenous group of diseases (Table 8.1). Important diseases, affecting chiefly young adults, are immune-mediated; others, affecting chiefly children, are inherited; and still others are caused by viruses, metabolic disorders, toxins, and blood-vessel diseases. The immune-mediated diseases are presented here. Diseases with other etiologies are covered in other chapters.

DISEASES WITH AUTOIMMUNE PATHOGENESIS

Multiple Sclerosis

Multiple sclerosis (MS) is a multifocal inflammatory demyelinating disease affecting chiefly young individuals between 20 and 40 years of age; it rarely occurs earlier or later in life. It is a major, chronic, disabling disease among young adults, affecting women more often than it does men. Its prevalence varies geographically: It occurs more often—averaging 90 to 100 cases per 100,000 population—in countries with temperate and cold climates. The clinical presentation of MS is greatly diverse and variable. It correlates well with the multiplicity of the lesions and their distributions at various anatomical sites within the brain and spinal cord. (see Chapter 2, for chemical composition and pathology of myelin).

Pathology

Grossly, multiple focal areas of demyelination, called *plaques,* are the pathologic hallmark of the disease. The location, number, size, and shape of the plaques vary greatly from case to case. Plaques typically occur within the white matter, but may also be found within gray structures, such as the cerebral cortex, thalamus, and basal ganglia. Preferential sites are the optic nerves and chiasma, the periventricular and periaqueductal regions,

TABLE 8.1.
Diseases of Central Myelin

Etiologies	*Diseases*
Autoimmune mechanism	Multiple sclerosis
Probably autoimmune mechanism	Postinfectious and postvaccination encephalomyelitis
	Acute hemorrhagic leukoencephalitis
Viruses	
JC virus	Progressive multifocal leukoencephalopathy
Measles virus	Subacute sclerosing panencephalitis
Rubella virus	Progressive rubella syndrome
Human immunodeficiency virus	Leukoencephalopathy
Acquired metabolic	Central pontine myelinolysis
	Marchiafava-Bignami disease
Vitamin B_{12} deficiency	Combined degeneration of the spinal cord
Inherited metabolic	Leukodystrophy
Vascular	Subcortical arteriosclerotic encephalopathy (Binswanger's disease)
X-irradiation	Leukoencephalopathy
Toxins	
Solvent: Toluene	Spongiform leukoencephalopathy
Carbon monoxide	Leukoencephalopathy
Drugs	
Amphotericin B	Multifocal leukoencephalopathy
Methotrexate	Necrotizing leukoencephalopathy
Chronic edema	Leukoencephalopathy
Immunosuppressed conditions	Multifocal necrotizing leukoencephalopathy

the floor of the fourth ventricle, and beneath the pia mater in the spinal cord. Acute plaques are poorly demarcated, soft, pinkish-yellow, and slightly granular. Chronic plaques are distinctly demarcated, firm, grayish, slightly retracted, and translucent or gelatinous (Figs. 8.1 through 8.4). Cerebral atrophy, not uncommon, is evidenced by a thinning of the cortical ribbon and corpus callosum, a reduction of the white matter, and the dilatation of the ventricles.

Histologically, three basic processes characterize plaque formation: inflammation, myelin breakdown, and astrocytic fibrillary gliosis.

Inflammation occurs with vasogenic edema and perivascular infiltrations with lymphocytes, chiefly T cells, some B cells, and macrophages (early in the course CD4 helper/inducer T-cell and later in the course CD8, cytotoxic/suppressor T-cells) (Fig. 8.5).

Myelin breaks down into neutral lipid globules, some of which immunoreact for myelin basic protein (MBP). The myelin globules are phagocytosed by macrophages and gradually removed to the perivascular and subarachnoid spaces (Fig.8.5).

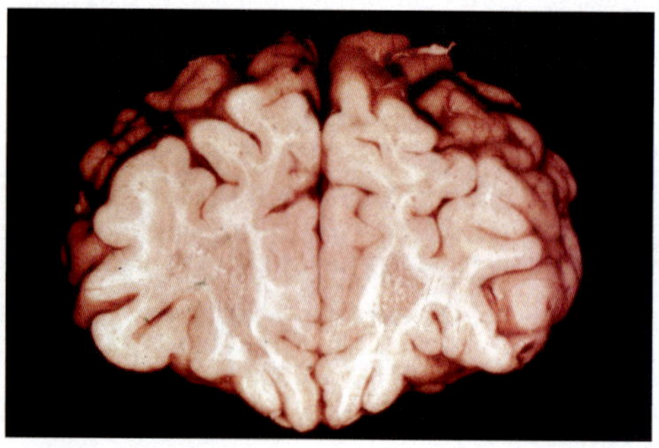

FIGURE 8.1
Acute MS plaques in cerebral hemispheric white matter are ill-defined, yellowish, and slightly granular.

Meanwhile, the astrocytes begin to proliferate, becoming plump with homogeneous eosinophilic cytoplasm and numerous fibrillary processes (Fig. 8.5). As the plaque matures, the edema and the inflammation resolve and the macrophages gradually disappear. The astrocytes produce more and more fibers and, ultimately, a dense and firm fibrillary gliosis (glial scar) fills the demyelinated plaque (astrocytic fibrillary gliosis)

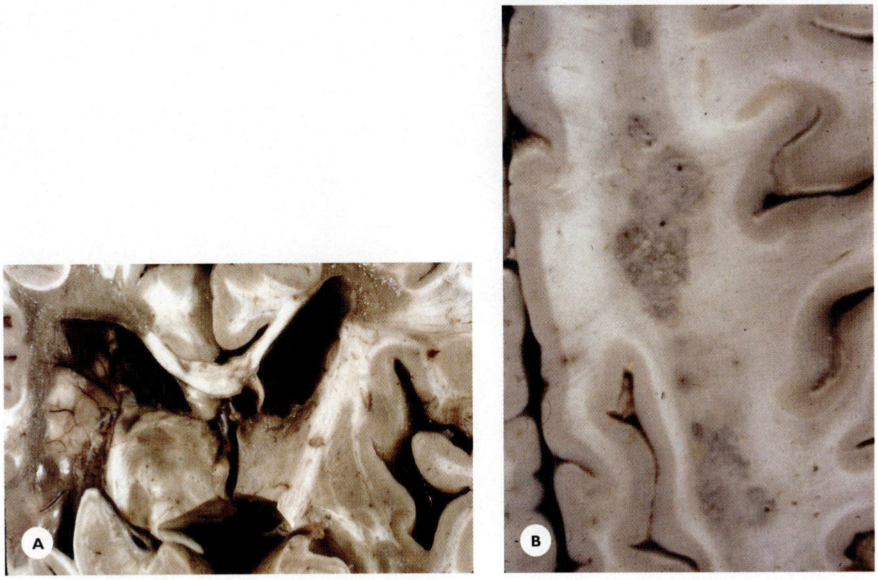

FIGURE 8.2
A. Chronic plaques around the lateral ventricles are sharply defined, gray, firm, translucent, and slightly depressed. Multiple small plaques are dispersed in the gray structures. **B.** Large confluent plaques in the central white matter.

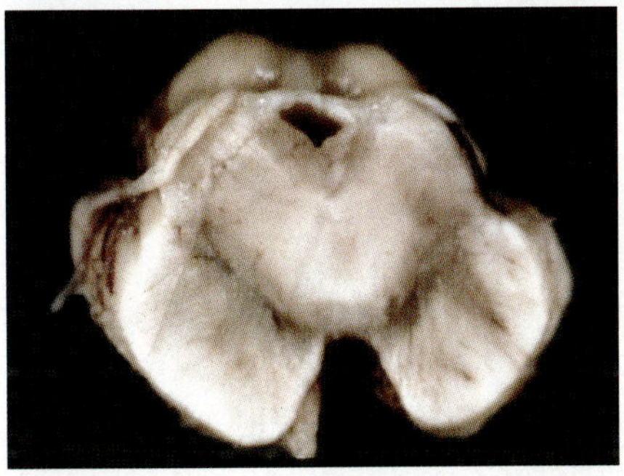

FIGURE 8.3
Midbrain showing chronic plaques around the aqueduct and in the tegmentum and basis.

(Fig. 8.6). These characteristic plaques prompted Charcot, a nineteenth-century French neurologist, to name the disease *sclerose en plaque* (sclerotic plaque or multiple sclerosis).

Concurrently, important alterations occur in the axons and oligodendrocytes and, to some extent, in the neurons:

In axonal changes, a variable number of nerve fibers are damaged, some reversibly and some permanently, probably by the inflammatory process and by being stripped of their myelin sheaths. They may be swollen, beaded, or thinned. In severe cases, they may be broken up (Fig. 8.7). Early damage to the axons is readily demonstrated by applying immunohistologic stain for β-amyloid precursor protein (β-APP). Disruption of structural integrity of the nerve fibers leads to wallerian degeneration in the distal segments.

In oligodendroglial changes, the number of oligodendrocytes within the plaques is variably reduced or totally absent (Fig. 8.8). Nevertheless, premyelinating oligodendrocytes and their migrating progenitor cells are evident in some plaques, as has been demonstrated using immunocytochemical techniques. These oligodendrocytes are credited with the potential of remyelinating the denuded nerve fibers under favorable conditions.

Within the plaques, the neurons may be unaffected, or they may show atrophy and some losses (Fig. 8.9). Neuronal losses outside the plaques have also been reported and are attributed to retrograde axonal degeneration.

There are three types of chronic plaques: an *inactive (burnt-out) chronic plaque* consists of a dense astrofibrosis with a reduced number of astrocytic nuclei, sparse or absent oligodendrocytes, and variably damaged nerve fibers.

An *active chronic plaque,* by contrast, shows marginal perivascular lymphocytic cuffings, ongoing myelin destruction, macrophages, and a variable number of oligodendrocytes.

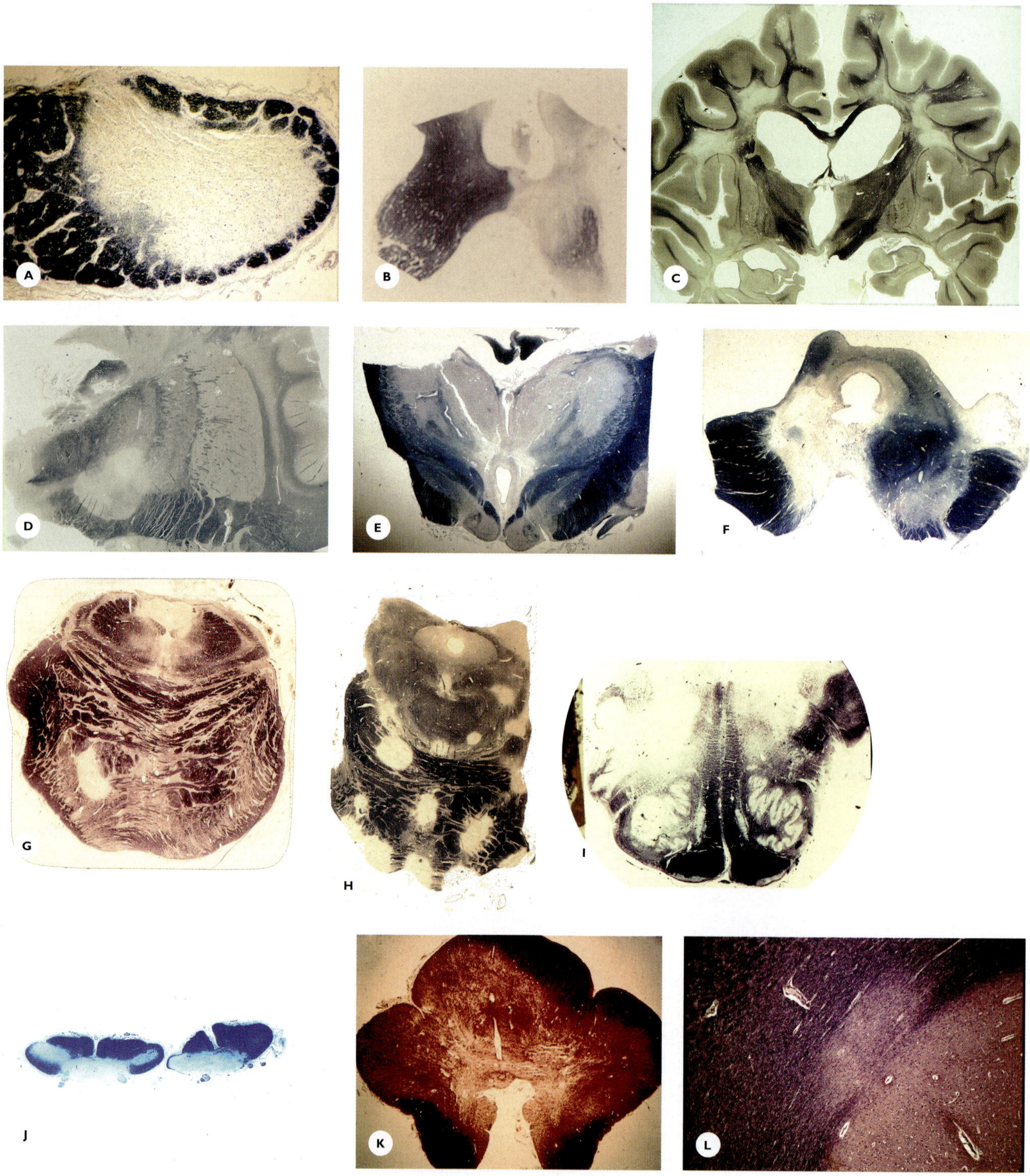

FIGURE 8.4

Variations in location, size, and shape of MS plaques (myelin stained sections): **A.** Optic nerve. **B.** Chiasma. **C.** Periventricular zones and central hemispheric white matter. **D.** Globus pallidus and sublenticular region. **E.** Thalamus and hypothalamus. **F.** Midbrain. **G.** Pons (note the tiny lesion in the MLF, pathologic correlate of internuclear ophthalmoplegia). **H.** Pons. **I.** Medulla. **J.** Spinal cord. **K.** Spinal cord. **L.** Subcortical white matter and cortex.

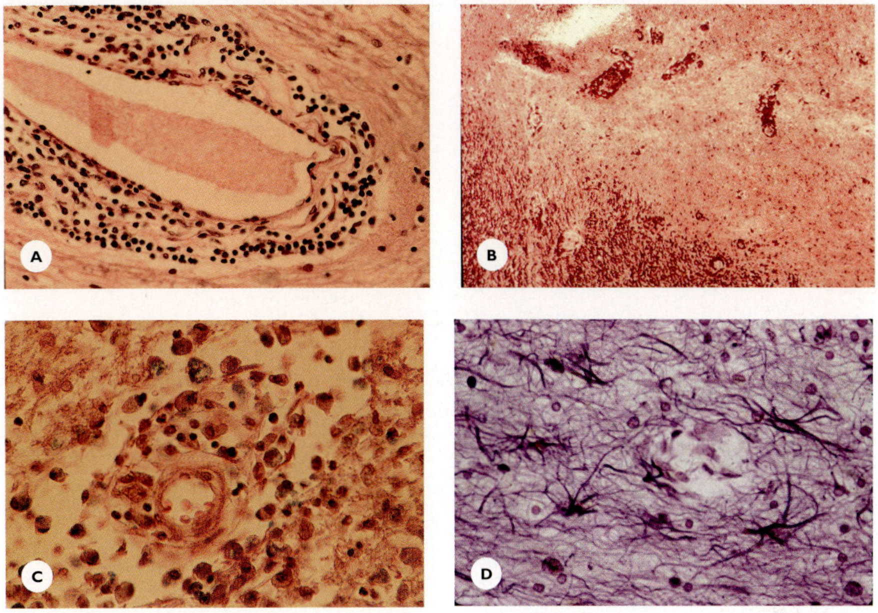

FIGURE 8.5
Histology of acute MS plaques: **A.** Perivascular lymphocytic infiltration (HE). **B.** Disintegration of myelin into oil-red-O–positive neutral lipid globules. **C.** Macrophages remove myelin debris (HE). **D.** Fibrous astrocytes produce fine fibrillary processes (Holzer stain).

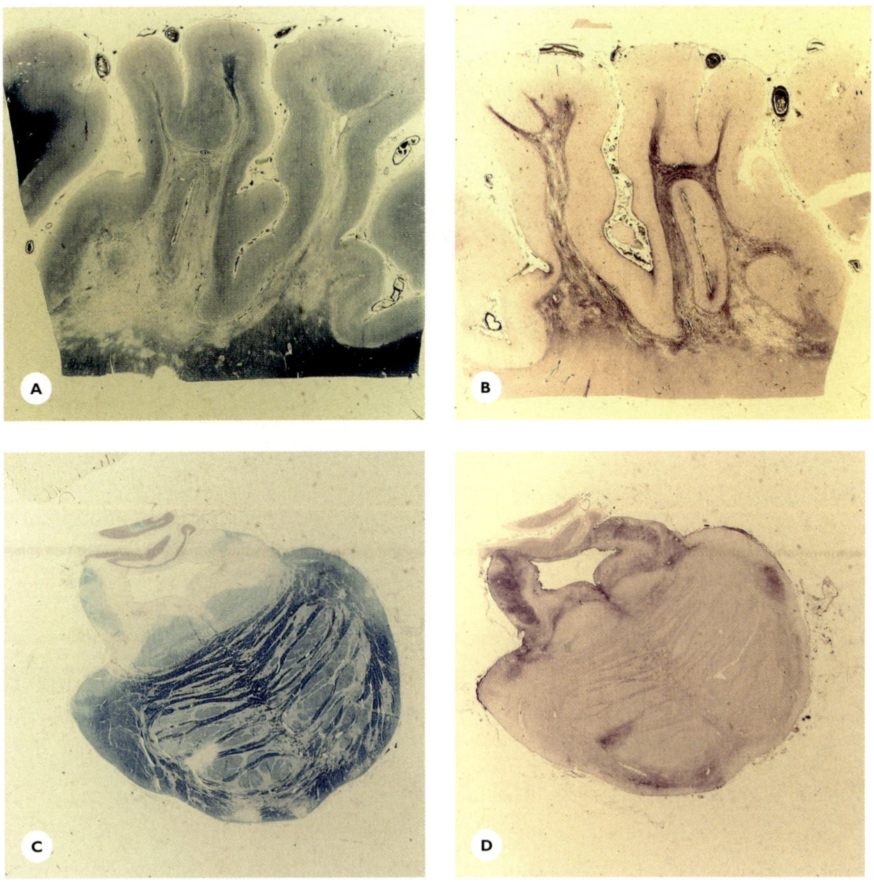

FIGURE 8.6
Chronic MS plaques. (**A**) Demyelination and (**B**) dense astrocytic gliosis in a subcortical plaque. **C.** Extensive demyelination in the tegmentum and small demyelinated foci in the basis of the pons and **D.** Dense astrogliosis within demyelinated areas (LFB-CV and Holzer stains).

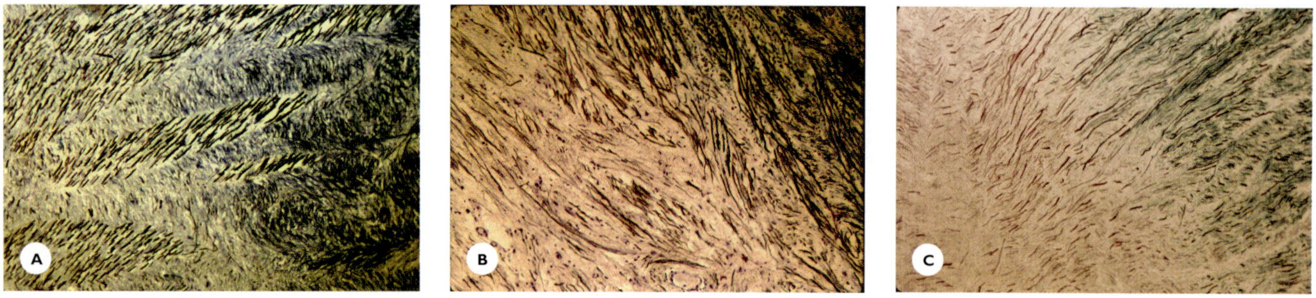

FIGURE 8.7
Nerve fiber changes within MS plaques. **A.** At the margin of a plaque, the myelin sheaths are sharply disrupted but a reduced number of nerve fibers is spared. **B.** Moderate and (C) total loss of nerve fibers in the center of a chronic plaque (Holmes stain).

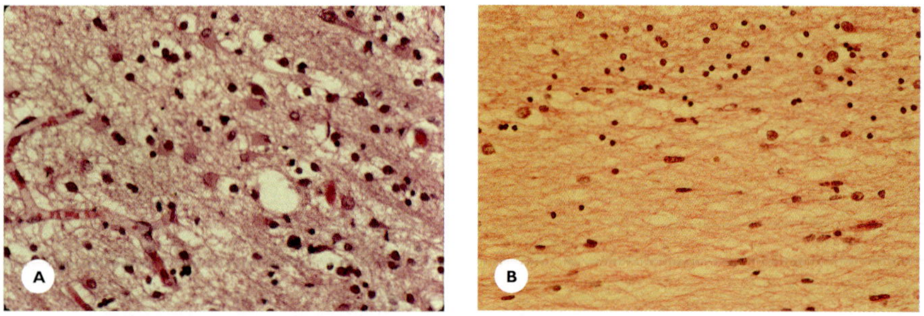

FIGURE 8.8
Oligodendrocytes within chronic MS plaques. **A.** Oligodendrocytes are sparse among large fibrillary astrocytes. **B.** Plaque depleted of oligodendrocytes (HE).

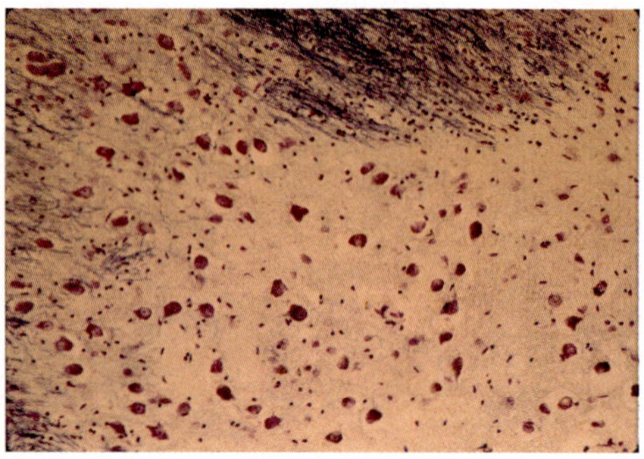

FIGURE 8.9
Preservation of neurons within MS plaque (LFB-CV).

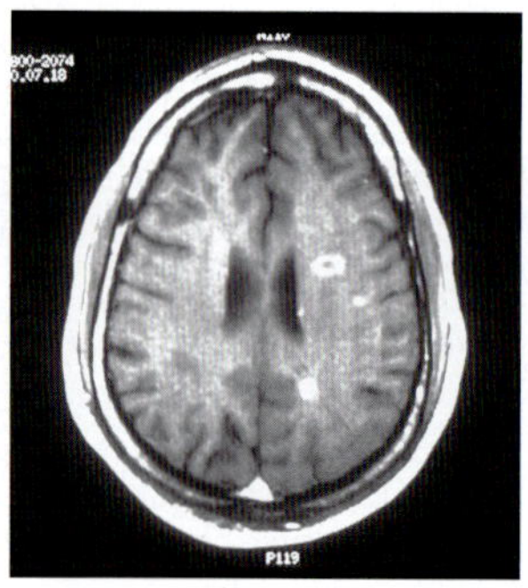

FIGURE 8.10
MRI of acute MS plaques in a 48-year-old man with relapsing MS. Gadolinium-enhanced T1-weighted axial image shows one ring-like enhancing and few homogenously enhancing lesions.

A *shadow or remyelinating plaque* shows reduced myelin density, thin and faintly staining myelin sheaths, and moderate to large number of oligodendrocytes.

Etiology

Despite a great interest in the disease and ample experimental and pathologic studies, the etiology remains elusive. A combination of genetic susceptibility and environmental factors are implicated in the etiology. Familial occurrences are recognized, and the disease has been reported in monozygotic and dizygotic twins. Certain major histocompatibility complexes (MHC)—HLA-DR2, HLA-A3, HLA-B7—are more frequent among MS patients than among the general population.

Individuals with HLA-DR2 on chromosome 6 are particularly susceptible to developing MS.

Epidemiologic data indicate a higher incidence of MS in certain geographic areas and among particular ethnic groups. The incidence is higher in northern Europe, the northern United States, and Canada. It is also higher in people of Anglo-Saxon and Scandinavian descent, and lower among Japanese and Chinese. In the United States, the incidence is lower among African American than it is among whites.

Exposure to an as yet unidentified infectious agent probably occurs during the early years of life. As mentioned, the incidence of the disease is higher in cold and temperate climates. Studies indicate that persons who migrate from a cold climates to a warm climate after 15 years of age keep the higher risk of their native locality. Conversely, persons who migrate before age 15 years acquire the lower risk of their new locality.

Pathogenesis

Current views favor an autoimmune-mediated reaction against the myelin (immunologic attack against self-antigen) involving both cellular and humoral immunity. This autoimmune mechanism is supported by similarities between the pathology of MS and the experimental allergic encephalomyelitis (EAE) induced by immunization with brain and spinal cord myelin extracts.

The cellular immune reaction is mediated by T lymphocytes. Simplistically, activated $CD4^+$ T lymphocytes possessing antigen-specific receptors cross the blood–brain barrier and react with myelin and/or oligodendroglia antigen. Cytokines released by T lymphocytes activate macrophages expressing MHC class II antigen. These macrophages present the myelin antigens to the T cells and, in time, remove the products of myelin disintegration. MBP, proteolipid protein, and myelin oligodendrocyte glycoprotein are major target antigens. The humoral immune reaction is mediated by activated B lymphocytes that secrete myelin-specific antibodies. Several pathogens have been postulated to trigger the immune reaction: measles virus, Epstein-Barr virus, human herpes virus 6, retroviruses, canine distemper virus, and Chlamydia pneumoniae. None has yet been confirmed.

An alternative view regarding the pathogenesis of MS implicates apoptotic oligodendroglial deaths and subsequent microglial activation as early events in plaque formation.

Clinical Features

The multiplicity of MS plaques and their locations at various anatomic sites account for the great variability of clinical symptoms and signs (Table 8.2). Visual impairment, varying from diminished visual acuity to total blindness in one or both eyes, orbital pain, and frontal headaches are often the presenting symptoms. However, any cerebral or spinal cord dysfunction may introduce the disease.

Among diagnostic tests, magnetic resonance imaging (MRI) is particularly valuable in supporting the diagnosis (Figs. 8.10–8.12). It shows the typical periventricular plaques and also plaques as small as 3 to 4 mm. Using contrast material, MRI identifies acute plaques and is helpful in monitoring therapeutic efficacy. MS plaques are hypointense (black holes) on T1-weighted images and hyperintense on T2-weighted images. Proton-density images better delineate the periventricular lesions,

TABLE 8.2.
Multiple Sclerosis: Common Symptoms and Signs

Ocular	Somatosensory
Optic/retrobulbar neuritis	Paresthesias, dysesthesias, sensory deficits, pain, Lhermitte's sign
Scotomas	Autonomic/endocrine
Temporal pallor of optic disc	Bladder, bowel, sexual, cardiovascular, temperature, eating, sleeping disorders
Diplopia	Speech/language impairment
Internuclear ophthalmoplegia	Cognitive decline
Nystagmus	Psychiatric
Cranial nerves	Behavioral changes
Facial numbness	Euphoria
Facial palsy	Depression
Trigeminal neuralgia	Fatigue
Vertigo	
Motor	
Weakness,	
Ataxia	
Tremor	
Spasticity	
Reflex changes	
Pathologic reflexes	

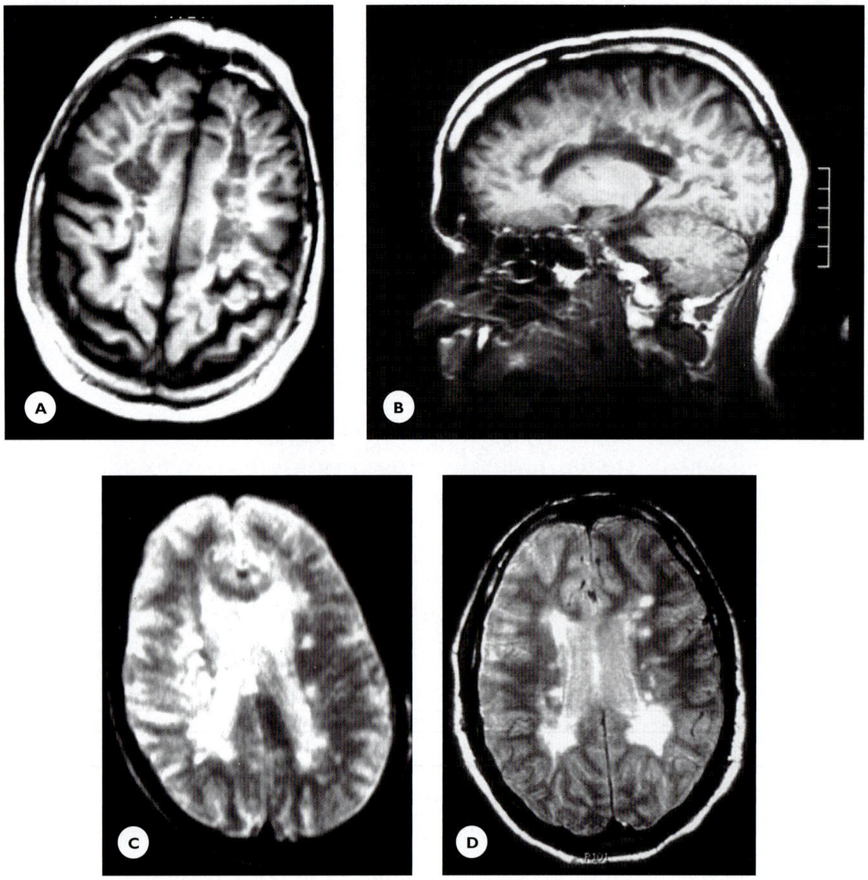

FIGURE 8.11
MRI of chronic MS plaques. Chronic lesions examined in axial planes. **A.** T1-weighted image shows extensive confluent hypointense lesions (black holes) in centrum semiovale. **B.** Parasagittal image shows lesions perpendicular to the ventricular surface (Dawson's fingers). **C.** On T2-weighted image, the lesions are hyperintense and the periventricular lesions are indistinct from the CSF. **D.** On proton density (PD) images, the hyperintense periventricular and small white matter lesions are distinct.

because the CSF is darker here than on T2-weighted images. The plaques are often oriented perpendicularly to the ventricular surface (Dawson's fingers). Magnetic resonance spectroscopy (MRS) is useful in demonstrating axonal injury. By measuring the concentration of *N*-acetyl aspartate (NAA), a neuron-specific marker, MRS monitors axonal dysfunction, which correlates with clinical disability. NAA levels are decreased in acute and chronic plaques. A temporary decrease in acute plaques is associated with reversible neurologic deficits. An increase in choline, a cellular membrane marker, indicates myelin breakdown.

Visual, somatosensory, and brainstem evoked potentials demonstrate a delay or a block in the conduction of nervous impulses and detect clinically silent plaques. CSF abnormalities are not specific, but an increase in γ-globulin fraction and the presence of oligoclonal IgG bands further support the diagnosis. An acute solitary plaque, by producing edema with mass effect, may mimic a space-occupying lesion requiring a diagnostic brain biopsy. The definite diagnosis of MS is based on (a) two or more episodes of neurologic deficits separated in time by at least 1 month, (b) two or more noncontiguous anatomic lesions on MRI, and (c) the absence of an alternative clinical diagnosis.

Although the course of MS is not predictable, two major forms are distinguished: remitting-relapsing and progressive—either from the onset (primary) or after a remitting-relapsing course (secondary). The outcome of an attack is defined by the anatomic and functional relationships between the myelin sheath and its axon, and between the myelin and the myelin-forming oligodendroglia. The severity and extent of axonal injury largely determines the degree of recovery or the persistence of neurologic deficits. Briefly, after the inflammation has resolved and the myelin debris has been removed, the conduction of the neural impulses is reestablished in the denuded nerve fibers. This results in remission with full or partial recovery of neurologic deficits. If remyelination of nerve fibers occurs, this also contributes to remission. New plaques, which may develop at any time throughout the course of the disease, account for relapses. New attacks of myelin destruction, with a further reduction in nerve fibers within and around an established plaque (active chronic plaque) account for the progression of existing neurologic deficits. The disability becomes permanent when the structural continuity of the nerve fibers is disrupted and wallerian degeneration develops.

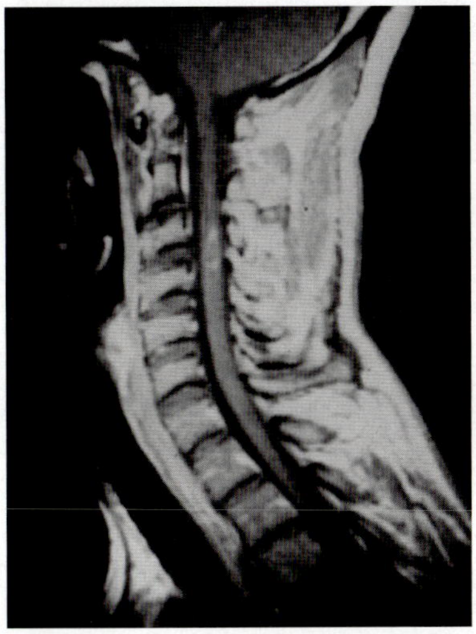

FIGURE 8.12
MRI of MS plaques in the spinal cord. Multiple small hyperintense lesions are present in several segments.

The average duration of the disease is 25 to 30 years. Approximately one-third of patients have a benign course, with little disability for 15 years. Death is usually due to an intercurrent infection.

Variants of Multiple Sclerosis

Neuromyelitis optica or Devic's disease is characterized by an acute inflammatory demyelination confined to the optic nerves and spinal cord, often the cervical segments. The demyelination, in severe cases, progresses to necrosis and even cavitation (Fig. 8.13).

Charcot classic type MS shows the typical clinical features and course of MS.

Marburg type MS has an acute onset and rapid progression. Death usually occurs within 1 to 6 months of onset.

Balo's concentric sclerosis is characterized by concentric zones of demyelination alternating with zones of intact myelin, believed to represent remyelination

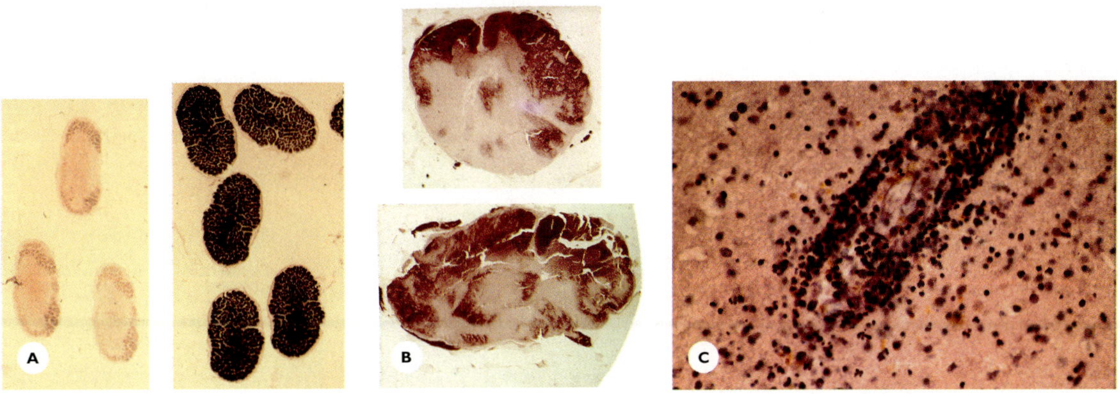

FIGURE 8.13
Neuromyelitis optica or Devic's disease. A 30-year-old woman presented with a history of headaches and rapidly progressing loss of vision in the left eye that began about 5 weeks following a difficult labor and a short febrile episode. Shortly after the onset of visual impairment, she developed paresthesias and weakness in all four extremities and urinary retention. After a short period of improvement, her condition deteriorated; she became quadriplegic and experienced respiratory difficulties. Six months after the onset of symptoms, she died. **A.** Extensive demyelination in left optic nerve. **B.** Extensive demyelination in the swollen cervical and thoracic cord (Weil stain). **C.** Massive perivascular lymphocytic infiltration (HE).

(Fig. 8.14). *Schilder's disease* refers to extensive demyelination in the cerebral hemispheres, with sudanophilic breakdown products (Fig. 8.15). The disease affects both children and adults.

The association of MS with *inflammatory demyelinating polyradiculopathy* is rare. A few cases have been documented using MRI, electrophysiologic studies, and nerve biopsy.

DISEASES WITH PROBABLE AUTOIMMUNE PATHOGENESIS

Acute Disseminated Postinfectious and Postvaccination Encephalomyelitis

Acute disseminated postinfectious and postvaccination encephalomyelitis develops 1 to 3 weeks following a viral or bacterial infection such as measles, varicella, rubella, influenza, mumps, infectious mononucleosis, or scarlet fever, or it develops following vaccination for rabies, smallpox, measles, typhoid, and paratyphoid.

The onset is acute with headaches, fever, meningeal signs, focal neurologic deficits, and often seizures. The disease resolves within several weeks, and the course is monophasic. The outcome varies from full recovery through variable residual neurologic impairment to death, which occurs in about 20% to 30% of cases.

Grossly, the brain and spinal cord are swollen and congested. The histology is characterized by perivenous inflammatory demyelination. Lymphocytes and lipid-laden macrophages fill the demyelinated zones (Fig. 8.16).

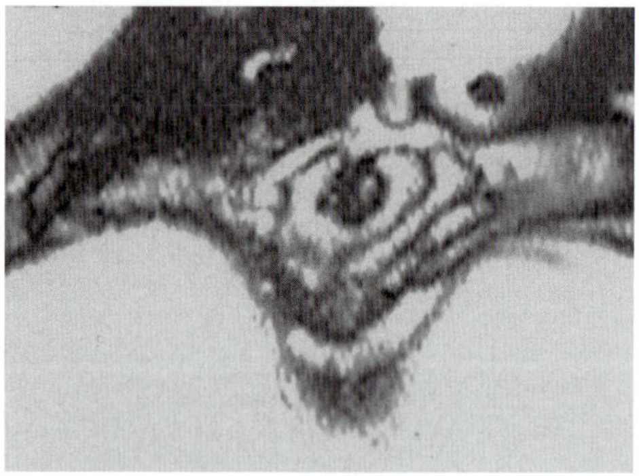

FIGURE 8.14
Balo's concentric sclerosis shows zones of myelin losses alternating with zones of intact myelin in a circular fashion (myelin stain).

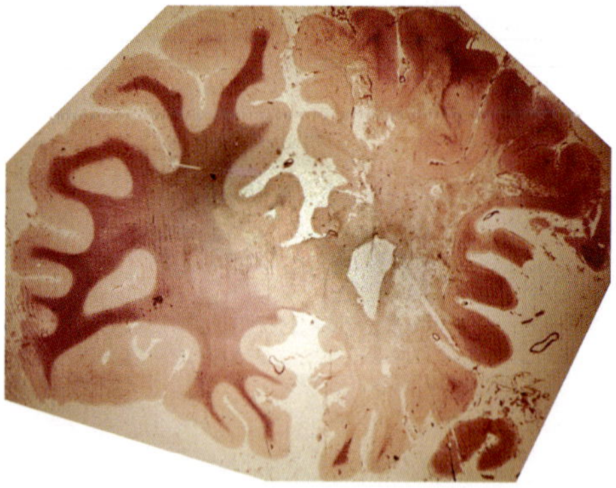

FIGURE 8.15
Schilder's disease in a 40-year-old woman. Extensive demyelination in one frontal lobe extends into the corpus callosum (PTAH).

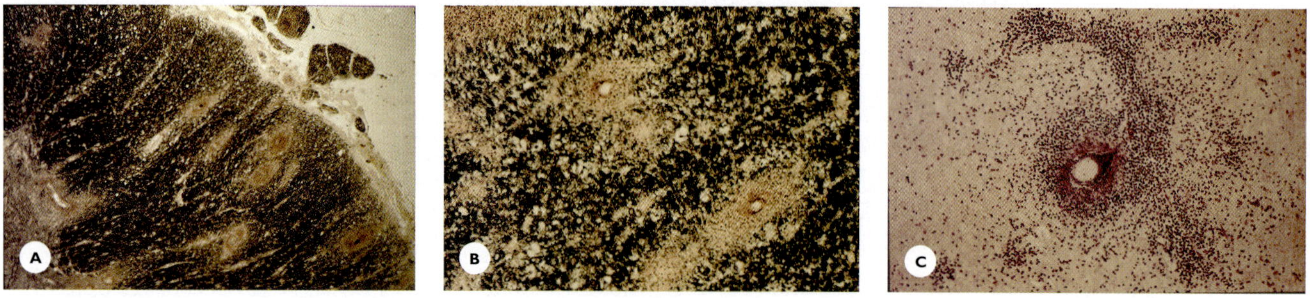

FIGURE 8.16
Acute disseminated perivenous encephalomyelitis. **A** and **B.** Spinal cord showing demyelination along radially oriented veins (myelin stain). **C.** Dense infiltrations with neutrophils, lymphocytes, and macrophages in the demyelinated zones (cresyl violet).

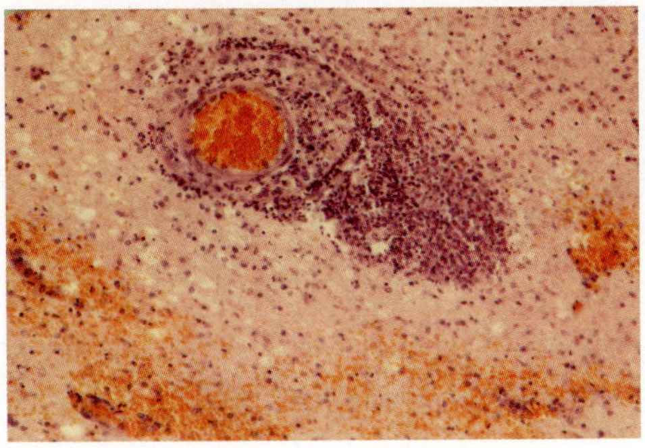

FIGURE 8.17
Acute hemorrhagic leukoencephalitis. A 42-year-old man, with a 3-week history of muscle and stomach aches and cough, suddenly developed headaches, neck pain, fever, and left hemiparesis. Four days later, he became hemiplegic and comatose. Six days after the headaches began, he died. Grossly, the hemispheric white matter displayed multiple petechial hemorrhages. Histologic section shows fibrinoid necrosis of a small vessel, dense perivascular and diffuse parenchymal infiltrations with neutrophils and lymphocytes, and small hemorrhages (HE).

Acute Hemorrhagic Leukoencephalitis

Acute hemorrhagic leukoencephalitis or Hurst's disease usually develops after a nonspecific upper respiratory infection. The onset is acute, the course fulminant, and the mortality high. Mental changes, focal neurologic deficits, and seizures are common.

Grossly, the brain is swollen and congested, and the white matter displays multiple confluent petechial hemorrhages. Characteristic histological features are fibrinoid necrosis of the arterioles and capillaries, ring- and ball-shaped petechial hemorrhages, and perivascular infiltrations with neutrophils, lymphocytes, and macrophages (Fig. 8.17).

BIBLIOGRAPHY

Cook, S. D. (Ed.). (2001). *Handbook of multiple sclerosis*, 3rd edition. New York: Marcel Dekker.

Ferguson, B., Matyszak, M. K., Esiri, M. M., & Perry, V. H. (1997). Axonal damage in acute multiple sclerosis lesions. *Brain 120*, 393–399.

Kidd, D., Barkhof, F., McConnel, R., et al. (2000). Cortical lesions in multiple sclerosis. *Brain 122*, 17–26.

Lucchinetty, C., Brück, W., Parisi, J., et al. (2004). Heterogeneity of multiple sclerosis lesions: implications for the pathogenesis and demyelination. *Ann Neurol 47*, 707–717.

Prineas, J. W., McDonald, W. I., and Franklin, R. J. M. (2002). Demyelinating diseases. In Graham, D. I., and Lantos, P. L. (Eds.), *Greenfield's Neuropathology*, 7th edition. London: Arnold.

Raine, C. S., & Wu, E. (1993). Multiple sclerosis: remyelination in acute lesions. *J Neuropathol Exp Neurol 52*, 199–204.

REVIEW QUESTIONS

1. Neurologic manifestations commonly encountered in patients with multiple sclerosis (MS) are:

   A. Paresthesias in extremities
   B. Internuclear ophthalmoplegia
   C. Difficulty with balance
   D. Sudden loss of vision
   E. Urinary retention

2. The histologic features of an acute MS plaque include all of the following *except*:

   A. Perivascular lymphocytic infiltrations
   B. Breakdown of myelin
   C. Axonal swelling
   D. Capillary proliferation
   E. Lipid-laden macrophages

3. Early axonal damage in MS plaque is best revealed in paraffin section with:
   A. Luxol fast blue
   B. Antibodies to β-APP
   C. Phosphotungstic acid hematoxylin (PTAH)
   D. Cresyl violet
   E. None of these

4. The current view on the pathogenesis of MS is:
   A. Reactivation of a dormant viral infection
   B. An autoimmune reaction to myelin
   C. Acute infection with papovavirus
   D. All of these
   E. None of these

5. The severity of neurologic deficits best correlates with:
   A. Virulence of an infective virus
   B. Degeneration of axons
   C. Loss of astrocytes
   D. Loss of oligodendrocytes
   E. Loss of myelin

6. The term *shadow plaque* refers to:
   A. Partially demyelinated plaque
   B. Remyelinating plaque
   C. Chronic inactive plaque
   D. None of these
   E. All of these

7. Potential risk factors for MS include:
   A. Familial occurrence
   B. Infection with varicella-zoster virus
   C. Association with HLA-DR2
   D. All of these
   E. None of these

8. Encephalitis that develops following smallpox vaccination is characterized by all the following *except*:
   A. It presents with perivenous demyelination.
   B. It presents with perivenous inflammation.
   C. It has a remitting-relapsing course.
   D. It has a monophasic course.
   E. It is more common in women.

9. Devic disease is characterized by demyelination predominantly in the:
   A. Pons and spinal cord
   B. Optic nerves and spinal cord
   C. Optic nerves and pons
   D. Pons and cerebellum
   E. Optic nerves and cerebral hemispheres

10. The MRI features of MS plaques include:
    A. They appear as hyperintense lesions on T2-weighted images.
    B. They appear as black holes on T1-weighted images.
    C. Acute plaques enhance with contrast.
    D. The lesions are not specific.
    E. Periventricular distribution is common.

(Answers are provided in the Appendix.)

CHAPTER 9

Hereditary Neurometabolic Diseases

Lysosomal Diseases
Peroxisomal Diseases
Leukodystrophies
Mitochondrial Diseases
Amino Acid Metabolic Diseases
Carbohydrates Metabolic Diseases
Copper Metabolic Diseases
Neuroaxonal Dystrophies
Miscellaneous Neurometabolic Diseases

Inherited neurometabolic diseases result from genetically determined defects in the biochemical processes of neural tissue, specifically, the deficient activity of enzymes or activator proteins. A group of diseases is caused by dysfunctions of the cellular organelles—lysosomes, peroxisomes, and mitochondria. The biochemical defects, the genes responsible, and their chromosomal loci have been defined, as have the types of mutations, in many diseases. The majority of diseases are inherited as an autosomal recessive trait; some are transmitted in an X-linked or autosomal dominant mode. Most diseases are panethnic, but some are prevalent in particular ethnic groups.

Inherited metabolic diseases chiefly afflict children. Some diseases manifest at birth, some develop during infancy or early childhood, and some occur from childhood to adulthood. The clinical course is progressive; the rate varies according to the disease. Malignant early childhood diseases progress relentlessly, and death occurs within several months or a few years. Children affected with more benign diseases survive into adolescence or adulthood and usually present with mental retardation, neurologic deficits, and seizures. Juvenile- and adult-onset diseases may have a protracted course.

The clinical presentation is highly variable. It may be limited to the nervous system, or it may be multisystemic, affecting the eyes, visceral organs, skin, muscles, blood vessels, and skeleton. Some diseases present with characteristic somatic abnormalities that aid in their diagnosis.

A definitive diagnosis rests on demonstrations of a specific enzyme deficiency. Enzyme assays are performed on plasma, leucocytes, and cultured skin fibroblasts. Prenatal diagnosis is possible using enzyme assays on cultured amniocytes at 18 to 20 weeks' gestation, or on chorionic villi at 10 weeks' gestation. A number of laboratory tests and ancillary procedures are useful in supporting the diagnosis (Table 9.1). Biopsies of peripheral nerves, muscles, skin, and rectal mucosa are useful in demonstrating deposits of abnormal metabolites. Neuroimaging is a mandatory complementary diagnostic tool. DNA studies are important to identify the mutant gene and type of mutation and to detect carriers of the disease.

Early diagnosis is imperative, because therapy using dietary restriction or enzyme replacement is effective in some diseases, provided it is begun very early in life. The therapeutic benefits of bone marrow and liver transplantation are variable. Unfortunately, for a number of devastating neurometabolic diseases, no curative therapy exists as yet. Genetic counseling is an important means of prevention, and gene and stem cell therapies may hold future promise.

The pathology presents a broad spectrum of changes affecting particular anatomic regions. Specific neuronal and glial changes, extensive neuronal losses, or widespread myelin degeneration are characteristic. Notably, concomitant histogenetic malformations and inflammatory reactions distinguish the pathology of some diseases.

Hereditary neurometabolic diseases are grouped into the following major categories:

- Diseases caused by malfunctioning of subcellular organelles: lysosomes, peroxisomes, and mitochondria.
- Diseases caused by defective metabolism of amino acids, carbohydrates, and copper
- Neuroaxonal dystrophies
- Miscellaneous diseases

TABLE 9.1.

Common Tests for Diagnosis of Hereditary Neurometabolic Diseases

Enzyme assays on leukocytes and skin fibroblasts
Blood and urine tests for abnormal metabolites
CSF examination
Blood smear for abnormalities of blood cells
Bone marrow aspirate for storage products
Biopsy of skin, sural nerve, muscle, conjunctiva, rectal mucosa
Neuroimaging
DNA study
Prenatal enzyme assay on amniotic cells or chorionic villi

LYSOSOMAL DISEASES

The lysosomes, membrane-bound cytoplasmic organelles, are rich in the hydrolytic enzymes that are essential for the degradation of complex lipids, complex carbohydrates, and mucopolysaccharides. Mutations in genes encoding these enzymes cause partial or complete loss of enzymatic activity, which then results in the accumulation and storage of the corresponding substrates within the lysosomal compartment. Lysosomal diseases are classified according to the chemical composition of the stored material:

- Neuronal lipidoses
- Neuronal ceroid lipofuscinoses
- Carbohydrate disorders

Neuronal Lipidoses

These diseases are inherited in an autosomal recessive mode except for the Fabry's disease, which has an X-linked recessive inheritance. They affect chiefly infants and children and may also occur in juveniles and adults. The diseases display both similar and distinctive clinical features. Generally, infantile diseases with onset at 6 months to 2.5 years manifest with loss of already acquired psychomotor skills, growth retardation, visual impairment, and often seizures. Death occurs within 1 to 3 years of onset. Juvenile diseases with onset at 4 to 8 years of age manifest with combinations of pyramidal, extrapyramidal, and cerebellar symptoms and signs; behavioral changes; and mental decline. The clinical course may range from 10 to 15 years. Adult-onset diseases present with psychiatric symptoms, cognitive decline, and variable neurologic signs. The clinical course is protracted, averaging 15 to 20 years. The diagnosis requires enzyme assays complemented by ancillary tests (see Table 9.1). In several diseases, magnetic resonance imaging (MRI) demonstrates abnormalities in basal

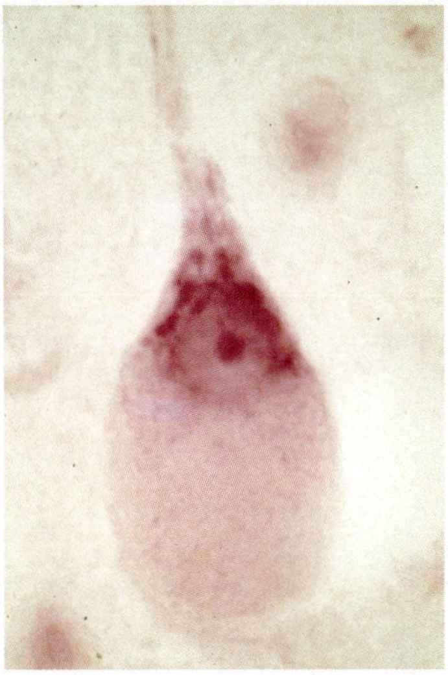

FIGURE 9.1
Ballooned cortical pyramidal neuron, a histologic hallmark of storage diseases. The perikaryon is large, pear shaped. The nucleus and some residual Nissl substance are displaced toward the apical dendrite.

ganglia and thalamus in the early stage and cortical and white matter atrophy in the late stage.

The lipids involved in neuronal lipidoses are the sphingolipids: sphingomyelin, cerebrosides, and gangliosides, all normal constituents of the neurons. They have in common a ceramide moiety (derived from the amino alcohol sphingosine) attached to a long-chain fatty acid. The deficiency of a specific enzyme blocks the degradation of its lipid, which then accumulates in excessive amounts in the perikaryon of the neurons, first hindering their function and eventually leading to their disintegration. The neuronal storage is widespread in the central, peripheral, and autonomic nervous systems. Ballooned neurons filled with storage material are histologic markers (Fig. 9.1). A number of diseases are multisystemic. In these, the retina and the visceral organs, chiefly the liver and spleen, participate in the storage process (Table 9.2).

GM2 Gangliosidosis

The gangliosides are glycosphingolipids consisting of ceramide, hexose molecules, sialic acid, and hexosamine,

TABLE 9.2.

Lysosomal Enzyme Deficiencies with Systemic Lipid Storage

Diseases	*Deficient Enzymes*	*Stored Products*
GM1 Gangliosidosis	β-Galactosidase	GM1 Galactoside Oligosaccharides Keratan sulfate
Niemann-Pick disease	Sphingomyelinase	Sphingomyelin
Gaucher's disease	Glucocerebrosidase	Glucocerebroside
Farber's disease	Ceramidase	Ceramide
Fabry's disease	α-Galactosidase	Trihexosyl glycolipids
Wolman's disease	Acid lipase	Triglycerides, cholesteryl esters

normally present in the plasma membrane of the neurons. Catabolic degradation of GM2 ganglioside to GM3 ganglioside requires two isoenzymes—hexosaminidase A (HexA) and hexosaminidase B (HexB) and an activator protein. HexA consists of an α-subunit and a β-subunit, and HexB consists of two β-subunits (Table 9.3).

The three genetic variants of GM2 gangliosidosis have similar clinical expression.

- *Tay-Sachs disease* or *variant B* is caused by mutations in the gene for the α-subunit of hexosaminidase A. The gene (HEXA) maps to chromosome 15.
- *Sandhoff disease* or *variant O* is caused by mutations in the gene for the β-subunits of hexosaminidase A and B. The gene (HEX B) maps to chromosome 5.
- *Variant AB* is caused by mutations in the gene of GM2 activator protein (GM2A), located on chromosome 5.

Tay-Sachs Disease

Tay-Sachs disease exemplifies GM2 gangliosidosis. The disease has a predilection for the Ashkenazi Jewish population. Distinct clinical features are a fine complexion; regression of psychomotor functions; visual impairment, rapidly progressing to blindness; a cherry red spot at the macula; startle reactions, particularly to sound; seizures; and macrocephaly in the late course of the

TABLE 9.3.
GM2 Gangliosidosis

Diseases	*Enzyme Deficiency*	*Gene Symbol*	*Gene Locus*
Tay-Sachs disease variant B	Hex A–α-subunit	HEX A	Chromosome 15
Sandhoff's disease variant O	Hex A–β-subunit Hex B–β-subunit	HEX B	Chromosome 5
Variant AB	GM2 Activator–protein	GM2 A	Chromosome 5

Hex A, hexosaminidase A; Hex B, hexosaminidase B.

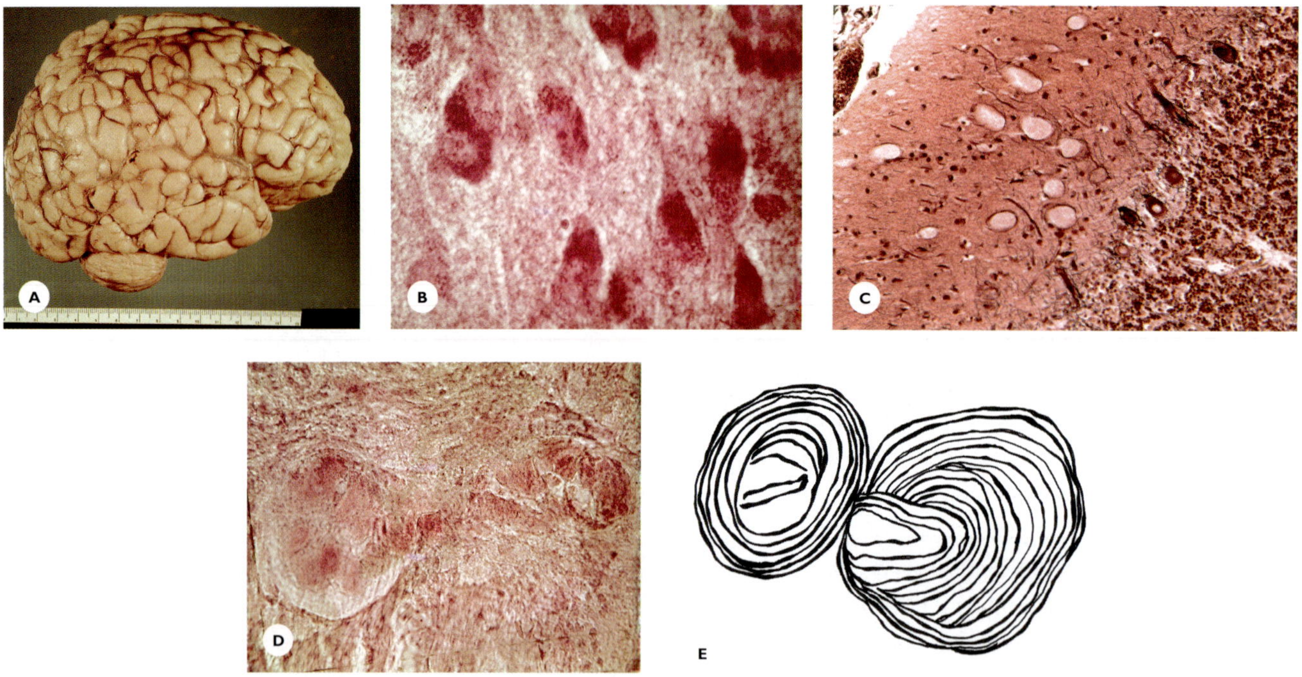

FIGURE 9.2
Tay-Sachs disease. A first-born infant girl of healthy Ashkenazi Jewish parents developed normally up to 6 months of age, when she became listless and unresponsive to her environment. A few months later, cherry red spot of the macula was diagnosed. She startled in response to all stimuli and developed seizures. She steadily regressed to a vegetative state and, at 20 months of age, she died. **A.** The brain is large, weighing 1,400 g. **B.** Frozen section of the cerebral cortex shows accumulation of glycolipids in the neurons (oil-red O stain). **C.** Cerebellum shows Purkinje cell losses and expansion of empty-appearing dendrites due to extraction of lipids during tissue processing (Bodian stain). **D.** Autonomic ganglia in rectal mucosa contain lipid material (Oil-red O). **E.** Schematic drawing of concentric lamellar bodies, the EM appearance of storage material.

disease. MRI may demonstrate hyperintensities in the basal ganglia and thalami in early stage of the disease. By the age of 18 to 36 months, the disease is inevitably fatal.

The rare late infantile, juvenile, and adult variants of GM2 gangliosidosis present with psychomotor regression; mental decline, slowly progressing to dementia; seizures; and neurologic deficits. The clinical course is protracted.

Pathology: Grossly, the brain is large and heavy, weighing 1,200 to 1,400 g (Fig. 9.2). The ventricles are enlarged, and the central hemispheric white matter is soft. Histologically, the neurons throughout the nervous system are markedly swollen, ballooned with the Nissl substance, and the nucleus displaced to the periphery. The stored material stains positively for lipids with oil-red O and Luxol fast blue, and for sugar with PAS reagent. Under the electron microscope, the stored material appears as concentric membranous cytoplasmic bodies (MCBs) with a homogenous or finely granular center (see Fig. 9.2). In time, the distended neurons burst and disintegrate, leaving empty spaces. Macrophages remove the debris while reactive astrocytes replace the neuronal losses. The hemispheric white matter shows variable degrees of failure of myelination and/or demyelination.

GM1 Gangliosidosis

GM1 gangliosidosis is a systemic disorder. The mutating gene coding for the enzyme β-galactosidase is located on chromosome 3. Deficiency of the enzyme results in the accumulation of GM1 gangliosides in the neurons. In the infantile form, the neuronal storage is associated with storage of oligosaccharides and keratan sulfate in the viscera and vascular endothelium. Facial dysmorphism, skeletal anomalies, and hepatomegaly are characteristic features, resembling Hurler's disease. Vacuolated lymphocytes occur in circulating blood. Oligosaccharides and keratan sulfate are excreted in the urine. The pathology is characterized by the presence of foamy macrophages storing PAS-positive material in the liver, spleen, lung, lymph nodes, and bone marrow. Neuronal storage of gangliosides is ubiquitous and is also present in the glial cells. In adults, the basal ganglia are chiefly affected.

Morquio B Disease

Morquio B disease is caused by a deficiency of the enzyme β-galactosidase. Formerly classified in the group of mucopolysaccharidosis, at present it is regarded as a variant of GM1 gangliosidosis.

Niemann-Pick Disease

Niemann-Pick disease, types A and B, are systemic lipidoses caused by a deficiency of the enzyme acid sphingomyelinase, encoded by a gene on chromosome 11. As a result, sphingomyelin accumulates in the neurons and visceral organs in type A, and only in the viscera in type B. Type A occurs in Ashkenazi Jewish population and affects chiefly children. A macular cherry red spot may be present. Foam cells are found in the bone marrow, and vacuolated lymphocytes are found in blood. The clinical course averages from 1 to 3 years.

Pathology: Grossly, the brain is atrophic. Histologically, ballooned neurons contain sphingomyelin, which in frozen sections stains positively for lipids and weakly with PAS (Fig. 9.3). Systemic pathology is characterized by the presence of foamy microphages in the liver, spleen, lung, lymph nodes, and bone marrow.

Gaucher's Disease

Gaucher's disease, a systemic lipidosis, is caused by deficient activity of the enzyme β-glucosidase, encoded by a gene located on chromosome 1. Subsequently, glucocerebrosides accumulate in the visceral organs and the brain. Among the three clinical phenotypes, the nervous system is affected in type 2 and type 3. Hepatosplenomegaly is evident in both. In infants, type 2 presents with bulbar symptoms, strabismus, and pyramidal and extrapyramidal symptoms. The clinical course averages 3 to 4 years. In juveniles and adults, type 3 presents with horizontal supranuclear gaze palsy, bulbar symptoms, cognitive decline, myoclonus, and seizures. The clinical course averages 10 to 15 years.

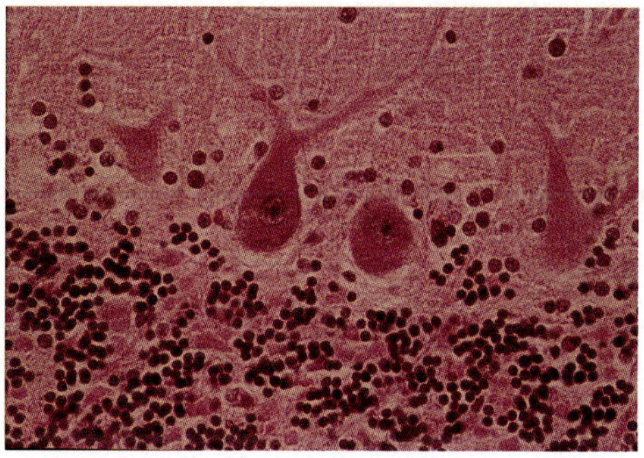

FIGURE 9.3
Niemann-Pick disease. Ballooned Purkinje cells in the cerebellum with distended dendrites (HE).

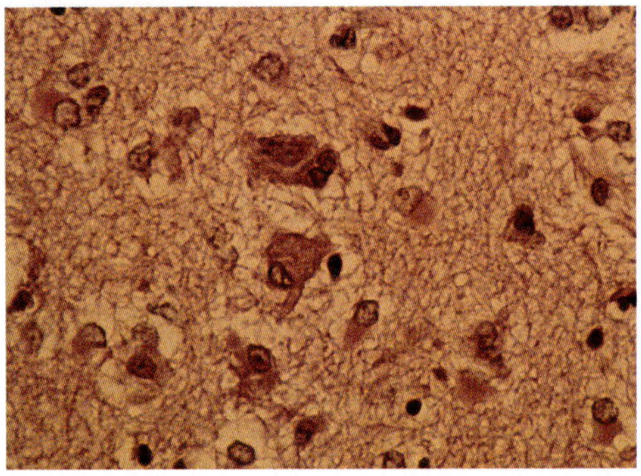

FIGURE 9.4
Gaucher's disease. Gaucher cell in the hemispheric white matter (HE).

Presence of Gaucher cells characterizes the pathology (Fig. 9.4). These cells of monocyte/macrophage origin are dispersed throughout the cerebral cortex, deep gray structures, and white matter. Neuronal losses are prominent. Gaucher cells are evident in the liver, spleen, lymph nodes, and bone marrow.

Farber's Disease

Farber's disease of infancy is caused by a deficiency of the enzyme ceramidase, encoded by a gene located on chromosome 8. Ceramide accumulates in the brain, visceral organs, skin, and lymph nodes. Cutaneous nodules, joint pain, hepatosplenomegaly, psychomotor regression, seizures, and a hoarse cry are characteristic clinical manifestations. The pathology is characterized by (a) widespread neuronal storage of PAS-positive ceramide; (b) foamy macrophages in viscera, lymph nodes, and bone marrow; and (c) granulomatous nodules of histiocytes, lymphocytes, and giant cells in the skin, joints, and various tissues.

Fabry's Disease

Fabry disease, an X-linked recessive lipidosis, results from a deficiency of the enzyme α-galactosidase, encoded by a gene on the long arm of the X-chromosome. Consequently, ceramide trihexoside and related glycolipids accumulate in various tissues. Clinically, the disease is characterized by angiokeratomas of the skin; cornea opacities; burning pain in extremities; gastrointestinal, renal, and cardiovascular disorders; and strokes.

The pathology consists of glycolipid storage in the neurons and glial cells in the central, peripheral, and autonomic nervous systems, and in macrophages in the vascular walls and affected organs.

Wolman's Disease

Wolman's disease, a rare autosomal disorder of infants, is caused by a deficiency of the lysosomal enzyme acid lipase. As a result, triglycerides and cholesteryl-esters accumulate in the visceral organs, lymph nodes, bone marrow, and adrenals, which often show cortical calcifications. The brain shows lipid-containing foamy cells in the choroid plexus and leptomeninges. Death occurs in the first year of life. A milder form of the disease affects adults and presents with hepatomegaly, premature atherosclerosis, and hyperlipoproteinemia.

Neuronal Ceroid Lipofuscinoses

This group of lysosomal diseases is distinguished by neuronal storage of glycoproteolipids that resemble ceroid and lipofuscin. Neuronal ceroid lipofuscinosis (NCL) may occur any time from infancy to late adulthood. In children, it is the most common lipid storage disease. The diseases are panethnic, with a worldwide distribution. The mode of inheritance is autosomal recessive. To date, eight mutant genes (CLN1 through CLN8) have been implicated in NCL, and six of them have been identified. The following classification is based on genotype and clinical phenotype correlation:

- The gene CLN1, located on chromosome 1, encodes the lysosomal enzyme palmitoyl protein thioesterase 1 (PPT1). Mutations in the gene result in four phenotypes: infantile, or *Haltia-Santavuori disease*, late infantile, juvenile, and adult types.
- The gene CLN2, located on chromosome 11, encodes the lysosomal enzyme tripeptidyl peptidase 1 (TPP1).

Mutations in the gene produce the classical *late infantile* or *Jansky-Bielschowsky disease.*

- The gene CLN3, located on chromosome 16, encodes a lysosomal membrane protein. Mutations in the gene produce the *juvenile* or *Batten-Vogt-Spielmeyer disease.*
- The gene CLN4 is a hypothetical gene for the *adult NCL* or *Kuf disease.*
- The genes CLN5 through CLN8 genes are implicated in the Finnish variant, the juvenile variant, and the Northern epilepsy syndrome with mental retardation. The genes encode lysosomal membrane proteins. Two of the proteins (CLN6 and CLN8) are probably localized to the endoplasmic reticulum.

Clinical Features

Cerebellar ataxia, seizures, and myoclonic jerks characterize all age-related variants. Infantile and late-infantile NCL present with psychomotor regression and visual failure progressing to blindness from macular and retinal degeneration. Behavioral changes, cognitive decline, visual impairment from pigmentary retinal degeneration, and vacuolated lymphocytes occur in juvenile NCL. Adult NCL may be of early onset (phenotype A), presenting with cognitive impairment, or it may be of late onset (phenotype B), presenting with behavioral and affective changes and motor deficits. Mixed forms may also occur. Vision is not affected in either. Low-frequency photic stimulation typically evokes myoclonic responses. Autosomal dominant inheritance has been reported in one family.

The diagnosis is confirmed with skin, conjunctival, or rectal biopsy. Histochemical stains reveal the storage material. Electron microscopic examination shows distinct ultrastructural patterns. Biochemical enzyme assays confirm lysosomal protease deficiencies in infantile and late infantile diseases. Genetic studies complement the diagnostic evaluation.

Clinical Course

The earlier the onset, the faster the progression and shorter the course, averaging from a few years to 10 years in infantile and late infantile, and ranging from 10 to 20 years in juvenile and adult NCLs.

Pathology

Grossly, cerebral and cerebellar atrophy is present in all clinical types, but the severity varies greatly, being very severe in the infantile and late infantile and only moderately severe in the juvenile and adult diseases (Figs. 9.5, 9.6, and 9.7).

Histologically, the neuronal storage is most prominent in the infantile and late infantile variants. Ballooned neurons dominate throughout the brain in the early stage. Severe neuronal losses in the cerebral and cerebellar cortex and deep gray structures dominate in the late stage (see Fig. 9.5). Astrocytosis parallels the neuronal losses. The white matter shows variable myelin degeneration and astrofibrosis. Neuronal storage and losses are moderate in the juvenile and adult variants.

The stored compound is composed of proteolipids combined with saccharides. The protein component consists of two fractions: (a) subunit C of the mitochondrial ATP synthase (SOMAS) and (b) saposin (SAP). The compound autofluoresces in ultraviolet light, stains positively with oil-red O, Sudan black B, and PAS. It displays various ultrastructural patterns, distinct for each major disease: granular deposits in early infantile, curvilinear bodies in late infantile, and fingerprint-like deposits in juvenile NCL. Storage without conspicuous cell losses occurs in the viscera, vascular endothelium, sweat glands, skin, and muscles.

Lysosomal Carbohydrate Diseases

Deficiencies of lysosomal enzymes necessary for the degradation of complex carbohydrates result in an accumulation of nondegraded products in various tissues and cells. Such products are the mucopolysaccharides, the mucolipids, the glycoproteins, and the glycogen. The diseases affect chiefly infants and children. Despite genetic and enzymatic heterogeneity, many diseases share facial and skeletal abnormalities, multiorgan manifestations, and urinary excretion of abnormal metabolites, mucopolysaccharides, mucolipids, and glycoproteins (Table 9.4).

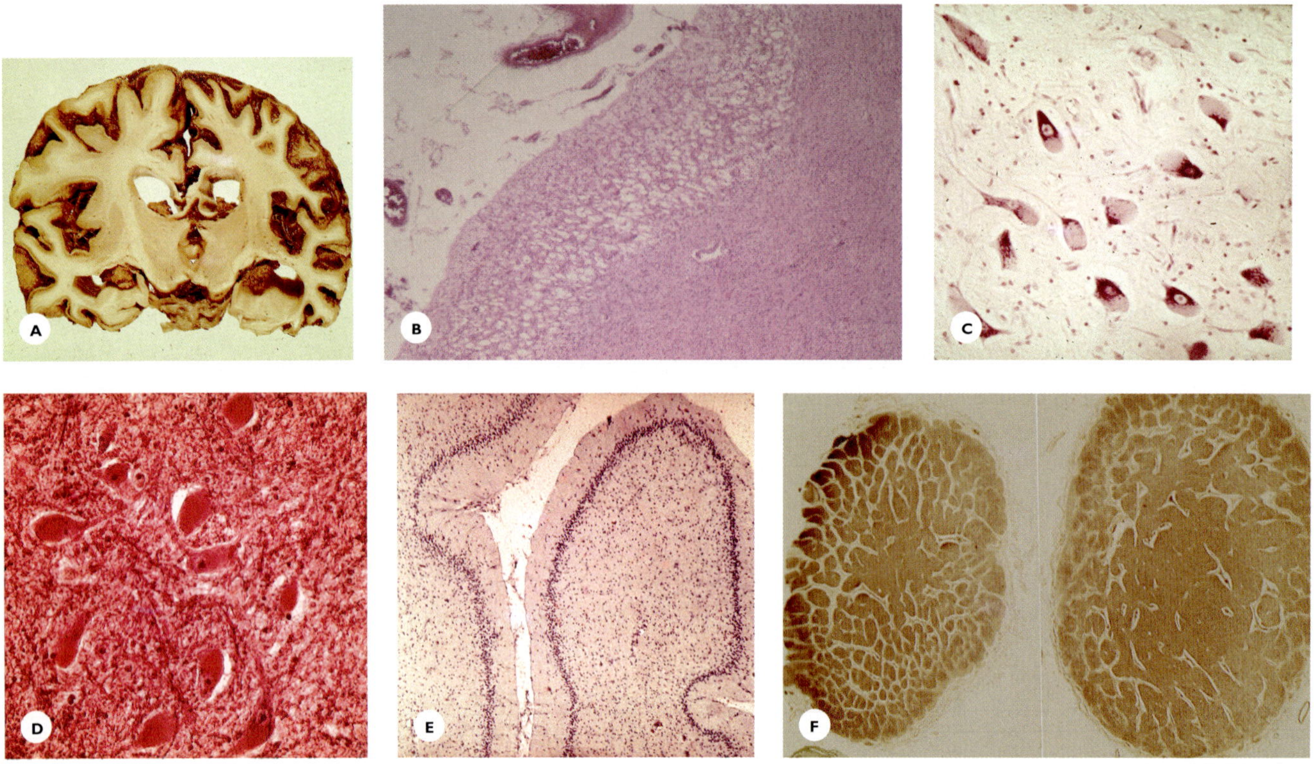

FIGURE 9.5

Late infantile neuronal ceroid lipofuscinosis. This boy's disease began at 3 years of age, when he had his first generalized tonic-clonic seizure and his gait became unsteady. At 4 years of age, he developed jerking movements in his body and extremities. He gradually lost his motor skills and language. By age 5 years, he was blind, unresponsive, unable to hold his head up or sit, and displayed constant myoclonic jerks. At age 6 years, he died. **A.** Transverse section of the brain at thalamus level shows severe generalized cortical and white matter atrophy and enlarged ventricles. **B.** The cerebral cortex, totally depleted of neurons, is spongy. **C.** The medullary neurons are swollen (Cresyl-violet) and **(D)** filled with PAS positive material (PAS stain). **E.** The cerebellar cortex is depleted of Purkinje cells and granule cells. Instead, a prominent astrocytic layer outlines the site of lost Purkinje cells (Cresyl-violet). **F.** Both optic nerves are degenerated (Weil stain).

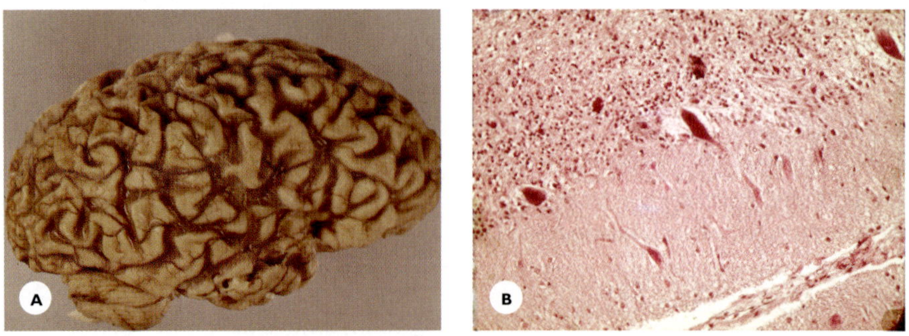

FIGURE 9.6

Juvenile neuronal ceroid lipofuscinosis. The disease of a 6-year-old girl began with failing eyesight. Over the years, her mental functions, motor skills, and speech progressively deteriorated. After an 8-year clinical course, she died. **A.** The brain shows a moderately severe cortical atrophy. **B.** The cerebellum shows Purkinje cell losses and storage of PAS-positive material in remaining Purkinje cell and dendrites (PAS stain).

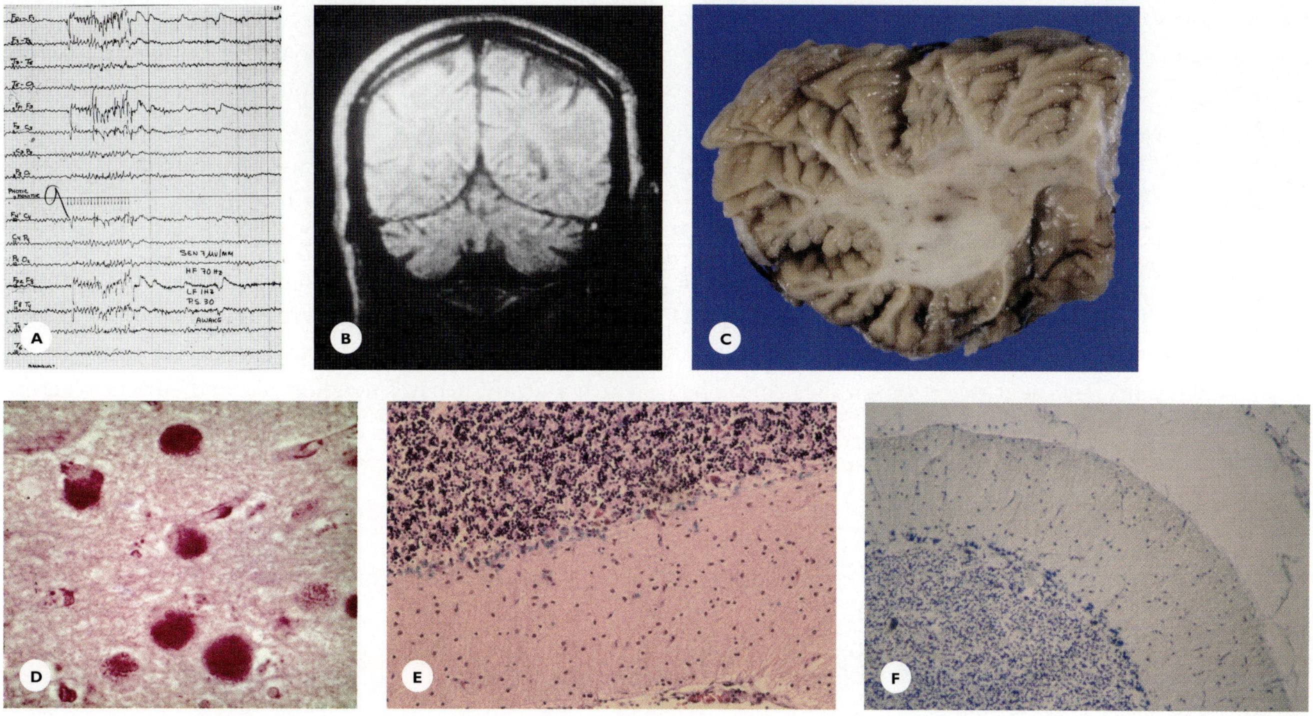

FIGURE 9.7
Adult ceroid lipofuscinosis. Difficulty walking was the presenting symptom in a 57-year-old man. Examination revealed a moderate weakness with increased extensor tone, brisk reflexes, and Babinski signs in the legs, and a mild dysmetria and coarse intention tremor in the arms and hands. Vision, sensation, and autonomic functions were normal. Over the years, his weakness slowly progressed and, by age 63, he was wheelchair bound. Around the same time, he had his first grand mal seizure and developed myoclonic jerks. EEG was abnormal with spike and photomyoclonic discharges, and MRI displayed severe cerebellar atrophy. Psychological testing revealed mild memory and cognitive deficits. Over the next few years, he became bedridden, dysphagic, and dysarthric and myoclonic jerks were constant. After a 13-year clinical course, he died at age 70 years. **A.** EEG shows photomyoclonic responses. **B.** MRI shows marked cerebellar atrophy. **C.** The cerebellar cortex is severely atrophic. **D.** The neurons in the hippocampus are distended with PAS-positive material. **E.** The cerebellar cortex shows Purkinje cell losses (HE) and **(F)** freely dispersed LFB-positive granules at the site of disintegrated Purkinje cells (LFB stain).

TABLE 9.4.
Lysosomal Diseases with Phenotypic Resemblance to MSP-I

GM1 Gangliosidosis
MLD with multiple sulfatase deficiency
Mucolipidosis
  MLII (I-cell disease)
  MLIII
Glycoproteinosis
  Mannosidosis
  Fucosidosis
Aspartylglucosaminuria
Sialuria
  Infantile

MSP, mucopolysaccharidosis; MLD, metachromatic leukodystrophy

Mucopolysaccharidoses

Mucopolysaccharides (MPS) or glycosaminoglycans (GAGs) consist of polysaccharide chains attached to a polypeptide core. Due to deficient activities of specific enzymes, MPSs accumulate in visceral organs and mesenchymal tissues and are excreted in urine. The mucopolysaccharides that are stored and excreted in urine are dermatan sulfate, heparan sulfate, and chondroitin sulfate.

Mucopolysaccharidoses, common lysosomal diseases, affect chiefly infants and young children and are transmitted in an autosomal recessive fashion except for Hunter's disease, which has an X-linked recessive inheritance. Characteristic facial and skeletal abnormalities, cardiomyopathy, hepatosplenomegaly, corneal opacity, hearing impairments, and mental retardation are prominent clinical features. Several types of MPSs are distinguished based on specific enzyme defects, stored products, and clinical expression.

Hurler's disease (MPS1) is the model of mucopolysaccharidoses. The disease is caused by a deficiency of the enzyme α-L-iduronidase, encoded by a gene located on chromosome. 4. The enzyme deficiency results in an accumulation of dermatan sulfate and heparan sulfate in affected organs, and their excretions in the urine. The physical appearance of the affected infant has been compared to that of a gargoyle: coarse facial feature, a large scaphocephalic head with frontal bossing, coarse hair, depressed nasal bridge, thick eyebrows, and a thick tongue protruding through an open mouth. Dwarfism is evident by 3 to 4 years of age (Fig. 9.8). Dorsolumbar kyphosis is present, and the hands and fingers are broad. Bony abnormalities and skeletal changes are referred to as *dysostosis multiplex*. Skull radiographs show enlargement of the sella. Mental retardation, corneal opacity, cardiomegaly, hepatosplenomegaly, and umbilical hernia

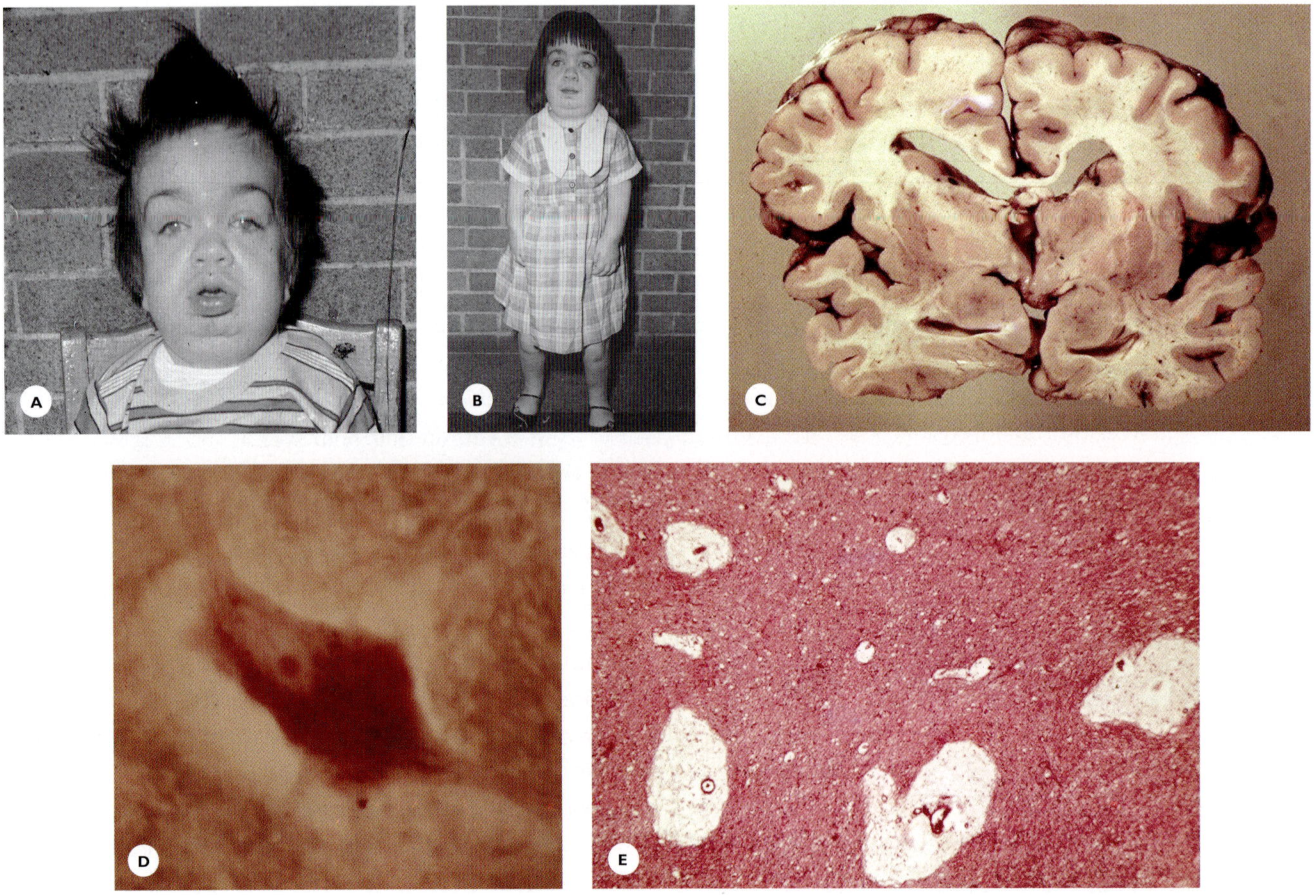

FIGURE 9.8

Hurler's disease. **A** and **B.** Pictures of a mentally retarded girl show the characteristic facial and skeletal features of the disease at ages 9 and 13 years. At age 13, she died of pulmonary infection. Note the short stature, large head, coarse facial features, thick tongue, and short neck. **C.** Transverse section of the brain shows dilated ventricles, focal thickening of the leptomeninges, and dilated perivascular spaces. **D.** Neuronal storage of PAS-positive material is moderate (PAS stain). **E.** The dilated pericapillary spaces are filled with a fine mesenchymal network (HE).

are commonly present. Recurrent infections, spinal cord compression, and peripheral nerve entrapment are frequent complications.

Grossly, the brain is large and shows leptomeninges thickened from deposits of mucopolysaccharides in vascular endothelium and fibrous tissue. The ventricles are enlarged due to communicating obstructive hydrocephalus. The histology is characterized by the neuronal storage of a mixture of gangliosides that stain positively for lipids and carbohydrates. Dilated perivascular spaces are filled with foamy macrophages (see Fig. 9.8).

Mucolipidoses

This group of autosomal recessive disorders is characterized by the combined storage of mucopolysaccharides and lipids (ML) in tissues and a lack of urinary excretion of mucopolysaccharides.

Type I ML (sialidosis I) affects chiefly juveniles and presents with cherry red spot at the macula, seizures, and myoclonic jerks.

Type II ML (sialidosis II) or I-Cell disease (I inclusion) affects infants and presents with features of Hurler's disease. The circulating lymphocytes are vacuolated, and the bone marrow shows foamy histiocytes. Sudanophilic inclusions are present in skin fibroblasts. The clinical course ranges from 1 to several years.

Type III ML is a milder form of type II ML.

Glycoproteinoses

This group of rare lysosomal disorders results from deficiencies of enzymes involved in glycoprotein degradation. Glycoproteins consist of oligosaccharide chains attached to a protein core. Defective degradation of glycoproteins leads to the neurovisceral storage of oligosaccharides, glycopeptides, and glycolipids, and the urinary excretion of abnormal oligosaccharides. The group encompasses the *mannosidosis*, the *fucosidoses, aspartyl-glycosaminuria*, and *Schindler's disease*. The diseases affect neonates, infants, and young children, but juvenile and adult forms also occur. The clinical expression, except for the Schindler's disease, resembles that of Hurler's disease: psychomotor retardation, facial and skeletal abnormalities, corneal opacity, deafness, angiokeratomas, and hepatosplenomegaly. Vacuolated lymphocytes in blood smear and foamy histiocytes in bone marrow occur in all diseases.

The brain may be atrophic or enlarged. The neurons, in paraffin sections, are vacuolated because the water-soluble stored material is extracted during processing. In frozen sections, the compound stains positively with PAS and lipid stains.

Schindler's disease presents with psychomotor retardation, visual impairment, various neurologic deficits, and myoclonus. The pathology is distinguished by the presence of neuroaxonal dystrophy in the cerebral white matter.

Glycogenoses

When the lysosomal enzymes necessary in catabolic metabolism of glycogen are deficient, glycogen is stored in the skeletal muscles, heart, and liver. The nervous system is involved in Pompe's disease or glycogenosis type II.

Pompe's disease is caused by acid maltase (α-1-4-glucosidase) deficiency and is inherited as an autosomal recessive trait. The disease affects infants, juveniles, and adults. The infantile form is most severe; the juvenile form is relatively benign, with a protracted course. In the adult form, no neuronal storage occurs.

In infants, the disease manifests soon after birth with progressive muscle weakness and firmness, cardiomyopathy, and macroglossia. Death, usually from cardiac failure, occurs within 1 to 2 years. A myopathic EMG pattern and the presence of discrete cytoplasmic vacuoles in the circulating lymphocytes are helpful diagnostic clues. The neuronal glycogen storage is ubiquitous and particularly prominent in the spinal cord and brain stem. Astrocytes store glycogen in the cerebral hemispheric white matter (Fig. 9.9).

PEROXISOMAL DISEASES

Peroxisomes, membrane-bound intracellular organelles, play important roles in various metabolic processes of the nervous system and the adrenals. Their major functions include (a) the synthesis of plasmalogen, an

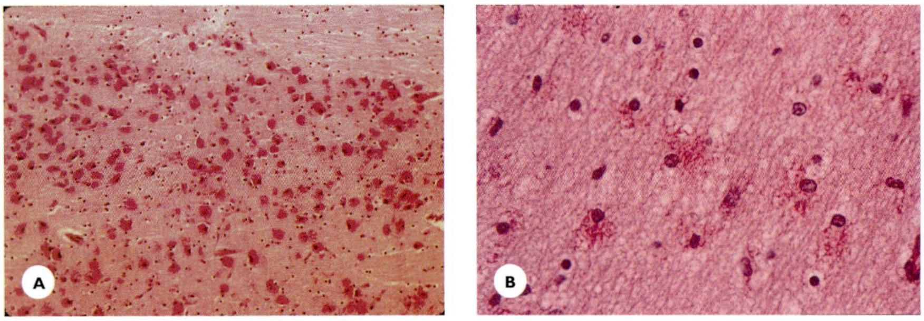

FIGURE 9.9
Pompe's disease. Glycogen is stored (**A**) in the neurons and (**B**) astrocytes (frozen section, PAS stain).

important membrane component of cells and myelin; (b) the synthesis of cholesterol and dolichols; (c) the oxidation of very long-chain-fatty acids (VLCFA); and (d) the oxidation of phytanic acid.

Neurologic diseases associated with peroxisomal disorders are caused either by the absence or reduced number and size of peroxisomes (disorder of biogenesis), resulting in generalized enzyme deficiencies; or by single-enzyme deficiencies of structurally normal peroxisomes. The diseases may occur from the neonatal period through adulthood and have a wide range of phenotypic expression. Adrenal insufficiency is an integral part of some.

The pathology in both generalized and single-enzyme deficiencies consists of extensive degeneration of myelin in the brain, spinal cord, or peripheral nerves. Concomitant congenital malformation and inflammatory reaction are noteworthy in some diseases.

Diseases Associated with Generalized Enzyme Deficiencies

Peroxisomal biogenesis disorders (PBD) are represented by Zellweger's disease or cerebrohepatorenal syndrome (ZS), neonatal adrenoleukodystrophy (NALD), and infantile Refsum disease (IRD). Each is inherited in an autosomal recessive mode. To date, mutations in 12 genes (*PEX*) (with gene products peroxins) have been associated with PBD. Mutations in *PEX1*, located on chromosome 7, and in *PEX6*, located on chromosome 6, are the most common.

Defective synthesis of plasmalogen and defective oxidation of VLCFA are major biochemical defects. A reduced plasmalogen level and high VLCFA levels in plasma and cultured skin fibroblasts, and the absence of peroxisomes in the liver are diagnostic laboratory findings. Prenatal diagnosis is possible by performing the tests on amniocytes or cultured chorionic villi. MRI of the brain is helpful in revealing cortical and white matter abnormalities.

Zellweger's Disease or Cerebrohepatorenal Syndrome

Neonates present with craniofacial dysmorphism, pigmentary retinopathy, cataract, sensorineuronal hearing impairment, hypotonia, failure to thrive, seizures, patellar calcification, and hepatomegaly. Death usually occurs within 5 to 6 months of onset.

The cerebral pathology is distinguished by developmental abnormalities, such as disorders of neuronal migration: pachygyria and microgyria along the Sylvian fissures, heterotopias of the Purkinje cells, and anomalous dentate and olivary nuclei. Other changes are variable neuronal losses, diminution and/or breakdown of myelin, lipid deposits within macrophages, and degeneration of the optic nerves. Common visceral changes include liver fibrosis, often progressing to cirrhosis; kidney cysts; and lipid-containing striated cortical cells in the adrenals.

Neonatal Adrenoleukodystrophy

NALD presents clinically with a regression of psychomotor development, visual impairment and retinal degeneration, sensorineuronal hearing loss, and seizures. Death usually occurs within 2 to 3 years of onset.

The pathology is distinguished by a widespread degeneration of myelin with sudanophilic breakdown products accompanied by perivascular lymphocytic infiltrations (see the section on leukodystrophies). The adrenals are atrophic. Cortical malformations are less evident.

Infantile Refsum's Disease

The principal manifestations of IRD are polyneuropathy, mental retardation, pigmentary degeneration of the retina, sensory neuronal hearing impairment, and hepatomegaly. Infants may survive into childhood or even adolescence. Due to defective oxidation, phytanic acid accumulates in the nervous tissue and the organs involved. Cortical anomalies are minimal or none.

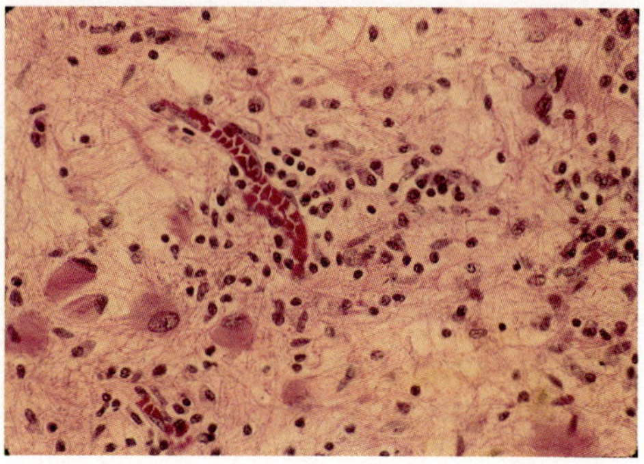

FIGURE 9.10
Adrenoleukodystrophy. Loose perivascular lymphocytic infiltrations and reactive astrocytes are present in the hemispheric white matter (HE).

Diseases Associated with Single-Enzyme Deficiencies

This group comprises the X-linked recessive adrenoleukodystrophies (X-ALDs) and the recessively inherited adult Refsum's disease (ARD). The X-linked leukodystrophies, the most common peroxisomal diseases, include childhood, juvenile, and adult adrenoleukodystrophies and adult adrenomyeloneuropathy (AMN). X-ALDs are caused by mutations in the gene *ABCD1*, which codes for a peroxisomal membrane protein (ALDP) located on chromosome Xg28. Due to defective oxidation, VLCFAs accumulate in the cerebral and spinal cord white matter and adrenocortical cells, and variably in other tissues. High levels of VLCFA in plasma and skin fibroblasts confirm the diagnosis. MRI T2-weighted images demonstrate hyperintense lesions in parieto-occipital white matter and magnetic resonance spectroscopy (MRS) shows increased levels of choline.

Childhood, Juvenile, and Adult Adrenoleukodystrophies

Childhood, juvenile, and adult adrenoleukodystrophies are characterized by mental regression progressing to dementia, motor disorders, visual and sensorineuronal hearing loss, and seizures culminating in a terminal vegetative state. Death occurs 2 to 3 years after onset in childhood cases. The clinical course is longer in juvenile and adult cases.

The cerebral pathology is characterized by a widespread, often symmetric, degeneration of myelin in the cerebrum and cerebellum, with sudanophilic breakdown products within macrophages. These may contain lamellar inclusions of VLCFA esters. The demyelination usually proceeds from the parieto-occipital regions to the frontal areas. Perivascular lymphocytic infiltrations in the demyelinated areas are diagnostic hallmarks. With time, a dense astrocytic fibrosis replaces the myelin (Fig. 9.10).

Adult Adrenomyeloneuropathy

Adult adrenomyeloneuropathy presents with a slowly progressive spastic paraparesis and peripheral neuropathy. It may be associated with cerebral ALD. Demyelination is prominent in the spinal cord, particularly in the posterior columns and pyramidal tracts, but lymphocytic infiltrations are rare or absent.

Adrenal insufficiency is variably present. Usually it is severe in AMN, in which the testes are also involved. The atrophic adrenal cortex contains ballooned eosinophilic cells, and some contain ultrastructural lamellar inclusions. Similar inclusions are found in the Leydig cells of the testes.

Dietary therapy with *Lorenzo's oil* is aimed at reducing the rate of synthesis of saturated VLCFAs. The therapy does not seem to be effective in reversing or halting the neurologic symptoms, but it may prevent their development in asymptomatic patients with Addison disease.

Adult Refsum's Disease

This disease presents in adulthood, but earlier onsets are not uncommon. Cardinal clinical features are slowly progressive sensorimotor neuropathy, retinitis pigmentosa, optic atrophy, ichthyosis of the skin and, later in the course, cerebellar ataxia. Additional features are cardiomyopathy, anosmia, and neuronal hearing impairment. Skeletal anomalies and cutaneous changes may occur.

The major biochemical defect is deficient α-oxidation of phytanic acid due to deficiency of the enzyme phytanoyl coenzyme A-hydroxylase (PHYH). The *PHYH* gene maps to chromosome 10.

Early diagnosis, by demonstrating elevated phytanic acid in plasma and deficiency of enzyme PHYH, is important. Dietary therapy eliminating dairy products and ruminant fats results in improvement, whereas undiagnosed cases have a poor prognosis.

The pathology of the peripheral nerves consists of a loss of myelinated fibers and axons, onion-bulb formations, and paracrystalline inclusions in Schwann cells.

LEUKODYSTROPHIES

Leukodystrophies, inherited metabolic diseases of the central myelin, have various etiologies: defective functions of the lysosomes or peroxisomes, deficient synthesis of myelin, and a disorder of amino acid metabolism (Table 9.5). The mode of inheritance varies: Some diseases are autosomal recessive, some autosomal dominant, and some X- linked recessive. The diseases share certain clinical and pathologic features, but each has its distinct characteristics.

TABLE 9.5.
Etiologies of Leukodystrophies

Lysosomal enzyme deficiencies Metachromatic leukodystrophy Multiple sulfatase deficiency Globoid cell leukodystrophy	**Peroxisomal enzyme deficiencies** Adrenoleukodystrophies neonatal childhood, juvenile, adult
Myelin synthesis deficiency Pelizaeus-Merzbacher disease	**Aspartoacylase deficiency** Canavan's disease
	Mutation in GFAP gene Alexander's disease

Clinical Features

Leukodystrophies affect chiefly infants and young children but may occur to adulthood. Common age-related clinical manifestations are:

- In neonates and early infancy, lack of psychomotor development, listlessness, failure to thrive, and hypotonia changing to hypertonia
- In late infancy, motor difficulties and mental regression
- In juveniles, behavioral changes, declining school performance, gradual loss of motor functions, loss of language and acquired mental skills progressing to dementia and eventually to a vegetative state
- In adults, behavioral changes, cognitive decline, and dementia

Visual impairment with optic atrophy and, less frequently, seizures may develop at any age.

MRI is essential to demonstrate white matter abnormalities. Other diagnostic tests include enzymatic studies and biopsies to demonstrate deposits of abnormal metabolites in cultured skin fibroblasts, sural nerve, or liver. Prenatal diagnosis rests on enzyme studies of amniocytes or chorionic villi.

Pathologic Features

Extensive, often symmetric loss of myelin in the cerebral and cerebellar hemispheres and the brainstem, with relative sparing of the arcuate fibers, are characteristic features common to all. In the affected regions, the axons are variably diminished in density, and the oligodendroglial cells are reduced in number. With time, a dense astrocytic gliosis develops in the demyelinated areas. The spinal cord and the peripheral nerves may also be involved.

Metachromatic Leukodystrophy, Sulfatide Lipidosis

Metachromatic leukodystrophy or sulfatide lipidosis is an autosomal recessive disorder affecting chiefly infants, but juvenile and adult variants are also known. It is caused by deficiency of the lysosomal enzyme arylsulfatase A (ASA). The ASA gene is located on chromosome 22. ASA normally degrades the myelin sulfatides to cerebroside and inorganic sulfate (Table 9.6). A deficiency of the enzyme ASA results in the excessive accumulation of sulfatides in the myelin, rendering it chemically unstable and prone to disintegration. *Grossly*, the cerebral and cerebellar white matter is diffusely soft in early stages and firm and yellowish in chronic stages. The subcortical white matter usually is spared, except in longstanding cases, in which it also degenerates (Fig. 9.11). A general autopsy may show a fibrotic gall bladder. Histologically, the myelin breakdown products contain large amounts of sulfatides which, in frozen sections, stain metachromatically brown with acidified cresyl violet, giving the name to the disease. Sulfatides may accumulate in the neurons of the cerebral gray structures, brainstem, spinal cord, and retina. Metachromatic myelin globules are demonstrated in the biopsied sural nerve. Sulfatides are also deposited in the tubular epithelium of the kidneys and mucosa of the gall bladder (see Fig. 9.11). Increased levels of sulfatides in the urine and the presence of metachromatic granules in the sediment are easily demonstrated.

Multiple Sulfatase Deficiency (MSD)

Multiple sulfatase deficiency (MSD), a rare autosomal recessive disorder, is caused by deficient activities of arylsulfatase A, B, and C. The mutating gene is located on chromosome 3. Due to these enzyme deficiencies

TABLE 9.6
Metachromatic Leukodystrophy

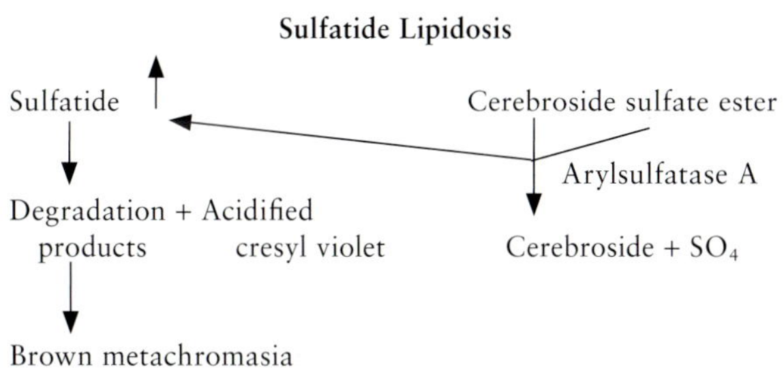

sulfatides, mucopolysaccharide sulfates, steroid sulfates, and gangliosides accumulate in the nervous system and various tissues.

The disease affects neonates, infants, and juveniles. Coarse facial features and skeletal anomalies resembling mucopolysaccharidosis, corneal opacity, deafness, and mental retardation are characteristic clinical features. The pathology combines the features of metachromatic leukodystrophy with those of mucopolysaccharidosis.

Krabbe's Disease

Krabbe's disease, or *globoid cell leukodystrophy*, an autosomal recessive disorder chiefly of infants, is caused by a deficiency of the lysosomal enzyme galactosyl ceramidase, which degrades the cerebroside (galactosyl ceramide) to ceramide and galactose. The mutant gene is located on chromosome 14. The enzymatic failure leads to an accumulation of galactosylceramide in globoid cells and an accumulation of toxic galactosylsphingosine (psychosine) in the white matter and oligodendrocytes, which accounts for the myelin degeneration and oligodendroglial loss. Globoid cells in the demyelinated areas are the diagnostic features of the disease. These large mono- or multinucleated macrophages contain galactocerebrosides that stain strongly with PAS reagent and weakly for lipids. The globoid cells have a tendency to cluster, particularly around blood vessels (Fig. 9.12).

Canavan's Disease or Spongy Degeneration

Canavan's disease, spongy degeneration of the neuroaxis, is an autosomal recessive disorder caused by deficiency of the enzyme *N*-aspartoacylase, encoded by a gene on chromosome 17. Subsequently, the amino acid *N*-acetyl aspartic acid accumulates in the cerebrospinal fluid (CSF) and brain and is excreted in urine. Onset is in early infancy; blindness and macrocephaly are characteristic clinical features.

The cerebral pathology is distinguished by (a) the lack of myelination, extensive vacuolation, and spongy degeneration of the white matter; (b) the presence of a few sudanophilic myelin breakdown products in some

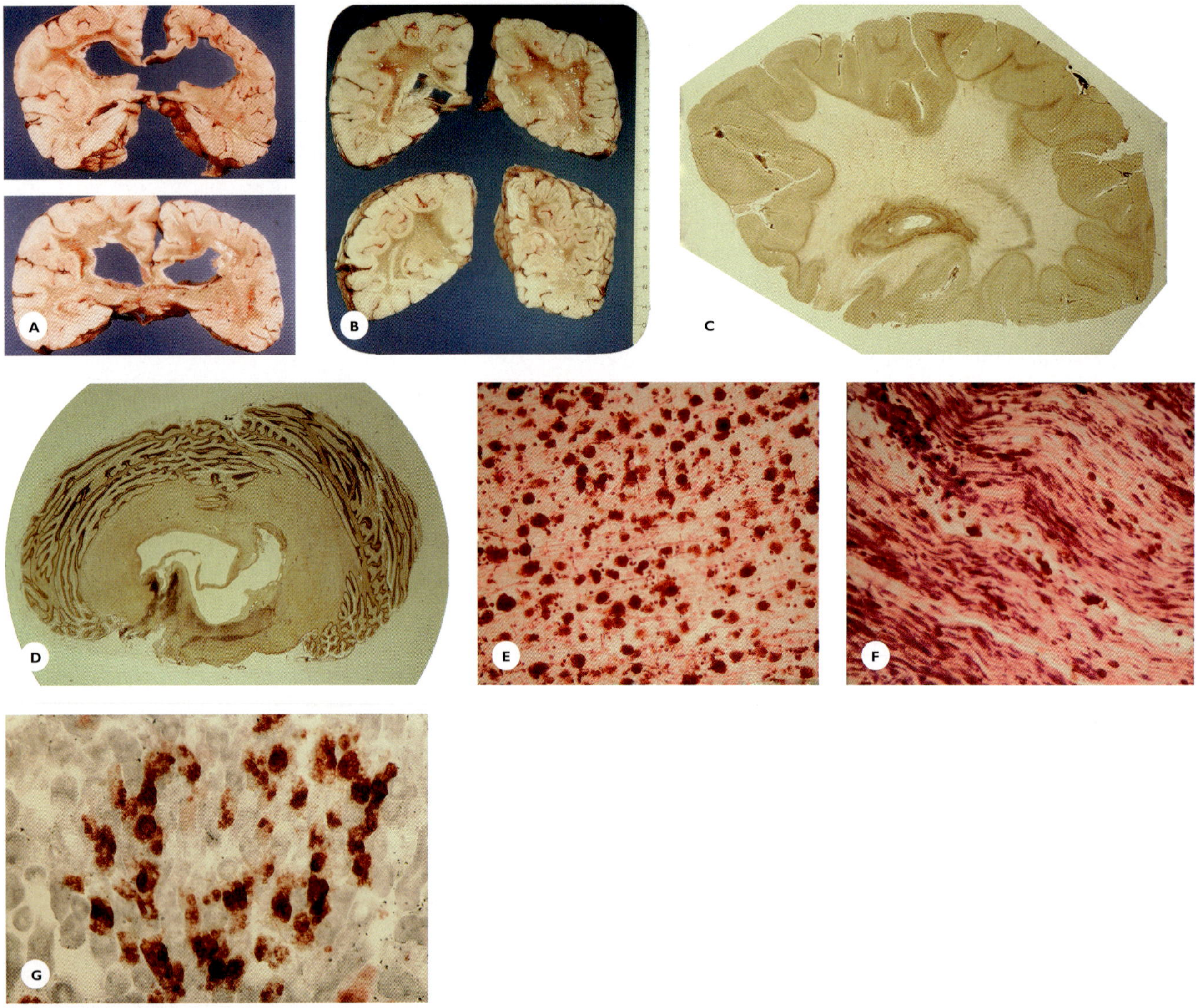

FIGURE 9.11

Juvenile metachromatic leukodystrophy. The disease of an 8-year-old boy began with a decline in his school performance, day-dreaming, and aimless scribbling. At age 11, he had his first grand mal seizure. Over the ensuring years, his mental and motor functions rapidly deteriorated. First, he became speechless and unable to stand or walk; then he became bedridden, with his extremities in flexion contractures. After a 12-year course, at age 20 years, he died. His younger sister developed a similar illness and died before him. **A** and **B.** On transverse sections the hemispheric white matter from the frontal to the occipital lobes is reduced in volume, sunken, yellow, and gelatinous. **C.** Occipital lobe shows total loss of myelin and relative sparing of arcuate fibers. **D.** Myelin loss is total in the cerebellum and almost total in the pons (Weil stain). **E.** Brown, metachromatically stained myelin breakdown products are abundant in the subcortical white matter. **F.** Peripheral nerve shows myelin degeneration with metachromatic granules. **G.** Metachromatic granules are present in tubular epithelium of kidney (acidic Cresyl-violet).

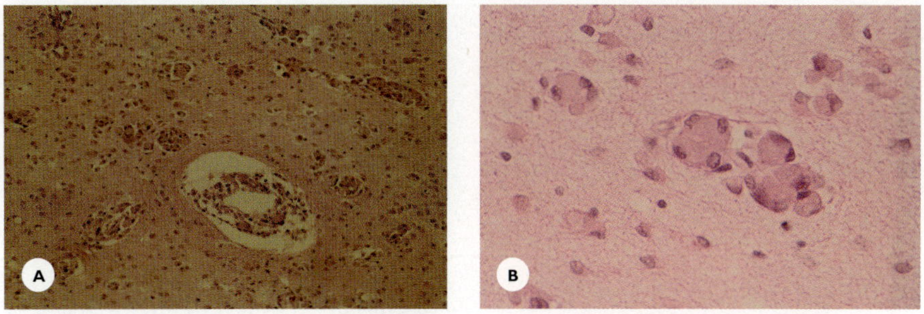

FIGURE 9.12
Globoid leukodystrophy. **A.** Single and clustered globoid cells are dispersed in the demyelinated cerebral hemisphere. **B.** Higher magnification view of multinucleated globoid cells (HE).

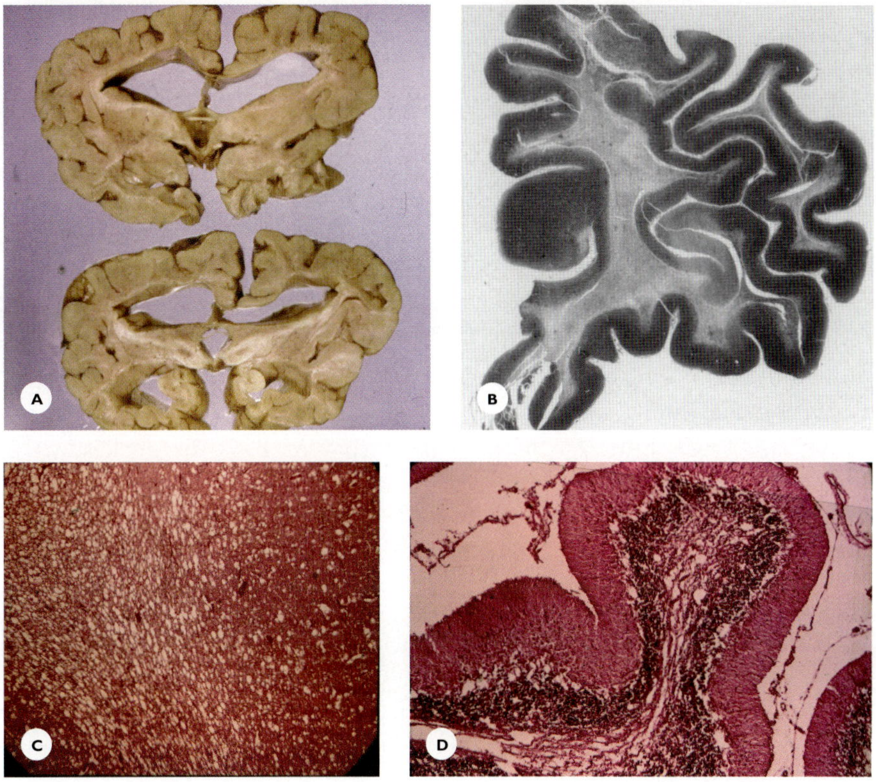

FIGURE 9.13
Canavan's disease in a 6-year-old profoundly retarded, blind, quadriplegic, macrocephalic boy. **A.** Transverse sections from the 1,465 g brain shows markedly reduced and soft hemispheric white matter. **B.** There is total absence of myelin in the frontal lobe (Weil stain). **C.** The white matter is vacuolated and spongy. **D.** The cerebellar white matter, and to some extent the cortex, are vacuolated and spongy (HE).

myelinated regions; and (c) the presence of large protoplasmic astrocytes in gray structures (Fig. 9.13).

Alexander's Disease

Alexander's disease may be sporadic or familial. Autosomal dominant inheritance has been demonstrated in familial cases. Alexander disease is associated with mutations in the gene coding for glial fibrillary acidic protein (GFAP), an intermediate filament protein of astrocytes. In infants, the clinical course ranges from a few weeks to several years. Older infants develop megalencephaly. The juvenile form, with onset between 4 and 10 years, has a slower course. Bulbar symptoms and signs are characteristic clinical manifestations. The rare adult form may present with motor dysfunction, palatal myoclonus, and abnormal eye movements. No specific laboratory test is available for the disease. MRI is helpful in demonstrating the white matter changes and a periventricular rim.

The pathology is characterized by bilateral widespread degeneration of myelin with frontal predominance and the presence of Rosenthal fibers. In infants, the myelin degeneration is extensive and may progress to cavitation. It is less severe in older children and adults. The arcuate fibers are preserved, and axonal damage is

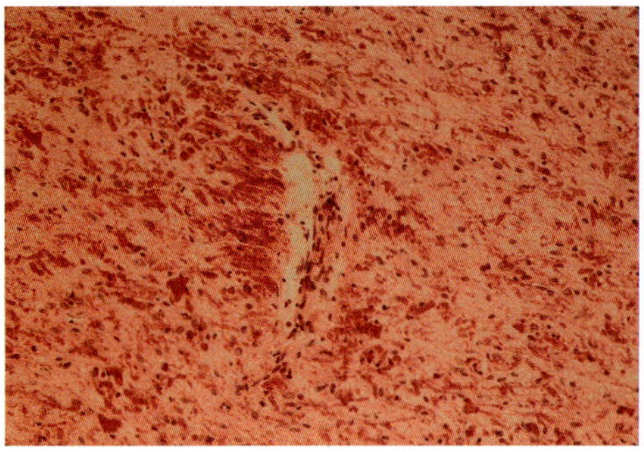

FIGURE 9.14
Alexander's disease. Rosenthal fibers are concentrated around a blood vessel and are also diffusely dispersed in the white matter (HE).

variable. The Rosenthal fibers are the diagnostic hallmark of the disease (Fig. 9.14). These are eosinophilic, rod-shaped structures of astrocytic origin situated around blood vessels, beneath the pia mater, and along the ependymal lining of the ventricles. They contain GFAP and two heat shock proteins (hsp)—α B-crystalline and hsp27.

Pelizaeus-Merzbacher Disease

Pelizaeus-Merzbacher disease, an X-linked recessive disorder, is caused by mutations in a gene on chromosome xg22 encoding myelin proteolipid protein. A deficiency of myelin proteolipid protein accounts for the defective myelination.

The disease presents in two forms: connatal and childhood. The connatal form manifests with psychomotor retardation, optic atrophy, and nystagmus. Death usually occurs by 2 years of age. The childhood form, presenting with spasticity, cerebellar symptoms, and optic atrophy, has a slower clinical course, extending into adulthood.

Grossly, the brain is atrophic. Histologically, the white matter in the brain and spinal cord shows failure of myelination, hypomyelination, and perivascular myelin islands, giving the characteristic tigroid appearance. The density of nerve fibers is relatively normal. The number of oligodendrocytes is variably reduced.

Adrenoleukodystrophies (ALDs)

Adrenoleukodystrophies (ALDs) (described in detail in section on peroxisomal diseases) are characterized by a failure of degradation of saturated very long-chain fatty acids (VLCFAs), which then accumulate in the cerebral white matter, adrenals, and practically all tissues. Neonatal ALD, is autosomal recessive and results from a disorder of peroxisomal biogenesis. Childhood, juvenile, and adult ALDs are X-linked recessive and result from single-enzyme defects. The pathology, common to all forms, is distinguished by lymphocytic perivascular infiltrations in the demyelinated areas (Fig. 9.10).

MITOCHONDRIAL DISEASES

A complexity of genetic defects, a unique mode of inheritance, a great variation in clinical expression, and a wide spectrum of pathology characterize mitochondrial diseases. Mitochondria, membrane-bound cellular organelles, are importantly involved in oxidative phosphorylation (OXPHOS) and, consequently, in supplying the energy essential for the functioning of cells in all organs. Diseases caused by defective oxidative phosphorylation are generally determined genetically, with both the mitochondrial (mtDNA) and the nuclear (nDNA) genomes involved. Mitochondrial DNA codes 13 proteins of the oxidative phosphorylation system and also a set of transfer RNA (tRNA) and ribosomal RNA. The rest of the proteins (more than 80) are encoded by nDNA. Mutations in either the mtDNA or the nDNA or both can cause diseases. Diseases with mutations in mtDNA are sporadic or transmitted maternally to offsprings of both sexes, but only the daughters transmit the disease to subsequent generations. Maternally inherited diseases are associated with mtDNA deletion, depletion, or missense mutation, and tRNA mutations. Diseases with mutations in nDNA are transmitted in a mendelian mode of inheritance: recessive, dominant, or X-linked. In addition, some diseases are caused by defects in intergenomic communication; that is, mutations in the nDNA gene affect the mtDNA gene, resulting in deletion or depletion of mtDNA. The inheritance of these diseases is also mendelian.

Clinical Features

Mitochondrial diseases occur from infancy to childhood, adolescence, and early adulthood. In children, the incidence is estimated at 1 per 11,000. Most diseases are multiple-organ disorders: the brain, retina, skeletal muscles, and heart are affected because of their high energy demand. Diseases with concurrent involvement of the brain and skeletal muscles constitute the group of encephalomyopathies. Commonly encountered manifestations are:

- Ocular—Optic atrophy, pigmentary retinopathy, bilateral extraocular muscle palsy progressing to ophthalmoplegia
- Neurologic—Combinations of movement disorders, cerebellar ataxia, hearing impairment, mental decline, seizures, episodic encephalopathy, and polyneuropathy
- Myopathic—Presence of ragged-red fibers
- Visceral/endocrine—Cardiomyopathy, liver and kidney dysfunctions, diabetes mellitus, and thyroid, parathyroid, and gonadal dysfunctions
- Metabolic—Elevated lactate and pyruvate levels in serum and CSF

Diagnosing mitochondrial diseases requires a panel of metabolic tests, neuroimaging, muscle biopsy, and genetic testing. Basic metabolic tests are for lactate and pyruvate in blood and CSF, amino acids in blood and urine, organic acids in urine, and carnitine in blood. Computed tomography (CT) scans and MRI are helpful in demonstrating calcifications and lesions in gray and white matter. The presence of ragged-red fibers (RRF) in muscle biopsy supports the diagnosis of a mitochondrial disease, but its absence does not rule it out. Testing for genetic mutations is carried out on blood leucocytes and on DNA in muscle fibers.

Pathology

Neuronal losses, gliosis, parenchymal necrosis, spongiosis, and calcifications are common. The distribution of these lesions, however, is fairly characteristic for a particular disease.

Mitochondrial myopathy is characterized by the presence of ragged-red fibers. These result from subsarcolemmal mitochondrial aggregates and are readily demonstrated in histologic sections stained with Gomori modified trichrome method. Histochemical examination shows absent cytochrome oxidase in the region of ragged-red fibers and increased succinic dehydrogenase activity. Electron microscopic study reveals paracrystalline inclusions from precipitations of mitochondrial proteins.

Classification

Two major groups of mitochondrial diseases are (a) those caused by mutations in mtDNA and (b) those caused by mutations in nDNA. Mutations in mtDNA are either primary or secondary to nDNA mutations (defective intergenomic communication). The mode of inheritance of the diseases is shown in (Table 9.7).

Encephalomyopathies Caused by Mutations in mtDNA

Kearns-Sayre Syndrome

Kearns-Sayre Syndrome (KSS), with onset in adolescence, is distinguished by progressive external ophthalmoplegia, pigmentary retinopathy, sensorineuronal hearing loss, cerebellar ataxia, heart block, mental regression, myopathy, and elevated CSF protein. Neuroimaging shows white matter hyperintensities on T2-weighted MRI and calcifications in the basal ganglia

TABLE 9.7
Mode of Inheritance of Mitochondrial Diseases

Maternal	*Mendelian*
MELAS	AD: PEO
MERRF	AR: MNGIE
LHON	AR: LS
LS	X-linked: LS
KSS*	

AD, autosomal dominant; AR, autosomal recessive; *sporadic mtDNA mutation.

on CT scan. Death occurs in the third or fourth decade. The disease is sporadic and is associated with duplications and deletions of mtDNA.

Characteristic pathologic changes are (a) widespread spongiform degenerations of the cerebral and cerebellar white matter, (b) prominent neuronal degenerations in the brain stem and cerebellum, (c) calcifications in the globus pallidus, thalamus, and substantia nigra, and (d) ragged-red fiber myopathy.

Mitochondrial Encephalomyopathy with Lactic Acidosis and Stroke-like Episodes

Mitochondrial encephalomyopathy with lactic acidosis and stroke-like episodes (MELAS) of children and young adults is defined by retinitis pigmentosa, recurrent attacks of focal neurologic deficits, seizures, migrainous headaches, progressive external ophthalmoplegia, intellectual deterioration, and myopathy. The disease is maternally inherited and is associated with point mutations in transfer RNA (tRNA) genes.

The pathology is characterized by solitary or multiple necrotic lesions in the cerebral cortex and white matter, mainly in the parieto-occipital lobes. Histologically, they resemble ischemic necrosis, although do not conform to arterial territories. Mineral deposits are seen in the basal ganglia, and ragged-red fiber myopathy is present.

Myoclonus Epilepsy with Ragged-Red Fibers

Myoclonus epilepsy with ragged red fibers (MERRF) affects children and adults. Cardinal clinical manifestations include short stature, seizures, polymyoclonus, optic atrophy, sensory-neuronal hearing loss, cerebellar ataxia, peripheral neuropathy, and myopathy. The disease is maternally transmitted and is associated with point mutations in tRNA gene.

The pathology consists of (a)neuronal degenerations and gliosis in the dentate nuclei and cortex of the cerebellum, inferior olivary nuclei, red nucleus, substantia nigra, globus pallidus, and Clarke nucleus of the spinal cord; (b) demyelination of the superior cerebellar peduncles and posterior columns and spinocerebellar tracts of the spinal cord; and (c) ragged-red fiber myopathy.

Leber's Hereditary Optic Neuropathy

The disease, maternally inherited, is associated with mutations of mtDNA. It affects chiefly male adolescents or young adults. It manifests with acute or subacute visual impairment and papilledema progressing to optic atrophy and blindness. Pyramidal and extrapyramidal symptoms, ataxia, polyneuropathy, and cardiac conduction defect may also occur.

Encephalomyopathies Caused by Defects in Intergenomic Communication

Mitochondrial Neurogastrointestinal Encephalomyopathy

Mitochondrial neurogastrointestinal encephalomyopathy (MNGIE), an autosomal recessive disorder, is associated with deletions of mtDNA. The disease affects adolescents and young adults. It presents with recurrent abdominal pain, vomiting, intestinal pseudo-obstruction, and diarrhea. External ophthalmoplegia, leukoencephalopathy on MRI, dementia, peripheral neuropathy, and ragged-red myopathy add to the clinical picture.

Autosomal Dominant Progressive External Ophthalmoplegia

Autosomal dominant progressive external ophthalmoplegia (AD-PEO) is associated with mtDNA deletion. Cardiomyopathy, ataxia, and peripheral neuropathy variably accompany the ocular disorder.

Encephalomyopathy Caused by Mutations in Both nDNA and mtDNA

Leigh Syndrome

Leigh syndrome (LS) or subacute necrotizing encephalomyopathy, is genetically heterogenous, caused by mutations in the nuclear gene coding for SORF1 and mutations in the mitochondrial gene coding for ATPase 6. The inheritance is mendelian—autosomal recessive or X-linked recessive—or maternal. The biochemical defect results from defects in the OXPHO system and the pyruvate dehydrogenase complex.

The disease commonly affects infants and young children, rarely adolescents or adults. It presents with feeding difficulties, vomiting, hypotonia, oculomotor abnormalities, blindness and optic atrophy, seizures, and failure of psychomotor development. Central respiratory abnormalities, hypertension, and bouts of fever are characteristic. The pyruvate and lactate levels are elevated in the CSF. In older children, pyramidal, extrapyramidal, and cerebellar symptoms and mental retardation occur in various combinations. The disease progresses to death within 1 to 2 years of onset. The course may be slower and remitting in older patients. Hyperintense symmetric lesions in the putamens and brainstem tegmentum on T2-weighted MRI are helpful diagnostic clues. Magnetic resonance spectroscopy (MRS) shows increased lactic acid in the affected regions.

The lesions are typically symmetrically situated in the basal ganglia, diencephalon, midbrain, tegmentum of the pons and medulla, and the spinal cord. The mammillary bodies are usually spared. Grossly, the affected regions are soft, brownish, often cystic and cavitated. The histology consists of spongiform degeneration of the neuropil, capillary endothelial hyperplasia and proliferation, and relative preservation of the neurons. Fat-laden macrophages are present in acute, and gliosis in chronic lesions. The optic nerves are often demyelinated.

AMINO ACID METABOLIC DISEASES

This group of inherited metabolic diseases results from enzymatic failure in the degradation of amino acids. Accumulated amino acids and their metabolites are toxic to neural tissue. With few exceptions, the diseases are autosomal recessive. Some diseases manifest at birth and have a rapidly progressive course; others, with a more benign course, present with seizures and mental retardation.

Newborns are routinely screened for major aminoacidurias in urine. Prenatal diagnosis is possible by demonstrating abnormal metabolites in amniotic fluid and deficient enzyme activity on cultured amniocytes or chorionic villi. Early diagnosis is important, because dietary restriction and enzyme replacement therapy are effective in several diseases. The pathology varies from predominantly white matter spongiosis to nonspecific neuronal losses in the cortex and deep gray structures.

Phenylketonuria

Phenylketonuria (PKU), one of the most common inherited metabolic disorders, is estimated at 1 per 10,000 to 15,000 births. The inheritance is autosomal recessive. The mutant gene maps to chromosome 12. Deficient activity of the hepatic enzyme phenylalanine hydroxylase, which converts the phenylalanine to tyrosine, results in an accumulation of phenylalanine in the plasma and excretion of phenylpyruvic acid in the urine. Blood phenylalanine levels may reach 1,200 μmol/L or more. Acceptable levels range from 180 to 900 μmol/L. The urine test is positive for phenylpyruvic acid when the color of the urine changes to green after adding 10% $FeCl_3$ to it. Early treatment with a phenylalanine-free diet prevents the development of neurologic complications. In untreated phenylketonuria, severe mental retardation, behavioral abnormalities, seizures, and motor dysfunctions are major neurologic complications. Patients usually have blond hair, fair skin, and blue eyes. Children of mothers with untreated PKU during pregnancy may have malformations such as microcephaly, agenesis of the corpus callosum, and cortical abnormalities.

A small brain, delayed and deficient myelination with spongiosis, and astrocytic fibrosis are characteristic pathologic features of untreated cases.

Maple Syrup Urine Disease

Maple syrup urine disease (MSUD) is a disorder of the branched-chain amino acids leucin, isoleucine, and valine and their corresponding keto-acids. Defective activity of the enzyme α-keto-acid dehydrogenase results in an accumulation of these amino acids and their keto-acids in the plasma, tissues, and CSF, and in their excretion in the urine. Leucin gives the characteristic maple syrup odor to urine.

The disease is inherited as an autosomal recessive trait. It manifests a few days after birth with vomiting, lethargy, myoclonic jerks, opisthotonus, episodes of apnea, and seizures progressing rapidly to coma and death. Edema, vacuolation, sponginess, and astrocytosis in the white matter are common cerebral findings. The brains of survivors show defective myelination and reduced numbers of oligodendrocytes.

Homocystinuria

In homocystinuria, homocysteine is not catabolized to cystathionine due to a deficiency of the enzyme cystathionine-β-synthase (CBS). As a result, homocysteine accumulates in the plasma and is excreted in the urine. The mutant gene for CBS maps to chromosome 21. The disease is autosomal recessive and develops gradually, affecting multiple organs. Characteristic features are arterial and venous thromboses, myocardial infarct, skeletal abnormalities, lens dislocation and myopia, and livido reticularis. Mental retardation, recurrent strokes, seizures, psychiatric symptoms, and focal deficits characterize the nervous system involvement. The cerebral pathology consists of vascular endothelial proliferation and arterial and venous infarcts.

Nonketotic Hyperglycinemia

Nonketotic hyperglycinemia, an autosomal recessive disorder, results from failure of glycine degradation caused by mutations in three proteins (P, H, T) of a mitochondrial enzyme complex. Protein P, most commonly involved, is coded by a gene on chromosome 9. Failure of degradation leads to elevated concentrations of glycine in the blood, CSF, and urine.

The disease affects neonates and rapidly progresses to coma and death. Survivors present with psychomotor retardation and seizures. The brain shows spongy degeneration of the white matter, especially prominent in the cerebellum. Malformations with cerebellar hypoplasia, agenesis of the corpus callosum, and cortical dysplasias have been reported in some cases.

Hyperammonemia

This urea-cycle disorder results from a failure of conversion of ammonia to urea. Subsequently, ammonia and glutamine are elevated, and urea nitrogen is decreased in the blood. The disease is associated with several enzyme deficiencies, mainly of ornithine transcarbamylase. Except for the ornithine transcarbamylase deficiency, which is X-linked inherited, all the other enzyme deficiencies are transmitted in autosomal recessive pattern.

Hyperammonemia presents shortly after birth with lethargy, vomiting, alkalosis, temperature abnormalities and, if not treated, death ensues from cerebral edema. Partial enzyme deficiencies are prone to cause episodic encephalopathies that can be precipitated by high protein intake, infection, and treatment with valproate.

The pathology consists of edema, variable neuronal losses in the cerebral cortex and deep gray structures, and the presence of Alzheimer type 2 glia. Cerebellar heterotopias, suggesting intrauterine damage, have been reported.

CARBOHYDRATE METABOLIC DISEASES

Galactosemia

This is a rare autosomal recessive disorder of newborns. Importantly, if diagnosed early, it is effectively treatable. Galactose in the normal metabolic pathway is converted to glucose in four steps, each step being catalyzed by a specific enzyme. In galactosemia, the conversion of exogenous galactose to glucose is blocked in step two due to a deficiency of the enzyme galactose-1-phosphate uridyl transferase (GALT). As a result, galactose-1-phosphate, a metabolite from step one, accumulates in erythrocytes, galactose accumulates in tissues and blood, and galactosyl is excreted in urine. The disease is diagnosed by measuring GALT enzyme content in erythrocytes and galactosyl in urine.

The disease presents soon after birth with prolonged jaundice, vomiting, diarrhea, hepatomegaly, and anemia. Untreated patients develop ocular, neurologic, visceral, and metabolic disorders; hepatomegaly progressing to nodular cirrhosis; kidney dysfunction; hypoglycemic episodes; and lenticular cataract. Mental retardation, seizures, extrapyramidal and cerebellar symptoms, and microcephaly are chief neurologic features. The dietary elimination of galactose (lactose-containing products) prevents the development of complications, provided it is initiated a few days after birth and continued throughout life.

The cerebral pathology is not specific; some changes relate to the toxic effect of galactose whereas others are complications of multiple metabolic derangements, including liver cirrhosis. Grossly, the brain is small, the cerebral and cerebellar cortex is thin, and the hemispheric white matter is diminished and firm. The histology is characterized by: variable neuronal losses in the cerebral and cerebellar cortex and subcortical gray structures, patchy myelin losses and astrogliosis in the white matter, and the presence of Alzheimer type 2 glial cells in gray structures. Basophilic mineral deposits may be found in basal ganglia (Fig. 9.15).

Polyglucosan Diseases

This group of carbohydrate metabolic diseases is distinguished by the presence of polyglycosan bodies. These

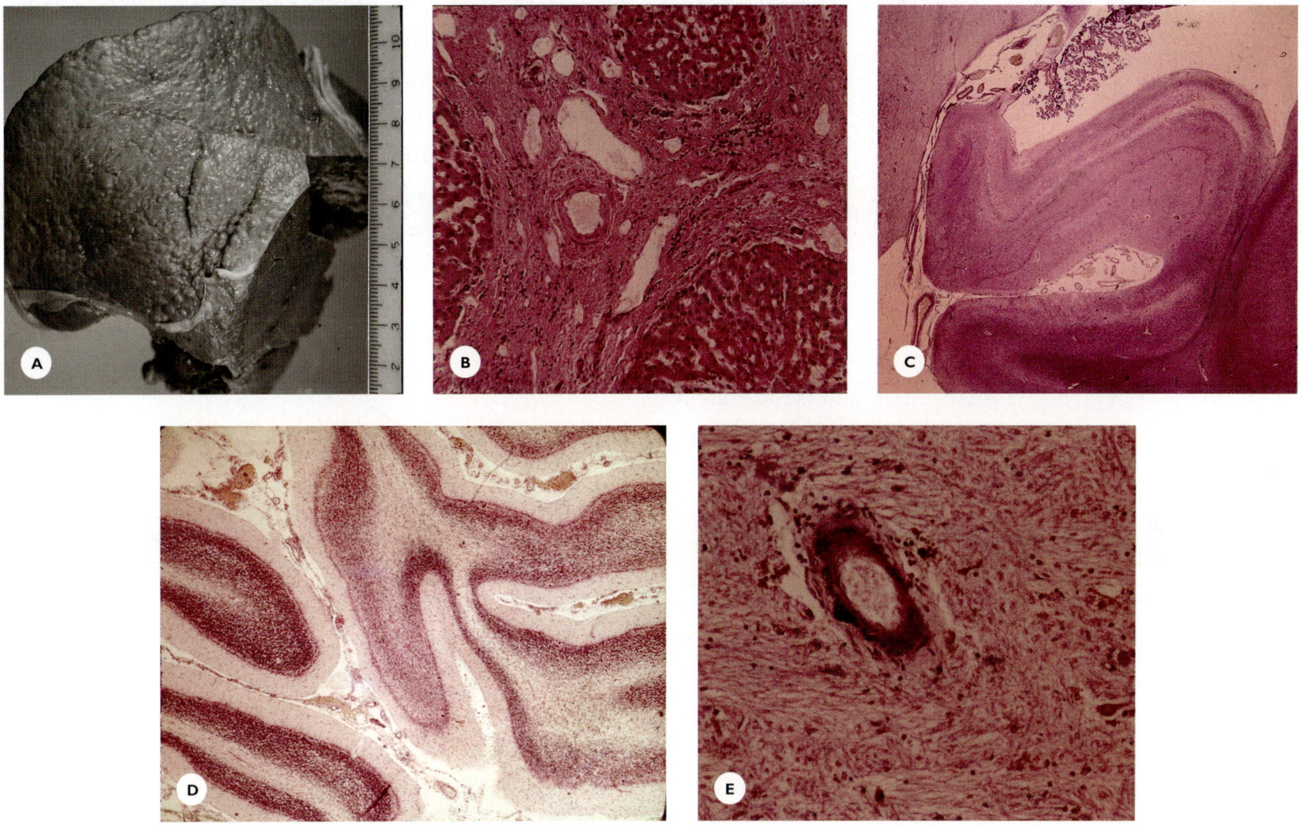

FIGURE 9.15
Galactosemia. A newborn boy was severely jaundiced, and his feeding was difficult because of frequent vomiting. In early childhood, his development was very slow and, after a few years, became arrested. At 7 years of age, he was physically underdeveloped and severely mentally retarded. Bilateral cataracts were diagnosed a few years later. He suffered from hypoglycemic episodes, frequent convulsions, and status epilepticus.

When he was 13 years old galactosemia was diagnosed in his newborn brother. An enzyme assay was performed on him at this time and confirmed his diagnosis of galactosemia. Dietary restriction of galactose was begun, but had no effect on his condition. At age 25 years, he died.

A. The liver is small and cirrhotic and shows (**B**) atrophy of the hepatic lobules and prominent perilobular fibrosis (HE). **C.** The hippocampus shows extensive neuronal losses. **D.** Severe Purkinje cell losses are present in the cerebellum (Cresyl-violet). **E.** Basal ganglia shows basophilic mineral granules in vessel's wall and parenchyma (HE).

round or spheroid filamentous aggregates, measuring 1 to 30 microns in diameter, occur in the central and peripheral nervous system and various organs. They have a basophilic core in hematoxylin-eosin (HE)-stained section, stain intensely with PAS and Alcian blue, and immunoreact for ubiquitin.

Lafora Disease with Myoclonic Epilepsy

Lafora disease with myoclonic epilepsy, a rare autosomal recessive disorder of juveniles, is caused by mutations in the gene *EPM2A*, located on chromosome 6. The disease presents with tonic-clonic seizures, widespread stimulus-induced myoclonic jerks, hearing impairment, ataxia, and mental regression. Over several years, the disease progresses to total disability. Death usually occurs in the third decade of life.

Grossly, the brain may show generalized atrophy. Histologically, polyglycosan bodies, also called *Lafora bodies*, are found in the perikaryon and dendrites of the neurons in the cerebral cortex, subcortical gray structures, cerebellar nuclei, and brainstem. Outside the nervous system, they occur in the ganglion cells of the retina, in the skeletal and cardiac muscles, in the liver, and in sweat glands in the skin. The presence of Lafora bodies in a biopsy of skin or liver confirms the diagnosis.

Adult Polyglycosan Body Disease

Adult polyglycosan body disease presents with upper and lower motor neuron deficits, sensory deficits, neurogenic bladder, and progressive dementia. Polyglycosan bodies are found in the brain, spinal cord, and peripheral nerves.

COPPER METABOLIC DISEASES

Defective metabolism of copper results in either excessive or insufficient copper in tissues. Both situations are harmful to nervous tissue, the former by being toxic and the latter by interfering with copper-dependent enzymatic activities.

Wilson Disease

Wilson disease or *familial hepatocerebral degeneration*, is caused by deficiency of a copper-transporting P-type ATPase encoded by the gene *ATP7B* on chromosome 13. As a result, copper is not incorporated into ceruloplasmin and is not excreted into the bile. Excess copper is deposited in the liver, brain, kidneys, and cornea.

Clinical Features

The disease is transmitted as an autosomal recessive trait and can occur from childhood through adolescence. Cardinal clinical manifestations are hepatic, neurologic, and psychiatric. Acute or chronic hepatitis and liver cirrhosis are common. During the course of the disease, splenomegaly, kidney dysfunction, and clotting abnormalities develop.

Neurologic manifestations are predominantly extrapyramidal: rigidity, dysarthria, dystonia, parkinsonian features, tremor, and choreiform and athetoid dyskinesias. Psychiatric manifestations include behavioral changes, schizophrenic-like symptoms, and memory and cognitive decline progressing to dementia. The presence of a Kayser-Fleischer ring, a diagnostic ocular sign, resulting from copper deposits in the Descemet membrane, appears as a greenish-brown ring in the limbus cornea. Diagnostic laboratory findings are low levels of ceruloplasmin and of total copper in the serum and increased urinary excretion of copper. In biopsied liver, the copper is greatly increased. T2-weighted MRI images reveal hyperintense lesions in the striatum, globus pallidus, and thalamus.

Pathology

Grossly, the brain is atrophic. The brunt of pathology is in the putamen and caudate, which are brownish, soft, and often cavitated. The histology is characterized by neuronal losses and a marked astrocytosis consisting chiefly of Alzheimer type 2 astrocytes. Macrophages are dispersed around the cavities; some contain lipids, and some contain pigments that stain positively for copper. A distinct finding is the presence of Opalski cells. These cells of macrophage/microglial origin are large, round, and have a small nucleus and finely granular eosinophilic cytoplasm. Similar, but less severe changes occur in the globus pallidus, thalamus, red nucleus, substantia nigra, and cerebellum. The cerebral cortex and white matter may show focal vacuolation and sponginess.

Menkes Disease

Menkes or *kinky hair disease*, an X-linked recessive disorder, is caused by a deficiency of P-type ATPase, encoded by the gene *ATP7A* located on the X-chromosome. Subsequently, the transport and distribution of intracellular copper are impaired and copper levels are reduced in the liver, brain, and plasma.

Clinical Features

The disease presents a few weeks after birth with feeding difficulties, lethargy, hypotonia, hypothermia, and seizures. Psychomotor development is markedly delayed, and death usually occurs within 1 to 2 years of onset. Somatic, vascular, and bony changes are characteristic. The infant's hair is short, stringy, wiry, often white, and, under the microscope, appears twisted. The skin is pale and thick or pasty. The blood vessels, as revealed by angiogram or at autopsy, are elongated, tortuous, and display focal luminal narrowing and dilations resulting from disruption and fragmentation of the elastic layer. The bone shows osteoporosis and an irregular lucent trabecular pattern on radiographs.

Pathology

Grossly, the brain is atrophic, particularly the cerebellum, and shows focal areas of necrosis. Subdural hematoma is common. The histology consists of neuronal losses, gliosis, and ischemic necrotic changes. The cerebellar pathology is distinguished by severe loss of Purkinje cells and granule cells. The dendrites of the remaining Purkinje cells are swollen and distorted and, under the electron microscope, display abnormal mitochondria.

NEUROAXONAL DYSTROPHIES

Neuroaxonal dystrophies, rare neurometabolic diseases, are characterized by the presence of axonal spheroids. These are round or ellipsoid homogenous structures, 50 to 100 microns in diameter, dispersed freely in the neural parenchyma. They stain brightly red with eosin, are argentophilic, and immunoreact for α-synuclein, amyloid precursor protein (APP), ubiquitin, and neurofilament. Their pathogenesis is undetermined. A suggested hypothesis is disruption of the axonal transport.

Two forms of neuroaxonal dystrophies are infantile neuroaxonal dystrophy and neuroaxonal dystrophy with iron deposition in the brain. Both occur sporadically or are inherited in an autosomal recessive mode.

Infantile Neuroaxonal Dystrophy

Infantile neuroaxonal dystrophy or *Seitelberger's disease* presents with mental regression, motor deficits, cerebellar symptoms, blindness from optic atrophy, seizures, and myoclonic jerks. Death occurs within 3 to 8 years of onset.

Grossly, the brain shows moderately severe generalized atrophy. Histologically, axonal spheroids are distributed widely in the gray matter of the cerebrum and spinal cord, in the peripheral nerves, and in the autonomic ganglia. Additional findings are moderate neuronal losses in the cerebral cortex, neuronal and myelin losses in the pallidum, and Purkinje and granule cell degenerations in the cerebellar cortex. The clinical diagnosis is supported by demonstration of axonal spheroids in sural nerve biopsy.

Neuroaxonal Dystrophy with Brain Iron Deposition

Neuroaxonal dystrophy with brain iron deposition or *Hallervorden-Spatz disease* is caused by mutations in the pantothenate kinase gene (*PANK2*) located on chromosome 20. The disease can occur from infancy through adulthood. Extrapyramidal symptoms and signs are in the foreground of the clinical picture: dystonic posturing, choreoathetotic movements, rigidity, and dysarthric speech. The movement disorders are associated with progressive mental deterioration. Specific diagnostic tests are not available. T2-weighted MRI is useful to show bilateral hypointensity (iron deposits) with a central hyperintense area (necrosis) in the globus pallidus and in the reticular zone of the substantia nigra.

Pathology: Grossly, the brain shows bilateral softening and rusty discoloration of the globus pallidus. The histology is characterized by necrosis of the globus pallidus, iron-containing pigments in the globus pallidus and reticular zone of the substantia nigra, and the presence of axonal spheroids in the cerebral cortex and deep gray structures. The affected areas show neuronal losses and astrogliosis (Fig. 9.16).

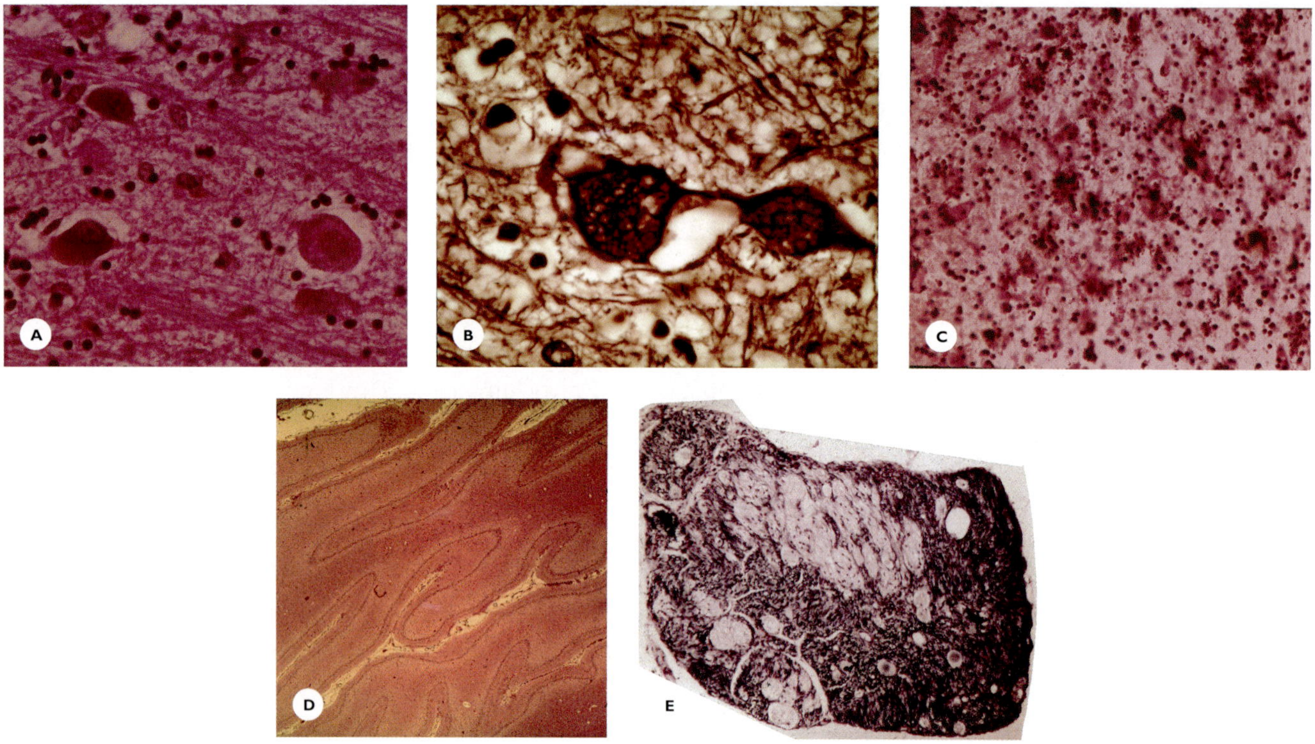

FIGURE 9.16

Neuroaxonal dystrophy with iron deposition. An infant girl developed normally until 1 year of age, when she began to stumble and gradually lost her ability to walk. At 3 years of age, she was speechless, had pale optic discs, searching nystagmus, and stiff extremities. Over the ensuing years, she developed seizures and myoclonic jerks. At nine and a half years of age, she died. Thalamus shows (**A**) eosinophilic (HE) and (**B**) argyrophilic axonal spheroids (Bodian stain). **C.** Basophilic-iron–positive granules are deposited in basal ganglia (HE). **D.** The cerebellum shows extensive Purkinje cell losses (HE). **E.** Peripheral nerve shows myelin degeneration and small axonal spheroids (LFB-CV).

MISCELLANEOUS NEUROMETABOLIC DISEASES

Niemann-Pick Type C Disease

Niemann-Pick type C disease (NPC), an autosomal recessive multiorgan disease, is caused by mutations in the gene *NPC1* located on chromosome 18, and less often by mutations in the gene *NPC2* located on chromosome 14. Abnormalities in intracellular cholesterol trafficking are major biochemical defects. Complex lipids accumulate in visceral organs, and glycolipids accumulate in the brain.

The disease can occur from the neonatal period through adulthood. The clinical presentation varies with age of onset. Hepatosplenomegaly is prevalent in neonates; psychomotor regression, vertical gaze palsy, and ataxia in young children; dysarthria, dysphagia, extrapyramidal disorders, behavioral changes, and intellectual decline in juveniles; and psychiatric symptoms and dementia in adults.

Grossly, the brain is atrophic. The histology consists of the following:

- The neurons are ballooned, containing storage material that stains with PAS and Luxol fast blue. A number of neurons display neurofibrillary tangles, similar to those in Alzheimer's disease.
- Axonal dystrophy in the form of axonal spheroids and focal swellings are prevalent throughout the cerebrum.

The liver, spleen, lymph nodes, and lungs show foamy cells that contain complex lipids.

Vanishing White Matter Disease

Vanishing white matter disease (VWD), an autosomal recessive leukoencephalopathy, is associated with defects in translation initiation factor eIF2B. The disease can be caused by mutations in any of five genes: *EIF2B1*, *EIF2B2*, *EIF2B3*, *EIF2B4*, and *EIF2B5*, located on chromosomes 12, 14, 1, 2, and 3, respectively.

The disease affects young children, but may also occur in juveniles and adults. It presents with progressive cerebellar ataxia, pyramidal signs, optic atrophy, seizures, and intellectual decline. In female patients, ovarian dysfunction has been reported. MRI demonstrates myelin losses and cystic cavitations in the white matter.

Grossly, the cerebral, cerebellar, and brainstem white matter are gelatinous, cystic, and cavitated. Histological changes in the white matter consist of pallor, thinning, vacuolation, and loss of myelin. Characteristically, the number of oligodendrocytes is markedly increased in some areas and reduced in others. Axonal losses are variable, and macrophage reaction and astrocytosis are not prominent.

Cockayne Syndrome

Cockayne syndrome, a rare autosomal recessive disorder, is caused by mutations in either the *CSA* or *CSB* gene. The disease manifests with dwarfism; microcephaly; facial dysmorphism with prognathism, malformed large ears, enophthalmos, and beaked nose; long extremities; and sensitivity to sunlight. Neurologic abnormalities are mental retardation, sensorineuronal hearing impairment, optic atrophy and pigmentary retinal degeneration, myoclonus, and pyramidal and extrapyramidal symptoms and signs.

Grossly, the brain is small, and the cerebral and cerebellar white matter is reduced. The histology is characterized by: (a) calcium deposits in the cerebral cortex, hemispheric white matter, basal ganglia, and cerebellum; (b) neuronal losses in the cerebral and cerebellar cortex; (c) an abnormal dendritic configuration of cortical neurons and Purkinje cells and the presence of binucleated neurons; (d) multifocal myelin losses in the cerebrum and cerebellum; and (e) bizarrely shaped binucleated astrocytes.

Congenital Disorders of Glycosylation

Congenital disorders of glycosylation (CDG), a group of autosomal recessive multisystem disorders, is caused by deficient activity of enzymes involved in glycosylation of proteins. Several carbohydrate-deficient glycoprotein diseases have been distinguished. Among them, CDG type Ia is the most common. It is caused by the deficient activity of the enzyme phosphomannomutase. The mutant gene maps to chromosome 16.

The disease affects chiefly infants and children and presents with many and various features:

- Somatic—Growth retardation, inverted nipples, abnormal fat pads
- Skeletal—Kyphosis, scoliosis
- Ocular—Strabismus, retinitis pigmentosa
- Neurologic—Mental retardation, hypotonia, cerebellar ataxia, stroke-like episodes, and polyneuropathy
- Visceral—Hepatic and renal dysfunctions
- Cardiac—Effusion
- Hematologic—Coagulopathy

MRI demonstrates cerebellar and pontine atrophy. Adult patients present with hypogonadism.

Grossly, the cerebellum and the pons are severely atrophic. Histology shows olivopontocerebellar hypoplasia or atrophy characterized by loss of the nuclei pontis and transverse pontine fibers, loss of Purkinje cells, and loss of neurons in the olivary nuclei. The liver shows cirrhosis, fibrosis, and fatty infiltration.

Abetalipoproteinemia

Abetalipoproteinemia or *Bassen-Kornzweig disease*, an autosomal recessive disorder of young adults, is caused by mutations in a gene on chromosome 9, which encodes the microsomal triglyceride transfer protein (MTP). The disease presents with malabsorption of fat, acanthocytosis (thorny erythrocytes), mental retardation, cerebellar dysfunction, peripheral neuropathy, and pigmentary retinopathy.

The pathology consists of axonal degeneration of the peripheral nerves, degeneration of the posterior columns of the spinal cord, and deposits of finely granular lipopigments in peripheral nerves, sensory neurons of the spinal ganglia, and skeletal muscles.

Tangier Disease

Tangier disease is characterized by the partial or total loss of circulating α-lipoproteins. It is caused by mutations in the ATP-binding cassette 1 (*ABC1*) gene located on chromosome 9. Cholesterol accumulates in bone marrow, lymph nodes, liver, and spleen. Patients present with large, orange-red tonsils and enlarged liver and spleen. Neurologic manifestations are a syringomyelia-like syndrome with loss of pain and temperature sensations, and polyneuropathy.

The pathology consists of myelin degeneration in the peripheral nerves and deposits of lipid droplets in the Schwann cells. The viscera, bone marrow, and lymph nodes show foam cells containing cholesterol esters.

Cerebrotendinous Xanthomatosis

Cerebrotendinous xanthomatosis, an autosomal recessive disorder, is caused by the defective metabolism of sterol. The disease occurs in young adults and manifests with polyneuropathy, cognitive impairment, ataxia, spasticity, and lipid deposition in large tendons. The pathology of neuropathy consists of demyelination, remyelination, and formation of onion bulbs.

BIBLIOGRAPHY

Golden, J.A., & Harding, B.N. (2004). *Pathology and genetics. Developmental neuropathology ISN*. Basel: Neuropath Press.

Lake, B.D. (1990). Metabolic disorders of the central and peripheral nervous system. In N.U. Filipe, B.P. Lake (Eds.), *Histochemistry in pathology*, 2nd edition. London: Churchill Livingstone.

Lyon, G., Adams, R.D., Kolodny, E.H. (1996). *Neurology of hereditary metabolic diseases of children*, 2nd edition. New York: McGraw-Hill.

Nyhan, W.L., & Ozand, P.T. (1998). *Atlas of metabolic diseases*. London: Chapman and Hall Medical.

Rosenberg, R.N., Prusiner, S.B., DiMauro, S., et al. (2003). *The molecular and genetic basis of neurologic and psychiatric diseases*, 3rd edition. Philadelphia: Butterworth Heinemann.

REVIEW QUESTIONS

1. The biochemical abnormalities in gangliosidosis GM2 are:
   A. Deficiency of hexosaminidase A
   B. Deficiency of hexosaminidase B
   C. Deficiency of an activator protein
   D. Deficiency of sphingomyelinase
   E. Accumulation of sphingomyelin

2. The gene associated with Tay-Sachs disease is best described as:
   A. It is the gene of an activator protein.
   B. It is the gene of α-subunit of hexosaminidase A (HEXA).
   C. It is the gene of α-subunit of hexosamidase B.
   D. It maps to chromosome 15.
   E. It maps to chromosome 10.

3. GM1 gangliosidosis in infants is best characterized by:
   A. Deficiency of β-galactosidase
   B. Dominant inheritance
   C. Mutant gene of missing enzyme maps to chromosome 5
   D. Facial dysmorphism and hepatomegaly
   E. Circulating vacuolated lymphocytes

4. Neuronal lipid storage diseases that manifest with extraneural lipid storage include:
   A. Niemann-Pick disease type A and B
   B. Gaucher disease
   C. Farber disease
   D. Fabry disease
   E. Niemann-Pick disease type C

5. Neuronal ceroid lipofuscinosis is a disorder of:

A. Peroxisomes
B. Amino acids
C. Mitochondria
D. Lysosomes
E. Copper metabolism

6. Clinical presentation of lipofuscinosis include:

A. Seizures
B. Cerebellar ataxia
C. Myoclonus
D. Facial anomalies
E. Macrocephaly

7. Batten-Vogt-Spielmeyer disease is described as:

A. The juvenile variant of lipofuscinosis
B. Pigmentary retinal degeneration as the ocular abnormality
C. The gene *CLN3* maps to chromosome 16
D. Conspicuous hepatosplenomegaly
E. Cherry-red spot of the macula as a common ocular finding

8. Hurler disease is best characterized by the following *except*:

A. It is a disorder of glycosaminoglycans.
B. It is X-linked inherited.
C. Facial and skeletal anomalies are common.
D. Obstructive hydrocephalus may be present.
E. Heparan sulfate and keratan sulfate are stored in viscera.

9. Pompe disease is best described as:

A. A disease affecting chiefly adults
B. Mucolipids accumulate in the neurons
C. Glycogen accumulates in the neurons and astrocytes only
D. Glycogen accumulates in neurons and muscles
E. Caused by acid maltase deficiency

10. Commonly encountered findings in Zellweger's disease are:

A. Craniofacial dysmorphism
B. Widespread inflammatory myelin degeneration
C. Polymicrogyria
D. Hypotonia, seizures
E. Neuronal storage of sphingolipids

11. Childhood adrenoleukodystrophy is best characterized by:

A. Deficiency of galactocerebrosidase
B. Defective oxidation of very long-chain fatty acids (VLCFA)
C. Autosomal recessive inheritance
D. Metachromasia of myelin breakdown products
E. Perivascular lymphocytic infiltrations in areas of demyelination

12. Metachromatic leukodystrophy is best described as:

A. A disorder of myelin sulfatides
B. It results from deficiency of enzymes arylsulfatase A, B, and C
C. The gene of arylsulfatase A maps to chromosome 22
D. Metachromasia of myelin globules is demonstrated with acidic Cresyl-violet
E. Globoid cells in demyelinated areas are characteristic.

13. Alexander disease is best described as:

A. Associated with mutations in the gene coding for glial fibrillary acidic protein (GFAP)
B. Loss of myelin in hemispheric white matter
C. Presence of Rosenthal fibers
D. Presence of corpora amylacea around blood vessels
E. Spongiform degeneration of cerebral cortex

14. Which of the following best characterize mitochondrial diseases?

A. Diseases caused by mutations in mDNA are transmitted maternally.
B. Lactate and pyruvate levels are decreased in CSF.
C. Lactate and pyruvate levels are increased in serum.
D. The muscles display ragged-red fibers.
E. All of these.

15. Leigh syndrome is best characterized by:
    - A. The disease chiefly affects adults.
    - B. The brunt of pathology is in the cerebral and cerebellar cortex.
    - C. The brunt of pathology is in the basal ganglia.
    - D. The disease is associated with mutations in nuclear DNA gene coding for SORF1.
    - E. The disease is associated with mutations in gene coding for ATPase 6.

16. Which of the following characterize phenylketonuria (PKU)?
    - A. Deficiency of acid dehydrogenase
    - B. Deficiency of phenylalanine hydroxylase
    - C. Diagnosis rests on urine test with 10% ferric chloride
    - D. Autosomal dominant disorder
    - E. Calcifications common in the basal ganglia

17. Myoclonic epilepsy or Lafora disease is best characterized by:
    - A. Ataxia, seizures, mental regression
    - B. Lewy bodies in substantia nigra
    - C. Lafora bodies in neuronal cytoplasm
    - D. Lafora bodies in skeletal muscles
    - E. Association with mutations in the gene *EPM2A* on chromosome 6

18. Which of the following characterize Wilson disease?
    - A. Extrapyramidal movement disorders
    - B. Increased serum ceruloplasmin
    - C. Decreased serum ceruloplasmin
    - D. Increased copper in serum
    - E. Greenish brown ring in limbus cornea

(Answers are provided in the Appendix.)

CHAPTER 10

Acquired Neurometabolic Diseases

Vitamin Deficiencies
Metabolic Encephalopathies
Calcium Metabolic Disorders
Neurologic Complications of Chronic Alcoholism
Toxic Diseases of the Nervous System

This group comprises diseases caused by vitamin deficiencies, encephalopathies associated with metabolic and endocrine diseases, mineral disorders, diseases associated with chronic alcoholism, and toxic disorders.

VITAMIN DEFICIENCIES

Vitamins play key roles in biochemical processes that are essential for normal functioning of neural tissue. Malabsorption due to gastrointestinal, pancreatic, and biliary diseases; malnutrition; long-term parenteral alimentation without vitamin supplementation; and the use of vitamin antagonist drugs are major causes of vitamin deficiencies. Vitamin deficiencies produce distinct clinical features and pathologic changes in the central and peripheral nervous system. Major vitamin deficiencies are summarized in Table 10.1. Two major diseases are presented here.

Vitamin B_1 (Thiamine) Deficiency

Thiamine pyrophosphate (TPP) is an important cofactor of the enzyme transketolase, which is involved in glucose metabolism. Deficiency develops in various clinical settings: malnutrition, malabsorption syndromes, chronic gastritis, gastrointestinal malignancies, persistent vomiting, and prolonged intravenous feeding without vitamin supplement. Alcoholics are at particular risk for the disease because of malnutrition; moreover, alcohol interferes with the metabolism, absorption, and storage of thiamine.

Wernicke's Encephalopathy

Wernicke's encephalopathy is a major complication of thiamine deficiency. The clinical presentation is highly characteristic and poses a medical emergency, because

TABLE 10.1.

Nervous System Manifestations in Major Vitamin Deficiencies

Vitamins	*Neurologic Features*
B_1 thiamine	Wernicke-Korsakoff encephalopathy Cerebellar atrophy Polyneuropathy
B_6 pyridoxine	Seizures in infancy Polyneuropathy
B_{12} cobalamine	Combined degeneration of spinal cord Polyneuropathy
Vitamin E, α-tocopherol	Spinocerebellar disorder Degeneration of posterior and lateral columns of spinal cord Axonal spheroids in cuneate and gracile nuclei of medulla
Folic acid	Polyneuropathy Myelopathy
Nicotinic acid; niacin	Polyneuropathy Myelopathy Encephalopathy Chromatolysis of neurons in cerebral cortex, brainstem, spinal cord Dementia

untreated cases have a poor, even fatal, outcome. The onset is acute or subacute. The following cardinal features occur in various combinations:

- Ocular—Retinal hemorrhage, pupillary changes, extraocular muscle palsy, gaze palsy and nystagmus
- Autonomic—Hypo- or hypertension, hypo- or hyperthermia, cardiac arrhythmias, respiratory failure
- Depression of alertness ranging from obtundation to coma
- Ataxia that is due to vestibular and/or cerebellar dysfunction

Blood transketolase activity is reduced and pyruvate level is elevated. MRI demonstrates the periventricular and thalamic lesions.

Pathology: The distribution of the pathologic process is distinctive and correlates well with the clinical presentation. The lesions are situated, usually symmetrically, in the walls of the third ventricle, extending into the mammillary bodies and dorsomedial nuclei of the thalami, and continuing caudally to the periaqueductal gray matter and floor of the fourth ventricle (Fig. 10.1, Table 10.2).

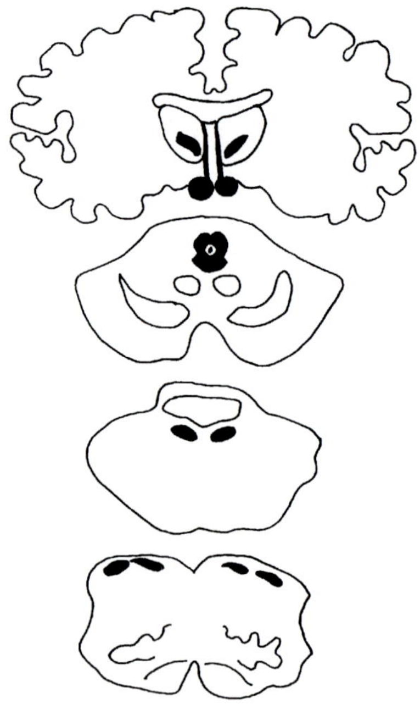

FIGURE 10.1
Wernicke-Korsakoff encephalopathy. Schematic drawing of distribution of lesions.

Grossly, the affected regions are soft, yellow to brown, finely granular, and contain petechial hemorrhages (Figs. 10.2 and 10.3). The histology is characterized by relative sparing of the neurons, destruction of myelin and, to a lesser degree, the axons; presence of lipid laden macrophages and astrocytic proliferation; prominent capillary endothelial hyperplasia; hemosiderin pigments; and fresh pericapillary hemorrhages (see Figs. 10.2 and 10.3). In chronic cases, the mammillary bodies are atrophic, spongy, and devoid of myelin and axons (Fig. 10.4).

Wernicke's encephalopathy is often associated with the *Korsakoff amnestic syndrome,* which is characterized by impairment of recent memory; that is, an inability to form lasting imprints of new information while at the same time the remote memory is retained. The memory impairment includes both verbal and nonverbal material. Learning is greatly impaired or impossible. The sense of time and sequences of events are disturbed. Confabulation is common. Other cognitive functions are variably impaired but less severely than the memory function. Such personality changes as apathy and loss of initiative and insight are frequent.

TABLE 10.2.
Wernicke-Korsakoff Encephalopathy

Clinical Features	*Site of Pathology*
Ocular: pupillary abnormalities: extraocular muscle palsy; gaze palsy: nystagmus	Brainstem tegmentum
Autonomic dysfunction: temperature; cardiocirculatory; respiratory	Hypothalamus Medulla: dorsal n. of vagus
Ataxia	Medulla: vestibular region Cerebellum
Depression of consciousness	Brainstem: periaqueductal gray
Altered mentation: global confusional state	Diffuse cerebral dysfunction
Amnestic syndrome for recent memory	Dorsomedial n. of thalamus Mammillary bodies

The Korsakoff amnestic syndrome usually becomes evident after recovery from Wernicke encephalopathy; less frequently, it occurs independently. It is attributed to lesions in the dorsomedial nuclei of the thalamus and/or the mammillary bodies, both important relay stations in the limbic lobe, which provides the anatomic substrate for memory and learning.

Vitamin B_{12} (Cobalamine) Deficiency

The intestinal absorption of vitamin B_{12} requires its binding to an intrinsic factor synthesized by the parietal cells of the gastric mucosa. An autoimmune gastritis, by interfering with the production or function of this intrinsic factor, is a major cause of the impaired absorption of vitamin B_{12}. Other causes are gastrectomy, enteritis, malabsorption diseases, malignancies, and fish tapeworm infestation.

Subacute combined degeneration of the spinal cord and megaloblastic (pernicious) anemia are major disorders associated with vitamin B_{12} deficiency. The

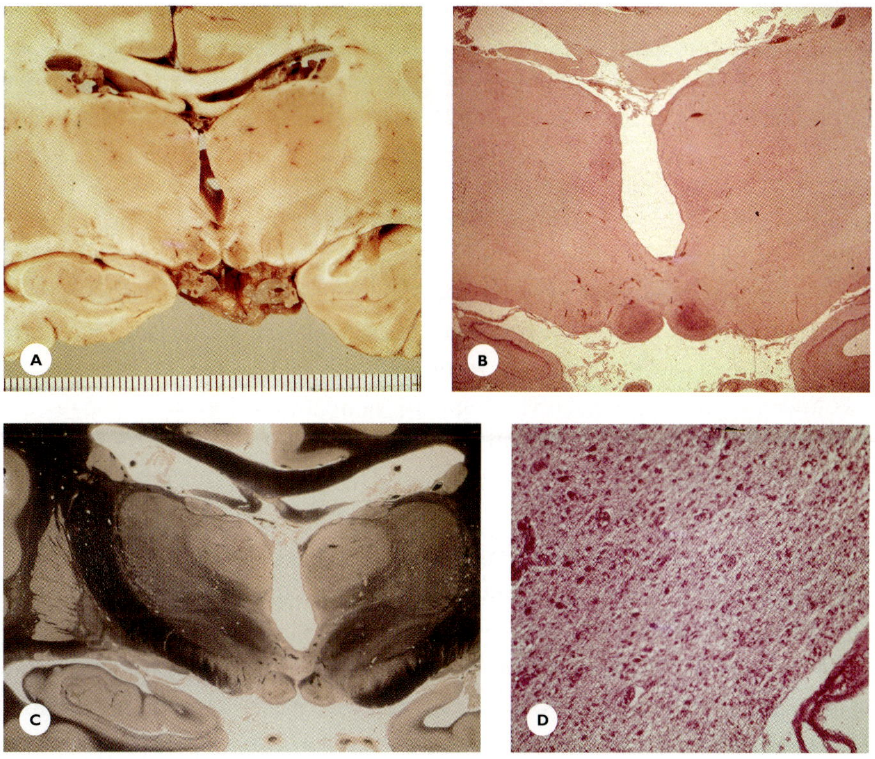

FIGURE 10.2
Wernicke-Korsakoff encephalopathy in a 48-year-old man, a heavy drinker. **A.** Transverse section at thalamus level shows brownish discoloration of the mammillary bodies and fresh petechiae in the floor of the third ventricle. Macrosections show (**B**) hypercellularity in mammillary bodies due to proliferated astrocytes and macrophages (Cresyl-violet), and (**C**) demyelination of stria medullaris and pallor of myelin in the thalami (Weil stain). **D.** Mammillary body contains macrophages and proliferated astrocytes (HE).

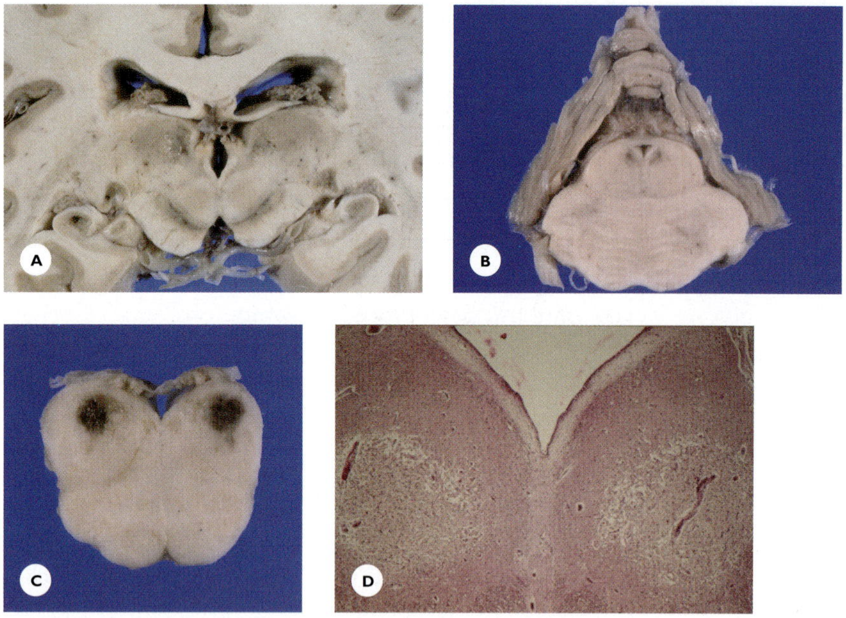

FIGURE 10.3
Wernicke-Korsakoff encephalopathy in an 87-year-old severely malnourished, anemic man. **A.** Transverse section at midbrain level shows hemorrhagic necrosis in dorsomedial aspects of pulvinars (habenular nuclei), grayish discoloration of ventricular wall and brownish-tan discoloration of lateral geniculate bodies, **B.** Upper pons shows hemorrhagic discoloration of locus ceruleus. **C.** Medulla shows symmetrically situated hemorrhages in the floor of fourth ventricle and (**D**) necrosis at the sites of hypoglossus nuclei (HE).

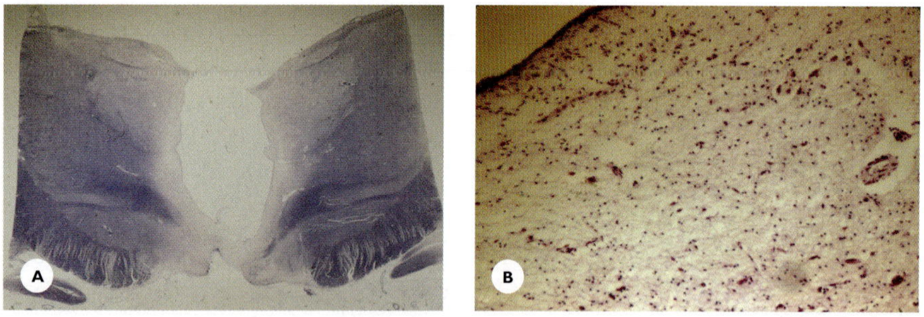

FIGURE 10.4
Chronic Wernicke-Korsakoff encephalopathy in an 80-year-old man, chronic alcoholic. **A.** Macrosection of the thalami shows severe atrophy of the mammillary bodies. **B.** Higher magnification view shows neuronal losses and mild astrocytosis in the wall of third ventricle (LFB-CV).

neurologic complication is attributed to the failure of a cobalamine-dependent enzyme necessary for the maintenance of myelin.

The disease has a subacute course, and manifests with paresthesias in the extremities, weakness and diminished or lost vibratory and position sensations in the lower extremities, positive Romberg sign, and a spastic ataxic (sensory) gait. Cerebral dysfunction, emotional lability, confusion, and intellectual decline may add to the clinical picture.

Pathology: Grossly, the spinal cord shows mild atrophy and grayish discoloration of the posterior and lateral columns. The histology is characterized by degeneration of myelin in the posterior and lateral columns, involving chiefly the corticospinal tracts. The degenerated tracts are vacuolated and spongy from the vacuolar distension of myelin (Fig. 10.5). In the acute stage, lipid-laden macrophages are numerous, but astrocytic reaction is not prominent in the chronic stage. Focal spongy myelin degenerations may also occur in the cerebral hemispheric white matter. Optic nerve degeneration is rare.

METABOLIC ENCEPHALOPATHIES

Hepatic Encephalopathy

Hepatic encephalopathy may develop acutely, complicating a fulminant hepatic failure or progress slowly, complicating chronic cirrhosis or a portocaval shunt. A disorder of nitrogen metabolism and elevated blood ammonia levels are implicated in the pathogenesis.

Acute hepatic encephalopathy presents with altered mentation, delirious state, seizures, and signs of raised intracranial pressure progressing rapidly to coma and death. Chronic hepatic encephalopathy presents with mild behavioral abnormalities, mental dullness, asterixis (flapping of outstretched hands), extrapyramidal symptoms (tremor, choreoathetosis), cerebellar ataxia, and dysarthria. In the terminal stage, altered mentation gradually progresses to stupor and coma. The blood ammonia level is elevated. EEG abnormalities consist of paroxysms of bilaterally synchronous slow or triphasic waves in the delta-range.

Pathology: Grossly, in acute hepatic encephalopathy, the brain is swollen (cytotoxic edema) and may have a greenish tint from bilirubin crossing the disrupted blood–brain barrier. In chronic encephalopathy, the brain is variably atrophic. Histologically, both acute and chronic encephalopathies are characterized by the presence of Alzheimer type 2 astroglia. These astrocytes have a large, round, less often lobulated or crescent-shaped vesicular nucleus with scanty chromatin and a prominent nucleolus. The perikaryon does not stain with eosin. They are usually immunonegative for GFAP but immunopositive for S-100 protein, and may contain glycogen inclusions (Fig. 10.6). These astrocytes are found in the deep cortical layers, basal ganglia, thalamus, and olivary and dentate nuclei. Additional characteristic features in chronic hepatic encephalopathy are necrosis and microvacuolation in the cerebral cortex at the junction with the white matter and in the basal ganglia and cerebellum.

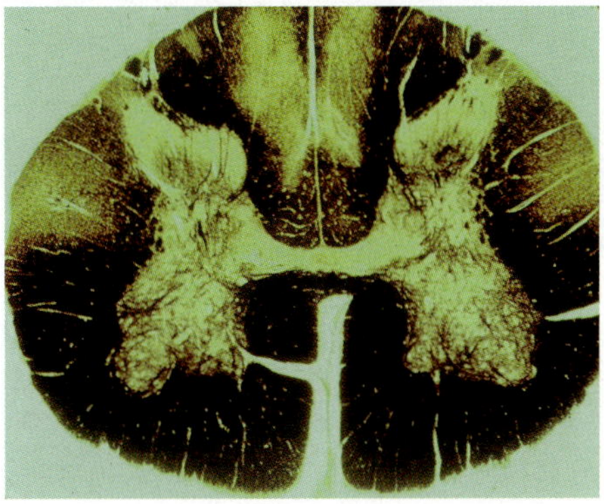

FIGURE 10.5
Subacute combined degeneration of the spinal cord in vitamin B_{12} deficiency. Macrosection of the lumbar spinal cord shows spongy degeneration of myelin in the posterior columns and corticospinal tracts of the lateral columns (Weil stain).

Hypoglycemic Encephalopathy

The brain's metabolism depends on a constant and adequate supply of glucose, because only small amounts of it are stored. A sudden drop in the blood glucose level to 30 to 40 mg/100 mL results in permanent brain damage within 1 to 2 hours. Major causes of hypoglycemic episodes are insulin overdose in diabetic patients,

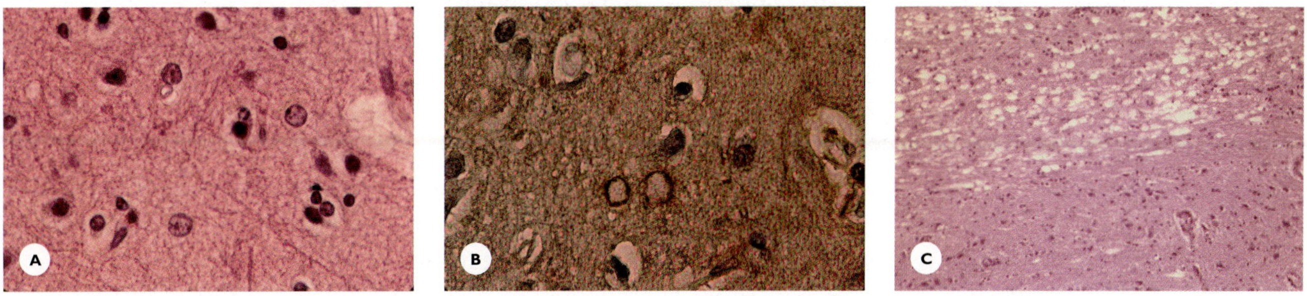

FIGURE 10.6
Hepatic encephalopathy in a 53-year-old chronic alcoholic man with severe liver cirrhosis. Alzheimer type 2 astrocytes in basal ganglia display (**A**) large vesicular nuclei, scanty chromatin, and prominent nucleoli (HE), and (**B**) positive immunostaining for S-100 protein (Immunostain). **C.** The subcortical white matter shows focal spongiosis (HE).

insulinoma of the pancreas islet cells, and liver, adrenal, pituitary, and thyroid diseases.

The clinical presentation varies with the severity and duration of hypoglycemia. It ranges from headaches, perspiration, nervousness, and tremulousness through confusion, myoclonic jerks, and seizures, to decerebrate rigidity and coma leading ultimately to death. Those who survive a severe and prolonged hypoglycemic episode usually are left with variable cognitive deficits and various neurologic symptoms and signs.

Similarities and differences can be seen between the pathogenesis and pathology of hypoglycemic and ischemic-hypoxic encephalopathies. In both conditions, the neurons are affected selectively, display similar morphology, and die by the process of excitotoxicity. But in hypoglycemic encephalopathy, the excitotoxicity is due chiefly to excessive accumulation of aspartate rather than of glutamate. Furthermore, hypoglycemic encephalopathy is associated with alkalosis due to an accumulation of ammonia and diminished production of lactate.

Pathology: Grossly, in chronic cases with long survival time, the cerebral cortex is atrophic and spongy, and the volume of the white matter is reduced. The histology of acute encephalopathy is characterized by selective neuronal necrosis. In hematoxylin-eosin (HE)-stained sections, the neurons appear shrunken, with angulated perikaryons that are depleted of Nissl substance and stain brightly red with eosin; The pyknotic nuclei stain homogeneously blue. Common sites of neuronal necrosis are: (a) the hippocampus, preferentially the neurons of the dentate gyrus, the C1 sector, and the subiculum; (b) the neocortical areas, (c) the caudate and the putamen; and (d) the Purkinje cells of the cerebellum, which usually are variably affected and often spared (Fig. 10.7). Chronic cases show variable neuronal losses, mineralization of some dead neurons, and replacement astrocytosis.

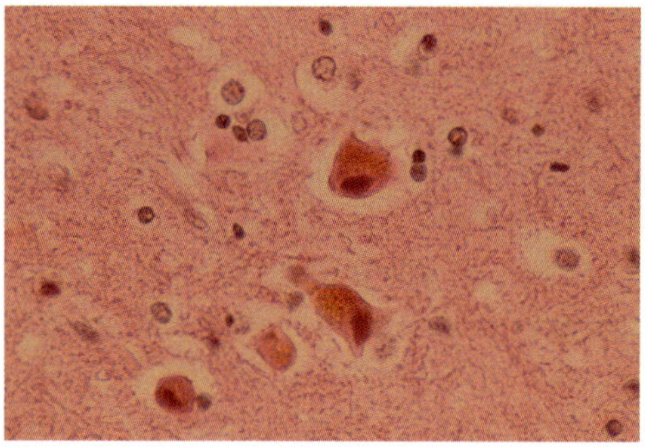

FIGURE 10.7
Hypoglycemic encephalopathy. A 68-year-old diabetic man, following administration of 11 units regular insulin, suffered a hypoglycemic episode with a blood glucose concentration of 28 mg/100 mL for approximately 8 hours. During this episode, he became comatose and, without regaining consciousness, died 15 days later. Eosinophilic neurons and mild astrocytosis (HE) are present in the thalamus.

Uremic Encephalopathy

Various neurologic complications develop in patients with renal failure and in patients receiving hemodialysis and peritoneal dialysis. Uremic encephalopathy presents with tremor, asterixis, myoclonic jerks, seizures, and stupor, which may progress to coma.

Neuropathologic findings include cerebral cytotoxic edema; neuronal losses in the cerebral and cerebellar cortex, deep gray structures and brainstem; perivascular demyelination; and occasional subdural hematoma.

Dialysis Encephalopathies

Dialysis encephalopathy (dementia) develops in patients on chronic hemodialysis and is attributed to aluminum toxicity.

Disequilibrium syndrome presents with headache, agitation, delirium, and seizures and usually develops toward the end of or after completion of dialysis. It is caused by water toxicity and brain edema.

Reye's Syndrome

This rare disease, predominantly of young children, usually develops acutely after a viral infection. Salicylate toxicity as a precipitating factor has been implicated in some cases. It manifests with fever, vomiting, enlarging liver, and rapidly progressing encephalopathy leading to death within days or a few weeks. High blood ammonia and low sugar levels are characteristic laboratory findings. Death occurs due to liver failure and raised intracranial pressure.

Grossly, the brain is swollen, displaying cerebellar and hippocampal herniations. The histology is characterized by fatty infiltration of the liver and cerebral cytotoxic edema, with neuronal and astrocytic swelling. Hepatic and cerebral mitochondrial dysfunctions are considered in the pathogenesis.

Hyperthermia

Excessive heat gain or insufficient heat loss lead to hyperthermia. Environmental exposure to high temperature (heat waves), exercises (marching, jogging), infection, and the neuroleptic malignant syndrome lead to hyperthermia. Old age, debility, use of anticholinergic drugs, and sympathetic autonomic failure predispose to insufficient heat loss.

Heat stroke refers to an elevated body temperature over 40°C. A rise in body temperature over 41°C is associated with a number of systemic and neurologic disorders: headache, vomiting, incoordination, acute respiratory distress with alkalosis, acute renal failure, electrolyte disorder, and intravascular coagulation. Confusion, depressed alertness, delirium, and seizures develop, and even death may ensue.

The pathology of heat-induced injury is characterized by selective degeneration of the Purkinje cells in both vermis and hemispheres. Replacement Bergmann glia expresses heat shock protein 70 during the acute stage. Purkinje cell degeneration is associated with the trans-synaptic loss of dentate neurons and pallor of efferent cerebellar pathways.

Late sequelae are cerebellar dysfunction due to cerebellar atrophy and occasional extrapyramidal syndrome, due to degeneration of the substantia nigra.

Multifocal Necrotizing Leukoencephalopathy

Multifocal necrotizing leukoencephalopathy (focal pontine leukoencephalopathy), a rare disease of undetermined pathogenesis, has been associated with immunosuppression, leukemia, use of cytotoxic drugs, and X-irradiation. The pathology is characterized by multiple small foci of parenchymal spongiosis and necrosis with calcification preferentially in the pons and also in the cerebral white matter. The cerebral lesions are microscopic, although pontine lesions may reach grossly detectable sizes (Fig. 10.8).

CALCIUM METABOLIC DISORDERS

Cerebral Calcification

Calcium deposits in the globus pallidus, less often in the Ammon horn and the dentate nucleus of the cerebellum, are frequent incidental autopsy findings, particularly in the brains of elderly individuals.

Striatopallidodentate calcification or *Fahr's disease* in some texts, refers to a distinct group of cerebral calcinoses. It commonly occurs in hypo- or hyperparathyroid disorders. It may also occur sporadically or be inherited in an autosomal dominant or autosomal recessive fashion. Characteristically, in the familial form, the serum calcium and phosphorous levels are normal, as is the endocrine function.

Cerebral calcinosis in young individuals may remain clinically asymptomatic for some time, then it presents with a wide range of symptoms: extrapyramidal such as, choreoathetosis, parkinsonian features, dystonia; cerebellar ataxias; seizures; mental retardation; intellectual decline and dementia. The calcifications are readily demonstrated on CT scan (Fig. 10.9).

Pathology: Calcifications, in addition to the basal ganglia and dentate nuclei, may involve the thalamus, internal capsule, cerebral and cerebellar cortex, and the white matter. In HE-stained sections, the calcium deposits appear as basophilic concretions varying in size from small globules to mulberry-like or larger coalescent masses. Some are dispersed in the tissue, and some are deposited within the walls of capillaries and small arteries (see Fig. 10.9). Their colloid matrix contains calcium, iron, aluminum, magnesium, phosphate, and bicarbonate.

NEUROLOGIC COMPLICATIONS OF CHRONIC ALCOHOLISM

Chronic alcohol (ethanol) abuse affects the nervous system, visceral organs, skeletal muscles and, in pregnant women, the fetus. Neurologic and psychiatric complications, acute or chronic, are frequent and comprise a wide

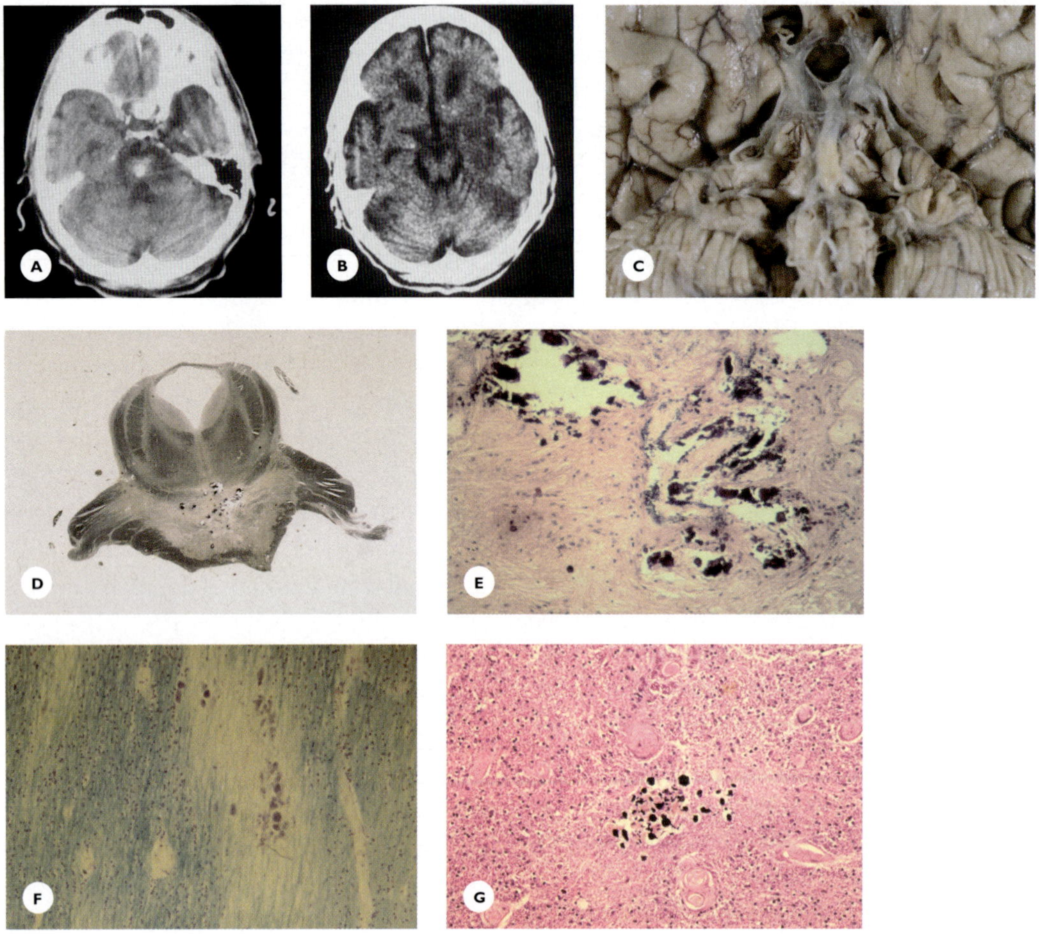

FIGURE 10.8

Multifocal necrotizing leukoencephalopathy. The disease of a 53-year-old man began with spasticity of his legs and difficulty walking. **A.** A CT scan of the head at age 55 years revealed a massive calcified lesion in the basis of the pons and enlarged fourth ventricle. At age 60 years, he underwent resection of a left maxillary "osteoma." His neurologic condition slowly progressed and, by age 66 years, he was spastic quadriparetic, dysarthric, dysphagic, and confused. One year later, he became bedridden, tube-fed, and incontinent. **B.** A CT scan at age 69 showed tiny calcified lesions in the hemispheric white matter and a large left maxillary tumor extending into the temporal fossa, diagnosed postmortem as an ameloblastoma. At age 72, he died, following a 19-year clinical course. **C.** Basal view of the brain shows severe atrophy of the pons. **D.** Macrosection of the pons shows extensive myelin destruction in pontine basis and multiple mineral deposits (myelin stain). **E.** Higher-magnification view shows large calcium-positive deposits in the parenchyma (von Kossa/HE). **F.** Cerebral hemispheric white matter shows multiple small areas of spongiosis with granular mineral deposits (LFB-CV). **G.** Spinal cord shows small basophilic mineral granules (HE).

range of clinical manifestations: ocular, motor, sensory, and autonomic; memory and cognitive deficits slowly progressing to dementia; and altered mentation ranging from delirium, hallucinosis, and stupor to coma.

Etiologies include malnutrition; vitamin deficiencies, particularly thiamine deficiency; metabolic derangements, mainly hepatic; and a direct toxic effect of alcohol on the neural tissue. Alcohol-associated central nervous system diseases may occur individually or in various combinations, and may be joined with peripheral neuropathy and myopathy.

Wernicke-Korsakoff encephalopathy, a serious complication of thiamine deficiency, is discussed in the section on vitamin deficiencies.

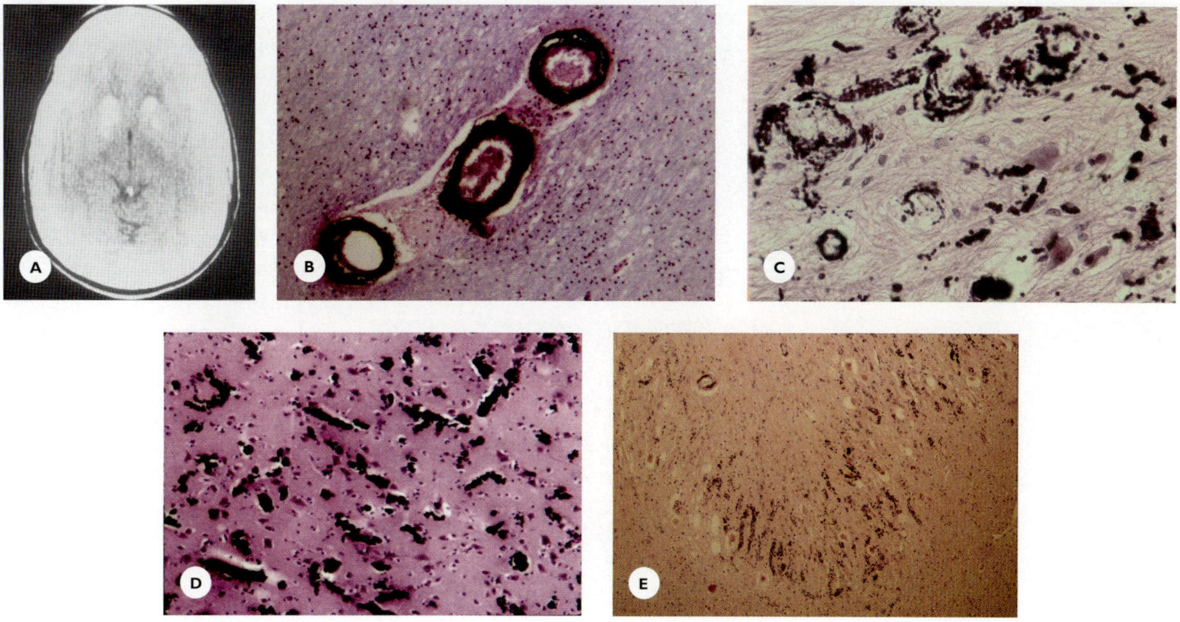

FIGURE 10.9

Cerebral calcinosis associated with hypoparathyroidism. A 19-year-old man developed tonic-clonic seizures and was diagnosed with hypoparathyroidism. He died of an acute viral infection, at age 38 years. **A.** A CT scan of the head reveals calcifications in the basal ganglia and frontal lobes. Basophilic (calcium and iron positive) granules are deposited in (**B**) walls of small arteries, (**C**) capillaries and parenchyma of basal ganglia (von Kossa), (**D**) cerebral cortex, and (**E**) dentate nucleus (HE).

Cerebellar atrophy, probably a complication of thiamine deficiency, presents with slowly progressive ataxia of the trunk and lower extremities and a broad-based irregular gait.

Grossly, the atrophy is typically confined to the superior vermis. In severe chronic cases, it involves the entire vermis and the hemispheres (Fig. 10.10). The histology is characterized by a degeneration of the Purkinje cells and, to a lesser degree, the granule cells. The molecular layer and the myelin core of the folia are atrophic. A prominent Bergmann astrocytic layer replaces the lost Purkinje cells. Axonal torpedoes of the degenerated Purkinje cells are common in the granular cell layer (see Fig. 10.10). The inferior olivary nuclei show neuronal losses (retrograde trans-synaptic degeneration) and gliosis.

Central Pontine Myelinolysis

Central pontine myelinolysis has been reported in malnourished chronic alcoholics. It also occurs in liver diseases, liver transplants, severe burns, and hyponatremia. A rapid correction of hyponatremia is suggested to be a major cause of the disease. The onset is acute, with para- or quadriparesis, dysarthria, and dysphagia resembling the locked-in syndrome. The prognosis is poor. Death may occur within a few weeks; a small number of patients may recover partially or completely. The diagnosis is supported by CT scan and MRI.

Pathology: Grossly, a triangular or butterfly-shaped grayish, soft, slightly granular lesion is situated in the center of the basis of the pons. The histology is distinguished by demyelination of the fiber tracts, most commonly the transverse pontine fibers. The axons are relatively preserved except in severe and chronic cases, and the neurons are spared (Fig. 10.11). Lipid-laden macrophages are numerous in the acute stage, and reactive astrocytes predominate in the chronic stage. Similar lesions may occur outside the pons, in the striatum, thalamus, lateral geniculate bodies, cerebral white matter, and cerebellum.

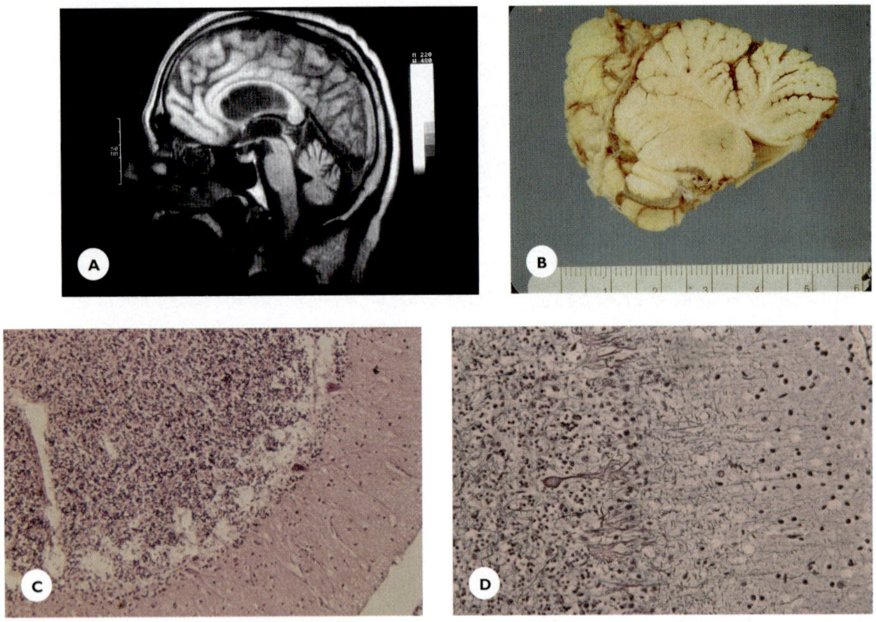

FIGURE 10.10
Alcoholic cerebellar atrophy. **A.** MRI of a chronic alcoholic man shows atrophy of the vermis, particularly the superior folia. **B.** Sagittal section of the vermis shows prominent atrophy of the superior folia in a 58-year-old alcoholic woman. Superior vermis shows (**C**) loss of the Purkinje cells and a prominent Bergmann astrocytosis (HE). **D.** Some basket cell fibers are preserved, and axonal torpedoes are present in the granular layer (Bodian stain).

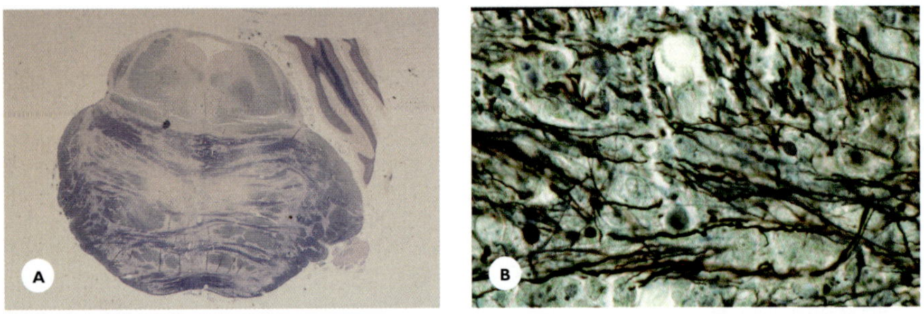

FIGURE 10.11
Central pontine myelinosis. An incidental autopsy finding in a 74-year old man with Alzheimer's disease. **A.** Macrosection shows demyelination in the center of the pontine basis. Higher-magnification view shows in the demyelinated area: (**B**) partial preservation of nerve fibers (Holmes stain).

Marchiafava-Bignami Disease

Marchiafava-Bignami disease, a rare condition in chronic alcoholics, presents with symptoms and signs of an interhemispheric disconnection syndrome. The pathology consists of demyelination of the genu and body of the corpus callosum, often extending symmetrically into the centum semiovale. The anterior commissure, optic chiasma, and middle cerebellar peduncles may also be involved (Fig. 10.12). MRI and CT scan make the diagnosis possible antemortem.

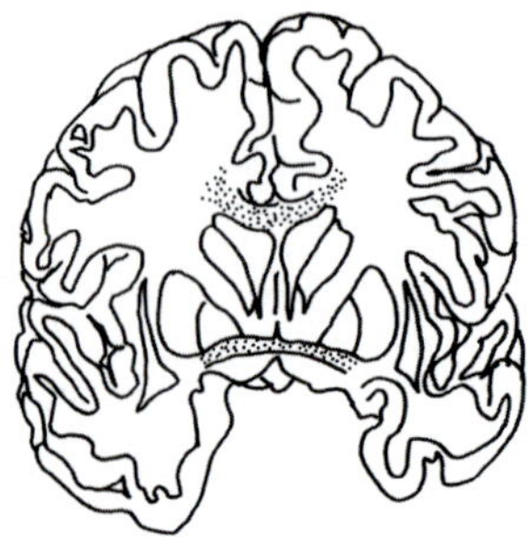

FIGURE 10.12
Schematic drawing of distribution of myelin degeneration in Marchiafava-Bignami disease.

Optic Neuropathy

Optic neuropathy due to nutritional deficiency presents with slowly progressive visual impairment, ultimately leading to blindness. Myelin and axonal degeneration of the optic nerves characterize the pathology (Fig. 10.13).

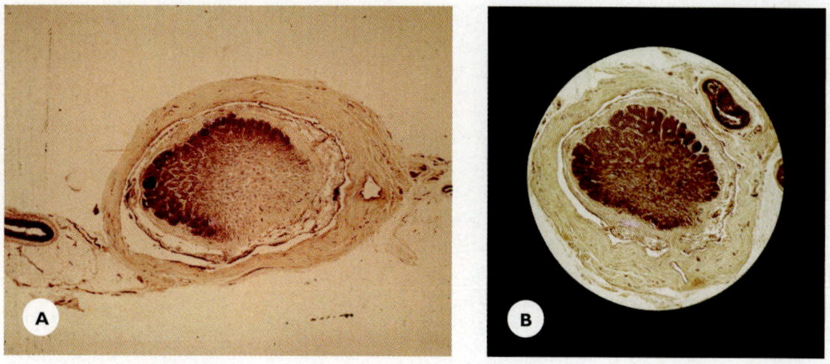

FIGURE 10.13

Optic nerve degeneration. The disease of a 48-year-old shipping clerk, a heavy drinker, began with progressively failing vision that, over several weeks, progressed to the point that he was unable to read the shipping labels. He developed Wernicke encephalopathy and died several months later. **A** and **B.** Both optic nerves show partial myelin degeneration (myelin stain).

TABLE 10.3.
Major Toxic Disorders of the Nervous System

Substances	*Neuropathology*
Carbon monoxide	Acute: congestion, edema, petechial hemorrhages Chronic: bilateral pallidal necrosis, cortical necrosis, leukoencephalopathy
Cyanide	Edema, petechial hemorrhages Necrosis: basal ganglia, hemispheric white matter, Purkinje cell degeneration
Methanol (methyl alcohol)	Retinal ganglionic degeneration, optic nerve degeneration, Putaminal necrosis, hemorrhagic leukoencephalopathy
Lead	Encephalopathy: edema, congestion, petechial hemorrhages, capillary, endothelial hyperplasia, motor neuropathy
Arsenic	Peripheral neuropathy, predominantly axonal Hemorrhagic leukoencephalopathy (hypersensitivity reaction)
Manganese	Bilateral pallidal degeneration, Subthalamic n. degeneration
Mercury (organic and inorganic)	Cortical neuronal degeneration: calcarine and motor cortex, Granule cell degeneration in cerebellar cortex
Aluminum	Cortical gliosis
Hexacarbon (sniffing glue)	Giant axonal neuropathy
Methotrexate (intrathecal)	Meningitis, meningoencephalitis, transverse myelitis, Disseminated necrotizing coagulative leukoencephalopathy
Vincristine	Cranial neuropathy, peripheral axonal neuropathy, Myelopathy with eosinophilic intracytoplasmic inclusions
Phenytoin	Cerebellar cortical degeneration, Peripheral, predominantly sensory neuropathy

Cerebral Atrophy

The brains of chronic alcoholics who had no other alcohol-related pathology may display a diminished volume of the cerebral white matter, especially of the frontal lobes, and neuronal losses in the frontal association cortex. The changes suggest a direct toxic effect of alcohol on the neural tissue and probably contribute to the cognitive decline (alcoholic dementia).

Fetal Alcohol Syndrome

Fetal alcohol syndrome consists of various abnormalities in the infants of mothers who consumed

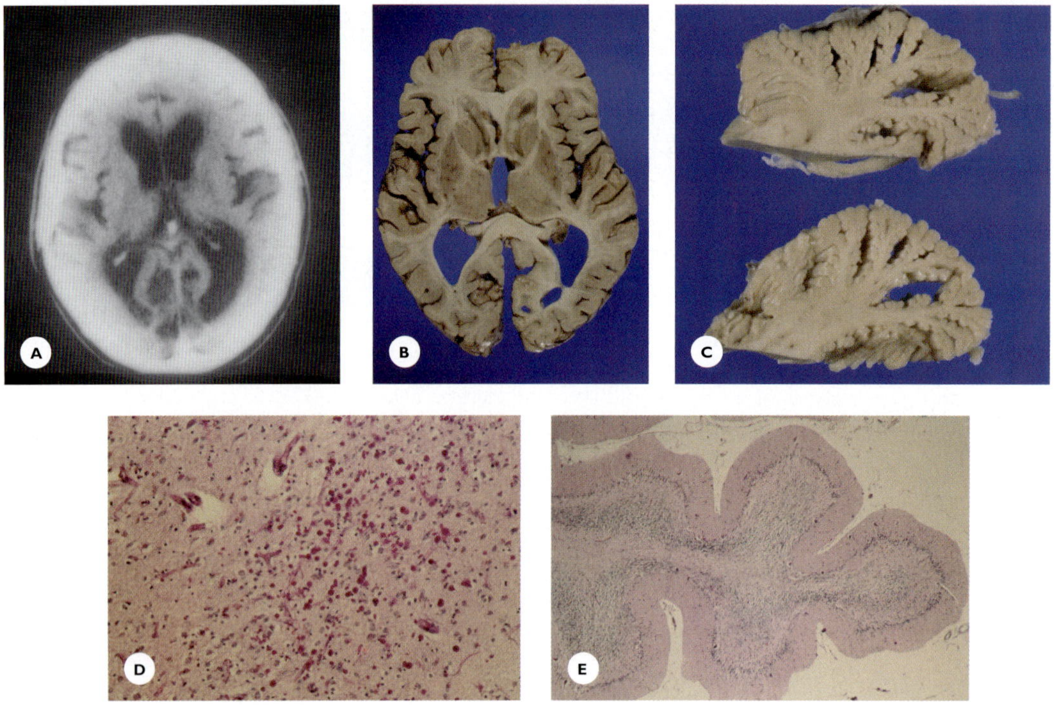

FIGURE 10.14
Mercury neurotoxicity. A 46-year-old chemical operator was exposed to organic mercury compounds for approximately 3 years. At age 50 years, he was evaluated for unsteadiness of gait, clumsiness of hands, and deteriorating eyesight. His neurologic deficits slowly progressed, along with mental decline. At age 74, he died. CT scan of the head at age 72 years shows (**A**) prominent calcarine and Sylvian fissures and marked atrophy of the medial aspects of the occipital lobes and insular regions. **B.** Horizontal slice of the brain shows cortical and white matter atrophy of the medial occipital lobes. **C.** The cerebellar cortex is severely atrophic. **D.** The striate cortex shows significant neuronal losses and abundance of corpora amylacea (PAS). **E.** The cerebellum shows diffuse losses of granule cells and only moderate Purkinje cell losses (HE).

excessive alcohol during pregnancy. Microcephaly, facial anomalies (short palpebral fissure, thin upper lip, incomplete jaw development), growth retardation, cerebellar dysgenesis, and neuroglial heterotopia are among the common anomalies.

TOXIC DISEASES OF THE NERVOUS SYSTEM

A great number of toxic substances, metals, industrial chemicals, and therapeutic agents have affinity for the central and/or peripheral nervous system, producing a variety of pathologic changes (Table 10.3). A case of mercury toxicity is illustrated in Figure 10.14.

BIBLIOGRAPHY

Anders, K. H., Becker, P. S., et al. (1993). Multifocal necrotizing leukoencephalopathy with pontine predilection in immunosuppressed, patients: a clinicopathologic review of 16 cases. *Human Pathol 24*, 897–904.

Antony, D. C., Montine, T. J., Valentine, W. M., & Graham, D. G. (2001). Toxic responses of the nervous system. In C. D. Klassen (Ed.), *Casarett and Doull's toxicology, the basic science of poisons*, 6th edition (pp. 14–19; 535–563). New York: McGraw-Hill.

Eto, K. (2000). Minamato disease Neuropathology *20*, 14–19.

Harper, C. (1998). The neuropathology of alcohol-specific brain damage, or does alcohol damage the brain? *J Neuropathol Exp Neurol 57*, 101–110.

Victor, M., Adams, R. D., & Collins, G. H. (1971). *The Wernicke-Korsakoff syndrome: contemporary neurology series.* Philadelphia, F. A. Davis.

REVIEW QUESTIONS

1. Patients with Wernicke encephalopathy present with all of the following *except*:

   A. Spastic paraparesis
   B. Mental changes
   C. Extraocular muscle palsy
   D. Nystagmus
   E. Cardiac arrhythmias

2. Which of the following statements concerning Wernicke encephalopathy are incorrect:

   A. The lesions are situated in the hypothalamus.
   B. The disease is caused by vitamin B_{12} deficiency.
   C. The lesions are common in the pontine basis.
   D. The lesions display petechial hemorrhages.
   E. The periaqueductal region often is involved.

3. The Korsakoff amnestic syndrome may coexist with Wernicke's encephalopathy. In this case, the lesions that account for the amnestic syndrome are situated in the:

   A. Ammon's horns
   B. Mammillary bodies and/or dorsomedial nuclei of the thalami
   C. Frontal lobes
   D. Left temporal lobe
   E. Both temporal lobes

4. Concerning subacute degeneration of the spinal cord, all of the following are correct *except*:

   A. It presents with spastic-ataxic paraparesis.
   B. It is caused by vitamin B_{12} deficiency.
   C. The Romberg sign is negative.
   D. Spongy degeneration occurs in the cerebral white matter.
   E. The posterior and lateral columns of the spinal cord show spongy degeneration.

5. Alzheimer's type 2 astrocytes are characteristic of:

   A. Hypoglycemic encephalopathy
   B. Central pontine myelinolysis
   C. Hepatic encephalopathy
   D. Alcoholic cerebellar degeneration
   E. None of these

6. Cortical cerebellar degeneration occurs in:

   A. Dilantin toxicity
   B. Mercury toxicity
   C. Chronic alcoholism
   D. None of these
   E. All of these

(Answers are provided in the Appendix.)

CHAPTER 11

Tumors of the Central Nervous System

General Aspects
Tumors of the Neuroepithelium
Tumors of the Meninges
Tumors of the Pituitary Gland and Sellar Region
Germ Cell Tumors
Tumors of the Cranial and Spinal Nerves
Maldevelopmental Tumors and Cysts
Hemangiomas
Lymphomas and Hemopoietic Tumors
Metastatic Tumors
Tumors of the Spinal Cord, Nerve Roots, and Meninges
Tumors of the Cranium and Spine
Primary Intracranial Tumors in Children
Hereditary Tumor Syndromes
Nervous System Complications of Radiation and Chemotherapy
Paraneoplastic Diseases

GENERAL ASPECTS

Primary brain tumors constitute approximately 2% of all malignancies and 20% of malignancies in children. Brain tumors among adolescents and young adults are the third most common cause of death due to cancer. The survival time in about one-third of patients is poor, averaging 5 years. The prognosis is unfavorable because a significant number of brain tumors grow infiltratively and diffusely, and therefore are not amenable to total resection and are prone to recur, and they are often located in functionally highly specialized or vital regions. Moreover, therapeutic options are limited.

Etiologies

Both genetic predisposition and environmental agents are factors in the etiology of nervous system tumors. Inherited predisposition is supported by occurrences of specific brain tumors in families and by occurrences in inherited tumor syndromes. Structural changes in chromosomes and genetic alterations have been identified in a significant number of tumors. Two major classes of genes implicated in tumor pathogenesis are the *oncogenes* and the *tumor suppressor genes*. Chief oncogenes are the epidermal growth factor receptor (EGFR) gene on chromosome 7, the platelet-derived growth factor (PDGF) receptor gene, and a group of genes on chromosome 12q. An important tumor suppressor gene is the p53 on chromosome 17p. Potential tumor suppressor genes are located on chromosomes 1p, 9p, 10, 17p, 19q, and 22q. Tumor suppressor genes are involved in normal cell-cycle control, DNA repair, apoptosis, and the inhibition of angiogenesis. The activation of oncogenes by duplication or amplification, point mutation, and rearrangement, and the inactivation of tumor suppressor genes by mutations, physical loss, or deletion are common genetic alterations in nervous-system tumorigenesis. Genetic alterations may be inherited, or they may be acquired by the action of environmental agents.

Among environmental factors, irradiation to the head has been established as a potential risk for tumor development. An association between head trauma and brain tumor, particularly meningioma, has been suggested. Epstein-Barr virus has oncogenic potentials and is associated with primary central nervous system (CNS) lymphomas in HIV-infected patients. The papovavirus SV40 is implicated in the pathogenesis of choroids plexus papilloma and choroid plexus carcinomas. An association between brain tumors in human and various chemicals has been suggested but not proven.

TABLE 11.1.
Age-Related Distribution of Common Intracranial Tumors

Tumors	*Average range of age (yrs)*
Optic nerve/chiasma astrocytoma Brainstem glioma Choroid plexus papilloma	0–15
Cerebellar astrocytoma Medulloblastoma	5–20
Craniopharyngioma	5–15
Ependymoma	5–45
Cerebral atrocytoma Oligodendroglioma	20–50
Pituitary adenoma Hemangioblastoma	20–60
Meningioma Schwannoma	20–65
Metastases	35–65

Clinical Features

Tumors of the nervous system are distinguished by their preference for particular age groups (Table 11.1) and gender and predilection for particular anatomic sites. Brain tumors occur at all ages, but the incidence is higher in childhood and late adulthood. With few exceptions, a male prevalence is noted. In children, they are more common in the infratentorial, and in adults, in the supratentorial compartment. Brain tumors can present with seizures, focal neurologic deficits, psychiatric symptoms, and symptoms and signs of raised intracranial pressure (ICP) (see Chapter 2).

Diagnosing brain tumors relies on their clinical presentation, supplemented with ancillary tests. Standard diagnostic aids are neuroimaging using computed tomography (CT) scan, magnetic resonance imaging (MRI), and angiography. Emerging new MRI techniques (such as fast fluid-attenuated inversion recovery [FLAIR] imaging, magnetization transfer imaging, diffusion/perfusion-weighted imaging, and MR spectroscopy) better define the neural tumors by distinguishing between benign and malignant features, outlining their metabolic activities and vascular supply, and differentiating between recurrence and radiation effect. Biochemical assays identify tumor-secreted hormones and circulating tumor markers. A cytologic study of the cerebrospinal fluid is indicated when subarachnoid dissemination of a tumor is suspected. Biopsy is valuable to confirm the neoplastic nature of a lesion and to determine its histology.

Pathologic Features

Brain tumors are graded on the basis of their histologic characteristics from 1 to 4, providing an approximate prognostic guide. Grade 1, a benign tumor, grows slowly. Grossly, it is circumscribed or encapsulated. Histologically, the tumor cells are well differentiated, resembling the cell of origin; mitosis is absent or very rare; blood vessels are scanty and normal.

By contrast, grade 4, a malignant tumor, grows fast, invading and destroying the local tissue. Grossly, it is ill-defined and is surrounded by edema. (The pathologic effects of edema are presented in Chapter 2 and summarized here in Table 11.2.) Histologically, the tumor cells are anaplastic (undifferentiated); pleomorphic, (varied in shape, size, and pattern); mitosis is common, often atypical; blood supply is rich with abnormal vessels; and hemorrhage and necrosis are common. Grade 2 tumors have one, and grade 3 tumors, three or four criteria of malignancy. Brain tumors are prone to disseminate and seed along the cerebrospinal fluid (CNF) pathways. A few metastasize outside the nervous system to lymph nodes, viscera, and bone marrow. Tumorous invasion of the veins and dural sinuses and shunting procedures are potential routes for extracranial metastases.

A correlation between the histologic appearance and biologic behavior of the tumors varies and often is poor. The biologic behavior takes into account the speed and pattern of growth, tendency to malignant transformation and recurrence, dissemination via CSF, and responsiveness to therapy. Estimated mean-survival with grade 2 tumors is 5 to 10 years; with grade 3, 2 to 3 years; and with grade 4, 1 to 1.5 years.

Diagnosing nervous system tumors in surgical or autopsy specimens requires a supplementation of standard histologic stains with immunohistologic techniques using antibodies to tumor-specific antigens (Table 11.3). The proliferative capacity of the tumor cells can be assessed by using monoclonal antibodies MIB-1 to the Ki-67 proliferation related nuclear antigen. A Ki-67/MIB-1 labeling index (LI) of greater than 7% to 8% indicates a higher grade of malignancy and poorer prognosis. Immunohistologic stain can be applied to detect mutations in the p53 suppressor gene. Electron microscopic examination is helpful in diagnostically doubtful cases.

TABLE 11.2.

Pathologic Changes Produced by Expanding Intracranial Lesions

Edema	Hydrocephalus
Herniations	Pituitary necrosis
Vascular lesions	Bony erosions

TABLE 11.3.

Major Tumor-Related Immunohistologic Stains

GFAP	*S-100 protein*	*Synaptophysin*
Astrocytic tumors Ependymoma Oligodendroglioma Neuronal/glial tumors	Astrocytic tumors Ependymoma Oligodendroglioma Neuronal/glial tumors Choroid plexus papilloma Neurinoma Neurofibroma	Neuronal/glial tumors Medulloblastoma Pineal gland tumor
Vimentin	***EMA***	***Cytokeratin***
Meningioma Hemangioblstoma Hemangiopericytoma Choroid plexus papilloma	Meningioma Choroid plexus papilloma	Craniopharyngioma Choroid plexus papilloma
Chromogranin	***AFP***	***PLAP***
Neuroendocrine tumor	Embryonal carcinoma	Germinoma

GFAP, glial fibrillary acidic protein; EMA, epithelial membrane antigen; PLAP, placental alkaline phosphatase; AFP, α-fetoprotein.

Classification

The first valid classification of brain tumors based on their histogenesis was published by Bailey and Cushing in 1929, and served as the basis for further classification. A newly revised classification of tumors of the nervous system was published by the World Health Organization (WHO) in 2000. Cytogenetic and molecular genetic features have become important in tumor characterization. It is anticipated that genetic profiling of the tumors will provide an improved prognostic guide and help in selecting appropriate therapy.

The tumors presented here are divided into 11 categories and graded according to the WHO. An overview of childhood tumors and hereditary tumor syndromes, harmful effects of tumor therapies, and paraneoplastic diseases complete the chapter.

TUMORS OF THE NEUROEPITHELIUM

During brain development, the primitive cells of the neuroepithelium proliferate and differentiate into neuroblasts and glioblasts, which then mature into neurons and glial cells. Tumors with neuroepithelial cell lineage constitute the largest group of intracranial tumors. The group includes gliomas, neuronal and mixed neuronal/glial tumors, embryonal tumors, and tumors of the pineal gland parenchyma. Their preferential sites are listed in Table 11.4.

Gliomas

This largest group of neuroepithelial tumors comprises the astrocytic, oligodendroglial, and ependymal tumors derived from the three types of glial cells: astrocyte, oligodendroglia, and ependymal glia, respectively.

Astrocytic Tumors

Astrocytic tumors constitute the largest group of intracranial tumors in both adults and children. Their locations, gross and histologic features, biologic behavior, and genetic alterations vary greatly. The WHO distinguishes four grades of astrocytic tumors based on their histologic characteristics (Table 11.5).

Astrocytic Tumors (Grades 2, 3, and 4)

Diffuse astrocytoma grade 2, anaplastic astrocytoma grade 3, and glioblastoma grade 4 constitute the largest group of primary intracranial tumors affecting individuals from early adulthood to late midlife. These tumors are apt to progress malignantly: Diffuse astrocytomas can progress to anaplastic astrocytomas and glioblastomas, and anaplastic astrocytomas to glioblastomas. A significant number of tumors are associated with specific molecular abnormalities. Common genetic alterations are mutations of tumor suppressor gene p53 and loss of chromosome 17q; and overexpression of several oncogenes and their receptors, such as EGFR, PDGF, fibroblast growth factors (FGFs), and vascular endothelial growth factor (VEGF) receptors. In an appreciable number of astrocytomas, the progression from a low grade to a higher grade is associated with the inactivation of specific tumor suppressor genes and losses of specific chromosomes.

Diffuse Astrocytoma (Grade 2)

This tumor typically occurs in the cerebral hemispheres of young adults, less often in the brainstem, cerebellum. and cerebral hemispheres of children and adolescents. The tumor grows slowly and diffusely infiltrates the local structures, gradually enlarging and deforming them. Clin-

TABLE 11.4.
Regional Distribution of Common Neuroepithelial Tumors

Cerebral Hemispheres	*Cerebellum*	*Optic Nerve/Chiasma Hypothalamus Brainstem*	*Ventricles*
Astrocytoma Glioblastoma Oligodendroglioma Ependymoma	Astrocytoma Medulloblastoma	Astrocytoma	Ependymoma Choroid plexus papilloma Astrocytoma

ically, it often presents with seizures for months or years before focal neurologic deficits and raised ICP develop. Postsurgical survival is variable, averaging 5 years.

Diffuse astrocytoma is characterized grossly by poor demarcation from the adjacent healthy tissue and histologically by the low cellularity of well-differentiated neoplastic astrocytes displaying minimal pleomorphism and few or no mitosis. Vascular supply is sparse, and necrosis is absent.

Genetic alterations are mutations in the p53 gene, loss of chromosome 17, and overexpression of the PDGF system. The inactivation of the cell-cycle regulatory system is implicated in the progression of a diffuse astrocytoma to an anaplastic astrocytoma.

TABLE 11.5.
Astrocytic Tumors

Astrocytic Tumors
Diffuse astrocytoma (grade 2)
Fibrillary
Protoplasmic
Gemistocytic
Anaplastic astrocytoma (grade 3)
Glioblastoma (grade 4)
Pilocytic astrocytoma (grade 1)
Subependymal giant cell astrocytoma (grade 1)
Desmoplastic infantile astrocytoma/ganglioma (grade 1)
Pleomorphic xanthoastrocytoma (grade 2)

The three subtypes of diffuse astrocytomas are (a) protoplasmic, (b) fibrillary, and (c) gemistocytic.

A *protoplasmic astrocytoma* has a homogenous, translucent, gelatinous appearance. It is composed of neoplastic astrocytes with small, round to oval nuclei, which are moderately rich in chromatin and are surrounded by scanty cytoplasm with few processes. GFAP expression is sparse. Microcytic and mucoid degenerations are common (Fig. 11.2).

The *fibrillary astrocytoma* grossly is firm—in places rubbery—and the cut surfaces are whitish-gray. The tumor is composed of small stellate and elongated neoplastic astrocytes with fine fibrillary processes forming a loose meshwork and bundles, leaving the pre-existing tissue relatively preserved. GFAP expression is variable. Entrapped neurons are easily detected between the tumor cells. In the white matter, the astrocytic bundles run along the fiber tracts. Microcystic degenerations may be present (Fig. 11.3).

The *gemistocytic astrocytoma* is soft and homogenous. It is composed of large, plump neoplastic astrocytes with abundant glassy eosinophilic cytoplasms and peripherally displaced nuclei (Fig. 11.4). GFAP expression is common.

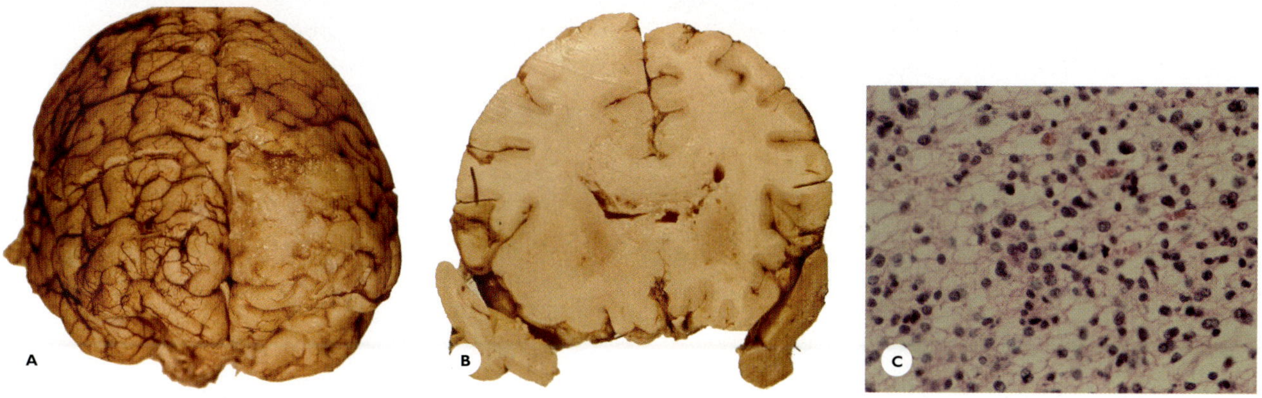

FIGURE 11.1
Diffuse protoplasmic astrocytoma. A well adjusted lively and sociable woman had her first tonic-clonic seizure at 33 years of age. One year later, she was evaluated for headaches and, around the same time, her behavior gradually changed: She became withdrawn, uncommunicative, spent the days in bed, neglected her appointments with her psychiatrist, and obstetrician. Following delivery of a healthy child, her condition rapidly deteriorated, she appeared catatonic, and died a few weeks later. **A.** The convolutional pattern of the left frontal lobe is effaced by a soft homogenous grayish mass lesion. **B.** The white matter of both frontal lobes, the corpus callosum, and the caudate are diffusely enlarged by a poorly demarcated, soft, gelatinous, pinkish-gray tumor that contains tiny cystic cavities. **C.** The tumor is moderately cellular, composed of neoplastic protoplasmic astrocytes showing mild nuclear pleomorphism (HE). Blood vessels are sparse; mitoses and necrosis are absent

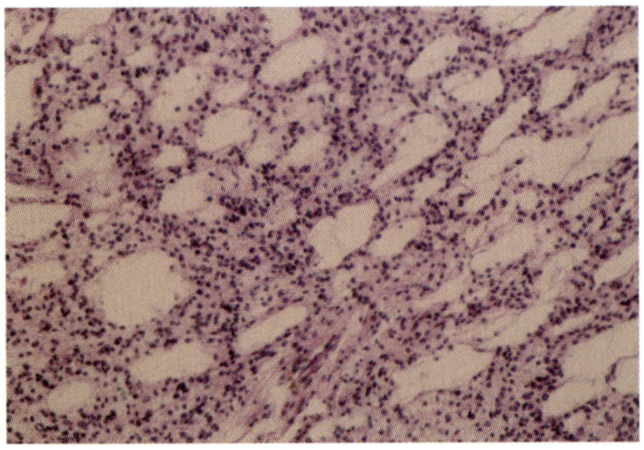

FIGURE 11.2
Microcystic degeneration in a protoplasmic astrocytoma.

Anaplastic Astrocytoma (Grade 3)

This tumor affects chiefly adults, and occurs in the cerebral hemispheres. Grossly, it is somewhat better demarcated, soft, and grayish-pink. Histologically, cellularity is high, and pleomorphism conspicuous. Hyperchromatic nuclei vary from small to large to multinucleated giant cells. Mitoses are frequent. Vascular proliferation usually is not prominent, and necrosis is absent (Figs. 11.5, 11.6, and 11.7). It may disseminate along the subarachnoid space (Fig. 11.8).

The genetic alteration is inactivation of the cell-cycle regulatory system, which includes the p16, cyclin-dependent kinase 4 (cdk4), cyclin D1 and retinoblastoma (Rb) proteins. Loss of the putative tumor suppressor gene on chromosome 19, amplification of the EGFR gene, and expression of VEGF gene are implicated in the progression to a glioblastoma.

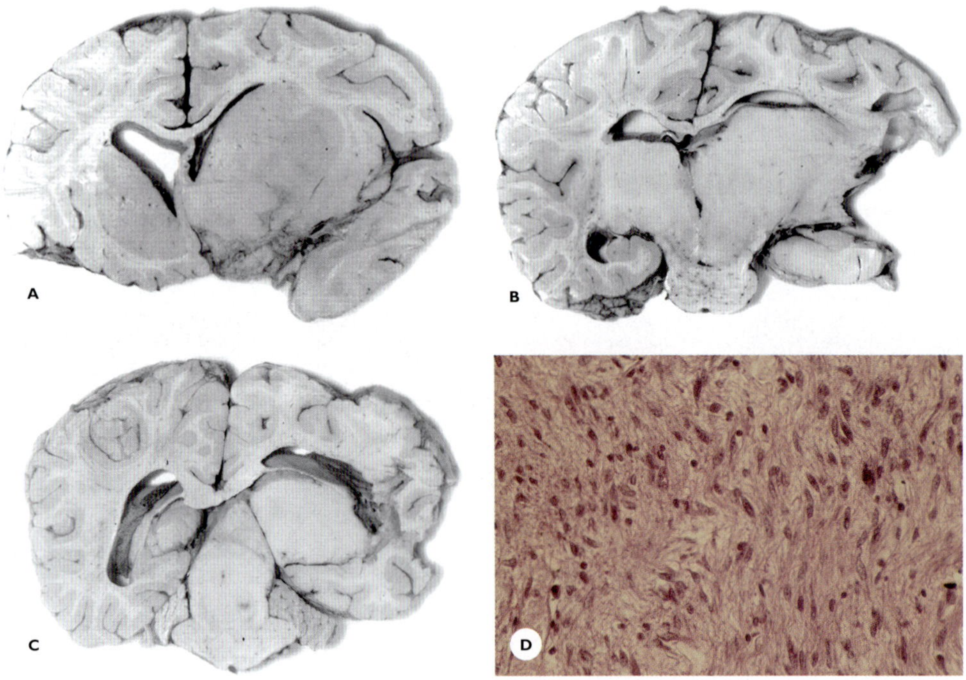

FIGURE 11.3
Fibrillary astrocytoma in an 11-year-old girl. **A** and **B.** A poorly demarcated, firm grayish tumor diffusely enlarges the right basal ganglia, both thalami, and upper brainstem and (**C**) extends extraparenchymally above the midbrain tectum. **D.** The tumor is composed of neoplastic astrocytes showing a mild nuclear pleomorphism and dense, elongated fibrillary processes which fill the intercellular spaces. The neuronal pattern of the infiltrated gray structures is generally preserved (HE).

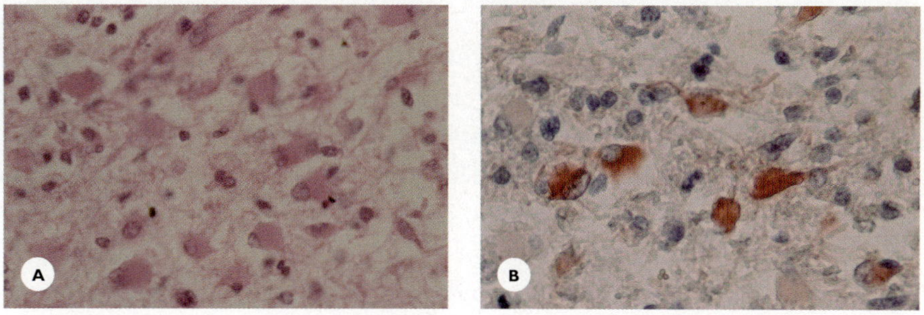

FIGURE 11.4
Gemistocytic astrocytoma in the wall of the third ventricle. **A.** It consists of large, plump, neoplastic astrocytes with glassy pink cytoplasm and eccentrically placed nucleus (HE). **B.** The cells strongly react for GFAP (immunostain).

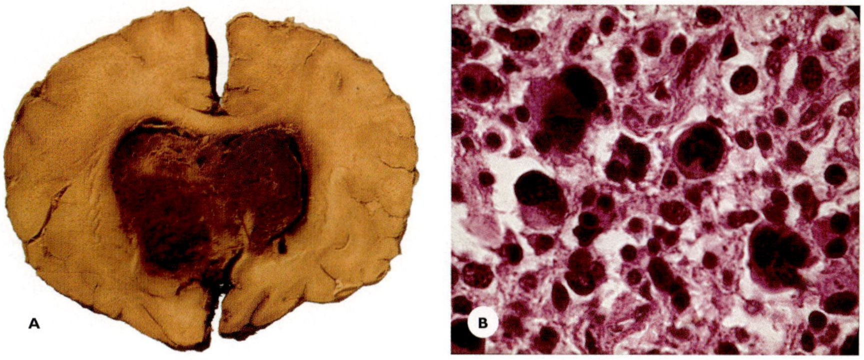

FIGURE 11.5
Anaplastic astrocytoma. A 35-year-old man, about 3 weeks prior to his death, developed severe, persistent headaches and gradually became confused and disoriented. Bilateral papilledema was the only significant neurologic finding. **A.** A large hemorrhagic tumor fills the anterior horns, destroys the septum and fornices, and extends into the walls of the third ventricle. **B.** It is highly cellular. The neoplastic cells have large hyperchromatic nuclei and variable amounts of cytoplasm. Bizarrely-shaped multinucleated cells are occasionally seen (HE).

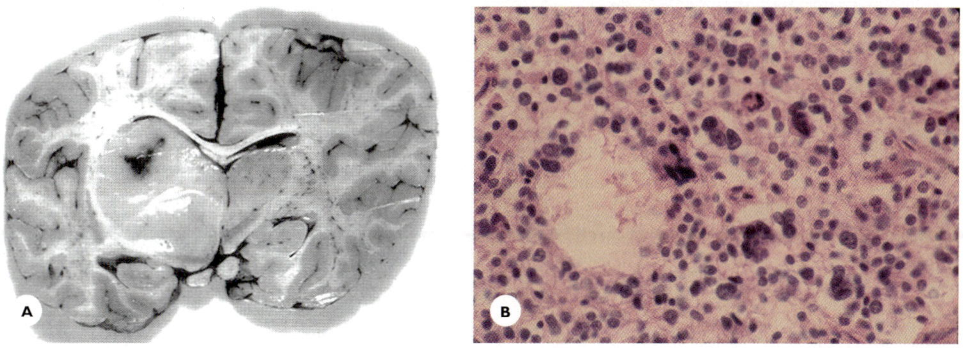

FIGURE 11.6
Anaplastic astrocytoma. A 7-year-old girl had a 3-week history of headaches, vomiting, right extremity weakness, and somnolence. Examination revealed bilateral papilledema, right hemiparesis, impaired touch and pain sensations, and asterognosis in the right hand, which was in an athetoid-like posture. **A.** A large, soft, grayish tumor diffusely enlarges the left thalamus. **B.** The tumor is highly cellular, with moderately large pleomorphic astrocytes. **C.** Intermixed are larger multinucleated cells (HE).

Glioblastoma (Grade 4)

Gliablastoma (GB), the most malignant fast-growing glioma, constitutes 50% to 60% of astrocytic tumors and 12% to 15% of all intracranial tumors. It occurs in mid and late midlife, the peak incidence being between 40 and 70 years of age. The average clinical course is 12 to 18 months (Fig. 11.9).

Glioblastoma arises either *de novo* from remnants of embryonal glial cells (primary GB) or from the malignant transformation of a low-grade or an anaplastic astrocytoma (secondary GB). These two subtypes of glioblastomas differ in their genetic alterations and clinical presentations. Primary glioblastoma chiefly affects older adults and presents with a short history of a few weeks to a few months. It rarely displays mutations in p53 tumor suppressor gene, but frequently displays the overexpression or amplification of the EGFR gene. Conversely, secondary glioblastoma affects younger adults and presents with a longer history of several months to years. It frequently displays mutations in p53 tumor suppressor gene and rarely overexpression of EGFR gene.

Grossly, glioblastoma is commonly situated in the cerebral hemispheres, preferentially in the frontal and temporal lobes. It appears circumscribed, but the borders are ill-defined. Some tumors tend to grow along the corpus callosum, into the opposite hemisphere in a butterfly pattern. Rarely, they are multifocal. Cut surfaces have a multicolored appearance; they contain pinkish-gray viable tissue, yellow necrosis, cystic degenerations, and rusty and reddish areas marking old and fresh hemorrhages. Being a fast-growing tumor, extensive edema and mass effects are prominent (Figs. 11.10, 11.11, 11.12, and 11.13).

Histologically, they are characterized by:

- High cellularity with a great degree of anaplasia and pleomorphism. Some cells are small, round to oval;

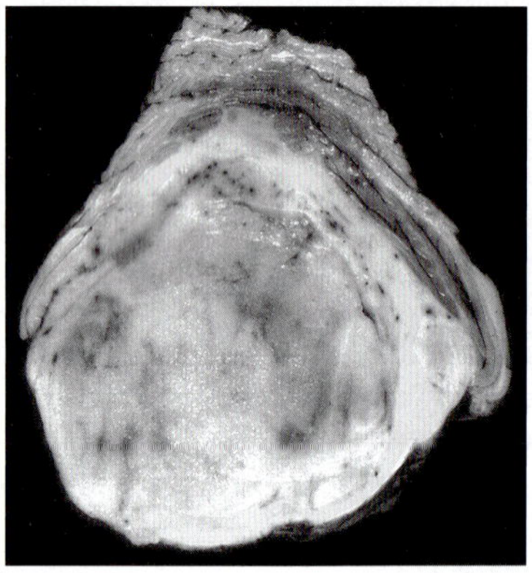

FIGURE 11.7
Anaplastic pontine astrocytoma in a 48-year-old woman. The tumor diffusely enlarges the pons and the tegmentum. It is grayish, soft, in places hemorrhagic.

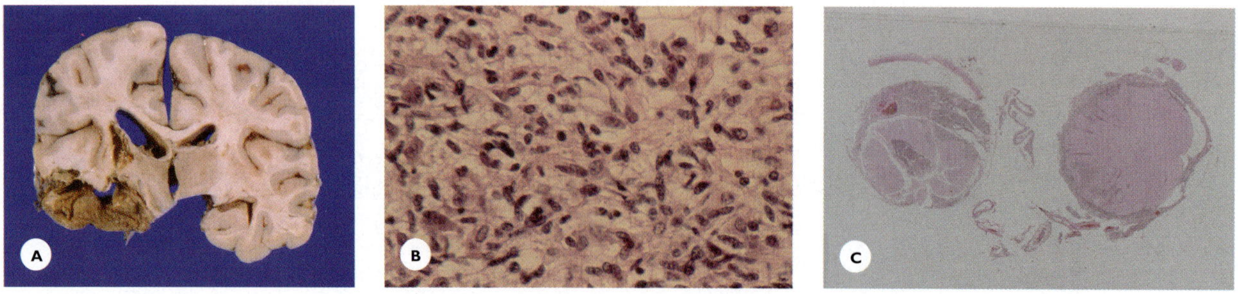

FIGURE 11.8
Anaplastic astrocytoma with subarachnoid dissemination. A 25 year-old man, following a one and a half year history of right-sided headaches and partial complex seizures with uncinate fits underwent a craniotomy for removal of a large right temporal lobe tumor diagnosed histologically as anaplastic astrocytoma. The surgery was followed by radiation and chemotherapy. One year later, he developed weakness in his legs and urinary retention. A myelogram showed diffuse obstruction of the subarachnoid space in the thoracolumbar region. Despite chemotherapy, he progressively deteriorated and died a few months later. **A.** Transverse section of the brain at thalamus level shows tumorous infiltration in the wall of a large residual cavity that communicates with the temporal horn. **B.** Ventricular wall shows a hypercellular and pleomorphic astrocytic tumor (HE). **C.** Massive tumorous infiltrations around the medulla and spinal cord, extending deeply into the parenchyma (HE).

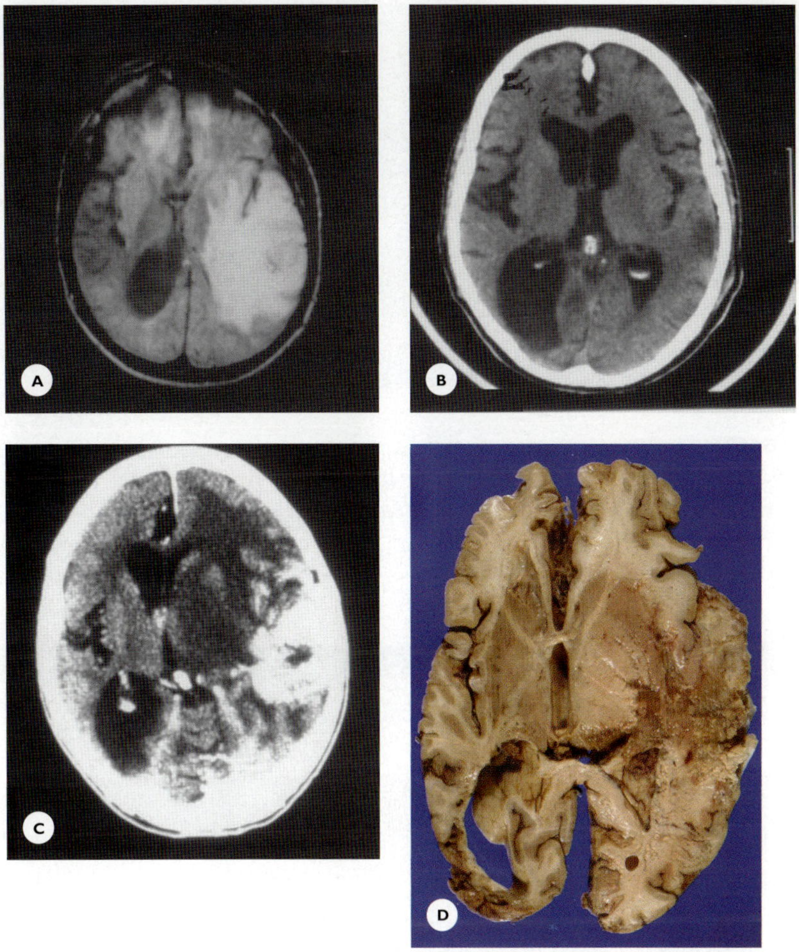

FIGURE 11.9
Glioblastoma, clinical presentation. A 57-year-old right-handed man experienced three episodes of incoherent speech for several hours within 1 month prior to hospitalization. His past medical history was significant for old head injuries. **A.** Contrast-enhanced T1-weighted MRI shows a left temporal tumor surrounded by massive edema. The tumor was resected and histologically diagnosed as glioblastoma. The surgery was followed by radiation therapy. **B.** A postoperative CT scan shows total resection of the tumor and resolution of the edema. **C.** Nonetheless, one year later, a CT scan shows recurrence of the tumor with massive edema. A few months later, he died. **D.** An extensive necrotic tumor occupies the left temporo-occipital region.

others are elongated, slender, or spindle-shaped; and still others are large, with one or multiple hyperchromatic nuclei. Giant monstrous cells are not uncommon. More mature astrocytes are sometimes present and express variably GFAP-immunoreactivity.

- High mitotic activity, often with bizarre mitotic figures.
- A rich vascular supply; the blood vessels display endothelial and adventitial proliferations and thrombotic occlusion. A glomeruloid appearance of proliferated capillaries is typical.
- Necroses are common and extensive. Smaller ones are surrounded by tumor cells in a pseudopalisading pattern (Figs. 11.14, 11.15, and 11.16)

Glioblastoma, when it reaches the subarachnoid space or the ventricles, may disseminate along the CSF pathways, forming small nodules or diffuse infiltrates. It seldom metastasizes outside the nervous system to the lymph nodes, lung, liver, and bone marrow.

Genetic alterations include loss of chromosome 10, amplification of EGFR oncogene and inactivation of the cell-cycle control system, and the expression of the VEGF receptor gene.

Variants of glioblastomas. *Giant cell glioblastoma* consists mostly of large bizarre-shaped glial cells. *Gliosarcoma* has a dense mesenchymal component.

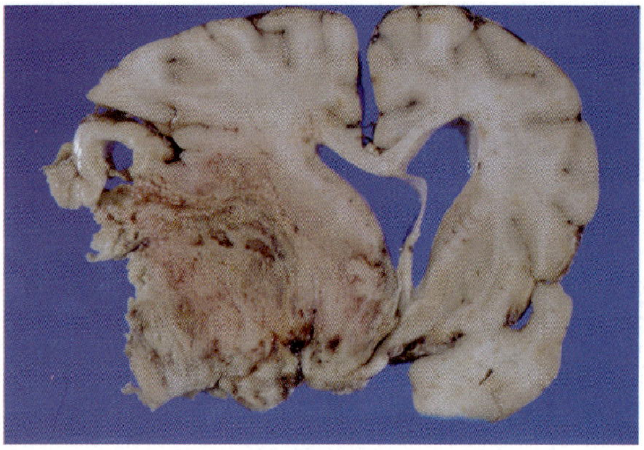

FIGURE 11.10
Glioblastoma. A large, left, poorly demarcated frontal tumor shows pinkish viable tumor, small cysts, areas of necrosis, and fresh hemorrhages. The left hemisphere is swollen, and the ipsilateral ventricle is compressed.

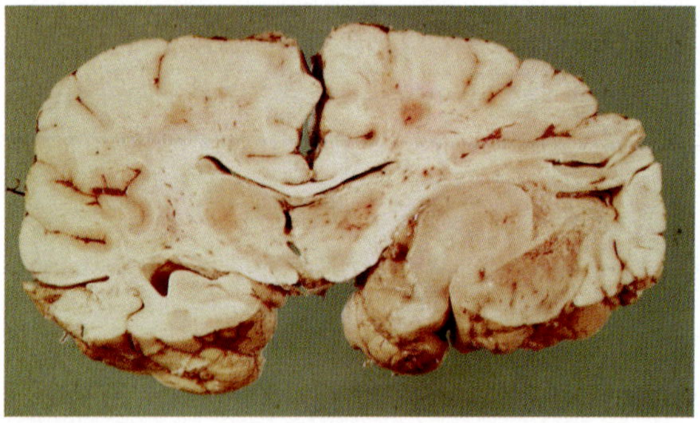

FIGURE 11.11
Glioblastoma. A 52-year-old man began to complain at times of smelling an acid-like odor or tasting something peculiar (uncinate fits). At other times, he complained of a floating sensation (vertiginous spells). His steadily deteriorating memory made him unable to function as a salesman. During this time, he received psychiatric treatment intermittently for depression. Examination prior to his sudden death at age 57 showed left hemiparesis, increased deep tendon reflexes, and Babinski sign. The right temporal lobe, including the uncus and the hippocampus, is tumorously enlarged. It contains grayish viable tumor, necrosis, and rusty areas from old hemorrhages.

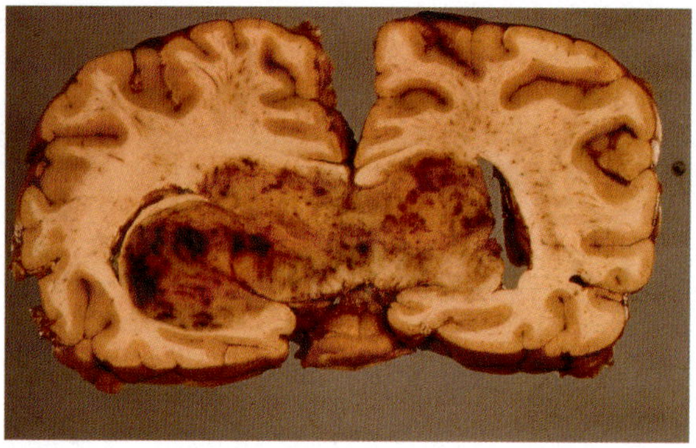

FIGURE 11.12
Glioblastoma. A 53-year-old woman with no previous psychiatric history was taken to a mental hospital following her knife attack on her husband. She had recently become more and more bizarre, complaining of severe headaches and inability to retain food. She had accused family members of trying to poison her. She also believed that her sister was turning her into a dog. During her examination, she was confused and incoherent. Her behavior rapidly changed from unresponsive to excitable and bizarre. During the third week of hospitalization, she was found stuporous. The following day, she died. A large glioblastoma is situated in the left posterior temporal lobe, extending into the right temporal lobe across the splenium in a butterfly pattern. It consists of grayish viable tumor and extensive yellow necrotic areas intermixed with old and recent hemorrhages.

Astrocytic Tumors (Grades 1 and 2)

Pilocytic Astrocytoma (Grade 1)

This slowly growing tumor affects chiefly children and adolescents. It occurs commonly in the cerebellum, optic nerves/chiasma, and hypothalamus/third ventricle and, less often, in the cerebral hemispheres. When situated in the optic nerves and chiasma, it may be associated with neurofibromatosis type 1 (NF1). Grossly, the tumor is fairly well circumscribed, soft, gray; it may adjoin a cyst or form a mural nodule within the cyst (Fig. 11.17). Histologically, the tumor is composed of elongated, mono- or bipolar pilocytes (*hair cells*), which form fascicles or a loose fibrillary matrix, and of small stellate cells with fine cytoplasmic processes. Microcysts, Rosenthal fibers, and eosinophilic bodies are characteristic features. The vascular supply is rich, and a variable degree of hyalinization and proliferation are present; these features do not necessarily predict a poor prognosis. Mitosis is uncommon. The tumor is apt to extend to the perivascular and subarachnoid spaces. Genetically, a gain on chromosome 6 to 10 is frequent; NF1-associated tumors may show a loss of chromosome 17q.

Subependymal Giant Cell Astrocytoma (Grade 1)

Subependymal giant cell astrocytoma (grade 1) is a slowly growing, well-demarcated tumor within the

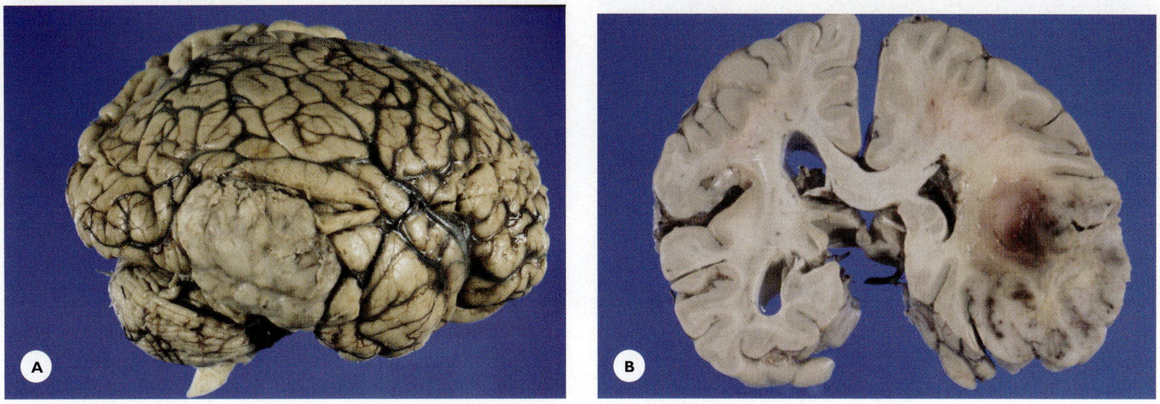

FIGURE 11.13
Glioblastoma. **A.** A grayish, firm, relatively circumscribed tumorous infiltration obscures the temporal convolutions. **B.** On transverse section, the tumor contains fresh hemorrhages and viable tumor in the cortex.

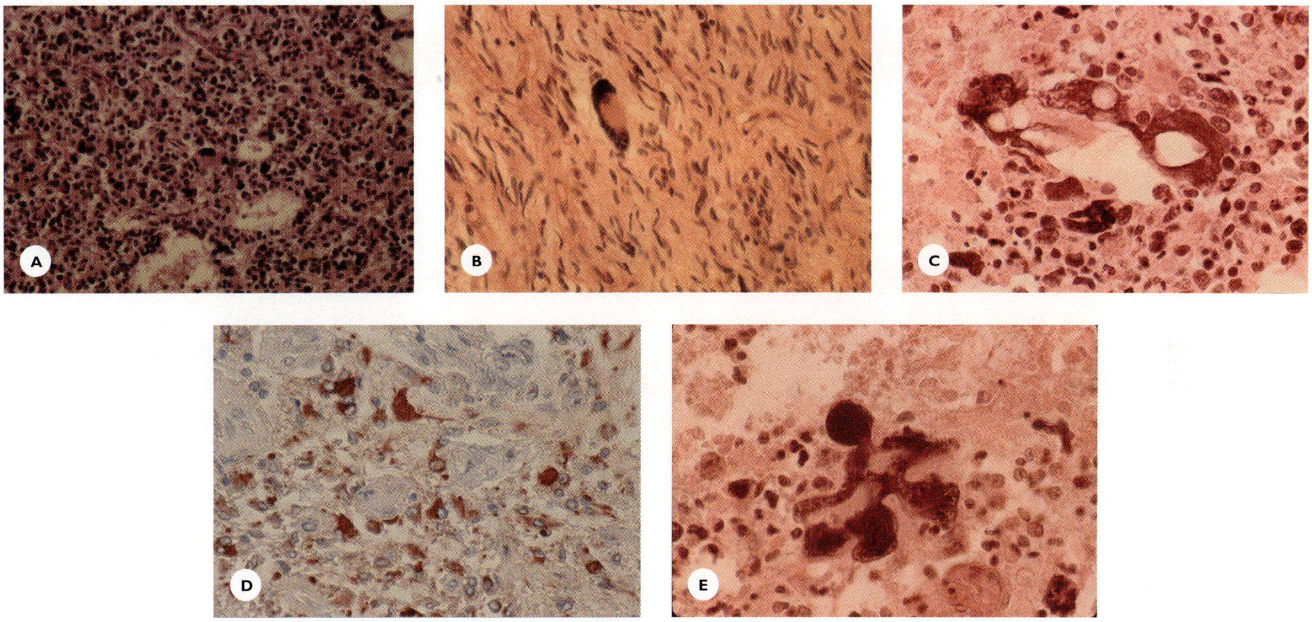

FIGURE 11.14
Glioblastoma, cytological features. **A.** Densely populated area of small, poorly differentiated glial cells (HE). **B.** Fusiform cells forming loose bundles displaying large atypical glial cells (HE). **C.** Giant mononucleated and multinucleated glial cells (HE). **D.** Some tumor cells express GFAP (immunostain). **E.** Atypical mitotic figure (HE).

lateral ventricles, often at the foramen Mono. It affects young children, and occurs commonly in the tuberose sclerosis syndrome (see Chapter 13). Histologically, the tumor cells vary in appearance: Some are large and globoid with abundant eosinophilic cytoplasm; others are small and fibrillated. Calcifications are common.

Pleomorphic Xanthoastrocytoma (Grade 2)

Pleomorphic xanthoastrocytoma affects children and young adults, and occurs in the cerebral hemispheres, rarely in the cerebellum. Grossly, the tumor is attached to the leptomeninges. It may contain a large cyst or form a mural nodule in a cyst wall. The histology is characterized by cellular pleomorphism with spindle cells and

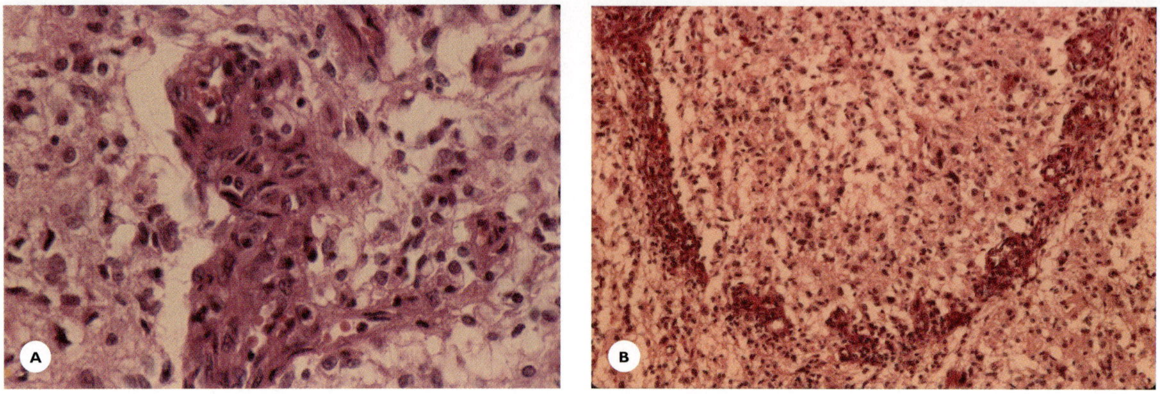

FIGURE 11.15
Glioblastoma, vascular features. **A.** Endothelial capillary hyperplasia. **B.** Glomeruloid capillary proliferation.

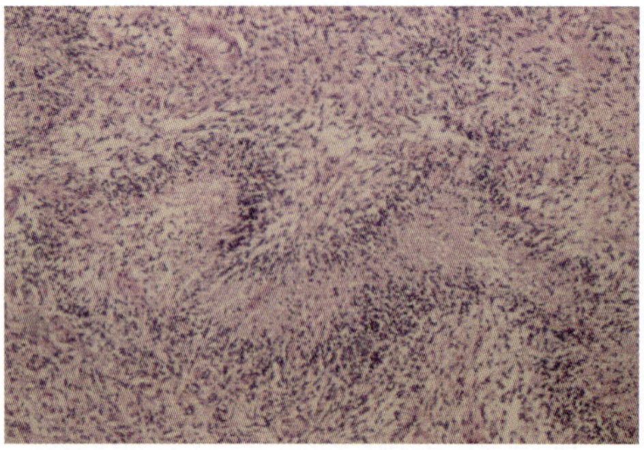

FIGURE 11.16
Glioblastoma, necrosis. Serpiginous areas of necrosis are surrounded by pseudopalisading tumor cells.

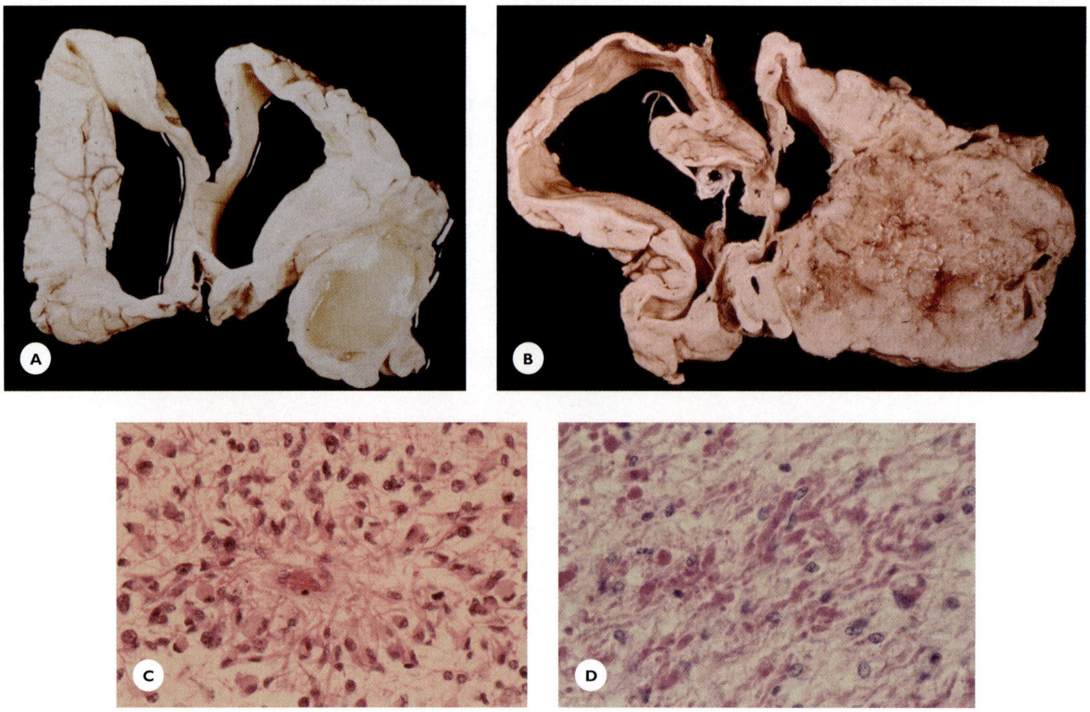

FIGURE 11.17
Pilocytic astrocytoma. A 2.5-year-old boy with unremarkable history developed infantile spasms and began to mentally deteriorate. At age 7, a large right temporoparietal mass lesion was diagnosed and parts of it—60 g—were resected. He received no radiation therapy. Following a temporary improvement, he developed seizures and slowly deteriorated. At age 13.5, following an 11-year clinical course, he died. **A.** A huge, fairly well-demarcated tumor occupies the temporal lobe and greater part of the hemisphere. **B.** Anteriorly it contains a large cyst. **C.** Astrocytes with uni- and bipolar processes form a fibrillary matrix around a capillary. **D.** Rosenthal fibers are abundant in some areas.

large mono- and multinucleated cells. Numerous cells contain lipid droplets, and a rich reticulin network separates the cells into small clusters.

Oligodendroglial Tumors

Oligodendroglioma (Grade 2)

This is a slowly growing, infiltrative tumor of adults, commonly situated in the cerebral hemispheres. It constitutes 5% to 10% of all gliomas. Seizures are often the presenting symptoms. Neurologic signs develop later in the course and indicate the location of the tumor. Average postoperative survival is 3 to 5 years, and recurrences are common.

Oligodendroglial tumors grades 2 and 3 that show a loss of chromosomal arms 1p and 19q respond favorably to radiation and chemotherapy, with survival reaching 10 to 15 years.

Grossly, oligodendroglioma is poorly demarcated, pinkish-gray in places gelatinous, and hemorrhagic. Gritty areas indicate calcifications, which are readily demonstrated on CT scan.

The histologic picture of a benign oligodendroglioma is generally uniform, consisting of well-differentiated neoplastic oligodendrocytes with round or oval nuclei, scanty or no stainable cytoplasm (perinuclear halo-fixation artifact), and a prominent cellular membrane (honeycomb cells) (Fig. 11.18). A rich vascular supply of thin-walled capillaries separates the cells into small groups. A variable number of tumor cells immunoreact for GFAP. In some tumors, the cells are arranged in parallel rows resembling palisading, or they form pseudorosettes around blood vessels. Often, they spread along the leptomeninges. Calcifications are prominent. Microcystic and mucinous degenerations and hemorrhages may occur (Fig. 11.19).

Variants of oligodendrogliomas. *Microgemistocytic oligodendroglioma* displays small cells with round eosinophilic cytoplasm and eccentric nucleus. They immunoreact for GFAP (see Fig. 11.19). *Anaplastic oligodendroglioma (grade 3)* is distinguished by increased cellularity, nuclear pleomorphism, mitotic activity, vascular proliferation, hemorrhages, and micronecroses. Leptomeningeal spread, subarachnoid dissemination, and metastasis outside the nervous system also occur.

Oligoastrocytoma contains well-differentiated neoplastic astrocytes and oligodendrocytes either diffusely intermingled or separated.

Ependymal Tumors

Ependymoma (Grade 1–3)

This tumor arises from the ependymal lining of the ventricular wall and either projects into the ventricular lumen or invades the parenchyma. It occurs from infancy to old age but predominates in children and adolescents. In children, it is more common in the fourth ventricle, accounting for 6% to 12% of intracranial childhood

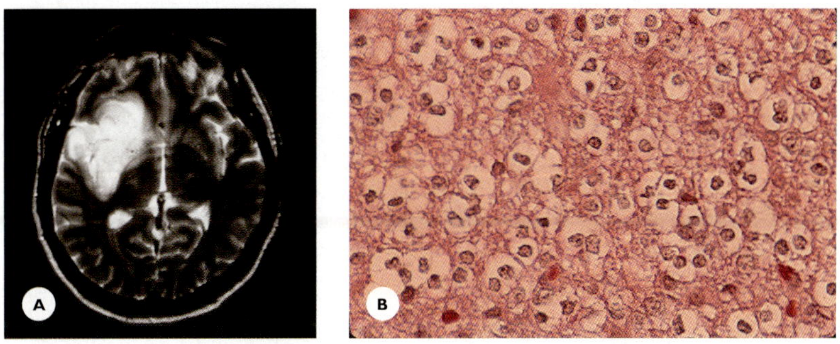

FIGURE 11.18
Oligodendroglioma. A 47-year-old man presented with a 2-month history of left-sided partial sensory seizures. Six months earlier, he experienced a short episode of left-sided weakness and loss of consciousness followed by confusion. **A.** Axial T2-weighted MRI shows a large inhomogeneous hyperintense right temporoparietal tumor extending into the basal ganglia. **B.** The partially resected tumor is composed of oligodendrocytes with round and oval nuclei and clear (halo) cytoplasm (fried egg appearance) (HE).

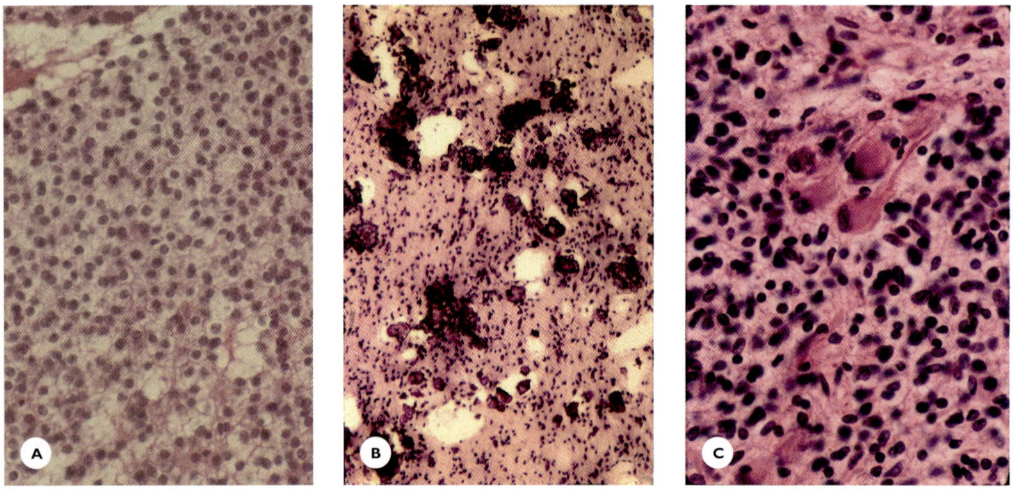

FIGURE 11.19
Oligodendroglioma showing (**A**) great uniformity of the tumor cells, (**B**) dense calcifications in the cerebral cortex, and (**C**) microgemistocytic components (HE).

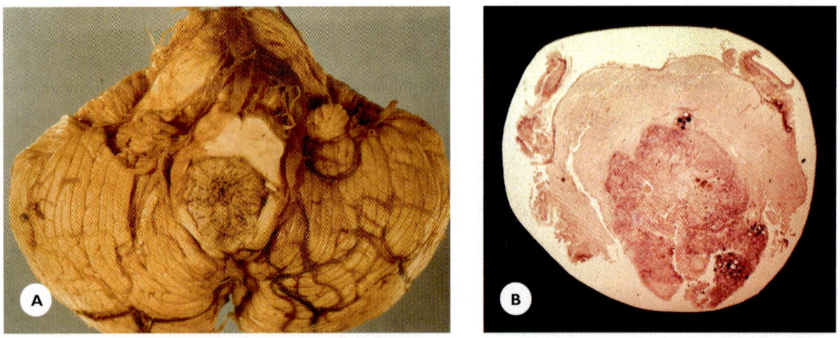

FIGURE 11.20
Ependymoma of the fourth ventricle in a 54-year-old man. He died following a 16-year clinical course. **A.** A circumscribed cherry-sized, firm, lobulated tumor fills the lumen of the fourth ventricle. **B.** Macrosection of the tumor at pontine level (cresyl violet).

tumors. It occurs in the cerebral hemispheres at any age, accounting for 5% to 6% of gliomas in all age groups.

Grossly, the tumor is fairly well demarcated and moderately firm; the cut surface is homogeneously gray and slightly granular (Fig. 11.20). Histologically, the tumor consists of medium-sized neoplastic ependymal glia with oval or round nuclei surrounded by a moderate amount of cytoplasm. Some cells have a columnar shape. The cells may form pseudorosettes around blood vessels, true rosettes lining small lumens, or small nests in a fibrillary matrix (Fig. 11.21). Rarely, the tumor contains hemorrhages, calcifications, and bony metaplasia. Genetic alteration includes loss of chromosome 22q, suggesting the presence of a tumor suppressor gene on that chromosome.

Subependymoma refers to a small nodule in the ventricular wall, usually benign and slowly growing. Histologically, nests of neoplastic ependymal cells are dispersed in a fibrillary matrix (Fig. 11.22).

Choroid Plexus Papilloma (Grade 1)

This benign tumor derives from the epithelial cells of the choroid plexus, and accounts for 0.5% of all intracranial tumors. It is more common in infants and children, and seldom is congenital. In children and adolescents, it has a predilection for the lateral ventricles; in adults, the fourth ventricle. Seldom, it occurs in the cerebellopontine angle. The detection of elements of the oncogenic papovavirus SV40 in some choroid plexus papillomas and carcinomas raises the possibility of the role of the virus in tumor pathogenesis.

Grossly, it is circumscribed and moderately firm, and the cut surface has a cauliflower- like appearance. When large enough, it occludes the ventricle, causing

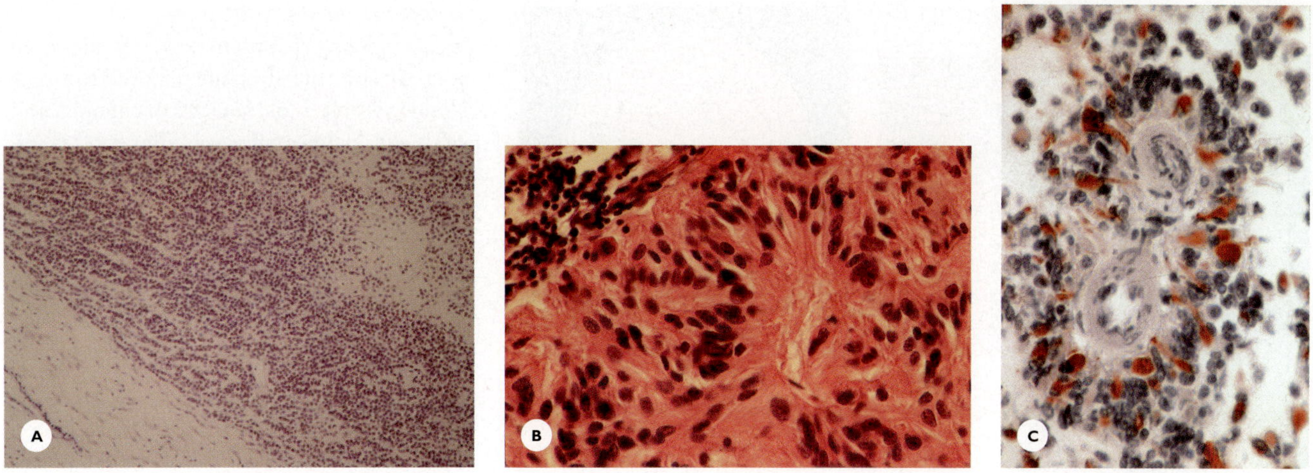

FIGURE 11.21
Ependymoma. **A.** Cuboidal ependymal cells fill the lumen of the lateral ventricle. The cells are uniform in appearance and are arranged in sheets or show no particular pattern (cresyl-violet). **B.** Papillary pattern (HE). **C.** Perivascular pseudorosettes. Some cells express GFAP (immunostain).

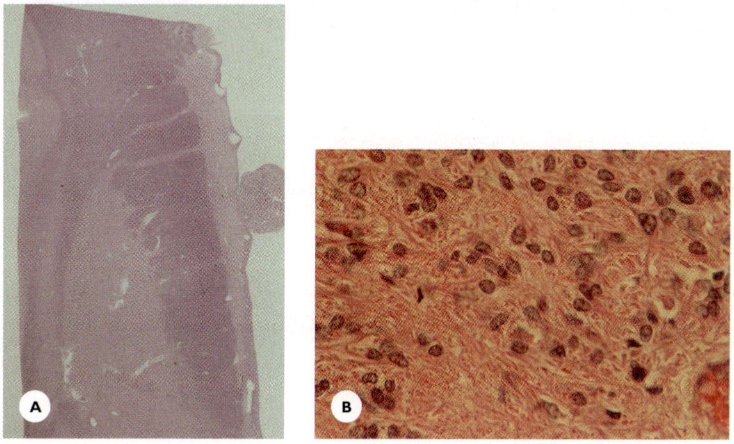

FIGURE 11.22
Subependymoma. **A.** A small tumorous nodule is attached to the wall of the lateral ventricle, incidental autopsy finding (HE) **B.** Nests of tumor cells are situated in a fibrillary matrix (HE stain).

hydrocephalus and raised ICP. Histologically, the tumor resembles a normal choroid plexus, but is more cellular, with cuboidal and columnar epithelial cells resting on a fine fibrovascular stroma. Hemorrhages and calcifications are common (see Fig. 11.23).

Choroid plexus carcinoma (grade 3), a malignant variant, shows cellular pleomorphism, mitoses, and necrosis. It is prone to invade adjacent structures and to disseminate along the CSF pathways (see Fig. 11.24).

Rare Variants of Glial Tumors

Gliomatosis refers to the diffuse and extensive infiltration of one or both cerebral hemispheres by neoplastic glial cells without forming a solid tumor.

Chordoid glioma of the third ventricle (grade 2) is a benign circumscribed tumor in adults. Histologically, it contains eosinophilic epitheloid cells that immunoreact for GFAP. The cells are arranged in cords or clusters.

Neuronal and Mixed Neuronal/Glial Tumors

This group comprises rare and slowly growing, relatively benign tumors (grade 1 to 2), affecting chiefly children and young adults. Seizures and symptoms and signs of increased ICP are common clinical manifestations.

Gangliocytoma (grade 1) and *ganglioglioma (grade 1, 2)* may occur at any site within the CNS, preferably in the temporal and frontal lobes. These tumors are gray, firm, and often cystic. Gangliocytomas are composed of

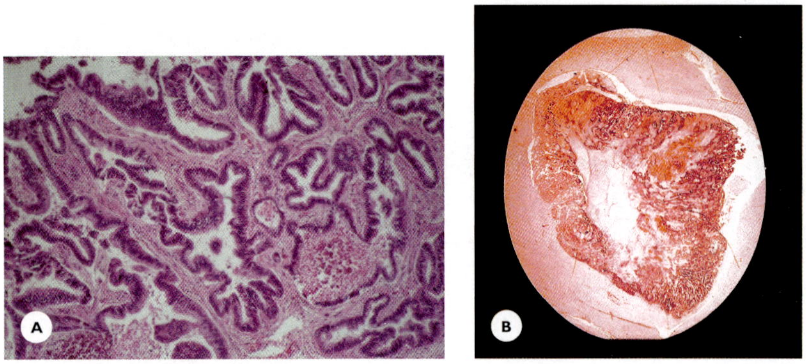

FIGURE 11.23
Choroid plexus papilloma **A.** A nut-sized amount of soft, bluish tissue removed from the cerebellopontine angle consists of cuboidal epithelial cells resting on fibrovascular core (extracerebral portion of the plexus of the fourth ventricle) (HE). **B.** Macrosection of a large choroid plexus papilloma in the lateral ventricle (HE).

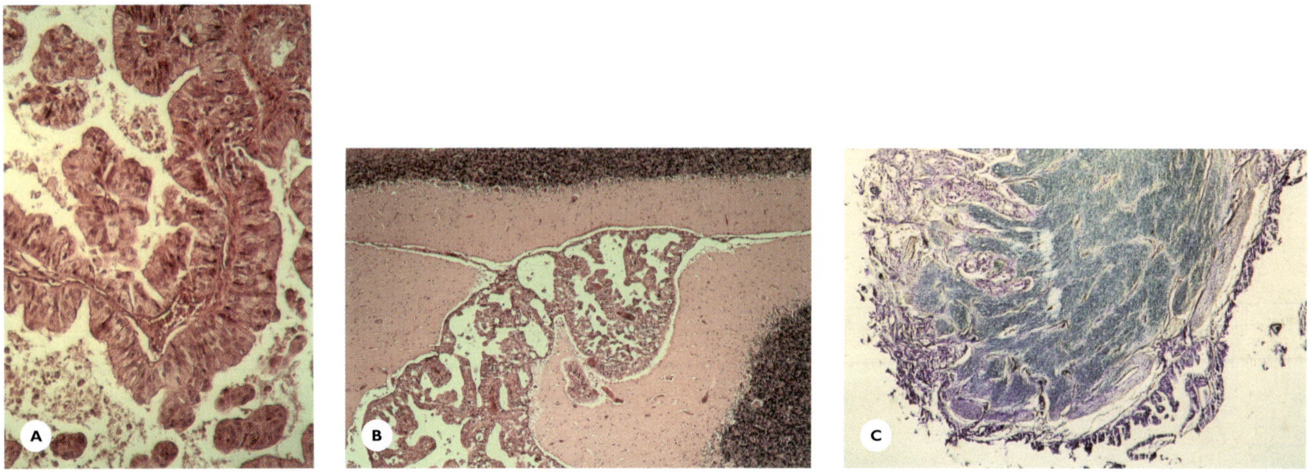

FIGURE 11.24
Choroid plexus carcinoma with extensive dissemination. **A.** Highly cellular tumor of pleomorphic columnar epithelial cells forming several rows on fibrovascular cores. **B.** Tumorous infiltration around the cerebellum (HE) and (**C**) optic nerve (LFB-CV).

atypical neoplastic neurons within a fibrillary matrix, whereas gangliogliomas contain a mixture of neoplastic neurons and glial cells, mostly astrocytes. The neuronal components immunoreact for synaptophysin and neurofilament proteins. Calcifications, eosinophilic globules, and perivascular lymphocytic infiltrations are common. Mitoses are rare, and necrosis is absent.

Central neurocytoma (grade 2) is situated in the lateral or third ventricle at the foramen Monro. It is a well-demarcated soft tumor composed of uniformly small neurocytes. Several architectural patterns are distinguished, resembling oligodendroglial and ependymal tumors. Calcifications are common, and hemorrhages may occur.

Dysembryoplastic neuroepithelial tumor (grade 1) is commonly situated in the cerebral cortex—often in the temporal lobe, less often in the cerebellum and pons. It has a mucinous or gelatinous appearance. It contains neoplastic neurons, astrocytes, and oligodendrocytes arranged in a nodular pattern. Pools of mucin, calcifications, and abnormal blood vessels are present.

Desmoplastic infantile astrocytoma ganglioglioma (grade 1) is a firm cystic tumor in the cerebral hemispheres. Usually, it infiltrates the leptomeninges and becomes attached to the dura. It has neoplastic neuronal and astrocytic elements arranged in a fascicular pattern within a dense reticulin network.

Dysplastic gangliocytoma of the cerebellum or *Lhermitte-Duclos disease (grade 1)* has neoplastic and maldevelopmental features. Grossly, the folia are thickened and histologically, the granular cell layer is replaced by dysplastic Purkinje cells. It is often associated with malformations, and it is a component of the Cowden syndrome, an autosmoal dominant disorder.

Embryonal Tumors

Embryonal tumors or primitive neuroectodermal tumors (PNET) arise from multipotential neuroepithelial cells that are capable of differentiation along neuronal and glial lines. These highly malignant (grade 4) tumors affect children from early infancy to adolescence. With the exception of medulloblastoma, they are rare.

Medulloblastoma (Grade 4)

This most important malignant tumor in children constitutes 16% to 20% of intracranial childhood tumors. In adults, it is rare. Situated in the cerebellum, it may arise from remnant cells of the external granular layer of the cortex, from embryonal cell nests in the superior medullary velum, or from subependymal matrix cells of the fourth ventricle. Familial occurrences (twins and siblings), coexistence with other brain tumors, and visceral malignancies and malformations are documented.

Medulloblastoma manifests with truncal ataxia and broad-based gait. Being fast-growing in the posterior fossa, it produces increased ICP, with headache, vomiting, and papilledema early in its clinical course. The tumor is inhomogeneously hyperintense on T2-weighted images and enhances with gadolinium on T1-weighted images. Postoperative survival averages 5 years.

Grossly, medulloblastoma is preferentially situated in the cerebellar vermis, extending into the fourth ventricle; less often into the hemispheres. Poorly demarcated, it is pinkish-gray and soft.

Histologically, medulloblastoma is densely cellular and composed of small cells with round, oval, or carrot-shaped hyperchromatic nuclei surrounded by scanty cytoplasm (blue cell tumor). The cytologic pattern varies from clusters separated by fine fibrovascular stroma, through pseudopalisading around necrosis, to pseudorosette formation. Mitotic activity is often high and apoptotic figures may be numerous. Medulloblasts may differentiate into neurons and glial cells. Neuronal differentiation is evidenced by immunoreactivity of tumor cells for neuron-specific enolase and synaptophysin. Glial differentiation is supported by the presence of GFAP-positive tumor cells. Necrosis, small cysts, and calcifications occasionally occur. Medulloblastoma may disseminate via CSF pathway to form small nodules and diffuse infiltrates in the ventricular wall and subarachnoid space (Fig. 11.25).

Genetic alterations include isochromosome 17q; losses of chromosomes 6q, 9q, 10q, 11, and 16q; trisomy-1q; and mutations of TP53 occur in a small number of tumors.

Histological Variants

Nodular medulloblastoma refers to the presence of "pale islands," consisting of tumor cells that display small nuclei, abundant cytoplasm, and a tendency to

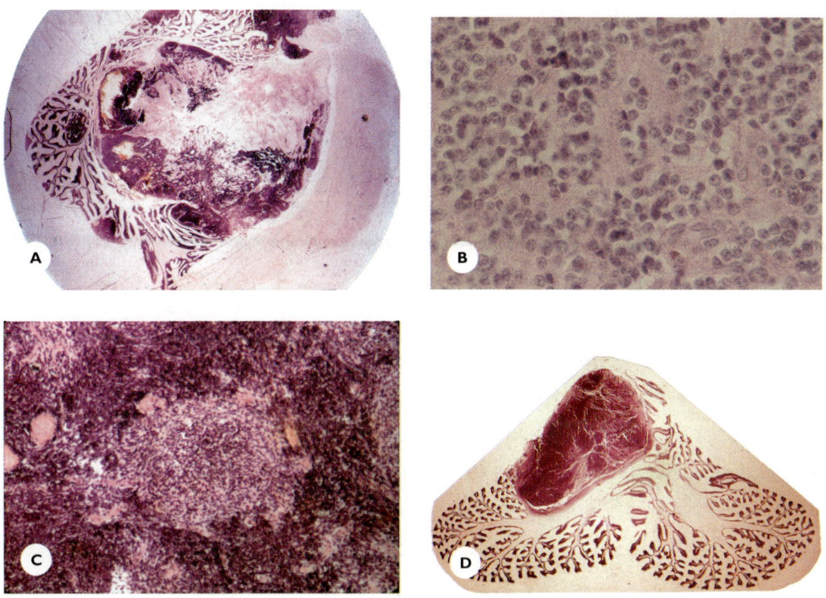

FIGURE 11.25
Medulloblastoma. **A.** Midsagittal section of the cerebellum shows a large tumor arising from the vermis and filling the lumen of the fourth ventricle. Small tumor nodules are present in the cerebellar cortex, indicating dissemination via CSF (cresyl violet). **B.** Highly cellular tumor consists of anaplastic cells with small round to oval hyperchromatic nuclei surrounded by scanty cytoplasm (HE). **C.** Pale island in nodular variant (HE). **D.** A desmoplastic variant in the cerebellar hemisphere (cresyl violet).

differentiate along neuronal line. This histologic pattern seems to be less aggressive and correlates with a longer survival.

Large cell/anaplastic medulloblastomas contain cells with large vesicular nuclei and pleomorphic anaplastic cells. Mitoses and apoptotic bodies are numerous. This histologic pattern seems to be more aggressive and correlates with shorter survival.

Desmoplastic medulloblastoma develops in the cerebellar hemispheres of children and young adults. Histologically, clusters of tumor cells are separated by a rich reticulin and collagenous network (see Fig. 11.25).

Medullomyoblastoma, lipomatous, and *melanotic medulloblastomas* contain striated muscle fibers, lipid cells, and melanotic cells, respectively.

Supratentorial Primitive Neuroectodermal Tumor (PNET)

PNET (grade 4) affects children and adolescents. It occurs anywhere in the cerebrum and in the pineal and suprasellar regions. The gross and histologic features resemble those of cerebellar medulloblastoma.

Other Embryonal Tumors

Central neuroblastoma (grade 4), an early childhood malignant tumor, occurs in the cerebral hemispheres. Histologically, it is composed of immature cells in various stages of neuronal differentiation.

Medulloepithelioma (grade 4), a rare malignant tumor of neonates and young children, occurs in the cerebrum, cerebellum, and brainstem. Grossly, this well-circumscribed tumor is soft and pinkish-gray, with hemorrhages and necrosis. Histologically, primitive epithelial cells are arranged in a tubular or papillary fashion that resembles the epithelial lining of the embryonic neural tube.

Ependymoblastoma (grade 4), a rare malignant tumor of neonates and young children, occurs in the cerebral hemispheres. Grossly, it is circumscribed, gray-pink, and moderately firm. Histologically, it is densely cellular with small cells forming rosettes around lumens. Mitoses are frequent. The cells may invade the leptomeninges.

Atypical Teratoid and Rhabdoid Tumors (Grade 4)

These malignant early childhood tumors have a widespread distribution in the brain and may also occur in the cerebellopontine angle. They display a mixed cellular composition, with rhabdoid cells (round or oval cells with eccentric nucleus and granular cytoplasm), neoplastic epithelial cells, and mesenchymal cells. Genetic alteration consists of a deletion on chromosome 22.

Tumors of the Pineal Gland Parenchyma

Tumors arising in the pineal parenchyma—the relatively benign pineocytoma (grade 2), the malignant pineo-blastoma (grade 4), and the mixed pineocytoma/pineoblastoma—constitute 1% of all primary intracranial tumors and 15% to 30% of all tumors in the pineal region. Clinically, these tumors are characterized as follows:

- Symptoms and signs of increased ICP are present due to occlusion of the aqueduct of Sylvius and subsequent hydrocephalus.
- Vertical gaze palsy (Parinaud syndrome), due to compression of the tectum of the midbrain.
- Hypothalamic and endocrine dysfunction, due to compression or infiltration of the wall of the third ventricle.

Pineocytoma and pineoblastoma are hypointense on T1- and hyperintense on T2-weighted images, and enhance with contrast. On CT scan, they are isodense or slightly hyperdense. Pineocytoma enhances homogenously and pineoblastoma inhomogenously. Survival with pineocytoma averages 5 years and with pineoblastoma, 3 years.

Pineocytoma (Grade 1)

This benign tumor originates from mature parenchymal cells with neuroendocrine and photosensory functions. More common in adolescents and young adults, it accounts for 15% to 30% of parenchymal tumors. It is slowly growing, grossly circumscribed, and may extend into the third ventricle (Fig. 11.26A). Histologically, the tumor consists of uniform cells with a small nucleus and a moderate amount of cytoplasm containing secretory granules. In silver-stained sections, the cells display short processes with club-like endings. They form

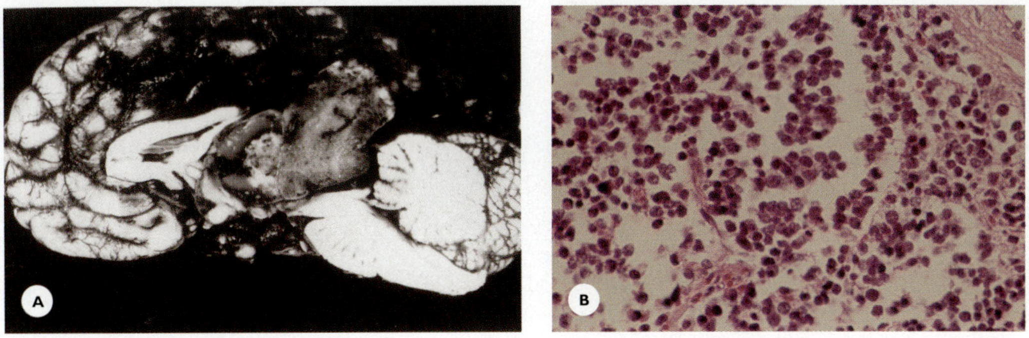

FIGURE 11.26A

A. Pineocytoma. An 11-year-old girl presented with a 1-week history of headaches, vomiting, and confusion. She had a stiff neck, papilledema, slowly reacting pupils, and vertical gaze palsy (Parinaud syndrome). She died of hypothalamic dysfunction 2 weeks following a shunting procedure. An egg-sized pineal gland tumor compresses the midbrain tectum and extends into the third ventricle. It is loosely attached to the wall of the ventricle. **B.** The tumor cells, resembling pineocytes, form groups separated by mesenchymal septa (HE).

rosettes around acellular areas or are separated into lobules by thin-walled vessels. They immunoreact for synaptophysin and retinal S antigen, and variably for neurofilament protein and chromogranin A.

Pineoblastoma (Grade 4)

This malignant tumor originates from immature neoplastic cells of the parenchyma and is more common in children and adolescents. It is fast growing, grossly soft, invasive, and may contain hemorrhages and necrosis. Histologically, pineoblastoma is highly cellular, comprised of small cells arranged in sheets or forming rosettes. The cells tend to seed within the subarachnoid space and metastasize outside the cerebrum. Their immunohistologic reactivities are similar to those of pineocytes (Fig. 11.26B).

Pineocytoma/Pineoblastoma

This pineal gland tumor of intermediate differentiation is rare, constituting about 8% of pineal tumors. It occurs in both children and adults. The tumor consists of a mixture of pineocytes and pineoblasts. It is moderately cellular, mitoses are common, and rosettes are absent.

Tumors in the Pineal Region

Apart from tumors arising within the pineal gland, the pineal region harbors a number of pathologically diverse tumors. They may arise from the leptomeninges, stromal astrocytes, ependymal cells, displaced germ cells, and primitive epithelial cells (Table 11.6).

TABLE 11.6.
Pineal Region Tumors

Pineal gland tumors	Germ cell tumors
Pineocytoma	Germinoma
Pineoblastoma	Embryonal carcinoma
Glioma	Yolk sac tumor
Meningioma	Choriocarcinoma
	Teratoma

TUMORS OF THE MENINGES

This group of primary intracranial tumors encompasses a variety of histologically diverse tumors arising from the meninges—most are benign, a few malignant. The group consists of meningothelial tumors, meningeal mesenchymal tumors, and primary meningeal melanocytic tumors.

Meningothelial Tumors

Meningiomas (Grades 1–3)

These generally benign tumors arising from the meningothelial cells of the arachnoidal cap cells occur in mid and late mid life, rarely in children. They constitute

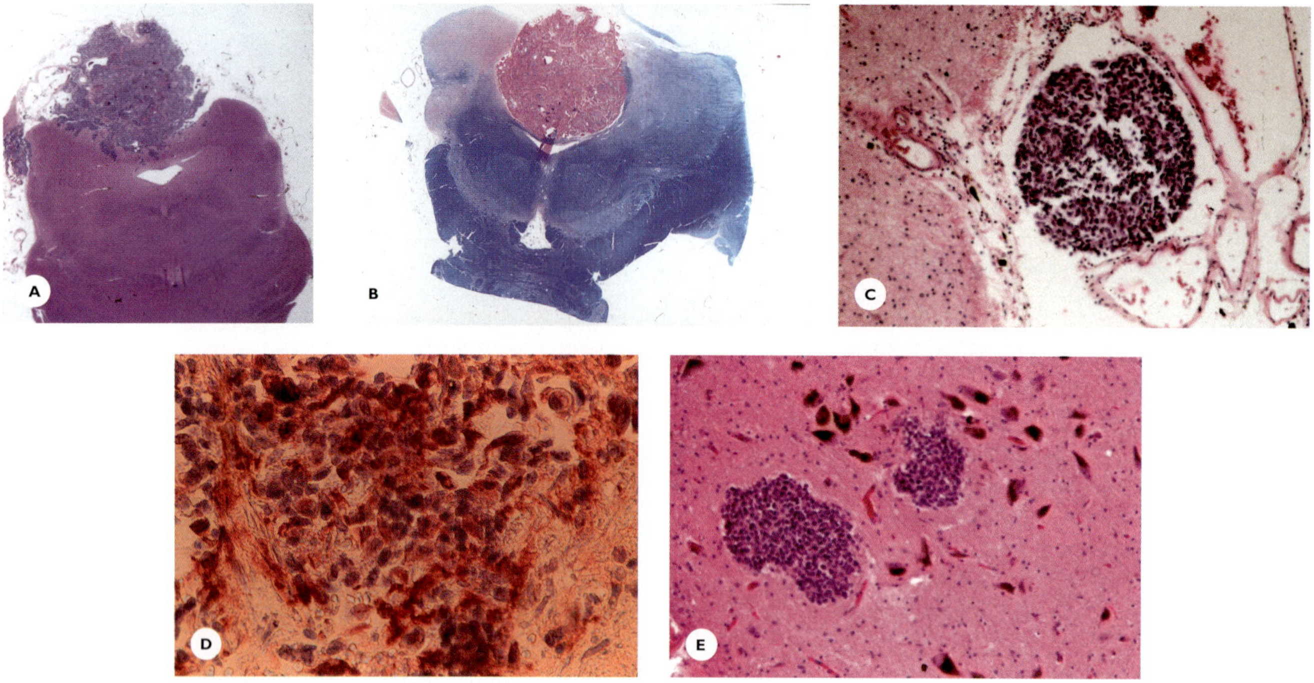

FIGURE 11.26B

Pineoblastoma in an adult male. **A.** Macrosection of the tumor (HE). **B.** The tumor fills the posterior part of the third ventricle (LFB-CV). **C.** Small seeding tumorous nodule in subarachnoid space consists of small cells with round-to-oval hyperchromatic nuclei (HE). **D.** The cells immunoreact for synaptophysin. **E.** Small tumorous nodules in the substantia nigra (HE).

15% to 25% of all intracranial tumors. A female predominance is attributed to the presence of progesterone receptors in the tumors. The majority of meningiomas are benign (80% to 90% are grade 1), a small number are atypical (5% to 15% are grade 2), and a smaller number are malignant (1% to 3% are grade 3). Preferential sites of meningiomas are the parasagittal region, the falx, and the lateral aspects of the hemispheres (plaque meningioma), and at the base the olfactory groove, the tuberculum sellae, and the sphenoid wing. They are less common in the posterior fossa and rare in the choroid plexus, pineal region, and orbit.

Head injury and therapeutic radiation to the head predispose to the growing of a meningioma. Solitary or multiple meningiomas occur in familial neurofibromatosis type 2 (NF2).

A number of cytogenetic and molecular genetic alterations have been identified in meningiomas. Mutations in NF2/merlin (schwannomin) gene protein on chromosome 22 and loss of DAL-1 gene protein on chromosome 18 occur in both benign and malignant meningiomas. Abnormalities of several chromosomes, including deletions of chromosomes 1, 10, 14, and loss of chromosome 9 have been implicated in meningiomas, particularly in malignant variants.

Clinical Features

Because meningiomas grow slowly and may become large before raising the ICP, partial or generalized seizures are often the presenting or only clinical manifestations for months or years. Focal neurologic symptoms and signs develop later and indicate the anatomic site. Bilateral parasagittal and falx meningiomas, by pressing on the leg area of the motor cortex, present with spastic paraparesis and urinary incontinence, mimicking a spinal cord lesion. On CT scan and MRI, meningiomas appear as extra-axial mass lesions compressing the brain substance. The surrounding edema and mass effect usually are not marked. CT scan readily identifies a calcified meningioma. On nonenhanced CT scan, a meningioma is iso- or hyperdense; it densely enhances with contrast media. It shows a dense homogenous enhancement on T1-weighted MR images, and is iso- or hyperintense on T2-weighted images.

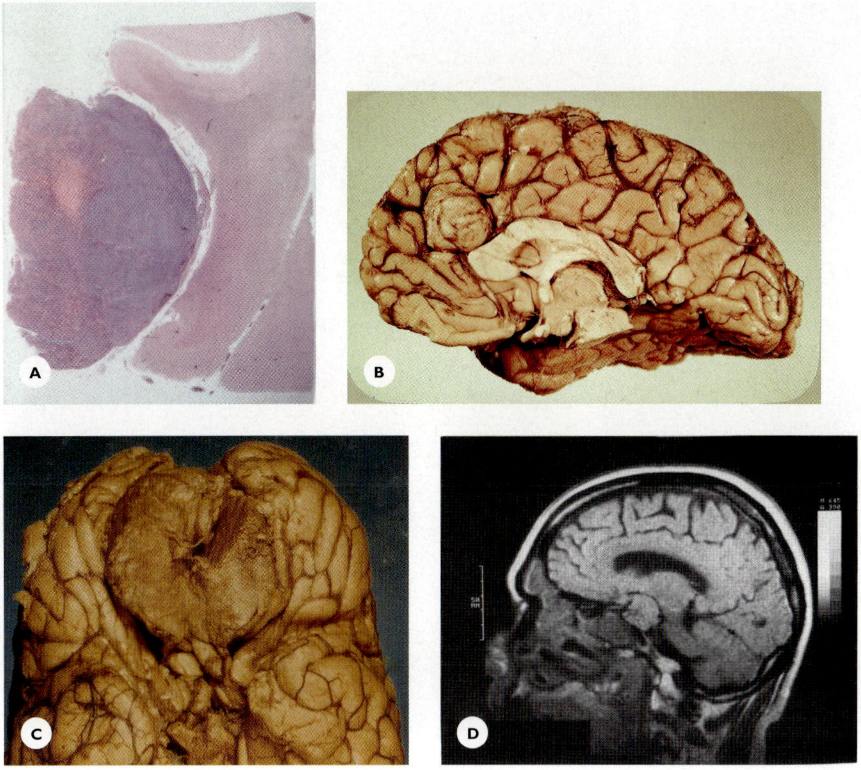

FIGURE 11.27
Meningiomas. **A.** A small, round encapsulated parasagittal meningioma is loosely attached to the leptomeninges. It indents but does not invade the underlying cortex (HE). **B.** A large, lobulated falx meningioma slightly indents the corpus callosum. **C.** A huge olfactory groove meningioma presented with psychiatric symptoms in a 43-year-old woman. The olfactory nerves are embedded in the tumor, and the chiasma and hypothalamus are displaced caudally. **D.** A left medial sphenoid wing meningioma on sagittal noncontrast T1-weighted MR image appears as an extra-axial isointense mass lesion. It is presented in a 58-year-old man with progressive loss of vision in the left eye.

Benign meningiomas, particularly when favorably located, can be totally excised and have an excellent prognosis. Atypical and chiefly anaplastic meningiomas are more aggressive, become invasive, and are prone to recur. Postoperative survival averages 2 years.

Pathology

Grossly, the meningioma is extra-axial; encapsulated; round, oval, or lobulated; and firm or moderately soft. It slowly indents and displaces the underlying neural tissue (see Fig. 11.27). Its blood supply is from the meningeal branches of the external carotid arteries. The cut surfaces are pinkish-gray, granular, or gritty. The tumor may invade the bone, producing osteolytic or osteoblastic lesions (Fig. 11.28). Histologically, several types are distinguished. The great majority are benign (WHO grade 1), with a low rate of proliferation index. The tumor cells immunoreact for epithelial membrane antigen (EMA) and vimetin, and inconsistently for S-100 protein.

Benign Meningiomas (Grade 1)

Meningothelial (Syncytial) Meningioma

The tumor cells have a round to oval nucleus with scanty chromatin, homogenous cytoplasm, and poorly defined cellular membrane. Some nuclei appear vacuolated from cytoplasmic invagination (pseudoinclusion). The cells form whorls separated by a fine reticulin network (see Fig. 11.28).

A *fibrous meningioma* consists of elongated and spindle-shaped cells forming interlacing bundles. Reticulin and collagenous fibers are abundant (see Fig. 11.28).

A *transitional (mixed) meningioma* contains elements of both meningoendothelial and fibrous meningiomas. Concentric whorls of crescent-shaped and

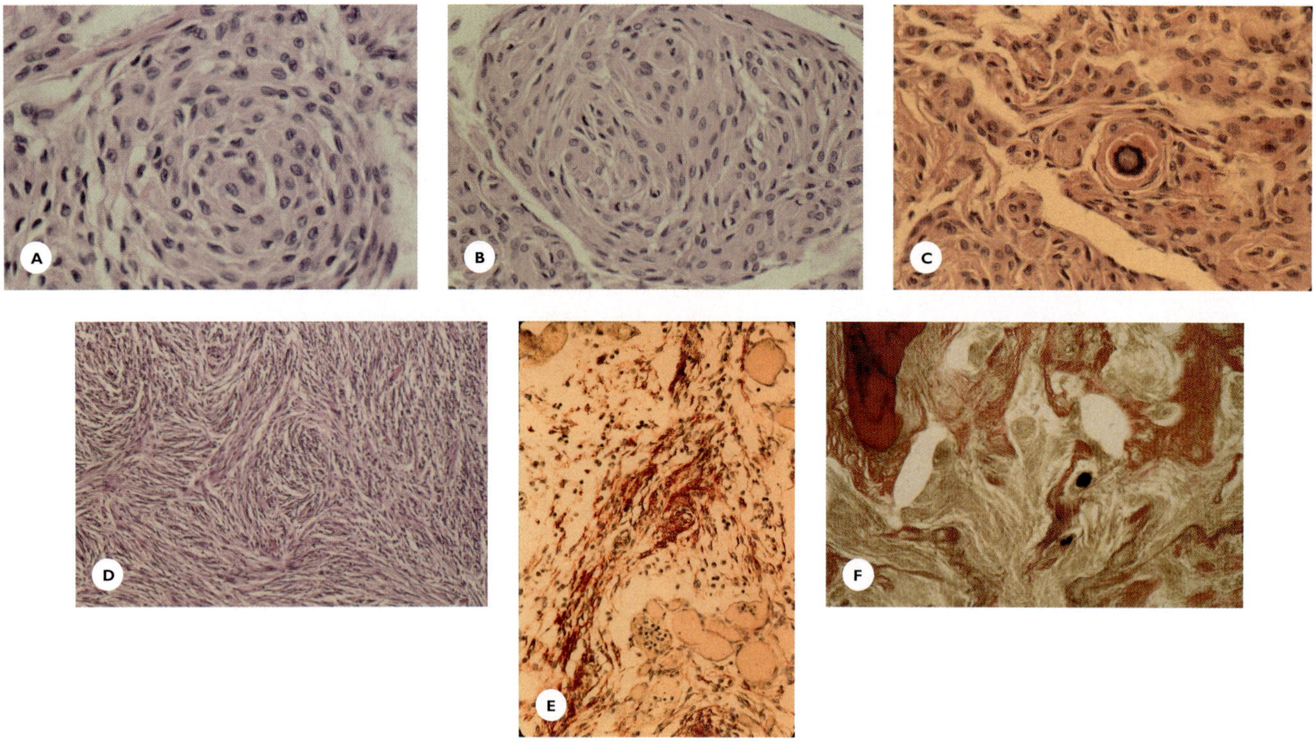

FIGURE 11.28
Meningiomas, histologic features. **A** and **B.** Meningothelial (syncytial) meningioma. Moderately large, oval nuclei are surrounded by round or polygonal cytoplasm with poorly defined borders. The cells typically are arranged in whorls (HE). **C.** The center of some whorls display a psammona body (HE). **D.** Fibrous meningioma consists of fibrillated spindle cells arranged in interlacing bundles (HE). **E.** The tumor cells immunoreact for vimentin (immunostain). **F.** Bony invasion by meningioma (van Gieson stain).

elongated cells are characteristic. The centers of the whorls often contain a *psammoma body*, which develops from calcium deposits in the degenerating tumor cells or from calcium deposits in the thickened, hyalinized walls of blood vessels.

A *psammomatous meningioma* displays numerous psammoma bodies and fewer neoplastic cells.

An *angiomatous meningioma* has a rich vascular supply, with thickened hyalinized blood vessels. Hemorrhages within the tumors are uncommon.

Microcystic meningiomas contain small mucinous cystic cavities.

Secretory meningiomas contain eosinophilic amorphous round to oval bodies.

Malignant Meningiomas

This small group encompasses the atypical and clear-cell grade 2, and the anaplastic and papillary grade 3 meningiomas. They all display increased cellularity, mitoses, and pleomorphism. Grade 3 meningiomas are prone to invade the brain, recur, seed via CSF, and metastasize to bones, lungs, and liver.

Clear-cell meningioma contains cells with clear cytoplasm containing glycogen.

In *papillary meningioma*, the cells and their processes are arranged around blood vessels in a papillary pattern.

Meningeal Mesenchymal Tumors

Hemangiopericytoma

This rare, malignant (grade 4) tumor, arising from pericites (periendothelial cells) of the blood vessels, is attached to the dura. It has a tendency to invade the brain, recur, and metastasize. It is most common in young adult men.

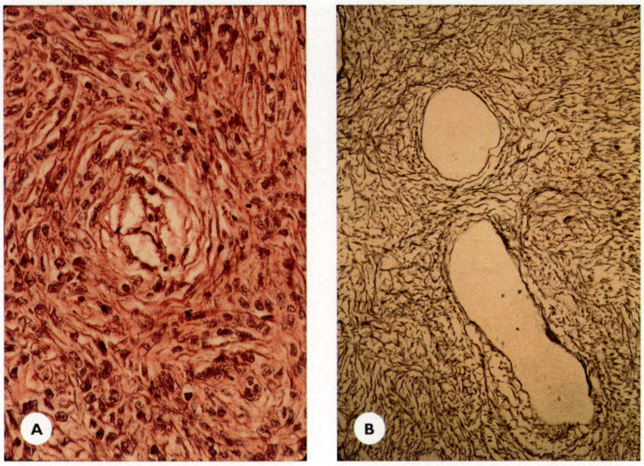

FIGURE 11.29
Hemangiopericytoma showing a high cellularity (**A**) with small elongated cells (HE) (**B**) in a rich reticulin network (reticulin stain).

Grossly, hemangiopericytoma is circumscribed, firm, round, oval, or lobulated. Histologically, it is highly cellular, composed of uniform polygonal cells arranged in sheets or small groups separated by a rich reticulin meshwork. The cells immunoreact for vimentin and CD34, but not for epithelial membrane antigen. Mitoses are frequent. A rich vascular supply consists of thin branching vessels (staghorn vessels) and sinusoids lined with endothelial cells (Fig. 11.29).

Meningeal Sarcomas

These rare and malignant tumors arise either from the dura or from the leptomeninges; seldom from pial or adventitial cells within the brain parenchyma. They may occur at any age.

Dural fibrosarcoma has a firm consistency and is composed of interlacing fascicles of fibroblasts.

Leptomeningeal sarcoma grossly appears demarcated, but not encapsulated, soft, grayish-pink with granular cut surfaces. It often contains hemorrhages, necrosis, and cysts. Histologically, the tumor invades the adjacent brain tissue and shows fascicles of fibroblasts separated by a rich reticulin stroma.

Primary meningeal sarcomatosis is more common in infants and children. Dense tumorous infiltrations with round or fusiform cells fill the subarachnoid space. The tumor may arise in multiple foci and spread diffusely. It may infiltrate the cranial nerve roots and brain parenchyma and, with time, can lead to hydrocephalus (Fig. 11.30).

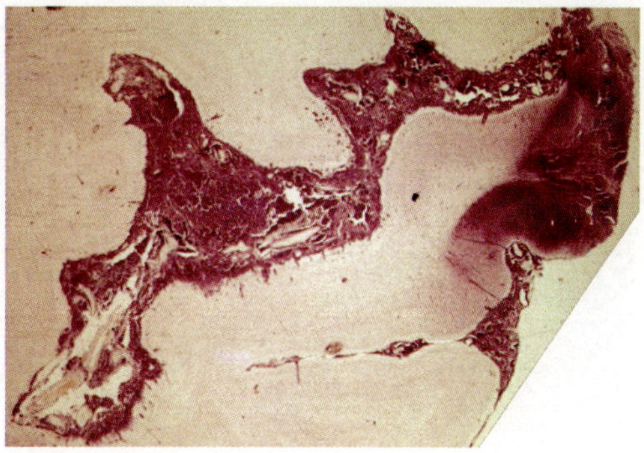

FIGURE 11.30
Primary meningeal sarcomatosis in a 15-year-old girl diffusely spreads into the subarachnoid space and invades the cerebral cortex (Cresyl violet).

Other Rare Mesenchymal Tumors

Dural fibroma, a benign tumor, is composed of fibrocytes and fibroblasts.

Malignant fibrous histiocytoma is a nonencapsulated, often hemorrhagic tumor made up of fibroblasts, histiocyte-like cells, and undifferentiated cells.

Primary Meningeal Melanocytic Tumors

Melanocytoma

Melanocytes are normally present in the pia mater and give a dark brown or dusky appearance to the leptomeninges. Very rarely, the melanocytes undergo tumorous transformation, producing solitary or multiple solid melanocytomas or diffuse leptomeningeal melanocytosis. The melanocytosis may be associated with cutaneous nevi (neurocutaneous melanosis, Touraine syndrome).

Grossly, the leptomeninges are dark brown or dusky. Histologically, the tumor consists of fusiform or polygonal melanin-containing cells (Fig. 11.31). Malignant transformation with dense cellularity, nuclear pleomorphism, giant cells, and high mitotic activity may also occur.

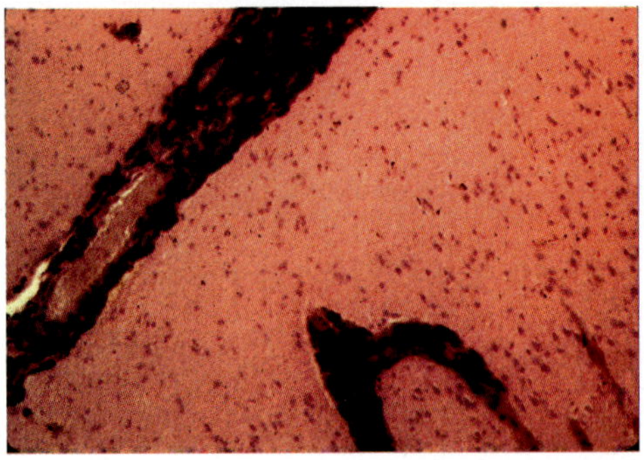

FIGURE 11.31
Meningeal melanocytosis. Melanin-containing cells infiltrate the leptomeninges and the parenchyma along the Virchow-Robin spaces (HE).

TUMORS OF THE PITUITARY GLAND AND SELLAR REGION

This group encompasses adenomas of the anterior pituitary (adenohypophysis), tumors of the posterior pituitary (neurohypophysis), and a variety of nonpituitary tumors in the sellar region.

Tumors of the Adenohypophysis

Adenomas arising in the anterior lobe of the pituitary gland constitute 10% to 15% of all intracranial tumors. Approximately two-thirds of pituitary adenomas secrete hormones, and the remaining one-third are hormonally inactive (null-cell adenomas). The tumors grow slowly, occur chiefly in adults between 30 and 60 years of age, and are more common in women than men. Endocrine symptoms due to hormonal overproduction stand in the foreground of the clinical picture and provide the basis for classification. The endocrine activities of the various adenomas and their corresponding clinical manifestations are listed in Table 11.7. Additional characteristic symptoms and signs result from compression or invasion of the adjacent structures and include headaches, bitemporal hemianopsia, hypothalamic dysfunction, cavernous sinus syndrome, hydrocephalus, and pituitary hypofunction. Enzyme assays and MRI make possible the early diagnosis of these tumors before they reach a size large enough to erode the sella, compress the chiasma, and destroy the pituitary gland.

TABLE 11.7.
Tumors of the Pituitary Gland

Hormones secreted by anterior pituitary adenomas
Prolactin: F: Amenorrhea
Galactorrhea
M: Hypogonadism
Growth hormone: acromegaly
ACTH: Cushing syndrome
TSH: Pituitary hyperthyroidism

Neurohypophysis
Astrocytoma
Granular cell tumor

Pituitary apoplexy due to a hemorrhagic infarction is a serious complication in about 1% to 2% of adenomas. It may be the first manifestation of the tumor, presenting acutely with headache, visual impairment, oculomotor palsy, and altered mentation.

Pathology

Grossly, the adenoma appears as a discrete, grayish-yellow, soft mass less than 1 cm in diameter (microadenoma). Some microadenomas show little tendency to grow, but others become invasive, destroy the sella and dura, and infiltrate the surrounding structures (macroadenoma). Massive hemorrhage and infarct may also occur (pituitary apoplexy).

Histologically, the tumor cells have small round or oval nuclei, which display stippled chromatin, a characteristic of hormone-secreting tumors. Mitoses and cellular pleomorphism may occur, but are not considered as evidence of aggressiveness. The cellular pattern may be uniform or may show a papillary, glandular, perivascular, or trabecular arrangement (Fig. 11.32). Hormone immunohistochemical studies identify the specific hormone produced by the adenoma. Null-cell adenomas are chromophobic and are immunonegative.

Tumors of the Neurohypophysis

Gliomas in this region are commonly astrocytomas, mostly of the pilocytic type.

Granular-cell tumor is generally benign, noninvasive, situated in the sella or supra- or parasellar region,

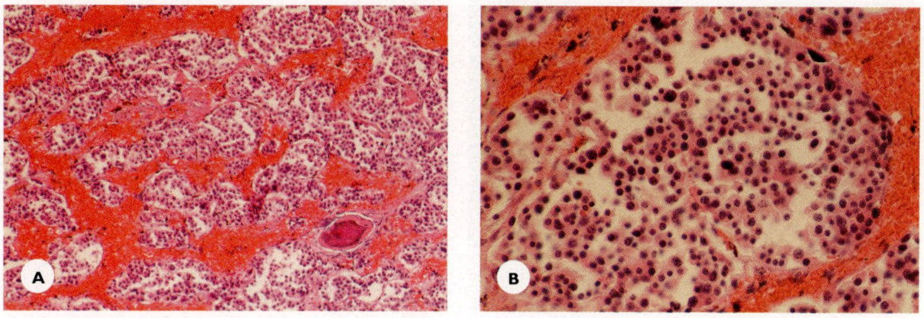

FIGURE 11.32
Pituitary chromophobe (null-cell) adenoma. **A.** The cells are separated into groups by sinusoidal tabeculae. **B.** They display a small nucleus, variable amount of cytoplasm, and slight pleomorphism.

TABLE 11.8.
Nonpituitary Tumors in the Sellar Region

Meningioma	Epidermoid, dermoid cysts
Craniopharyngioma	Teratoma
Germinoma	Lipoma
Glioma	Chordoma
Hamartoma	Metastasis

or in the third ventricle. Its cellular origin is controversial, as reflected by the various names given to it: choristoma, referring to the nests of large, granulated, dusty cells in the infundibular region; granular cell myoblastoma, implying a mesenchymal origin; and pituicytoma, suggesting an origin from the neurohypophysis. The tumor occurs most frequently in middle-aged women and presents with visual impairment, enlarged sella, and endocrine disturbances.

Grossly, the tumor is circumscribed, firm, and lobulated. Histologically, it consists of large, polygonal-shaped cells, loosely arranged in sheets. Their perikaryons contain eosinophilic and PAS-positive granules and an eccentric nucleus. Hormonal immunohistochemistry studies are negative.

Nonpituitary Tumors in the Sellar Region

A variety of tumors occur in the supra- and parasellar region. The common ones are listed in Table 11.8

GERM CELL TUMORS

A group of rare and malignant intracranial tumors arise from germ cell nests displaced during embryogenesis. Histologically, these cells are analogous to the gonadal germ cells. The group includes the germinomas, teratomas, embryonal carcinomas, endodermal sinus tumors, and choriocarcinomas.

Germ cell tumors commonly occur in children and adolescents and are preferentially situated in the pineal and suprasellar regions. They tend to disseminate along the CSF pathways and seldom metastasize extracranially via the bloodstream.

Pineal region tumors present with signs and symptoms of increased ICP, vertical gaze palsy, and hypothalamic and endocrine disturbances. Tumors in the suprasellar region produce diabetes insipidous, visual impairment, and hypopituitarism. On T1-weighted MR images, they appear isointense and densely enhanced with contrast. Elevated serum levels of α-fetoprotein and human chorionic gonadotropin complement the diagnosis.

Germinoma

Germinomas are the most common of germ cell tumors, constituting half of the tumors in the pineal region with a male predominance. (Suprasellar germinoma affects males and females almost equally.) Grossly, the tumor is pinkish-gray, soft, friable, variably demarcated, and often invades the adjacent structures. Histologically, the tumor consists of two types of cells:

- Large polygonal cells have round or spherical nuclei surrounded by abundant cytoplasm. Mitoses are common. The tumor cells are separated in lobules by thin fibrous septa.
- Lymphocytes, the second cell type, form variable collections between the lobules (Fig. 11.33). It is believed that they represent host reaction to the tumor.

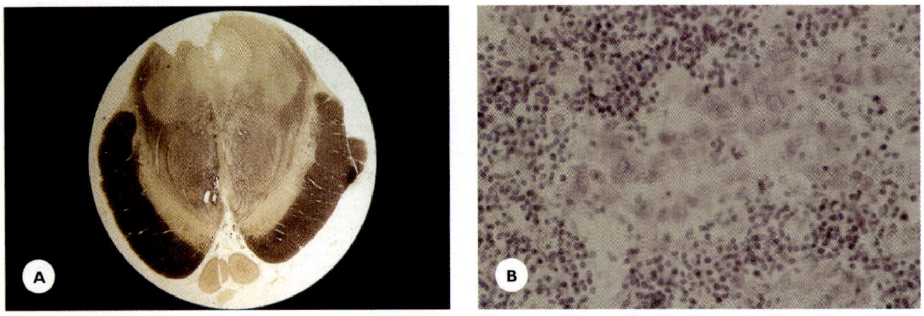

FIGURE 11.33
Germinoma. **A.** The tumor in the pineal region infiltrated the midbrain (myelin stain). **B.** Moderately large tumor cells with clear cytoplasm and prominent nucleus are separated into lobules by fibrous septa that contain large collections of lymphocytes (Cresyl-violet.)

Immunohistochemistry for α-fetoprotein and human chorionic gonadotrophin confirms the germ cell origins of the tumors. Immunoreactivity for placental alkaline phosphatase identifies the malignant cells. The tumors are radiosensitive; some have a more favorable clinical course than do other germ cell tumors.

Teratoma

The teratoma is common among children; it has a male predominance. Unlike the germinoma, on MR images a teratoma appears inhomogenous due to the presence of cysts and hemorrhages.

The tumor is composed of an admixture of tissues derived from all three germinal layers of the embryonic disc: ectoderm, mesoderm, and endoderm. Some teratomas are composed of well-differentiated, mature tissue resembling benign adult organs (mature variant) and others of immature tissue resembling fetal tissue (immature variant). Teratomas commonly are situated in the pineal region, less often in the suprasellar region, and rarely within the parenchyma. Grossly, they are cystic, often hemorrhagic, and contain calcifications. Histologically, they contain a mixture of epithelial, mesenchymal, and glandular elements.

Embryonal Carcinoma, Endodermal Sinus (Yolk Sac) Tumor, and Choriocarcinoma

These are highly malignant, but fortunately rare. Choriocarcinoma has a tendency to bleed.

TUMORS OF THE CRANIAL AND SPINAL NERVES

Various tumors arise from the peripheral nerve sheaths: the schwannomas, neurofibromas, perineurinomas, and malignant peripheral nerve sheath tumors.

These tumors, solitary or multiple, may occur from childhood to old age; they present most often in adults, rarely in children. They may involve the sensory, motor, and autonomic nerves anywhere along their course: roots, trunks, large and small branches, and cutaneous and visceral twigs. The majority of them are benign and slowly growing. The schwannomas and neurofibromas are particularly important because of their role in the hereditary neurofibromatosis syndromes (see Hereditary Tumor Syndromes).

Schwannomas (Grade 1)

Schwannomas, or neurinomas arising from Schwann cells, are slowly growing, benign tumors. Their preferential sites are the cranial and spinal nerve roots. Among the peripheral nerves, the large branches of the extremities are often involved. Multiple schwannomas are the hallmark of neurofibromatosis type 2.

Schwannomas of the Cranial Nerve Roots

These tumors constitute about 8% of intracranial tumors. Any cranial nerve can be involved, but the acoustic nerve is by far the most commonly affected. (Fig 11.34)

Acoustic schwannoma arising in the vestibular division of the nerve root occurs in adults between the ages of 40 and 60 and has a female predominance. The tumor grows in the cerebellopontine angle and presents with tinnitus, hearing impairment, dizziness, and unsteady gait. As the tumor grows, cerebellar symptoms, facial and trigeminal, and pyramidal signs develop, along with symptoms and signs of raised ICP. The tumor enlarges and erodes the acoustic meatus. Contrast-enhanced T1-weighted MRI detects small schwannomas

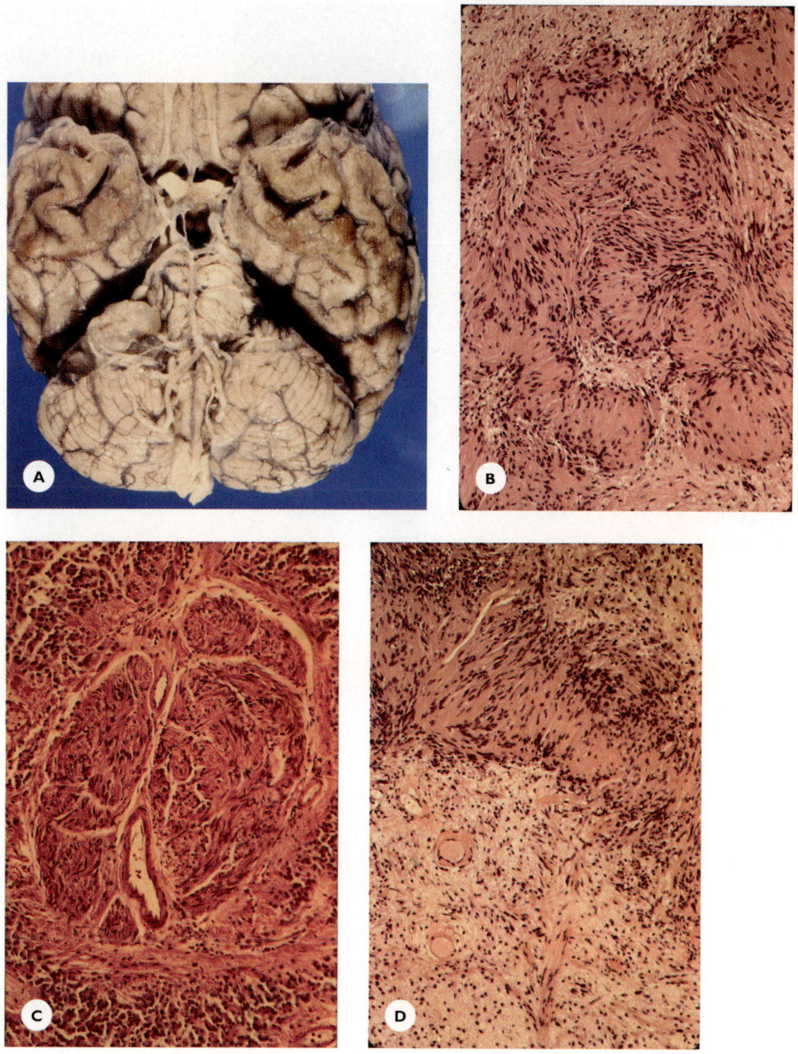

FIGURE 11.34
Acoustic neurinoma. **A.** Cherry-sized encapsulated tumor in the right cerebellarpontine angle. The tumor displays histologic features of Antoni types A and B. **B.** Spindle-shaped bipolar cells form fascicles and show palisading, with alternating zones of nuclei and processes. **C.** Verocay body, Antoni type B. **D.** Small stellate cells are situated in a loose matrix (HE).

as densely enhancing mass lesions. They are variably hyperintense in T2-weighted images. The tumors also enhance densely on CT scan. Patients with bilateral acoustic tumors must be evaluated for evidence of neurofibromatosis type 2.

The *trigeminal schwannoma* is situated in the middle fossa. In the early stage, it may mimic a trigeminal neuralgia.

Schwannomas of the Spinal Nerve Roots

The tumors constitute about 15% to 30% of spinal tumors. They are more common on the sensory roots, preferentially occurring on the cauda equina.

Clinically, they present with pain and sensory and motor deficits in a radicular distribution. If they reach a large size, symptoms and signs of spinal cord compression develop. *Hourglass* or *dumbbell schwannoma* refers to extension of the tumor through the intervertebral foramen into the mediastinum or peritoneal cavity.

Intraparenchymal schwannomas are rare in the brain or spinal cord. They derive from Schwann cells of the nerves that supply small arteries or from ectopic Schwann cells.

Grossly, schwannomas are encapsulated, moderately firm, round or lobulated light tan tumors with the nerve stretching over the capsule. (Figs. 11.34 and 11.35) Cut surfaces contain small cysts and old and fresh hemorrhages.

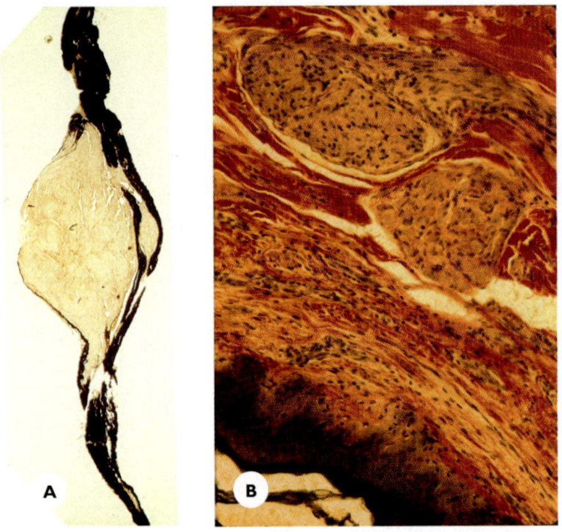

FIGURE 11.35
A. Peripheral nerve neurinoma (myelin stain). **B.** Intradermal neurinomas (van Gieson stain).

Histologically, two patterns are distinguished. The *Antoni type A* schwannoma consists of spindle-shaped cells with bipolar processes and small elongated nuclei arranged in interwoven fascicles. The cells immunoreact for S-100 protein. Mitosis is unusual. The nuclei tend to align in rows, giving the tumor a palisading pattern. Palisades around eosinophilic fibrillary areas form the characteristic *verocoy bodies* (Fig. 11.34). The *Antoni type B* schwannoma has a loose structure, with small stellate and fusiform cells situated in a mucoid matrix. Necrosis, cysts, hemorrhages, and hyalinized blood vessels are common (see Fig. 11.34).

Neurofibromas (Grade 1)

These slowly growing benign tumors derive from fibroblasts, Schwann cells, and pericites. Neurofibromas predominate in neurofibromatosis type 1. The two forms of neurofibromas are the cutaneous and the plexiform.

Cutaneous neurofibromas form multiple small nodules and lead occasionally to local elephantiasis. *Plexiform neurofibromas* affect the somatic and autonomic nerves at any site along their course.

Grossly, the tumors enlarge the nerves in a fusiform, cylindrical, or globular fashion. Histologically, they contain bipolar cells arranged in bundles and separated by dense collagenous fibers. Nerve fibers may be detected within the tumors. Neurofibromas may undergo malignant transformation.

Perineurinomas (Grade 1)

These rare, benign tumors derive from perineural cells and present in two forms, intraneural and soft-tissue perineurinomas.

The *intraneural perineurinoma* most often affects the peripheral nerves of the extremities of young adults. Grossly, it appears as a focal enlargement of the nerve. The histology is characterized by onion bulb formation; that is, a concentric arrangement of perineural cells around the myelin and axon. The cells immunoreact for epidermal membrane antigen (EMA) and are negative for S-100 protein.

The *soft-tissue perineurinoma* occurs in the subcutaneous tissue of the extremities, most often in women. The cells form bundles, interwoven fascicles, and whorls.

Malignant Peripheral Nerve Sheath Tumors (Grades 3–4)

These grade 3 and 4 tumors, previously called *neurogenic sarcoma*, are malignant schwannomas that may arise primarily from peripheral nerves or secondarily from neurofibromas. They involve large- and medium-sized nerves. Grossly, the tumors appear as a fusiform or globoid enlargement of the nerves. Histologically, they are highly cellular, with spindle-shaped cells forming interlacing bundles. Mitoses are frequent, and necroses and hemorrhages are common. Metaplasia with bone, cartilage, and muscles may occur (Fig. 11.36).

MALDEVELOPMENTAL TUMORS AND CYSTS

This group comprises a variety of solid and cystic mass lesions arising from tissues misplaced during embryonic development or from remnants of embryonic tissue. These relatively benign lesions occur in children and adults and are situated in the supra- or infratentorial compartments. They manifest with focal symptoms and signs relating to their location and, as their size gradually increases, raised ICP develops.

Craniopharyngioma

Craniopharyngioma occurs at any age, although more often in children, accounting for 5% to 10% of childhood intracranial tumors. It is a slowly growing tumor that originates from remnant epithelial cells of the craniopharyngeal duct (Rathke pouch). It is situated in the suprasellar region, less often in the sella, and may extend into the third ventricle.

Clinically, the tumor presents with visual impairment, endocrine and hypothalamic dysfunction, and symptoms and signs of raised ICP. Cognitive decline and personality changes are not unusual. The sella turcica may be enlarged, and calcifications are present on radiograph. CT scan and MRI show mixed signal intensities due to cystic and solid components and calcifications. The solid component enhances with contrast in CT and T1-weighted MR images.

Grossly, most craniopharyngiomas are cystic with a thick, machine-oil–like contents. The solid portion of the tumor forms nodules in the cyst's wall (Fig. 11.37). Histologically, the tumor consists of multistratified squamous epithelial cells. Two types are distinguished:

- The adamantinomatous type, in which the cells form strands and cords, and calcifications, amorphous masses of keratin (wet keratin), and cholesterol clefts are characteristic (see Fig. 11.37A,B).
- The papillary type, in which the cells rest on a fibrovascular stoma. This type lacks calcifications and cholesterol crystals. Glial reaction and Rosenthal fibers are conspicuous around the tumor, which

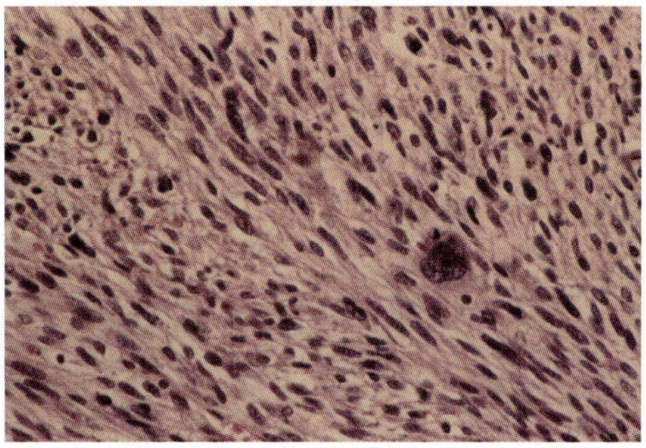

FIGURE 11.36
Malignant peripheral nerve tumor. The tumor shows great hypercellularity, with spindle-shaped cells forming bundles, nuclear pleomorphism, and multinucleated giant cell.

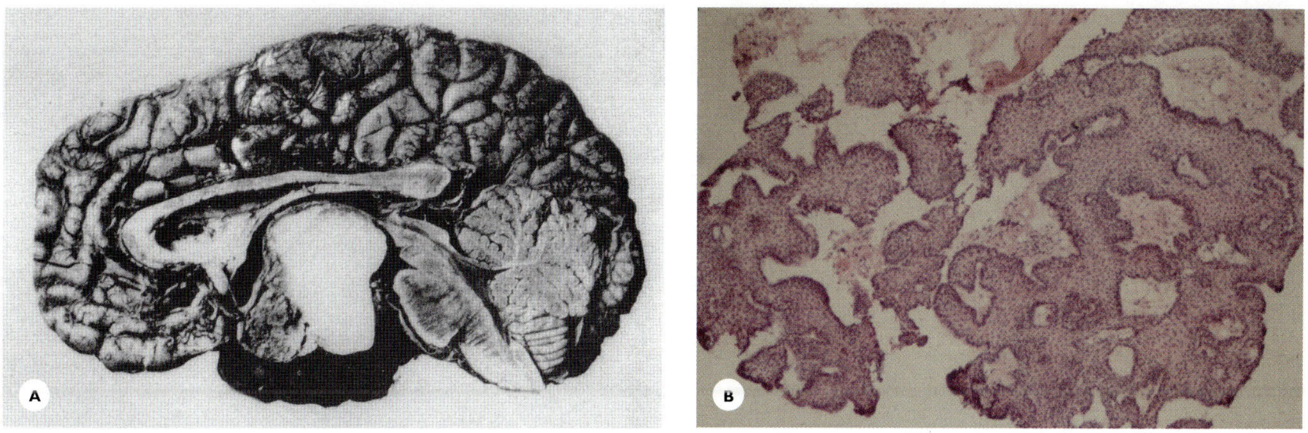

FIGURE 11.37A
Craniopharyngioma. A 55-year-old woman presented with headaches and declining memory of 3 years' duration and excessive daytime sleepiness of 1 year's duration. On examination, the optic discs were pale, and the visual acuity severely diminished. She lay motionless and speechless with a vacant expression, resembling *akinetic mutusim.* Her temperature was intermittently elevated, and she needed to be spoon-fed. **A.** Sagittal section of the brain shows a large cyst with small tumorous mural modules. The cyst is loosely attached to the infundibulum, compresses the diencephalons, and obliterates the third ventricle. The lumen is filled with machine-oil–like material. **B.** The mural nodules consist of squamous epithelial cells arranged in small islands (adamantinomatous pattern) (HE).

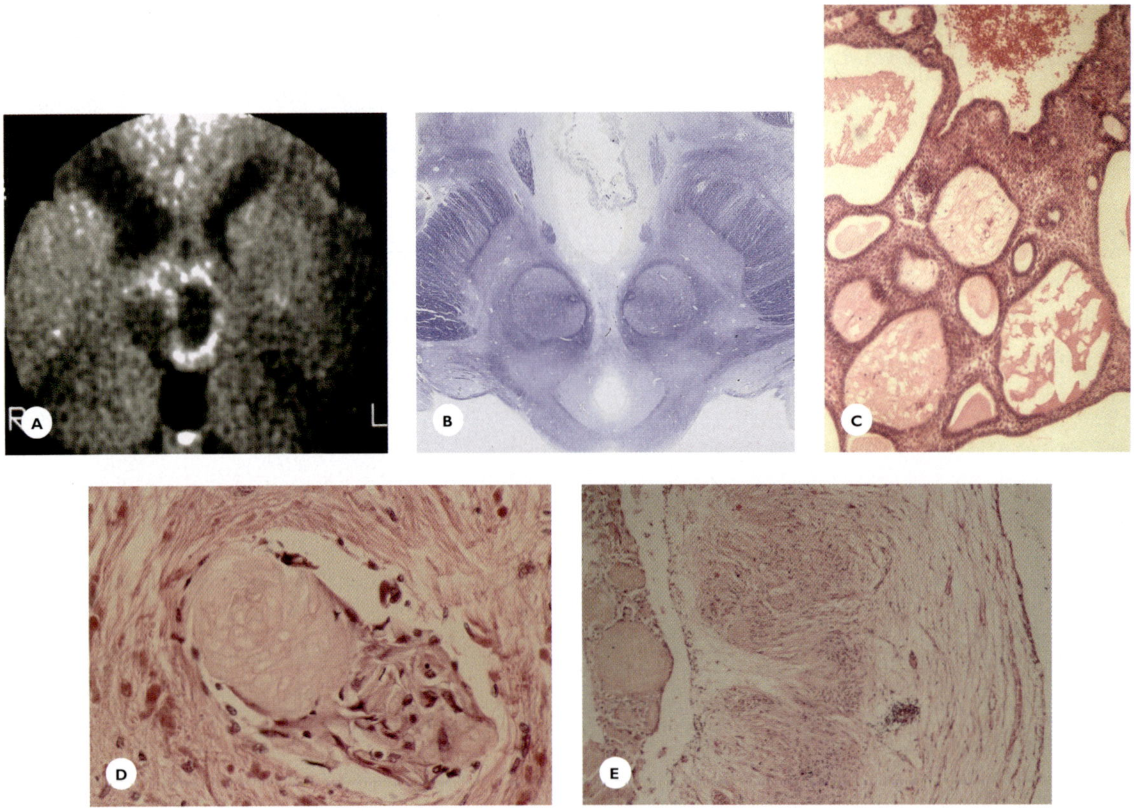

FIGURE 11.37B
Craniopharyngioma in a 75-year-old man. **A.** A contrast CT scan shows a large cystic mass within the third ventricle. **B.** Macrosection of the craniopharyngioma within the third ventricle (LFB-CV). The mural nodules contain (**C**) squamous epithelial cells and (**D.**) homogenous keratin material. **E.** The cyst wall is loosely attached to the ventricular wall; it contains astrocytic fibers and Rosenthal fibers (HE).

adheres to the neural parenchyma and sometimes invades it.

Epidermoid Cysts

This tumor-like lesion occurs chiefly in adults, usually in the cerebello-pontine angle, the parasellar region, or in the diploe of the skull.

Grossly, the cyst wall is smooth or nodular and contains white, glossy material resembling mother of pearl (*pearly tumor*) (Fig. 11.38). Histologically, the fibrous capsule is lined with stratified squamous epithelial cells, and the tumor contains concentrically arranged keratin from the desquamation of squamous epithelial cells. If the capsule breaks, the contents evoke a granulomatous aseptic meningitis and ependymitis with foreign-body giant cells (see Fig. 11.38).

Dermoid Cysts

Dermoid cysts occur in young individuals. Usually, they are situated in the posterior fossa, at the base of the brain, or in the region of anterior fontanel.

Grossly, the dermoid cyst is a well-delineated mass lesion with soft yellow content. Histologically, the cyst wall contains squamous epithelial cell, hair, and skin appendages.

Colloid Cyst of the Third Ventricle

A colloid cyst occurs in adults. Its size varies from a few millimeters to 3 to 4 cm.

The smooth cystic wall attaches to the choroid plexus, and may adhere to the fornices and the wall of the third ventricle. The content is mucinous (Fig. 11.39). The cyst intermittently blocks the foramen Mono and

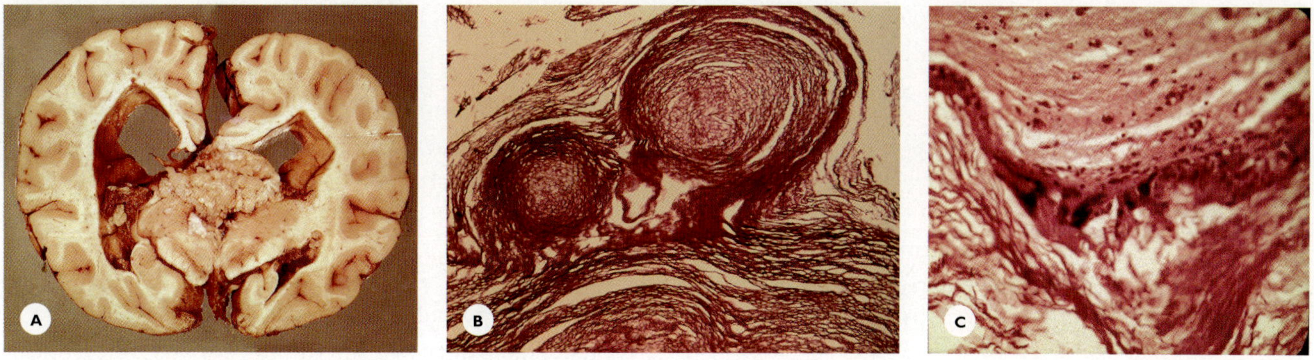

FIGURE 11.38
Epidermoid cyst in a 33-year-old mentally retarded epileptic man. **A.** A large cystic tumor situated in the pineal region compresses the tectum and the aqueduct. It breaks into the third and enlarged lateral ventricles. Small fragments of glossy material are deposited on the ventricular wall. **B.** The cyst wall consists of squamous epithelial cells, and the lumen contains keratin arranged in concentric lamellae. **C.** The ventricular wall shows epedymitis with foreign-body giant cells.

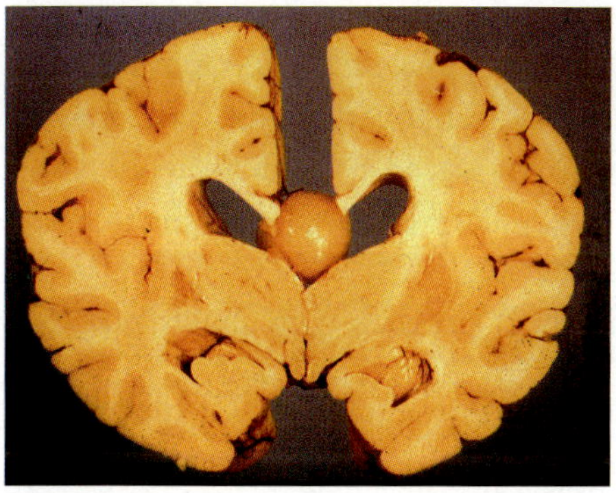

FIGURE 11.39
Colloid cyst of the third ventricle. A 35-year-old woman who suffered from severe headaches died suddenly. Transverse section at the thalamus level shows a cherry-sized colloid cyst blocking the foramen Monro. The lateral ventricles are moderately dilated. Separation of corpus callosum is artifactual.

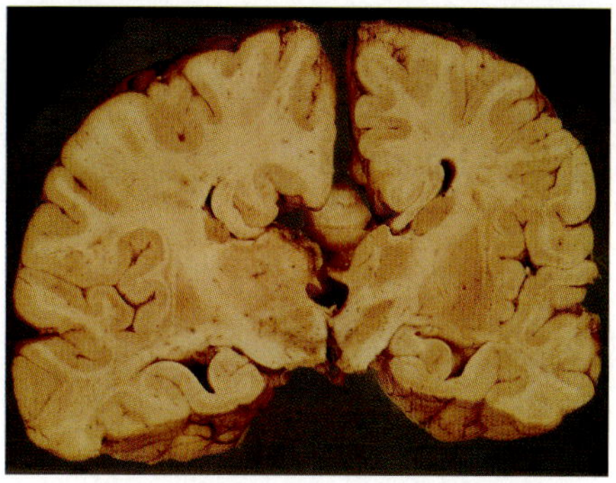

FIGURE 11.40
Lipoma associated with agenesis of the corpus callosum.

gradually leads to hydrocephalus. Clinically, the colloid cyst presents with headaches, often precipitated and aggravated by head movements. Due to obstruction of the foramen Mono and a sudden rise of ICP, death may occur suddenly. Histologically, the cyst wall contains cuboidal and columnar epithelial cells and mucin-producing cells.

Lipoma

This is a rare benign tumor generally is situated over the corpus callosum or quadrigeminal plate, less often in the region of the tuber cinereum or cerebellopontine angle. It often coexists with the agenesis of the corpus callosum and convolutional malformations. Grossly and histologically, the lipoma resembles normal adipose tissue and may also contain variable amounts of connective tissue and blood vessels (Fig. 11.40).

Arachnoid Cysts

These cysts result either from a congenital splitting of the arachnoid membrane or from an irritation of the leptomeninges by inflammation or hemorrhage. They occur in both children and adults. Common sites are along the sylvian fissure, in the cerebellopontine angle, and over the cerebellar hemispheres. Clinically, they may present with seizures, focal deficits and, in infants, with hydrocephalus. They may also remain asymptomatic, to be diagnosed incidentally on neuroimaging or at autopsy (Fig. 11.41). The cyst wall consists of collagenous tissue lined with arachnoid cells. The underlying brain may be indented and gliotic.

Hypothalamic Harmartomas

These circumscribed, firm tumors are composed of neurons, glial cells, and myelinated and unmyelinated fibers. They usually attach to the infundibulum or mammillary bodies.

HEMANGIOMAS

The group of hemangiomas comprises tumors of the blood vessels and malformative vascular lesions.

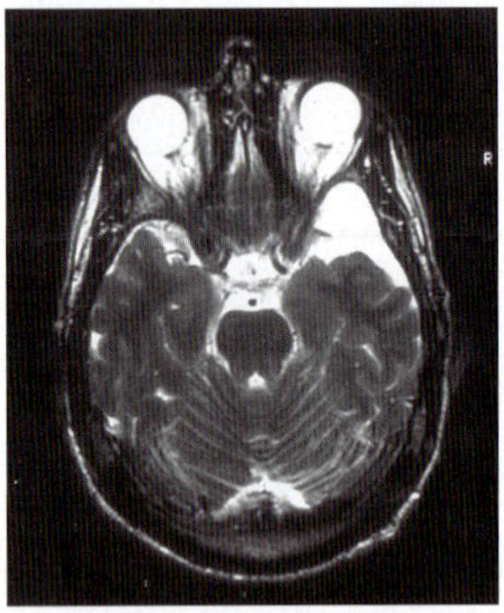

FIGURE 11.41
Arachnoid cyst at the temporal pole, an incidental MRI finding in a 47-year-old man.

Tumors of the Blood Vessels

Vascular tumors are rare, constituting only 1% to 2% of intracranial tumors. The group includes the capillary hemangioblastoma, the hemangiopericytoma, and the angiosarcoma.

Capillary Hemangioblastoma

This benign vascular tumor affects adults aged 20 to 50 years. The majority of the tumors are sporadic, few are familial, and about 25% of them are the diagnostic hallmark of the dominantly inherited von Hippel Lindau syndrome. The mutant gene maps to chromosome 3p25–26. The tumor, single or multiple, typically occurs in the cerebellum, seldom in the cerebrum, brainstem, or spinal cord. Extracerebral manifestations are various combinations of retinal angiomatosis, pheochromocytoma, congenital pancreatic and renal cysts, pancreatic islet cell tumor, renal carcinoma, and cystadenoma of epididymis. An erythropoietin hormone produced by the cells of capillary hemangioblastoma causes secondary polycythemia.

Clinically, it presents with slowly progressive cerebellar symptoms and raised ICP. Visual impairment from a retinal hemangioma may either precede or follow the cerebral symptoms.

Grossly, the tumor is a reddish mural nodule in the wall of a large cyst, which contains xanthochromic fluid (Fig. 11.42). Histologically, hemangioblastoma has two components: a capillary network lined with endothelial cells and large foamy stromal cells. These cells immu-

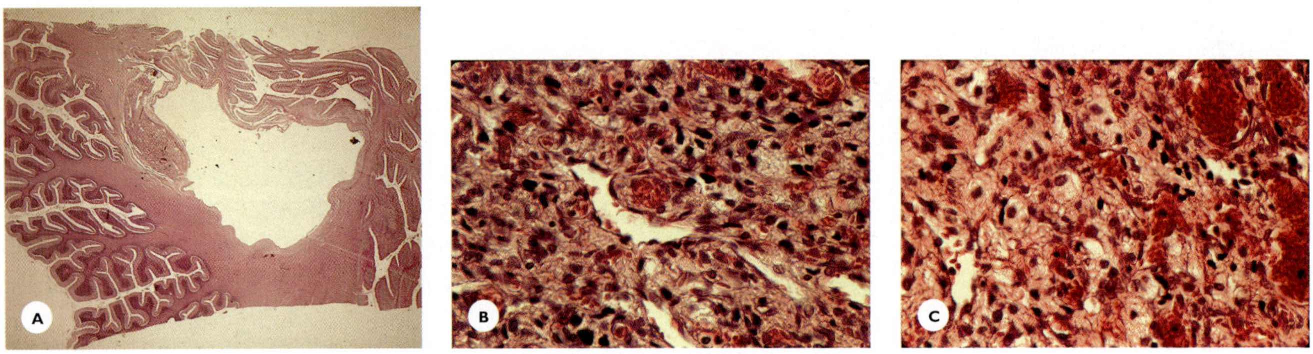

FIGURE 11.42
Capillary hemangioblastoma. **A.** Macrosection of the cerebellar hemisphere shows a large cyst with a small tumorous mural nodule. **B.** The tumor consists of endothelial cells lining capillary channels and (C.) large foamy stromal cells that contain lipid (HE).

noreact for vimentin and may contain lipid droplets (see Fig. 11.42).

Hemangiopericytoma

This malignant tumor of adults is described in the section, Tumors of the Meninges.

Anagiosarcoma

This malignant tumor of the brain and meninges consists of vascular channels lined with atypical endothelial cells displaying frequent mitoses.

Malformative Vascular Lesions

These circumscribed mass lesions of vascular channels are characterized by:

- An absence of proliferative tendencies; they may, however, expand by dilatation of vascular channels
- Single or multiple presentation
- Sporadic or familial occurrence

Clinically, vascular malformations usually manifest in adults and present with seizures and headaches. Progressive or fluctuating neurologic deficits follow. Serious complications are recurrent parenchymal and subarachnoid hemorrhages.

Cavernous angioma is a group of sinusoidal collagenous vascular channels separated by gliotic tissue. It is preferentially situated in the cerebral hemispheres and pons (Fig. 11.43).

The *arteriovenous angioma* is a conglomeration of arteries and veins of various sizes commonly situated in the cerebral hemispheres, often in the distribution of the middle cerebral artery. The vascular walls degenerate and proliferate, leading to luminal stenosis and thrombotic occlusion. The intervening neural tissue undergoes ischemic necrosis and eventually becomes gliotic. Distant ischemia develops from the "stealing" of blood from neighboring tissue (see Fig. 11.43).

The *venous angioma* consists of clusters of tortuous veins separated by gliotic tissue.

Capillary telangiectases consist of a group of dilated, varicose capillaries separated by normal tissue. Found in the pons, medulla, and cerebral white matter, they may produce slowly progressing neurologic deficits. Often they are incidental findings at autopsy (see Fig. 11.43).

LYMPHOMAS AND HEMATOPOIETIC TUMORS

This group encompasses the malignant primary lymphomas of the CNS and tumors derived from neoplastic plasma cells and histiocytes.

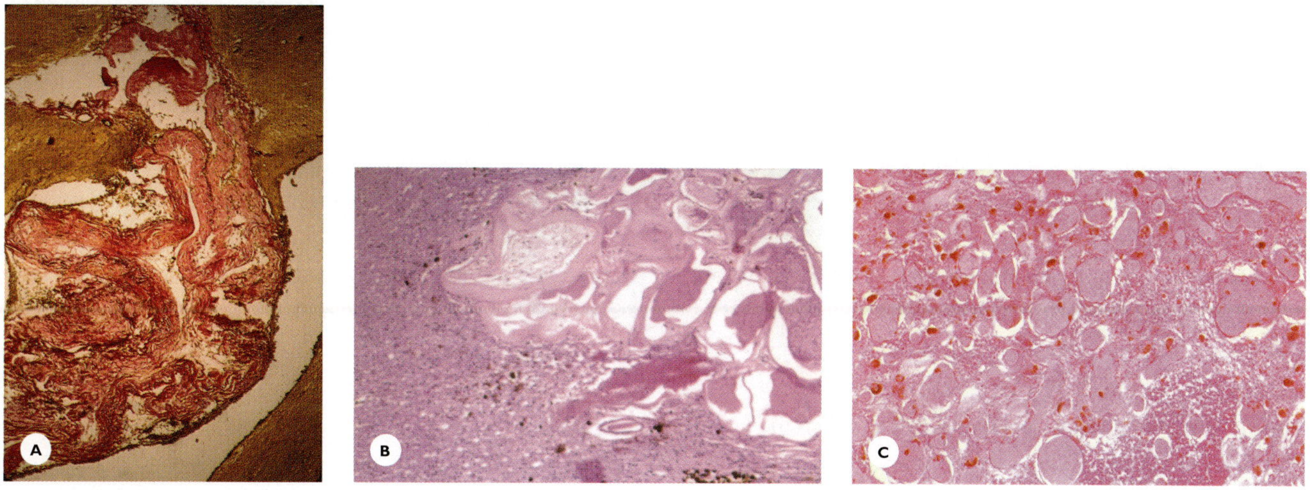

FIGURE 11.43
Vascular malformations. **A.** Cavernous angioma (van Gieson). **B.** Arteriovenous malformation. Hemosideum pigments are scattered around the lesion. **C.** Capillary telangiectasis (HE).

Primary Central Nervous System Lymphomas

Primary CNS lymphomas (PCNSLs) account for only for 2% to 3% of all intracranial tumors but their incidence is rising. About 80% to 90% of PCNSLs are B-cell lymphomas, the majority of which are large B-cell variants with a high grade of malignancy. The rest are T-cell lymphomas.

PCNSLs affect both immunocompetent and immunocompromised individuals. The incidence is as high as 5% to 10% in patients with AIDS. It also affects patients with organ transplants, patients receiving long-term steroid therapy, and those with congenital immunodeficiency syndrome. The incidence of lymphomas in AIDS patients increases with the duration of antiretroviral therapy and the decline of CD4 counts. AIDS- and organ transplant–related lymphomas are strongly associated with a latent Epstein-Barr virus infection.

PCNSLs can occur at any age from childhood on. The peak incidence is in the fifth and sixth decades in immunocompetent patients, and in the third and fourth decades in immunosuppressed patients. The clinical history is short, only a few weeks or months. General manifestations are headaches, neuropsychiatric symptoms, cognitive decline, altered mentation, and seizures. Focal neurologic signs indicate the location of the tumor. A cytologic study of the CSF using immunohistochemical markers and neuroimaging are the appropriate diagnostic tests.

Neuroimaging demonstrates the tumors around the lateral ventricles, in the corpus callosum, and in basal ganglia. On CT scan, in immunocompetent patients, lymphomas are hyperdense, occasionally hypo- to isodense relative to gray matter, and homogenously enhancing with contrast media (Fig. 11.44). In immunocompromised patients, they are hypodense and show ring-enhancement after contrast administration.

On T1-weighted MR images, lymphomas are iso- to hypointense and show homogenous enhancement. On T2-weighted images they are isointense- to moderately hyperintense. Single photon emission tomography (SPECT) and positron emission tomography (PET) are useful in differentiating lymphomas from toxoplasmosis, a common complication in AIDS patients. Lymphomas are sensitive to steroid therapy; they regress and may become temporarily undetectable in neuroimaging.

In the general population, the mean survival of lymphoma patients is 1 to 2 years; and in immunocompromised patients, it is 3 to 6 months.

Grossly, PCNSLs are often multiple, preferentially situated in the supratentorial compartment, rarely in the cerebellum and brainstem. They are often deep-seated in the periventricular regions, corpus callosum, and basal ganglia. Their margins are indistinct; cut surfaces are gray or brown, firm or soft, friable or granular, and may contain hemorrhages and necrosis. Periventricular and meningeal spreads are usual.

Histologically, PCNSLs diffusely spread and extend beyond their macroscopic appearance. Typically, the cells are arranged around blood vessels and are encircled by reticulin fibers (Fig. 11.45). A panel of immunohistochemical stains using B- and T-cell markers identifies the cell of origin.

Plasmacytoma

Tumors deriving from neoplastic plasma cells occur in middle-aged and elderly persons. They present as solitary or multiple lytic skull lesions (multiple myelomas) and dural infiltrations. The infiltrations may extend into the dural sinuses or may spread along the cranial nerves.

Langerhans' Cell Histiocytosis

The term *Langerhans' cell histiocytosis* refers to three conditions: *Hand-Schüler-Christian disease, Letterer-Siwe disease*, and *eosinophilic granuloma*. The lesions consist of a mixture of histiocytes, large histiocyte-like Langerhans' cells, monocytes, macrophages, and eosinophils. CNS involvement has a predilection for the hypothalamus, pituitary stalk, and orbit. Clinical presentations are diabetes insipidus, exophthalmus and, on neuroimaging, lesions in the base of the skull.

METASTATIC TUMORS

Metastases to the nervous system are serious, even fatal, complications of malignancies of any organ of the body. Carcinomas are the most common malignancies to metastasize to the brain, followed by hemapoietic malignancies. Sarcoma metastasis is rare. Dissemination

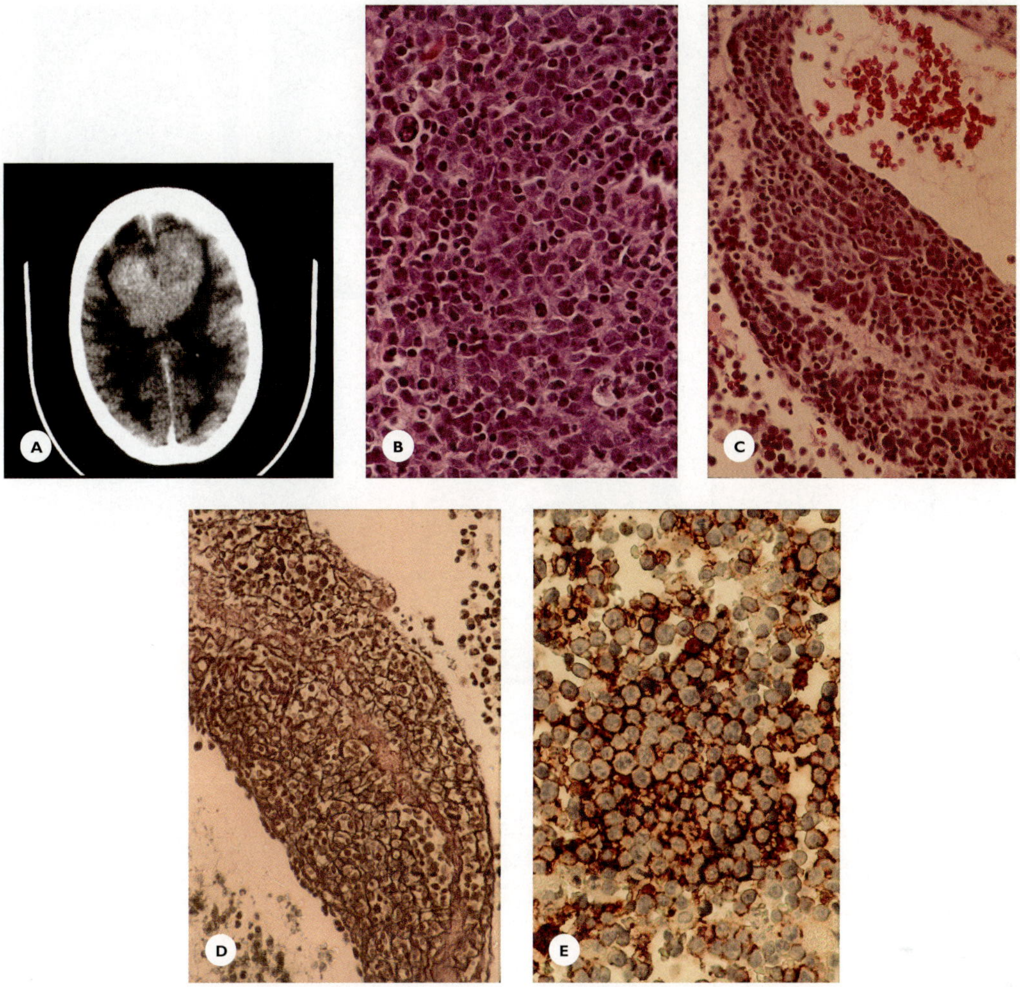

FIGURE 11.44
Primary large B-cell lymphoma. A 48-year-old man with no previous psychiatric history presented with confusion and bizarre behavior of 9 days' duration. He became irritable, agitated, sleepless, and incontinent. One day, he was found taking a shower with his clothes on. No evidence of trauma, immunodeficiency state, or systemic lymphomas was found. He was HIV-negative. On examination, his state of alertness fluctuated; one minute he was alert and responded appropriately, the next minute, he was unresponsive. His speech was slurred, at times, incoherent. He was picking at his clothes and bed sheet. He was able to stand with assistance. Reflexes were hyperactive, Babinski sign was present bilaterally, and muscle strength was good. He died 2 months after the initial symptoms. **A.** Contrast-enhanced CT scan shows bilateral hemispheric mass lesions in the genu and body of corpus callosum and periventricular white matter. Biopsy of the tumor shows (**B**) large B-cell lymphoma with (**C**) perivascular arrangement of tumor cells (HE stain). **D.** Concentrically arranged reticulin fibers encircle the tumor cells (reticulin stain), which (**E**) immunoreact for CD2O B-cell marker.

occurs by the bloodstream, less often by direct invasion from neighboring malignancies in the nasopharynx, facial sinuses, orbit, inner ear, or parotid gland. Common sites of metastases are the brain parenchyma and the meninges, less often the spinal cord and peripheral nerves. An estimated 20% to 30% of cancer patients develop intracranial metastases, accounting widely for 13% to 39% of intracranial tumors. They are most common in middle-aged and elderly patients.

Carcinomas

Carcinoma of the lung is the most common primary malignancy to metastasize to the brain, followed by carcinomas of the breast, kidney, gastrointestinal

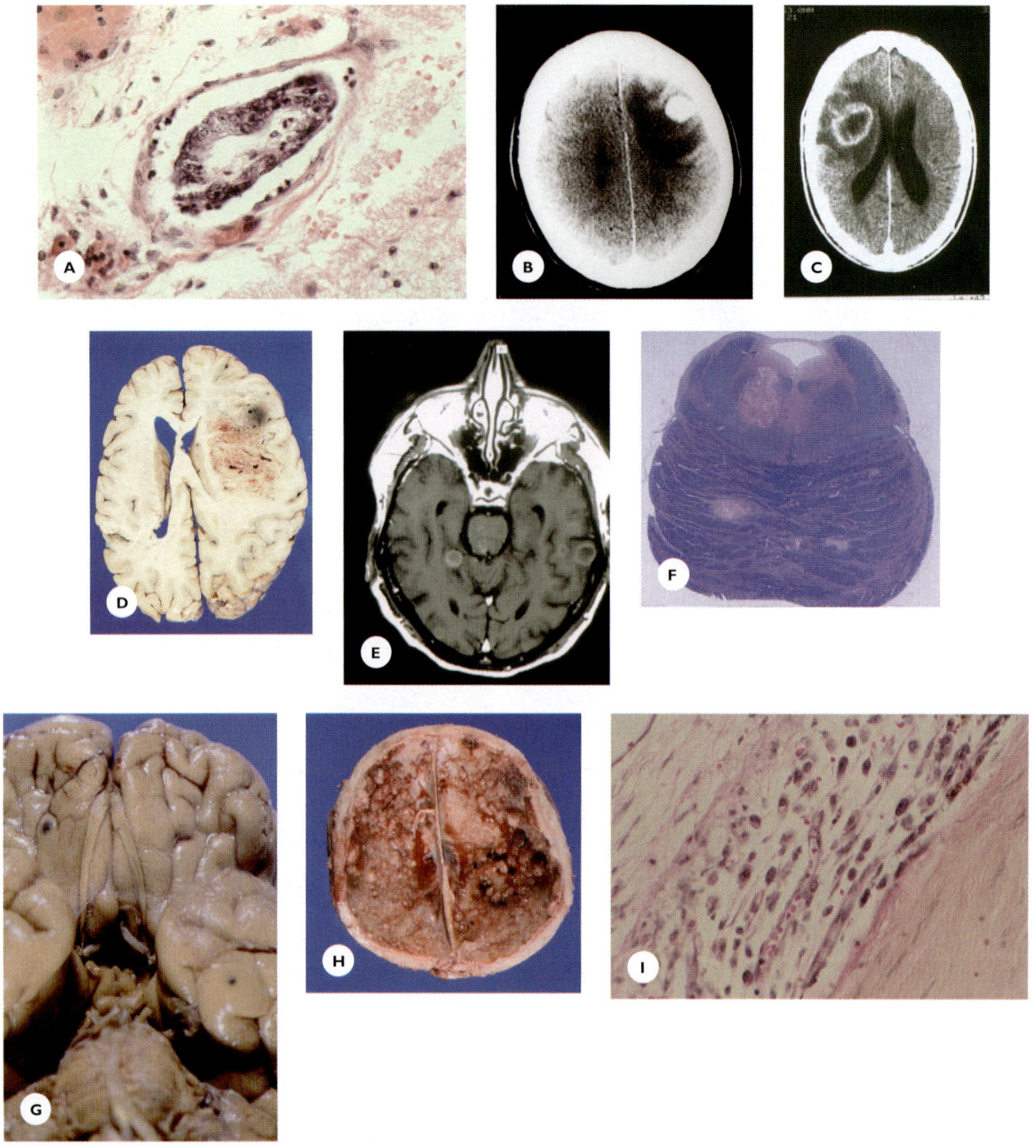

FIGURE 11.45

Metastatic cerebral tumors. **A.** Tumor embolus in a leptomeningeal capillary from pulmonary carcinoma. **B.** Solitary metastatic carcinoma from the lung. The tumor presented approximately one and a half years after resection of a left lower lobe adenocarcinoma in a 66-year-old man. Contrast-enhanced CT scan shows a circumscribed, round, hyperdense mass in the right frontocentral region at the junction of the cortex and white matter, surrounded by massive edema. **C.** On contrast-enhanced CT scan, a solitary carcinoma metastasis in the right central region from the lung appears as a ring-enhancing lesion. **D.** Horizontal section of the brain shows a necrotic and hemorrhagic tumor surrounded by edema. **E.** Multiple, widely dispersed bronchogenic carcinomas. Contrast-enhanced T-1 weighted MRI of a 55-year-old man showing small ring-enhancing lesions in cerebral and cerebellar hemispheres and pons. **F.** Macrosection of the pons demonstrates several small, circumscribed metastatic tumors (LFB-CV). **G.** Multiple tiny metastases from skin melanoma resected 9 years prior to patient's death. **H.** Dural and bony metastases from prostate carcinoma in a 77-year-old man. The tumor was diagnosed 2 years prior to patient's death and was treated with radiation and chemotherapy. **I.** Dural spread of acute myelocytic leukemia in a 52-year-old man.

tract, prostate, and thyroid gland. Skin melanoma and choriocarcinoma are less common malignancies, but they have a high tendency to spread to the brain.

Metastases can present before or simultaneously with the primary malignancy and, importantly, they can also appear months or years after the surgical resection of their source. Being fast-growing tumors, edema and raised ICP develop early in the clinical course. Highly vascular tumors—such as melanoma, choriocarcinoma, and renal carcinoma—are prone to bleed, mimicking a stroke. The prognosis is generally poor. There are few exceptional case reports of long survival following resection of primary and metastatic tumors.

The location, number, and size of metastases vary greatly. They may occur at any site in the cerebrum, preferentially at the junction of the cortex and white matter (see Fig. 11.45). The choroid plexus, the pineal, and the pituitary glands are less common sites. Prostate carcinoma spreads commonly to the skull and dura (see Fig. 11.45). Metastases can be solitary, but they are more often multiple, varying from as many as 10 to 15 or more. Their sizes range from microscopic clusters of malignant cells to large masses.

Grossly, the tumors are fairly well circumscribed but poorly demarcated, contain hemorrhages and necrosis, and are surrounded by extensive edema. Histologically, the picture varies from well-differentiated tumors resembling the primary tumor to anaplastic tumors. These may pose diagnostic difficulties, particularly when the primary malignancy is clinically not evident. Immunohistochemical studies for epithelial markers (cytokeratin, epithelial membrane antigen) support the carcinomatous origin of the metastasis.

Meningeal carcinomatosis or carcinomatous meningitis usually results from the spread of an intraparenchymal carcinoma to the leptomeninges. The meninges are seldom the primary sites of metastases. Contrast-enhanced MRI and cytologic study of the CSF confirm the diagnosis.

Hematopoietic Metastases

Lymphomas

The nervous system is involved in about 10% of non-Hodgkin's lymphomas and only rarely in Hodgkin's disease. Lymphomas can disseminate to the leptomeninges, diffusely or focally filling the subarachnoid space and infiltrating the cranial and spinal nerve roots. They can form nodules in the dura that compresses the adjacent tissue, and can also produce intracerebral mass lesions.

Leukemic Meningitis

Invasion of the leptomeninges in acute and chronic leukemias is high, averaging from 10% to 40%. It is noteworthy that prophylactic CNS therapy has led, in some instances, to the development of CNS tumors, particularly in young children.

Leukostasis

Occlusions of small parenchymal blood vessels by leukocytes occur in acute leukemias and in the blast crisis of chronic leukemias. Hemorrhages and infarcts are serious complications. Subdural and subarachnoid hemorrhages complicate thrombocytopenia.

TUMORS OF THE SPINAL CORD, NERVE ROOTS, AND MENINGES

Tumors within the spinal dural sac may arise in the spinal cord, nerve roots, and meninges. Their gross and histologic features generally resemble those of their intracranial counterparts.

Intramedullary Tumors

Gliomas with ependymomas and astrocytomas, are most frequently encountered within the spinal cord.

Ependymoma constitutes more than half of intramedullary tumors. It is common in adults and may occur in any segment of the cord. The well-demarcated solid tumor is situated around the central canal (Fig. 11.46).

Myxopapillary ependymoma arises within the conus or filum terminale and is situated between the nerve roots of the cauda equina. Histologically, the tumor is composed of cuboidal and columnar ependymal cells arranged around blood vessels or aligned along the fibrous stroma in a papillary fashion. Mucoid degeneration is prominent (see Fig. 11.46).

Astrocytoma diffusely enlarges the cords of children and adults, usually in the cervical and thoracic

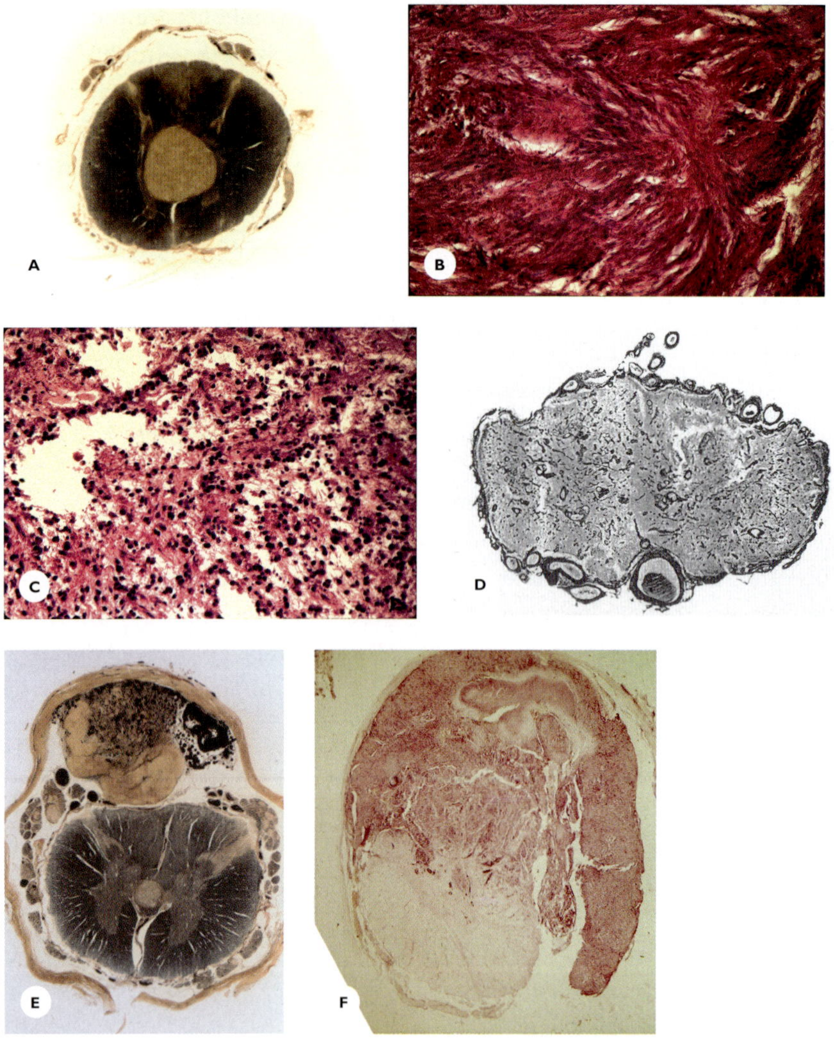

FIGURE 11.46
Spinal cord tumors **A.** Intramedullary ependymoma (myelin stain). **B** and **C.** Histology of mixopapillary ependymoma (HE). **D.** Intramedullary angiomatosis (Perdrau stain). **E.** Schwannomas of the nerve roots (myelin stain). **F.** Carcinoma metastasis (cresyl violet).

regions. The histologic features vary from benign to malignant. The tumor may be associated with syringomyelia.

Oligodendroglioma occurs rarely in the spinal cord and affects adults. Unlike its cerebral counterpart, calcification is uncommon.

Neuronal tumors, such as *gangliocytoma* and *ganglioglioma*, are rare.

Capillary hemangioblastoma has the histologic features of its cerebellar counterpart and occurs in von Hippel-Lindau syndrome.

Angiomatosis may produce massive hemorrhages or a slowly progressive necrotizing myelopathy. Angiomatosis of the leptomeninges may also be present (see Fig. 11.46).

Spinal enterogenous cyst, a rare intra- or extramedullary lesion. may present from childhood to old age. The cyst wall is lined with columnar epithelial cells resembling intestinal epithelium.

Metastatic tumors are rare, but meningeal malignancies may extend into the cord along the perivascular spaces (see Fig. 11.46).

Nerve Root Tumors

Schwannomas and *neurofibromas* commonly occur in adults. They preferentially arise in the sensory nerve roots and are positioned laterally to the cord (see Fig. 11.46). They may grow through the intervertebral foramina into the extraspinal compartment as a *dumbbell tumor.* Solitary or multiple, they are components of neurofibromatosis type 1 and type 2 syndromes.

Meningeal Tumors

Meningioma, derived from meningoendothelial arachnoidal cells, affects adults. Like its intracranial counterparts, it is more common in women. The thoracic region is the favored site, where the tumor is situated near the nerve roots.

The *hemangiopericytoma of the spinal dura*, a rare tumor of mesenchymal origin, occurs in adults. It is highly malignant, with a tendency to metastasize.

Other Intradural Tumors

Paraganglioma, a rare benign tumor in adults, is attached to the filum terminale and cauda equina. Histologically, its lobular pattern of round, uniform cells is similar to that seen in tumors in other places.

Lipoma and *dermoid cyst* are more common in children. They are situated in the lumbosacral region and are often associated with malformations of the spine.

Carcinomas and *lymphomas* can metastasize to the dura and leptomeninges; from there, they may invade the spinal cord (see Fig. 11.46).

Dissemination from primary intracranial tumors (medulloblastoma, glioblastoma, oligodendroglioma, germinoma, and choroid plexus papilloma) occurs via the CSF. The seeded tumor cells infiltrate the nerve roots and may extend into the spinal cord along the perivascular spaces (see Fig. 11.7).

TUMORS OF THE CRANIUM AND THE SPINE

This group encompasses several rare benign and malignant tumors of the bone, cartilage, and blood vessels that can compress or invade the adjacent neural tissue.

Benign tumors are the osteoma, chondroma, hemangioma, and the sacrococcygeal teratoma.

Malignant tumors are the osteosarcoma and chondrosarcoma.

Chordoma, a rare, slowly growing tumor, chiefly of adults, originates from remnant cells of the notochord and is situated over the clivus or in the sacrococcygeal region. It tends to invade the adjacent structures and metastasize to the lungs and lymph nodes.

Metastatic tumors are commonly from prostate and breast carcinomas. Multiple bony lesions occur in hematopoietic malignancies (myelomas) and Langerhans' histiocytosis.

PRIMARY INTRACRANIAL TUMORS IN CHILDREN

This section presents a brief overview of childhood tumors and reiterates some particular features of individual tumors. The histopathologic features of the tumors are covered in the appropriate sections.

In the pediatric age group, *intracranial tumors* are the most common tumors after leukemias. They are a major cause of cancer-related death in children. They may present at any time from birth on. Fetal tumors can be detected by the third trimester using ultrasonography; investigations are usually prompted by a sudden increased rate of uterine growth.

Signs of hydrocephalus—enlarging head, bulging fontanels, vomiting—and failure to thrive are common clinical manifestations in neonates and infants, whereas older children present with headaches, seizures, visual impairment, and focal neurologic deficits.

About 50% of tumors in children occur in the infratentorial compartment. The benign and relatively benign gliomas and the malignant embryonal tumors predominate. Their regional distribution is shown in Table 11.9. The malignant gliomas, meningiomas, and neurinomas rarely affect children.

Childhood tumors pose therapeutic challenges. The selection of appropriate therapy—surgery, radiation, and chemotherapy—is aimed not only at obtaining maximal therapeutic efficacy but also at avoiding any

TABLE 11.9.
Distribution of Intracranial Childhood Tumors

Cerebellum	*Ventricles*	*Sellar Region*	*Pineal Region*
Pilocytic astrocytoma Medulloblastoma Dermoid cyst	Ependymoma Choroid plexus Papilloma Carcinoma	Craniopharyngeoma Germinoma	Pineoblastoma Pineocytoma Germinoma Teratoma
Optic Nerve/Chiasma Hypothalamus	*Cerebral Hemispheres*		*Brain Stem*
Pilocytic astrocytoma	Diffuse astrocytoma Desmoplastic infantile astrocytoma/ganglioglioma Pleomorphic xanthoastrocytoma	Medulloepithelioma Central neuroblastoma Teratoid/rhabdoid tumor	Fibrillary astrocytoma

toxic damage to the maturing nervous tissue. Therapeutic decision-making takes several factors into account: patient's age, extent of tumor resection, histopathologic characteristics, and response to particular therapies.

A number of genetic alterations have been found in various pediatric tumors. One objective is to find consistent genetic alterations that can be applied as reliable prognostic and therapeutic guides.

Congenital Tumors

Teratomas, often in the pineal region, are the most common congenital tumors. Other common tumors are glioblastomas, lipomas, plexus papillomas, and craniopharyngeomas. Lipomas, situated in the midline and associated with agenesis of the corpus callosum, are often clinically silent. Glioblastomas and plexus papillomas may produce marked hydrocephalus.

The prognosis for congenital tumors is generally poor. Some fetuses are stillborn. In the majority of cases, survival ranges from a few weeks to 1 year, seldom longer.

Gliomas

Astrocytic Tumors

In the group of gliomas, *pilocytic astrocytoma* (grade 1) of the cerebellum is the most common tumor, accounting for 25% of all intracranial tumors in children. When totally resected, the prognosis is excellent, with a 15- to 20-year survival rate. A malignant variant occasionally develops following radiation therapy for a benign astrocytoma.

Desmoplastic infantile astrocytoma and *desmoplastic infantile ganglioglioma* (grade1), large cystic tumors of the cerebral hemispheres with dural attachment, have a generally good prognosis following surgery.

Subependymal giant cell astrocytoma (grade 1), a histologically benign tumor in the wall of the lateral ventricle, occurs in the setting of tuberous sclerosis complex.

Pleomorphic cystic xanthoastrocytoma (grade 2), a less common tumor of the cerebral hemispheres, has a favorable prognosis, but may occasionally recur and may undergo malignant transformation.

Low-grade diffuse astrocytoma (grade 2) of the cerebral hemispheres has a better prognosis and less frequent malignant progression than does the adult counterpart.

Anaplastic astrocytoma (grade 3) and *glioblastoma multiforme* (grade 4) account for about 7% of pediatric tumors each. Anaplastic astrocytomas that show gains of chromosome 1q lead to a shorter survival.

Ependymoma (grade 2), the second most common childhood glioma, is a relatively benign tumor of the fourth ventricle; it constitutes 6% to 12% of pediatric tumors. The prognosis is influenced by its amenability to total resection.

Choroid plexus papilloma (grade 1), a rare tumor, has a good prognosis when totally resected. Prognosis is better with diploid papilloma than it is with aneuploid, which is aggressive. The prognosis for its malignant variant, the choroid plexus carcinoma, is poor. Both tumors have a tendency to disseminate via CSF.

Oligodendroglioma accounts for only 1% to 2% of pediatric tumors. Unlike the adult counterpart, no particular genetic alteration is associated with prognosis.

Embryonal Tumors

Tumors in this group represent the most malignant childhood tumors, corresponding to WHO grade 4. Except for the medulloblastoma, the tumors are rare.

Medulloblastoma, situated in the cerebellum, usually in the midline, accounts for about 20% of all intracranial tumors in young patients. Subtotal resection, the presence of subarachnoid dissemination at the initial evaluation, certain histologic subtypes (large cell/anaplastic), and genetic alterations (myc17p) make the prognosis worse. Some patients treated with combined radiation and chemotherapy following total or subtotal resection may have a better outcome; survival may reach 5 years.

Craniopharyngeoma

This benign maldevelopmental tumor in the suprasellar region constitutes 5% to 10% of childhood tumors. Patients with a totally surgically resected tumor have a good prognosis, with an average 10 years of survival. Subtotal resection has a high recurrence rate.

Tumors of the Meninges

Meningiomas in children are rare, constituting only 3% of pediatric brain tumors; no female predominance is noted. They are more common during the second decade of life but may occur at any age, including in fetuses and infants. In a significant number of children, meningiomas are associated with neurofibromatosis type 2 (NF2), often in the absence of a family history. Ionizing radiation is a potential risk for the development of a meningioma that may occur many years later. Meningiomas in children may reach large sizes, may be cystic, and may be situated within the brain, ventricles, or in the posterior fossa. The various histologic types encountered in adults, including malignant variants, also occur in children. A *sclerosing variant*, consisting of collagen admixed with spindle cells, is particular to childhood meninginomas.

A correlation between histologic grading and prognosis is unpredictable. Benign meningiomas may recur, whereas malignant grade 2 and 3 meningiomas may have a relatively favorable course. Sporadic and NF2-associated meningiomas showing 1p and 14q deletions have a malignant course.

Germ Cell Tumors

Germinomas constitute 2% to 3% of childhood tumors. Situated in the pineal or suprasellar regions, they have a tendency to disseminate via CSF. They are radiosensitive, which makes the prognosis more favorable: Post-operative survival averages 5 years.

Teratoma, when totally resected, has a good prognosis.

Other germ cell tumors, such as embryonal carcinoma, choriocarcinoma, and malignant teratoma have a poor prognosis.

Pineal Gland Tumors

Pineoblastoma (grade 4) is the most common pineal gland tumor in children. Mixed tumors with intermediate differentiation are rare. Pineoblastoma tends to disseminate within the subarachnoid space and metastasize extracranially. Chromosomal imbalance has been reported in a small number of cases. Pinecytoma is rare.

HEREDITARY TUMOR SYNDROMES

The concurrence of nervous system tumors with ocular, cutaneous, visceral, and skeletal disorders, in various combinations, characterizes these genetically determined syndromes. The pathology of the tumors is presented in appropriate sections.

Neurofibromatosis Type 1 (NF1) and Neurofibromatosis Type 2 (NF2)

NF1 and NF2 share several features; both are inherited in an autosomal dominant fashion. About 50% of cases, however, occur sporadically because of a high rate of spontaneous mutations. Tumors of the peripheral nerves are the diagnostic hallmarks of both syndromes. Clinically, they may present from early childhood to adulthood. The expressivity varies from a monosymptomatic abortive form to a broad range of manifestations including seizures, mental retardation, and systemic disorders. T2-weighted MRI may show hyperintense lesions in the white matter and basal ganglia, corresponding to heterotopia and failure of myelination.

The two syndromes differ in genetic profiles, histologic tumor types, and systemic manifestations.

Neurofibromatosis Type 1

Neurofibromatosis type 1 or Recklinghausen's disease is one of the most common genetic diseases. The gene product—neurofibromin—is encoded by chromosome 17.

Nervous System Tumors

Typical peripheral nerve tumors are the fusiform and plexiform *neurofibromas*. They may involve the small cutaneous and visceral branches and the larger peripheral nerves anywhere along their course. Cutaneous tumors become apparent in childhood or adolescence as simple or multiple nodules or pendular masses.

A characteristic additional CNS tumor in children is the *optic nerve or chiasma glioma*, usually a pilocytic astrocytoma. Less common tumors are the cerebral and cerebellar astrocytomas and the spinal cord gliomas.

Systemic Disorders

Café-au-lait pigmentations of the skin are characteristic. They may be present at birth or develop during childhood, and their number increases with age. *Skinfold freckling* usually occurs in adults. *Lisch nodules*, benign hamaratomas of the iris, occur in adults. *Pheochromocytoma*, *malignancies of various organs*, and *hematopoietic diseases* are visceral manifestations. *Dysplasias*, *short stature*, *macrocephaly*, and *thinning of long bones* are skeletal abnormalities.

Neurofibromatosis Type 2

The defective gene of this less common hereditary tumor syndrome maps to chromosome 22. The gene product is meslin or schwannomin.

Nervous System Tumors

Characteristic nerve sheath tumors are the *schwannomas* (neurinomas) of the cranial and spinal nerve roots and peripheral nerves. Bilateral acoustic neurinomas are hallmarks of the syndrome. Additional CNS tumors are the meningiomas, single or multiple, spinal ependymoma, and astrocytoma. Heterotopia and cerebral calcifactions add to the pathology.

Systemic Disorders

Café-au-lait skin pigmentations are less common than in NF1. *Posterior subcapsular cataract* is the ocular abnormality.

Von Hippel-Lindau Syndrome

This is a multisystem disorder with an autosomal dominant trait. The gene of the syndrome is located at chromosome 3p25-26. Capillary hemangioblastoma preferentially in the cerebellum is the diagnostic hallmark of the disease (see section on hemangiomas). Retinal angioma, pheochromocytoma, variable visceral tumors and cysts and secondary polycythemia complete the syndrome.

Tuberous Sclerosis Complex (TSC)

This autosomal dominant disorder is caused by the inactivation of one of two genes: *TSC1* or *TSC2*. The *TSC1* gene product—hamartin—is encoded by chromosome 9. The *TSC2* gene product—tuberin—is encoded by chromosome 16. A significant number of sporadic cases are caused by mutations in the *TSC2* gene.

The syndrome presents in early childhood, usually with seizures. Seizures, mental retardation, and sebaceous adenomas of the face are principal features. A retinal phakoma (glial nodule), when present, is usually asymptomatic.

The cerebral pathology consists of histogenetic malformations of the neurons and glial cells including (a) cortical tubers, (b) subependymal glial nodules, and (c) glial heterotopia in the white matter. (See Chapter 13.) These malformative lesions are capable of tumorous proliferation. Giant-cell subependymal astrocytoma is characteristic.

Hamartomas of the kidneys and rhabdomyoma of the heart are typical visceral manifestations.

Miscellaneous Hereditary Tumor Syndromes

Medulloblastomas may occur with colorectal polyps (Turcot syndrome) and nevoid basal cell carcinoma (Gorlin syndrome).

Glioblastomas may occur with colorectal polyps.

Astrocytomas and *primitive neuroectodermal tumors* (PNET) may occur with breast carcinoma, adrenocortical carcinoma, sarcoma, and leukemia (Li-Fraumeni syndrome).

NERVOUS SYSTEM COMPLICATIONS OF RADIATION AND CHEMOTHERAPY

Radiation and chemotherapy are common treatment modalities for nervous system malignancies both in adults and children. In addition to their beneficial effects, they may injure the nervous tissue, chiefly the white matter, producing a leucoencephalopathy or a myelopathy. Moreover, radiation has oncogenic potentials and is apt to produce secondary malignancies, whereas chemotherapy carries the risk of hematologic complications.

X-Irradiation

Radiation-induced cerebral changes may develop acutely during radiation exposure, or they may be delayed, developing slowly over several weeks, months, or even years later. Radiation damage usually occurs with a total dose of over 6,000 rads.

Acute Radiation Effect

Acute cerebral changes result from vasogenic edema due to an increased permeability of the capillary endothelium and the escape of fluid and protein into the white matter. The associated encephalopathy responds to corticosteroid therapy and is transient.

Early Delayed Radiation Effect

Early changes present several weeks after radiation and consist of variable losses of myelin and axons and hyalinization of vascular walls.

Late Delayed Radiation Effect, Coagulative Leukoencephalopathy

Late changes present from several months to several years after radiation and may also develop following radiation to neighboring extracranial malignancies. They may progress and produce a mass effect that clinically and radiologically mimics tumor recurrence. In adults, the encephalopathy presents with cognitive decline and focal neurologic deficits. In children, late sequelae are learning difficulties, subnormal IQ, endocrine dysfunction, and vascular insults.

Gross pathology is typically confined to the cerebral hemispheric white matter and the periventricular zones. The affected regions are soft and granular and contain small cavities, fluid-filled cysts, and dusky areas of old and fresh hemorrhages. The cortex and arcuate fibers are usually spared.

The histology is characterized by extensive coagulative necrosis, demyelination, and axonal losses. Prominent vascular changes include fibrinoid necrosis, hyalinization, fibrosis, and thrombotic occlusions. Perivascular mononuclear infiltrates are usually not conspicuous. Hypertrophied and bizarrely-shaped astrocytes are present in the demyelinated areas. Oligodendroglial cells are variably lost. The cerebral cortex may show neuronal losses and vascular changes, and the cerebellar cortex may show Purkinje and granule cell losses (Fig. 11.47).

Postradiation Neoplasms

Radiation-induced neoplasms are confined to the radiation field and may arise many years after radiation. Common neoplasms in children and adults are meningiomas, benign or malignant gliomas, and sarcomas.

Chemotherapy

Multidrug chemotherapeutic regiments administered for the treatment of malignant gliomas and metastatic malignancies, in addition to affecting the bone m arrow, may produce a coagulative necrotizing leukoencephalopathy.

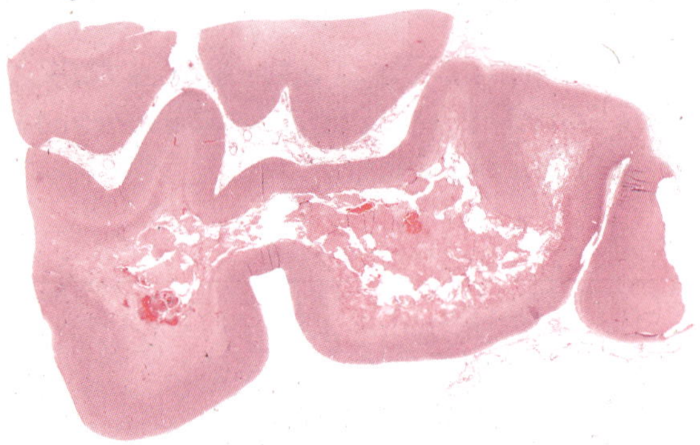

FIGURE. 11.47
Late delayed radiation leukoencephalopathy in a 64-year-old man. Following a resection of a primary lymphoma, he received first a total dose of 5,000 rads and, 2 years later, a total does of 3,800 rads. Macrosection from the cerebral hemisphere shows cavitated white matter, areas of coagulative necrosis, and preservation of the cortex (HE).

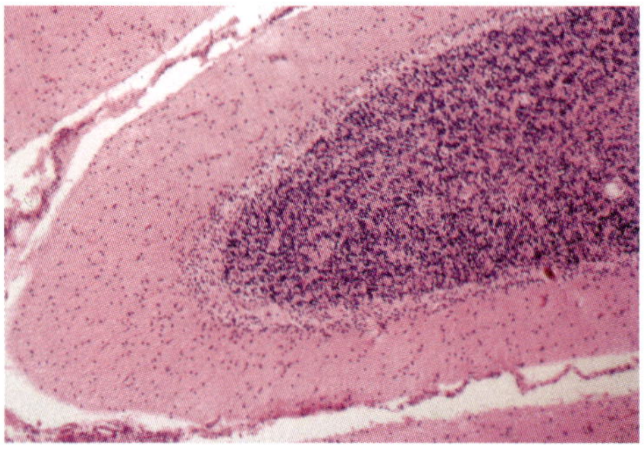

FIGURE 11.48
Cerebellar degeneration associated with a hepatocellular carcinoma that metastasized to the pancreas and the lung. The cortex shows extensive Purkinje cell loss and Bergmann astrocytosis (HE).

The degeneration of myelin is accompanied by a loss of oligodendrocytes and extensive axonal changes.

Methotrexate Leukoencephalopathy

Methotrexate is widely used for treatment of CNS lymphomas and acute leukemias in children. Administered intravenously or intrathecally, it may produce a necrotizing leucoencephalopathy confined to the central hemispheric white matter and periventricular zones. The blood vessels display necrotizing angiopathy, and the white matter shows coagulative necrosis.

PARANEOPLASTIC DISEASES

Paraneoplastic diseases, a group of neurologic disorders, are associated with malignancies in various visceral organs. Notably, they occur in the absence of metasis to the nervous system (the remote effects of malignancies). An estimated 1% to 3% of patients with various cancers develop paraneoplastic complications. These may present concurrently with the malignancy or may follow it, and importantly, may also precede it. Paraneoplastic diseases can be associated with almost any malignancy, but are most commonly associated with small-cell cancer of the lung and cancers of ovaries and breast. The diseases can affect the central and peripheral nervous systems, retina, and neuromuscular junction.

Paraneoplastic diseases are immune-mediated; antibodies initiated by the tumor react with antigens expressed by both the tumor and neurons. The presence of specific antibodies in the serum and CSF of these patients points to a particular malignancy—a helpful clue to the clinician, especially when the primary tumor is not clinically evident. About 50% to 60% of patients carry antibodies.

Subacute Cerebellar Degeneration

This disease is commonly associated with ovarian and breast carcinomas, small-cell lung carcinoma, and Hodgkin disease. Anti-Yo antibodies in patient's serum and CSF react with Purkinje cells. The histopathology consists of degeneration of the Purkinje cells, and some loss of granule cells and Bergmann astrocytosis. Concomitant changes are perivascular lymphocytic infiltrations and microglial proliferations in the brainstem and spinal cord (Fig. 11.48).

Encephalomyelitis and Limbic Encephalitis

This disease is associated with small-cell carcinoma of the lung and carcinoma of the testes. The histopathology, confined to the mesial temporal lobe, brainstem, and spinal cord, consists of neuronal losses, perivascular lymphocytic infiltrations, and microglial proliferation.

Lambert-Eaton Syndrome

LES or pseudomyasthenia is associated with small-cell lung carcinoma. The disease consists of proximal muscle weakness which, unlike that in myasthenia gravis, improves temporarily with exercise. LES is caused by the diminished release of acetylcholine due to antibodies directed against voltage-gated calcium channels in the presynaptic terminals.

Other Diseases

Sensory neuropathy can be associated with any malignancy, but more often with small-cell lung carcinoma. The histology consists of axonal degeneration and perivascular mononuclear infiltrations in the spinal ganglia, nerve roots, and peripheral nerves.

Opsoclonus/myoclonus—sudden irregular eye movements and muscle jerks—in adults is associated with small-cell carcinoma of the lung and carcinoma of the breast. In children these signs are associated with neuroblastoma.

Retinopathy is often associated with small-cell lung carcinoma.

BIBLIOGRAPHY

Eberhart, C.G. & Burger, P.C. (2003). Anaplasia and grading in medulloblastomas. *Brain Pathol 13*, 376–385.

Kleihues, P. & Cavenee, W.K., eds. (2000). *Pathology and genetics of tumours of the nervous system*. Lyon, France: World Health Organization IARC Press.

Kleihues, P., Louis, D.N., Scheithauer, B.W., et al. (2002). The WHO classification of tumors of the nervous system. *J Neuropathol Exp Neurol 61*, 215–225.

Lamszus, K. (2004). Meningioma pathology, genetics, and biology. *J Neuropathol Exp Neuro 63*, 275–286.

McLendon, R.E., Bigner, D.D., Bigner, S.H. & Provenzale, J.M. (2000). *Pathology of tumors of the central nervous system A guide to histologic diagnosis*. New York: Oxford University Press.

Perry, A. & Dehner, L.P. (2003). Meningeal tumors of childhood and infancy. An update and literature review. *Brain Pathol 13*, 386–408.

Pollack, I.F. & Mulvihill, J.J. (1997). Neurofibromatosis 1 and 2. *Brain Pathol 7*, 823–836.

Rickert, C.H. (1999). Neuropathology and prognosis of foetal brain tumors. *Acta Neuropathol 98*: 567–576.

Rickert, C.H. (2004). Prognosis-related molecular markers in pediatric central nervous system tumors. *J Neuropathol Exp Neurol 63*, 1211–1224.

REVIEW QUESTIONS

1. Potential risk factors for developing an intracranial tumor are:
   A. Familial occurrences
   B. Insecticides
   C. Irradiation to the head
   D. Immunosuppressed states
   E. Infection with hepatitis B virus

2. Genes implicated in neurotumorigenesis are:
   A. Epidermal growth factor (EGF) receptor gene
   B. Apolipoprotein E (APOE) gene
   C. p53
   D. All of these
   E. None of these

3. Characteristically, a diffuse astrocytomas, grade 2:
   A. Affects chiefly children
   B. Commonly occurs in the cerebral hemispheres
   C. Often presents clinically with seizures
   D. May progress into an anaplastic astrocytoma or a glioblastoma
   E. Is rarely associated with mutations in p53 gene

4. Histologic features characteristic of a glioblastoma are:
   A. Rich vascular supply
   B. Rosenthal fibers
   C. Pseudopalisading tumor cells around necrosis
   D. High mitotic activity
   E. Diffusely positive immunostaining with glial fibrillary acidic protein (GFAP)

5. Primary (*de nevo*) glioblastoma differs from secondary glioblastoma in that:
   A. It affects chiefly elderly individuals.
   B. It has a shorter clinical history.
   C. It is frequently associated with mutations in p53 gene.
   D. All of these.
   E. None of these.

6. Intracranial tumors that are particularly common in children are:
   A. Meningeoma
   B. Astrocytoma
   C. Brainstem glioblastoma
   D. Ependymoma
   E. Medulloblastoma

7. Features characteristic of medulloblastomas are:
   A. They account for 16% to 20% of all intracranial tumors in children.
   B. They grow slowly.
   C. They commonly occur in the cerebellar hemispheres.
   D. They have a tendency to disseminate via CSF.
   E. They may occur in twins.

8. Features characteristic of pilocytic astrocytomas are:
   A. They account for 20% to 25% of all intracranial tumors in children.
   B. They occur in the cerebellar vermis.
   C. They grow slowly.
   D. They are referred to as "blue cell tumors."
   E. They are often cystic.

9. All the following statements concerning oligodendrogliomas are correct *except*:
   A. They grow slowly.
   B. They contain psammona bodies.
   C. Calcifications are common.
   D. They may metastasize outside the nervous system.
   E. Tumors with loss of chromosomal arms 1 p and 19 q respond favorably to radiation and chemotherapy and have a longer survival.

10. Clinical features suggestive of pineal gland tumors are:
    A. Occurrences in the second and third decades of life
    B. Tendency to disseminate via CSF
    C. Hearing impairment
    D. Vertical gaze palsy
    E. Elevated α-fetoprotein in the serum

11. Features characteristic of meningeomas are:
    A. Fast growing, invasive tumors
    B. Slowly growing encapsulated tumors
    C. May develop after therapeutic radiation to the head
    D. Preponderance in males
    E. Commonly cystic

12. Characteristic features of germinomas include:
    A. They are usually situated in the pineal regions.
    B. They are radiosensitive.
    C. They have a tendency to disseminate via CSF.
    D. They are usually situated in the suprasellar region.
    E. None of these.

13. Neurofibromatosis type 1 is characterized by:
    A. Neurofibromas
    B. Optic nerve glioma
    C. Bilateral acoustic neurinoma
    D. Café-au-lait spots
    E. Autosomal recessive inheritance

14. Pituitary adenomas may present with all the following *except*:
    A. Amenorrhea
    B. Impotence
    C. Hemorrhage into the tumor
    D. Cortical blindness
    E. Visual field defect

15. Extracerebral manifestations associated with capillary hemangiomas in von Hippel-Lindau syndrome are:
    A. Retinal angiomatosis
    B. Cardiac rhabdomyoma
    C. Pheochromocytoma
    D. Secondary polycythemia
    E. Syringomyelia

16. All the following statements are correct concerning primary cerebral lymphomas *except*:

    A. They are often encountered in immunocompromized individuals.
    B. They are associated with the JC virus.
    C. Most tumors are large B-cell variant.
    D. They are poorly demarcated.
    E. They are often multifocal.

17. Commonly encountered tumors in the spinal cord are:

    A. Ependymoma
    B. Astrocytoma
    C. Ganglioglioma
    D. Teratoma
    E. Myxopapillary ependymoma

18. Neurologic diseases that are associated with carcinomas in the absence of metastases to the nervous system include:

    A. Eaton-Lambert syndrome
    B. Combined degeneration of the spinal cord
    C. Limbic encephalitis
    D. Subacute cerebellar degeneration
    E. Leigh disease

19. Cerebral lesions produced by X-radiation are:

    A. Cortical calcifications
    B. Caseaus necrosis of the white matter
    C. Sarcoma
    D. Coagulative necrosis of the white matter
    E. Vascular hyalinosis

20. Metastatic tumors are characterized as:

    A. Often multiple
    B. Grossly, fairly well circumscribed
    C. The most common CNS tumors
    D. All of these
    E. None of these

(Answers are provided in the Appendix.)

CHAPTER 12

Traumatic Injuries of the Central Nervous System

Blunt Head Injuries
Missile Head Injuries
Secondary Injuries
Clinical Presentation of Cerebral Injuries
Spinal Cord Injuries
Other Injuries

Head injuries are the major cause of death in young adults and account for one-third to one-half of traumatic deaths. An estimated 200 cases per 100,000 population occur annually, and the ratio of men to women is 2 : 1. About half of the survivors are left with variable degrees of neurologic disabilities. Often, no direct correlation can be made between the severity of a head injury and its outcome. An injury that appears mild or moderate may have a poor prognosis because of widespread damage to the axons that is only demonstrable histologically and because of complications from vascular or circulatory disorders and raised intracranial pressure (ICP). Genetic factors may also influence the outcome of a head injury.

Head injuries may be divided into primary and secondary. Primary injury relates directly to the trauma; secondary injury refers to the complications that may occur during the acute stage. Primary injuries are further divided into blunt, missile, and other.

BLUNT HEAD INJURIES

The major causes of blunt head injuries are motor-vehicle accidents, sports-related accidents, personal violence, physical abuse of children, blows to the head, and falls. The brain is injured either by direct contact injury to the head or by acceleration/deceleration movements of the head at the time of impact, causing motion of the brain within the skull. Sudden acceleration of the unsupported head usually results from a blow by a heavy object. Sudden deceleration of the moving head occurs in falls. These two mechanisms may act together (Table 12.1). Traumatic injury to the neurons is attributed, at least partly, to ionic fluxes. Damage to the cellular membrane at the time of injury allows an influx of sodium, chloride, water, and calcium into the neuronal

TABLE 12.1.

Mechanisms and Types of Cerebral Injuries

Contact Head Injury	*Acceleration/Deceleration Injury*
Epidural hematoma	Subdural hematoma
Intracerebral hematoma	Diffuse axonal injury
Contusion	Contusion
Laceration	Concussion

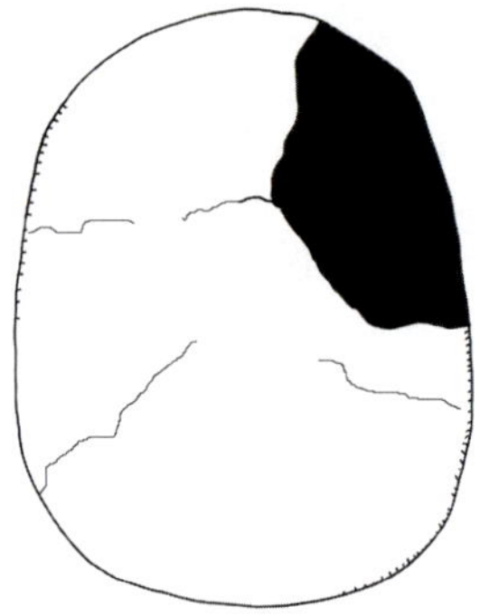

FIGURE 12.1
Epidural hematoma. Schematic drawing shows an epidural hematoma attached to the inner table of the calvarium.

compartment and an efflux of potassium into the extracellular compartment. These ionic exchanges, perpetuated by the release of excitatory neurotransmitters, disrupt neuronal functions and may even lead to neuronal disintegration.

The major types of blunt injuries are skull fractures, intracranial hemorrhages, and cerebral parenchymal injuries. These may occur singly or in combinations.

Skull Fractures

Skull fractures occur in several forms: linear, depressed, bursting, radiating, and circumferential. They predispose to several complications: infection, escape of cerebrospinal fluid (CSF) into the nasal cavity (rhinorrhea) and ear (otorrhea), entry of air into the subdural space, and cranial nerve injuries.

Intracranial Hemorrhages

Intracranial hemorrhages may occur in the epidural, subdural, and subarachnoid compartments and within the brain parenchyma.

Epidural hematoma (EDH) occurs in 2% of severe head injuries. An epidural hematoma forms between the inner table of the calvarium and the dura, usually in the frontotemporal region (Fig. 12.1). It is commonly an arterial bleed that results from tearing of meningeal arteries, often of the middle meningeal artery, by a linear fracture across its cranial groove. In children, it may occur without a skull fracture. Being an arterial bleed, it has a rapidly progressing course. Brain edema, increased ICP, and cerebral herniations rapidly develop. If the blood is not evacuated, mortality is 100%.

In *subdural hematoma* (SDH), the hematoma forms between the inner surface of the dura and the arachnoid, generally in the fronto-parietal regions, but it may cover the entire hemisphere. It results from tearing of the veins at the point where they enter the superior sagittal sinus (bridging veins). Here, unsupported by the brain parenchyma, they are prone to tearing by motions of the brain that occur in blows to the head, falls, and traffic accidents. SDH is a common finding in physically abused children (shaken baby syndrome). Importantly, it can result from minor injuries and, in about 20% of cases, no clinical evidence of injury exists. Alcoholism, hematologic disorders, anticoagulant therapy, ventricular shunting, and old age predispose to SDH.

It is customary to distinguish acute, subacute, and chronic stages of SDH (Figs. 12.2 and 12.3). In the acute stage, days 1 to 4, the blood is partially clotted. The associated brain edema produces herniations that pose a surgical emergency. In the subacute stage, days 5 to 14, the hematoma gradually liquefies. In the chronic stage, after the second week, encapsulation begins, with fibroblast and capillary proliferation along the inner surface of the dura and proceeding toward the center. Newly formed, fragile blood vessels are the source of rebleeding into the hematoma (see Fig. 12.3).

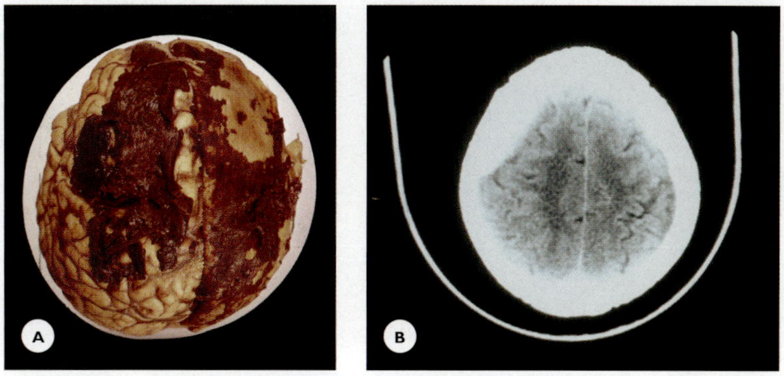

FIGURE 12.2

Acute subdural hematoma. A 50-year-old man became comatose 3 days after he was lightly hit on the head with a volleyball. He died 2 days later of a pontine hemorrhage (Düret hemorrhage) due to raised ICP. **A.** Clotted blood covers the undersurface of the left leaflet of the dura and lateral aspect of the cerebral hemisphere. **B.** Nonenhanced CT scan of the head from a different patient shows an acute subdural hematoma as a hyperdense, crescent-shaped lesion.

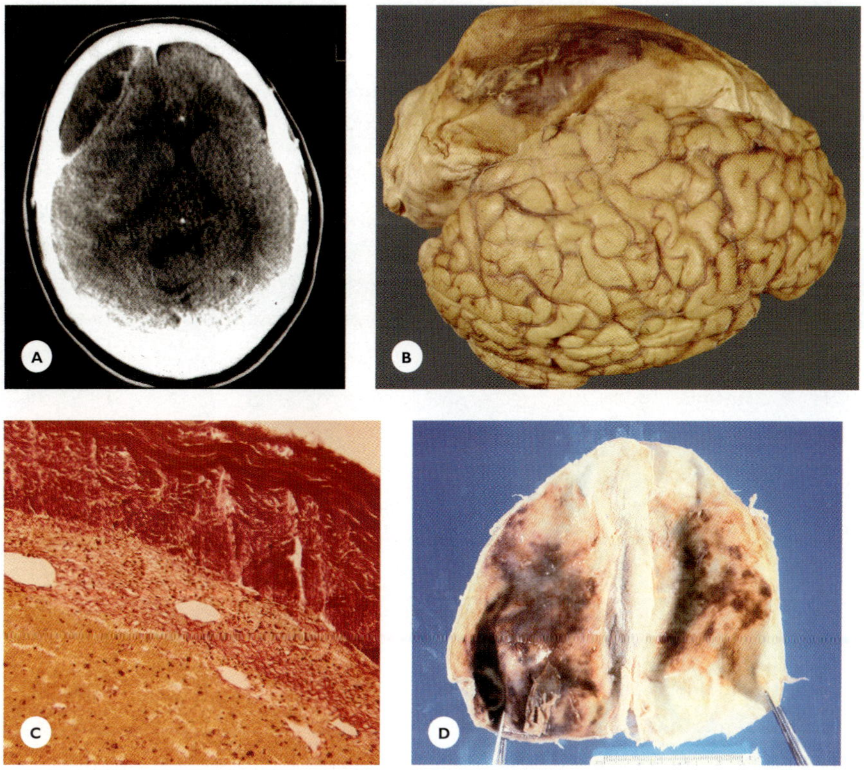

FIGURE 12.3A

Chronic subdural hematomas. **A.** Nonenhanced CT scan of a chronic hypodense subdural hematoma in a 63-year-old man who presented with headaches and had suffered a minor, forgotten head injury 6 weeks earlier. **B.** Chronic encapsulated hematoma in a 76-year-old alcoholic man. **C.** Granulation tissue of the capsule adheres to the inner surface of the dura (Van Gieson stain). **D.** Calcified subdural hematomas in a 58-year-old epileptic man.

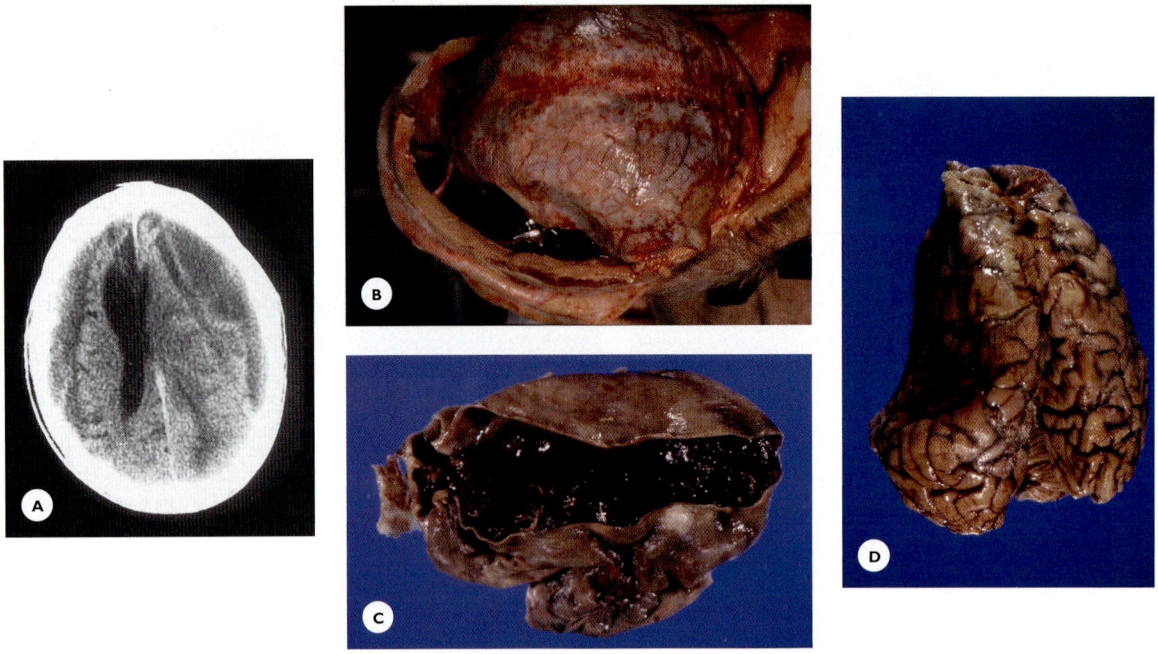

FIGURE 12.3B

Rebleeding within chronic subdural hematoma. **A.** Nonenhanced CT scan of the head of a 66-year-old severely demented man shows a small right and a large left chronic subdural hematoma with severe mass effect. **B.** Large amount of fresh blood has accumulated in the subdural space. **C.** The thick capsule of the left chronic hematoma contains fresh, partially clotted and liquefied blood. **D.** Marked deformation of the left hemisphere.

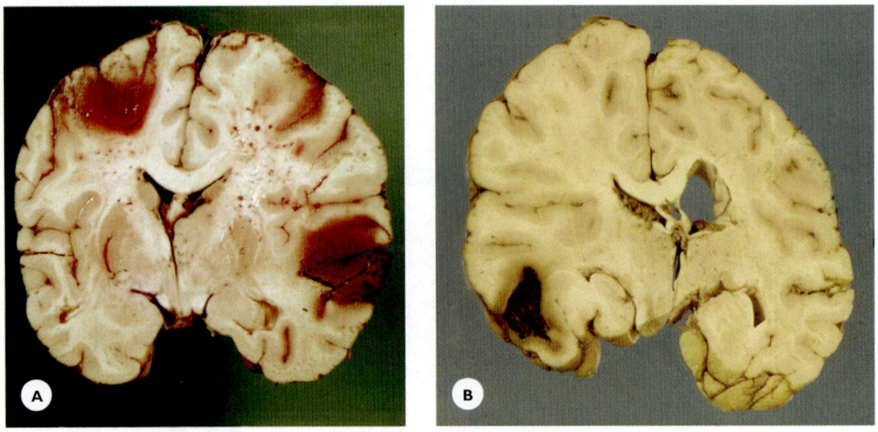

FIGURE 12.4

Parenchymal hemorrhages. **A.** Multiple hemorrhages. The right temporal hematoma is associated with contusion. **B.** Solitary temporal lobe hemorrhage. Note the extensive edema, ventricular compression, and the deep groove around the hippocampus indicating hippocampal herniation.

Subarachnoid hemorrhage (SAH) results from tearing of leptomeningeal blood vessels and *parenchymal hemorrhage (PH)* from shearing of the small or laceration of the large vessels by irregularities of the cranium. The hemorrhages, solitary or multiple, are often situated in the frontal or temporal lobes and may be continuous with a subdural hematoma (burst lobe) (Fig. 12.4).

Cerebral Parenchymal Injuries

Parenchymal injuries are focal, diffuse, or both. Focal injuries—contusion and laceration—generally result from contact head injuries. Diffuse injuries result from acceleration of the head.

Contusions are bruises in the crest of the convolutions, characteristically, in the frontal and temporal

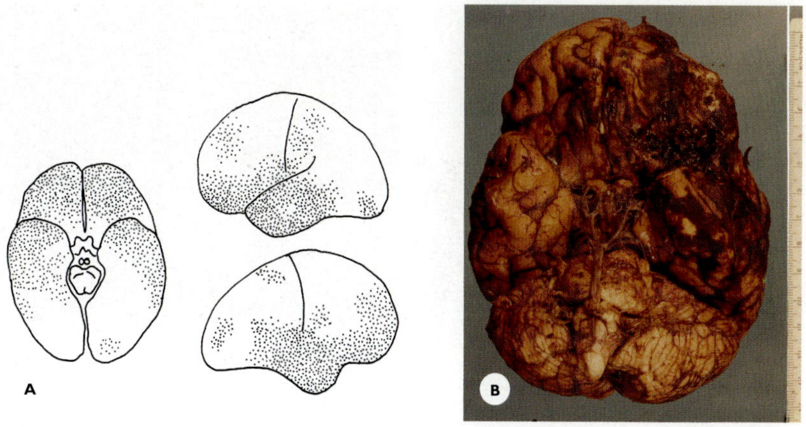

FIGURE 12.5
Acute contusion. **A.** Schematic drawing shows the sites of predilection of the contusions. **B.** Extensive subarachnoid hemorrhage and hemorrhagic necrosis of the frontoorbital and temporomesial cortex.

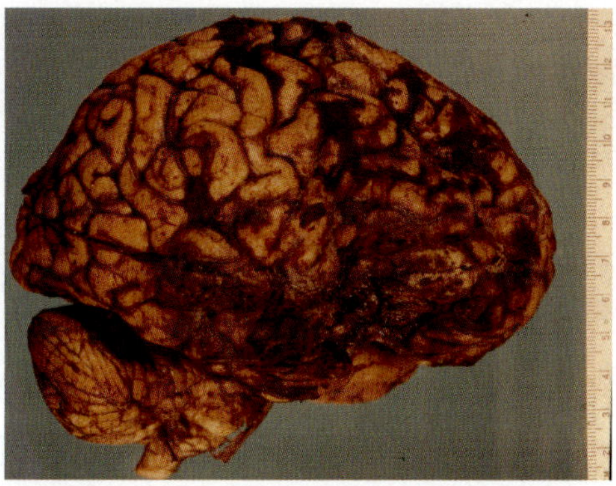

FIGURE 12.6
Acute contre-coup contusion. A 47-year-old epileptic woman fell during a seizure and sustained a fracture of the left temporal bone. Two days later, she died. Right side of the brain shows extensive frontal and temporal hemorrhagic necrosis and multifocal subarachnoid hemorrhages.

poles, orbital surfaces, and basal and lateral temporal regions. A stroke to a stationary head results in a "coup contusion" at the site of impact. When a moving head strikes a stationary object, the contusion is usually on the side opposite to the impact—a "contre-coup" contusion. Grossly, in acute contusions, the convolutions are hemorrhagic; in chronic contusions, they are yellow, depressed, soft, and necrotic. On cut section, the contusions are wedge-shaped cortical and subcortical defects with the apex toward the depth of the convolutions. The subcortical white matter is soft and, in severe cases, cavitated (Figs. 12.5 through 12.9). Histologically, the cortex in the crest of the convolutions is disrupted and partially missing. The margins of the defect contain fibrous astrocytes, macrophages, and hemosiderin pigments. The white matter is partially or completely demyelinated and, in severe cases, undergoes cystic necrosis that may extend deeply into the hemisphere.

Lacerations are tears in the dura, leptomeninges, and brain parenchyma caused by bony fragments or foreign bodies. Fracture dislocation of the base of the skull results in laceration of the brainstem and, in severe cases, pontomesencephalic or pontomedullary separations occur.

In *diffuse axonal injuries* (DAI), shearing of the axons results from movements of the brain during acceleration/deceleration of the head, as occurs in traffic accidents and falls and in shaken babies. The axonal disruption may continue even for a few hours after the accident.

In a few cases, the axonal injuries are grossly identified as minute hemorrhages in the dorsal aspect of the corpus callosum and fornices and the lateral aspect of the rostral brainstem. More often, however, they are discrete histologic findings diffusely distributed in the cerebral and cerebellar white matter and brainstem. They appear as eosinophilic and argyrophilic balls (blobs) of axoplasm extruded from the sheared ends of axons (Fig. 12.10). They can be identified a few hours after injury by using antibodies to amyloid precursor protein (APP), which accumulates in the disrupted axons (see Fig. 12.10). In the chronic stage, microglial clusters indicate the sites of axonal injuries.

DAIs are particularly important because they constitute the pathologic substrate of a broad spectrum of clinical symptoms that occur in the absence of a clinically or radiologically identifiable lesion.

Concussion is attributed to a transient biochemical dysfunction of the neurons that causes no structural alteration.

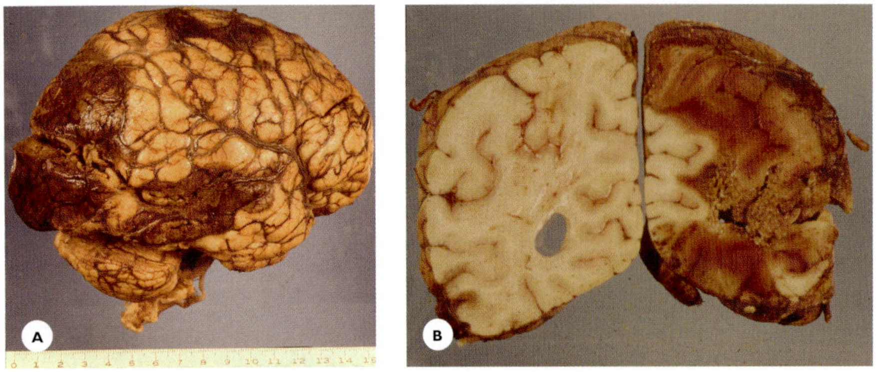

FIGURE 12.7
Subacute contusions. **A.** In lateral aspects of temporal and occipital lobes. **B.** Note the extensive necrosis and hemorrhagic discoloration of the hemispheric white matter.

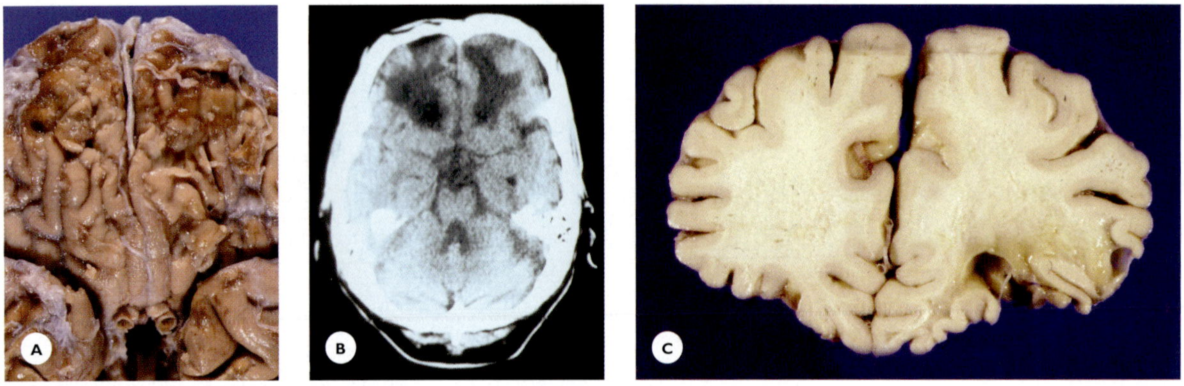

FIGURE 12.8
Chronic contusion. **A.** The fronto-orbital cortex is yellow, soft, and depressed. **B.** CT scan of orbital contusions in a different case. **C.** Transverse section shows wedge-shaped defects in fronto-orbital convolutions.

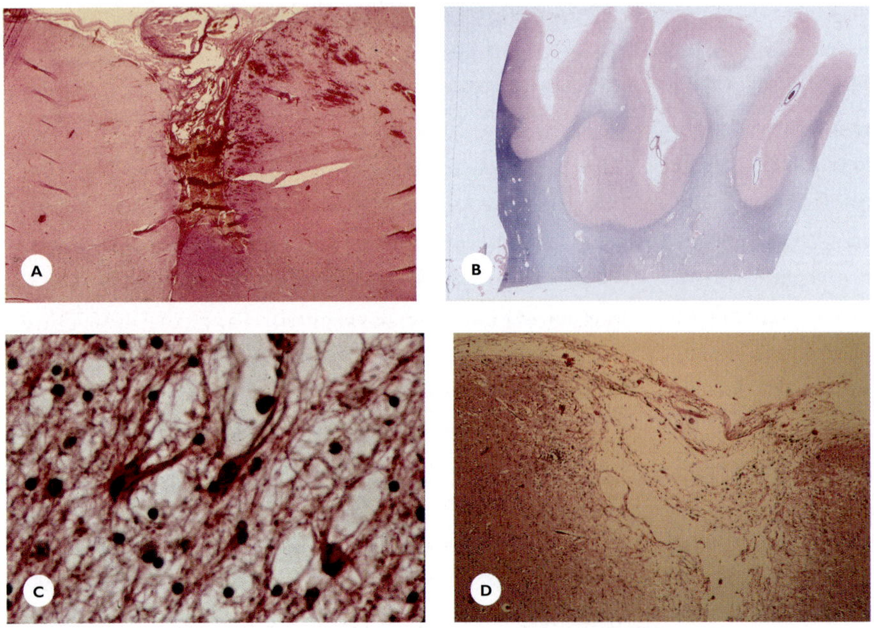

FIGURE 12.9
Histology of contusions. **A.** Acute contusion shows subarachnoid and cortical pericapillary hemorrhages. Pallor of staining of the adjacent convolution is likely from ischemic-hypoxic injury (HE). **B.** Chronic contusion shows disruption of the cortical ribbon in the crest of convolutions. The subcortical white matter is partially demyelinated (LFB-Eosin) and shows. **C.** large bizarre-shaped astrocytes (HE). **D.** Wedge-shaped cortical defect. The residual tissue and walls of the defect consist of a loose glial-mesodermal meshwork and collections of hemosiderin pigments (HE).

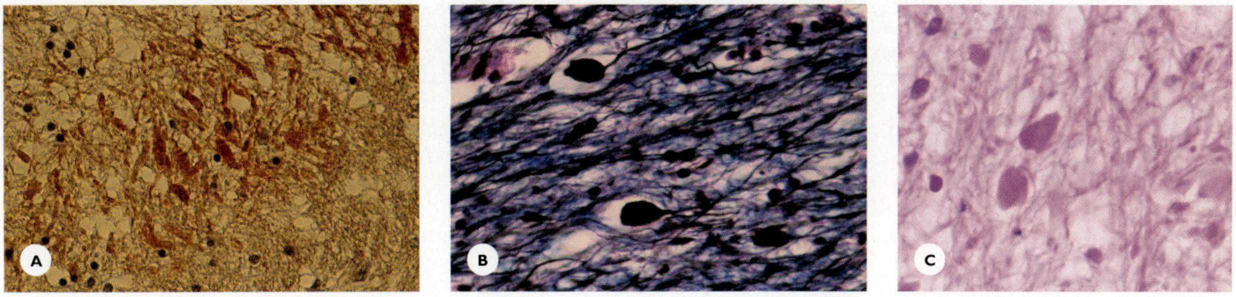

FIGURE 12.10

Shearing axonal injury. A 40-year old man survived 6 days following a head injury from a fall. Corpus callosum shows (**A**) injured axons staining positively for β-amyloid precursor protein (β-APP) (immunostain). Hemisphere white matter shows (**B**) axonal spheroids (Holmes stain). **C.** Axonal spheroids are present in medullary pyramids (HE).

TABLE 12.2.

Neuropathology of the Battered Child

Neuropathology of the Battered Child
Skull fracture
Subdural hematoma
Parenchymal hematoma
Cerebral contusion
Axonal shearing injury
Retinal hemorrhage

Injuries in Children

The types of injuries observed in battered children are summarized in Table 12.2.

MISSILE HEAD INJURIES

Missile injuries, caused by bullets and shrapnel, are either penetrating or perforating injuries (Fig. 12.11). In the former, the missile remains in the cranial cavity; in the latter, it traverses it. The exit wound is larger than the entrance wound. Both injuries carry a high risk of infection.

SECONDARY INJURIES

Acute cerebral injuries are apt to induce vascular/circulatory disorders and cerebral edema and are potential sources of infection.

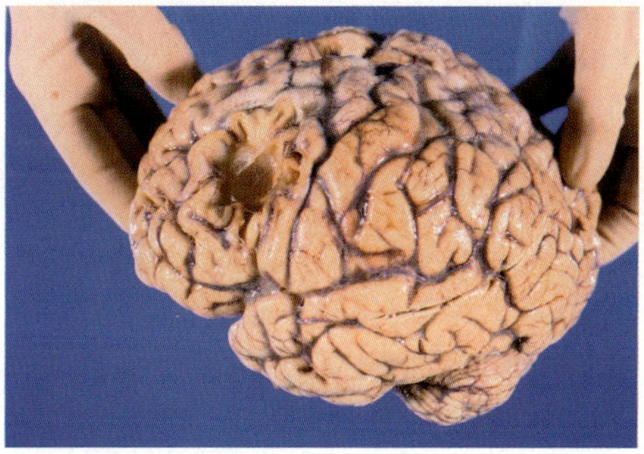

FIGURE 12.11

Shrapnel injury. A 68-year-old man had, at age 23, sustained shrapnel injury to his left forehead. The lateral aspect of the left frontal lobe contains a large, round cortical and white matter defect with irregular margins.

Vascular/Circulatory Disorders

Vasodilatation is due to impaired autoregulation. In *ischemic-hypoxic encephalopathy*, the lesions vary from discrete ischemic neuronal necrosis to multiple focal and laminar neuronal losses, preferentially in the hippocampus, cerebral cortex, basal ganglia, and cerebellar cortex. Less common ischemic complications are multiple focal or diffuse white matter degenerations.

Edema

Diffuse vasogenic edema results from an increased permeability of the capillary endothelium and an escape of protein and fluid into the white matter. An increase in brain volume and gradual rise of ICP decrease the cerebral perfusion pressure, leading to global ischemia and eventually to brain death.

Local edema, confined to a hematoma or a parenchymal lesion, when severe, presents a life-threatening situation. It leads to herniations and subsequent brainstem and medullary compression.

Infection at the site of a penetrating injury is a potential source of meningitis and abscesses.

CLINICAL PRESENTATION OF CEREBRAL INJURIES

The clinical presentation of head injuries depends on the type, location, and extent of the pathologic lesions and also on the presence of any secondary injury.

Acute Injury

Alterations of consciousness and neurologic deficits are the distinguishing clinical features of acute cerebral injuries. Concussion, the mildest injury, with no structural alteration, causes a loss of consciousness that usually lasts from seconds to a few minutes at most. Moderate and severe structural injuries cause a depression of consciousness ranging from drowsiness and obtundation to deep coma that may last from hours or days to months, even years.

The level of consciousness is determined using the Glasgow Coma Scale (GCS). The GCS assesses the patient's eye blinking and motor and verbal responses to stimuli. Scores of 15 to 13 indicate mild injuries, and scores below 8, severe injuries.

Among diagnostic tests, computed tomography (CT) scan is the method of choice to demonstrate hemorrhages. Acute epidural hematoma between the skull and the dura appears as an extra-axial hyperdense bioconvex lesion, whereas subdural hematoma between the dura and the cerebral cortex is crescent-shaped (see Fig. 12.2). Magnetic resonance imaging (MRI) demonstrates axonal injuries as tiny hemorrhages in the callosum and rostral brainstem. The determination of specific brain proteins (S-100 protein, neuron specific enolase [NSE], and glial fibrillary acidic protein [GFAP]) in the serum may provide prognostic information. High concentrations of these proteins suggest severe brain damage and poor outcome.

TABLE 12.3.
Sequelae of Traumatic Cerebral Injuries

Somatic complaints
Cranial nerve deficits
Seizures
Motor, sensory deficits
Language impairment
Normal-pressure hydrocephalus
Diabetes insipidus
Inappropriate antidiuretic hormone (ADH) secretion
Affective, behavioral changes
Personality changes
Cognitive decline
Dementia

Sequelae of Cerebral Injuries

An estimated 10% of head injuries are fatal. Infants and young children suffering from shaken baby syndrome have a high mortality rate, averaging 20% to 25%.

In survivors, the outcome varies widely from complete recovery to a prolonged coma or a persistent vegetative state. Between these extremes, a variety of neurologic and psychiatric symptoms may occur, some permanent and some reversible. Gradual recovery of consciousness is usually associated with amnesia and confusion of variable duration. *Retrograde amnesia* refers to memory loss for events that occurred before the trauma, and *anterograde amnesia* for events that occurred after awakening.

The major sequelae of moderate and severe cerebral injuries are seizures; normal-pressure hydrocephalus; variable neurologic deficits; hypothalamic–endocrine dysfunction; cognitive decline, ranging from memory impairment to dementia; and behavioral and affective changes (Table 12.3). Children present with learning disabilities and behavioral changes.

Concussion often is followed by headaches, dizziness, tinnitus, memory impairment, and fatigue. *Skull fractures* may injure cranial nerves 1, 3, 7, and 8.

SPINAL CORD INJURIES

The major causes of spinal cord injuries are fracture dislocation, subluxation from sudden flexion or hyperextension of the spinal column, and prolapsed intervertebral disc. These injuries occur in traffic and sports-related accidents, falls, and diving in shallow water. Penetrating injuries are caused by stabbing, gunshots, and missiles.

Compression, contusion, laceration, hemorrhage (hematomyelia), and complete transection from crush injury are major pathologic changes (Figs. 12.12 and 12.13). Extensive parenchymal necrosis, edema, hemorrhage, and axonal disruption with retraction balls characterize the acute stage of severe injuries. In the chronic stage, a mesoglial scar develops and wallerian degeneration takes place in the descending and ascending fiber tracts. In some cases, a cavity remains after the removal of tissue debris (posttraumatic syringomyelia). Schwann cell proliferation in the damaged nerve roots produces traumatic neurinomas.

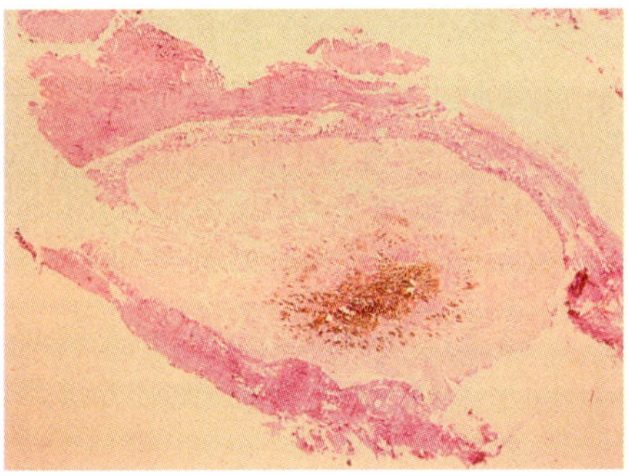

FIGURE 12.12
Transverse section of the spinal cord showing total necrosis and hemorrhages in a 27-year-old man involved in an automobile accident (HE).

The clinical course and outcome vary with the extent and anatomic level of the lesions. About 40% of patients with severe injuries die within 24 hours of the accident. Acute injuries cause a spinal shock with paralysis, anesthesia, and loss of reflexes below the level of the lesion, and loss of autonomic and sphincter functions. The spinal shock, gradually resolves, within 3 to 4 weeks. The return of functions depends on the extent of the lesions. Complete transection of the spinal cord results in loss of motor, sensory, and autonomic functions below the lesion. Incomplete transection produces various spinal cord syndromes, which often are not sharply defined. Minor injuries produce spinal cord concussion, in which the neurologic deficits resolve within minutes or hours.

OTHER INJURIES

Vascular Injuries

Vascular injuries, occurring alone or in conjunction with cerebral injuries, are arteriovenous fistula, dissection of carotid and vertebral arteries, arterial and venous thrombosis, and pseudoaneurysm. Carotid-cavernous fistula results from the laceration of the internal carotid artery within the cavernous sinus by skull fracture or penetrating missile. Dissection of the cervical arteries is caused by a fracture of the cervical spine or by spinal

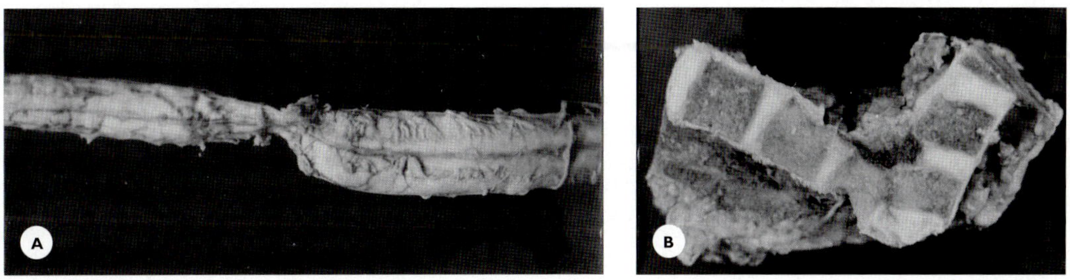

FIGURE 12.13
Crush injury (**A**) of the thoracic cord was caused by (**B**) fracture dislocation of the vertebrae due to neoplastic infiltration.

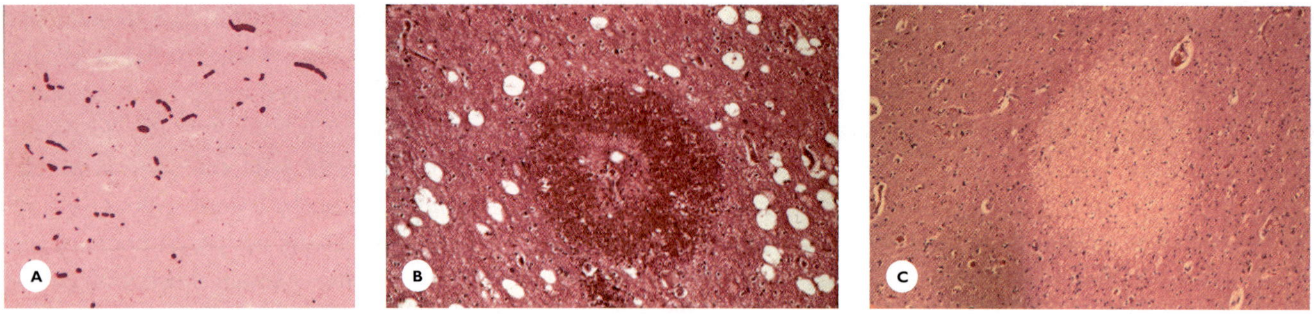

FIGURE 12.14
Fat embolization to the brain. A 77-year-old woman fell and fractured her femur. Within a few hours, she had lost consciousness and, 3 days later, she died. **A.** Fat emboli occlude distended capillaries in the cerebral hemispheric white matter (oil-red-O stain). **B.** Pericapillary ball hemorrhage and (**C**) microinfarct in the white matter (HE).

manipulative therapy. Hemorrhagic or thrombotic occlusion of the dissected artery carries the risk of cerebral infarction.

Pituitary necrosis and hemorrhage results from injury to the pituitary stalk.

In *subdural hygroma*, an accumulation of CSF in the subdural space results from tearing of the arachnoid.

Boxing Injuries

Dementia pugilistica (punch-drunk syndrome) develops in about 2% of boxers. Progressive dementia and parkinsonian syndrome characterize the clinical picture. Widespread neuronal losses, neurofibrillary tangles, and degeneration of the substantia nigra characterize the pathology.

Fat Embolization

The brain and lungs are common sites of fat embolization. The emboli originate from bone marrow fat that enters into the circulation through damaged blood vessels at the site of a long-bone injury. Occlusions of the small arteries and capillaries result in petechial hemorrhages and small perivascular infarctions, chiefly in the hemispheric white matter (Fig. 12.14).

Air and Gas Embolization

Air emboli to the brain and spinal cord may complicate cardiovascular, thoracic, abdominal, and pelvic surgeries; neurosurgical and radiologic procedures; labor; abortion; and subatmospheric decompression. The pathologic changes are small hemorrhages and infarctions in the gray and white matter. Nitrogen gas embolism in underwater divers and caisson workers usually affects the spinal cord.

Lightning and Electrical Injuries

A lightning strike can cause prolonged or permanent central nervous system injuries, including hemorrhages, often in the basal ganglia and brainstem; infarction; and post hypoxic-ischemic encephalopathy. Electrical trauma commonly causes peripheral nerve injuries.

Radiation Injuries

For a discussion of radiation injuries, see Chapter 11.

BIBLIOGRAPHY

Graham, D.I., Adams, J.H., Nicoll, J.A.R., et al. (1995). The nature, distribution and causes of traumatic brain injury. *Brain Pathol 5*, 397–406.

Graham, D.I., Maxwell, W.L., & Nicoll, J.A.R. (1997). Neurotrauma: axonal damage in short surviving head injury and the influence of Apolipoprotein E on outcome, *Brain Pathol 7*, 1285–1288.

Katayama, Y., Maeda, T., Koshinaga, M., et al. (1995). Role of excitatory amino acid-mediated ionic fluxes in traumatic brain injury *Brain Pathol 5*, 427–435.

McArthur, D. L., Hovda, D. A. (Eds). (2004). Symposium: traumatic brain injury. *Brain Pathol 14*, 183–222.

Vos, P.E., Lamers, K.J.B., Hendriks, J.C.M., et al. (2004). Glial and neuronal proteins in serum predict outcome after severe traumatic injury *Neurology 62*, 1303–1310.

REVIEW QUESTIONS

1. Concerning acute subdural hematomas, all of the following are correct *except*:
   A. They are caused by trauma, hematologic diseases or bleeding within metastases.
   B. They arise from tearing of bridging veins.
   C. They arise from tearing of middle meningeal arteries.
   D. They are commonly situated over the fronto-temporal and parietal regions.
   E. They are often bilateral.

2. An acute epidural hematoma carries the risk of:
   A. Cerebellar tonsillar herniation
   B. Brainstem hemorrhage
   C. Uncal hippocampal herniation
   D. All of these
   E. None of these

3. When the temple is struck with a heavy object, one can expect:
   A. A skull fracture at the site of impact
   B. A coup contusion
   C. A contre-coup contusion
   D. All of these
   E. None of these

4. The histopathology of cerebral contusion is characterized by:
   A. Loss of cortex in the crest of convolutions
   B. Sparing of the external cortical layer
   C. Wedge-shaped destruction of the cortex and white matter
   D. All of these
   E. None of these

5. Histologic changes that account for the persistent vegetative state that may occur following a severe head injury are:
   A. Multiple small infarcts
   B. Hypothalamic neuronal losses
   C. Axonal shearing injuries
   D. Cribriform state of the white matter
   E. Pontine basis hemorrhage

6. Boxing injuries may manifest with:
   A. Dementia
   B. Alzheimer fibrillary tangles
   C. Parkinsonism
   D. All of these
   E. None of these

7. Cerebral complications of long-bone fractures are:
   A. Fat emboli
   B. Petechial hemorrhages in the white matter
   C. Pericapillary infarcts
   D. All of these
   E. None of these

8. Being struck by lightning may cause:
   A. Cerebral hemorrhage in the basal ganglia
   B. Cerebral infarct
   C. Cerebral hemorrhage in the brain stem
   D. Ischemic encephalopathy
   E. None of these

(Answers are provided in the Appendix.)

CHAPTER 13

Congenital Malformations of the Central Nervous System

Neural Tube Defects: Dysraphic Disorders
Malformation of Prosencephalon: Holoprosencephaly
Malformations of Cerebral Hemispheres
Malformations of the Midline Structures and Ventricles
Malformations of the Cerebellum
Malformations of the Brainstem
Disorders of Brain Weight
Meningeal and Vascular Anomalies
Phakomatoses: Ectomesodermal Dysgenetic Syndromes
Congenital and Neonatal Hydrocephalus
Chromosomal Disorders

Congenital malformations of the central nervous system (CNS) constitute one-third of all congenital malformations and account for 75% of fetal deaths and 40% of deaths during the first year of life. Malformations have many causes: genetic mutations, chromosomal aberrations, maternal disease states, and maternal exposure to teratogens (Table 13.1). Some malformations are associated with hereditary metabolic diseases (Table 13.2). Genetic defects, chromosomal aberrations, and known teratogens are responsible for about 25% of malformations. The etiology of the rest remains unknown. Malformations of the CNS are often multiple, some are features of particular syndromes, and others are associated with malformations of various organ systems.

The development of the CNS depends on genetically regulated sequences of interdependent events: simplistically—induction, proliferation, differentiation, and migration. When these sequences are disrupted, certain events fail to occur or take an abnormal course: These result in malformations. The gestational age when a disruption occurs is critical in determining the pattern of a malformation; that is, different etiologies can produce the same kind of malformation by acting at the same gestational age (Table 13.3). The earlier the disruption, the more severe the malformation. A malformation may also occur secondarily as a result of a destructive process, commonly a hypoxic-ischemic insult or an infection. When these occur at a very early stage of development, they are not traceable, because the immature nervous tissue is not able to react and repair: Macrophage reaction does not occur until the second

TABLE 13.1.
Major Etiologies of CNS Malformations

Chromosomal alterations	Teratogenic drugs
Genetic mutations	Anticonvulsants
Maternal diseases	Warfarin
Infection	Retinoid
Viral	
Cytomegalovirus	Alcohol consumption
Varicella	Illicit substance abuse
Ionizing radiation	Cocaine
Metabolic diseases	Industrial chemical
Diabetes mellitus	Methylmercury
Phenylketonuria	

TABLE 13.2.
Malformations Associated with Hereditary Metabolic Diseases

Peroxisomal disorders
- Cortical dysplasia

Congenital disorder of glycosylation
- Pontocerebellar hypoplasia/atrophy

Nonketotic hyperglycinemia
- Agenesis of corpus callosum
- Cortical dysplasia
- Cerebellar hypoplasia

trimester, and astrocytic repair only begins during the second half of the gestational period. Thus, differentiation between primary and secondary malformation is difficult; still, it is important for genetic counseling because primary malformations carry the risk of recurrence.

Most fetuses with major malformations are stillborn or die during the neonatal period. Those who survive for some time are seriously incapacitated, ranging from unresponsiveness throughout their entire life to profound mental retardation, muteness, severe motor deficits, and seizures. Minor anomalies manifest with mental retardation, behavioral changes, motor disorders, and seizures.

The antenatal detection of major malformations is possible with maternal ultrasound examination. Chromosomal aberrations are diagnosed by the karyotyping of cultured amniocytes performed from 12 weeks' gestational age. DNA studies for the diagnosis of inherited diseases are carried out on chorionic villi from as early as 8 weeks gestational age. Magnetic resonance imaging (MRI) and computed tomography (CT) scan make the early postnatal diagnosis of a number of malformations possible.

TABLE 13.3.
Approximate Timing of Major Developmental Events

Major Events	*Gestational Age*
Development of neural plate	18 days
Development of neural tube	23 days
Closure of neural tube	23–26 days
Development of primary vesicles and cleavage of prosencephalon appears	4–8 weeks
Cerebellar primordium	4 weeks
Cerebellar development completed	24 weeks
Beginning of migration of neuroblasts	4 weeks
Completion of migration	20 weeks
Corpus callosum develops	12 weeks
Opening of foramen Magendie	12 weeks
Opening of foramina Luschka	16 weeks
Sylvian fissure appears	14 weeks
Rolandic and calcarine fissures appear	24–26 weeks
Secondary and tertiary sulci appear	7–9 months

NEURAL TUBE DEFECTS: DYSRAPHIC DISORDERS

The nervous system develops from the neural plate, a derivative of the ectodermal layer of the embryonic disc. The neural plate folds into the neural tube, which closes by the third gestational week (Fig. 13.1). The anterior part develops into the brain, and the posterior part develops into the spinal cord. Disorders of closure of the neural tube and its mesenchymal coverings—the future meninges, skull, and spinal column—constitute the group of neural tube defects (NTDs) or dysraphic disorders, the commonest malformations of the nervous system. The prevalence is estimated at 0.5 to 2 per 1,000 births. NTDs are associated with genetic risk factors, maternal diabetes mellitus, and the use of the anticonvulsants valproic acid and carbamazepine. The malformations may involve either the brain or the spinal cord, or both, with their coverings. Diagnosis, early in pregnancy, is possible using ultrasound and by determining the α-fetoprotein in the amniotic fluid or maternal serum. Elevated levels support the diagnosis.

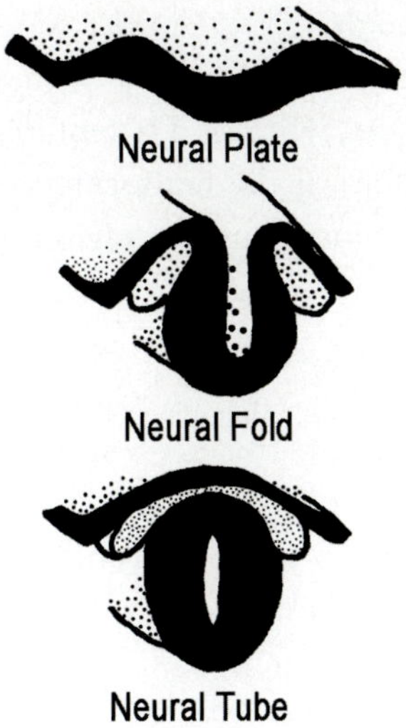

FIGURE 13.1
Schematic drawing of neural tube development.

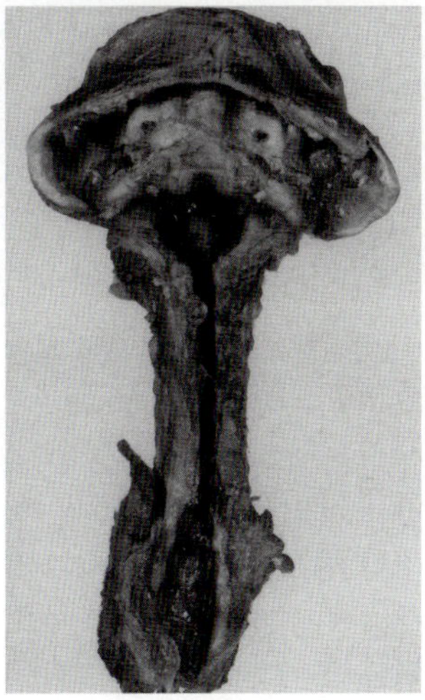

FIGURE 13.2
Anencephaly and amyelia in a stillborn fetus. Posterior view. The calvarium is partially absent. The skull base is covered with brown soft tissue (area cerebrovasculosa), the spinal canal is open, and the spinal cord is absent.

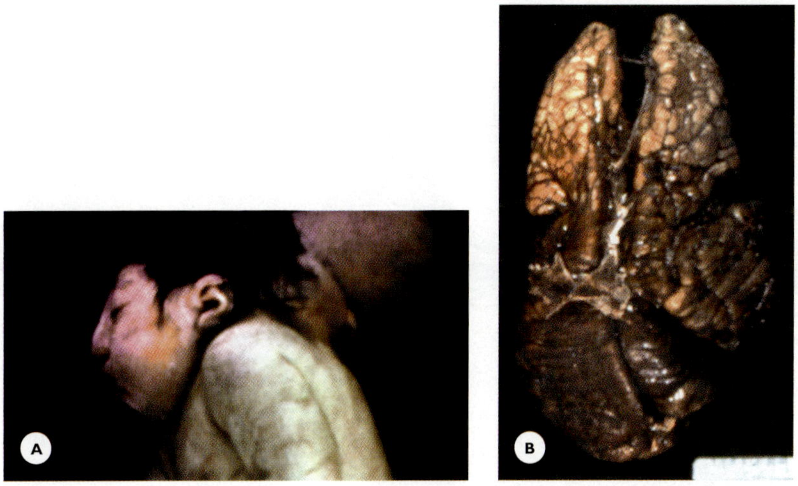

FIGURE 13.3
Occipital meningoencephalocele in a newborn. **A.** Lateral view of the head. The skin-covered encephalocele is almost as large as the head. **B.** A deep indentation on the dorsal aspects of the cerebral hemispheres is caused by the margin of the bony defect. The encephalocele contains the occipital lobes, portions of the brainstem, and the cerebellum.

Cranial and Cerebral Defects

Anencephaly, an extreme form of a dysraphic state, often leads to spontaneous abortion. The cranial vault is absent. The brain is absent or rudimentary; instead, a friable red mass of tissue contains thin-walled vascular channels and neural elements (area cerebrovasculosa) (Fig. 13.2). The anencephaly is associated with total or partial absence of the spinal cord, facial anomalies, and malformations of the visceral organs. *Meningoencephalocele* consists of the protrusion of the meninges and portion of the brain through a congenital defect in the skull, commonly in the occiput. The protruded portion may include the occipital lobes, cerebellum, and portion of the brainstem (Fig. 13.3). Less common sites are the parietal and frontal regions and the cranial base.

Chiari Malformations

Chiari type 1 and Arnold-Chiari type 2 malformations are covered under congenital hydrocephalus in a later section.

Chiari type 3 malformation consists of herniation of the cerebellar hemispheres through a craniovertebral defect into an occipitocervical encephalocele.

Spinal and Spinal Cord Defects

Dysraphic disorders of the spine and spinal cord comprise a broad spectrum of malformations, ranging from total absence of the cord to asymptomatic bony defects and cord anomalies. Familial occurrences are common. The clinical manifestations vary from mild motor and sensory deficits to paraplegia with severe sensory impairment and loss of sphincter control.

Amyelia, total absence of the spinal cord occurs with anencephaly (see Fig. 13.2). The cord is replaced with a mixture of fibrous tissue, blood vessels, and neural elements (area myelovasculosa).

Meningocele and *meningomyelocele* consist of herniations of the meninges or meninges, spinal cord, and nerve roots through a defect in the vertebral arch. The herniated structures are covered with a thin skin or vascular membrane, which is a potential source of infection. Common sites of the malformations are the lumbosacral and the thoracolumbar regions (Fig. 13.4). The myelocele may be associated with neuroenteric or enterogenous cysts, epidermoid cysts, and teratomas.

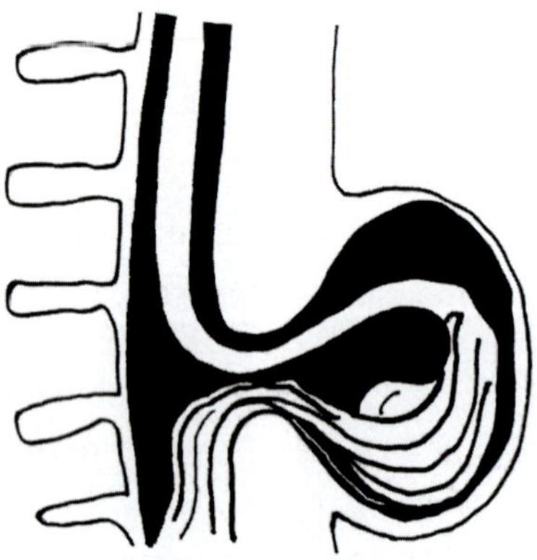

FIGURE 13.4
Schematic drawing of a lumbar meningomyelocele. The cystic sac covered with skin contains the spinal cord, meninges, and nerve roots.

In *tethered spinal cord*, the conus is fixed to a bony defect by a fibrous band that prevents the normal upward movement of the cord.

Spina bifida occulta is the mildest dysraphic disorder; the vertebral arches are absent or unfused, but the spinal cord and meninges are normal. The skin overlying the bony defect is usually pigmented and hairy. Fatty tissue may be present under the skin or in the extra- or intradural spaces.

Diastematomyelia refers to two half cords, separated by a bony spur or a fibrous septum extending from the vertebrae into the spinal canal. The lumbosacral segments are the usual sites. The ventral horns of the hemicords face each other, and each half has ventral and dorsal horns and roots. They may be contained within two separate or a single dural sac (Fig. 13.5).

Diplomyelia refers to two whole spinal cords within a single dural sac (Fig. 13.6).

Hydromyelia results from dilatation of the central canal, usually in the lumbosacral segments. It may be associated with other dysraphic disorders (Fig. 13.7).

Syringomyelia is a tubelike cavity (syrinx) extending over several segments of the cervicothoracic cord. On transverse sections, the cavity extends from one dorsal horn to the opposite dorsal horn, crossing the midline in the anterior commissure (Fig. 13.8). It contains xanthochromic fluid that gradually expands the cavity and compresses the surrounding structures. Often

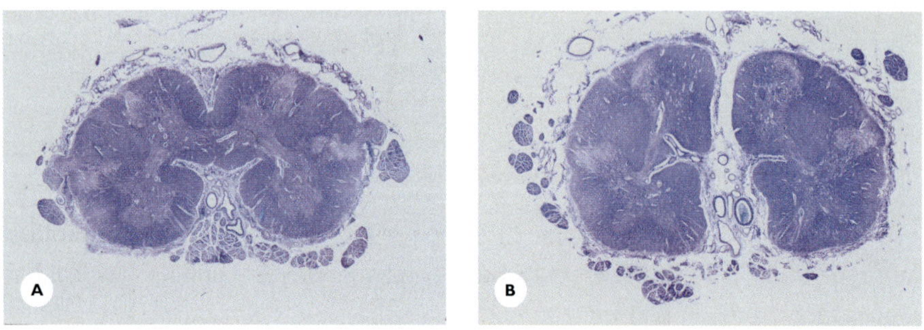

FIGURE 13.5
Diastematomyelia. **A** and **B**. The sacral cord splits gradually into two hemicords, the ventral horns facing each other (LFB-CV). The hemicords, separated by a fibrous band, share a common dural sac.

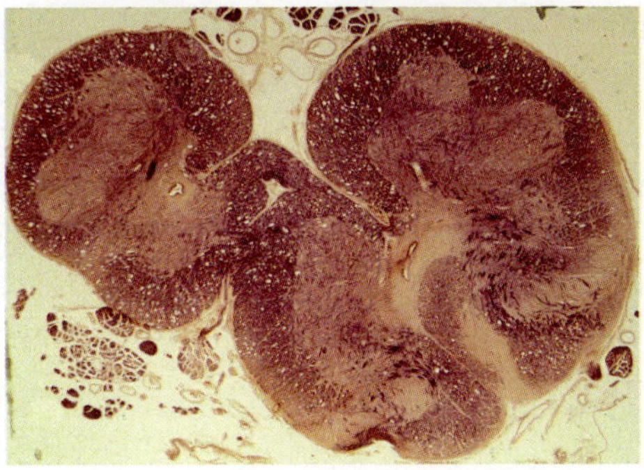

FIGURE 13.6
Diplomyelia. The cord is split into two cords. Each cord has a central canal, two ventral and two dorsal horns (Weil stain).

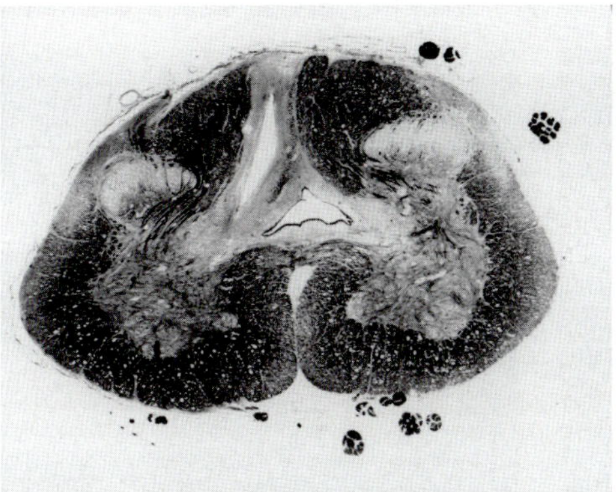

FIGURE 13.7
Hydromyelia in a 4-year-old girl with partial cerebellar agenesis. Transverse section of the lumbar cord shows an enlarged central canal. A small slit is present in the posterior column (Weil stain).

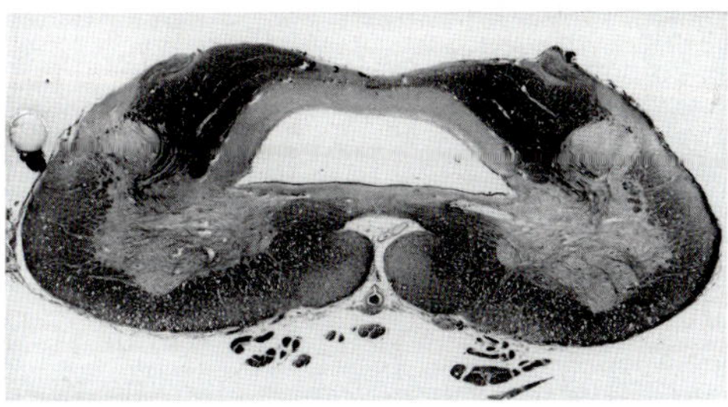

FIGURE 13.8
Syringomyelia. The cavity merges with the central canal and extends across the spinal cord. It is lined with gliotic tissue (Weil stain).

it merges with the central canal. Syringomyelia may coexist with gliomas and vascular tumors, Arnold-Chiari malformation, and kyphoscoliosis.

Syringomyelia is defined by a dissociated sensory impairment, such as loss of pain and temperature sensations with the preservation of vibratory, positional, and touch sensations in the upper extremities in a segmental distribution. As the disease progresses, the sensory deficits are associated with weakness and atrophy of the muscles and diminished or absent tendon reflexes in the corresponding segments. Later in the course, spasticity, weakness, and sensory ataxia develop in the lower extremities due to pressure on the corticospinal tracts and posterior columns. Charcot joints may also occur.

A *neurenteric (enterogenic) cyst*, intraspinal and extramedullary in the cervicothoracic region, is lined with epithelial cells resembling the gastrointestinal mucosa.

MALFORMATION OF THE PROSENCEPHALON: HOLOPROSENCEPHALY

Following the closure of the neural tube, the next major event is the formation of the three primary vesicles of the brain: the prosencephalon or forebrain, the mesencephalon or midbrain, and the rhombencephalon or hindbrain. The prosencephalon cleaves into the two telencephalic vesicles, which then develop into the two cerebral hemispheres and the two lateral ventricles (Fig. 13.9). A failure of this cleavage results in holoprosencephaly—a cerebrum that is undivided into hemispheres and has a single ventricular cavity.

Clinical features: Holoprosencephaly is associated with a broad spectrum of craniofacial anomalies, including microcephaly, hypo or hypertelorism, flat nose, harelip, and cleft palate, and ocular anomalies ranging from cyclopia to microphthalmia (Fig. 13.10). The malformation occurs sporadically or is inherited in an autosomal dominant, autosomal recessive, or X-linked fashion. Some cases are associated with chromosomal aberrations such as trisomy 13 and 18 and triploidy. Among environmental factors, maternal diabetes mellitus, infection, irradiation, and excessive alcohol

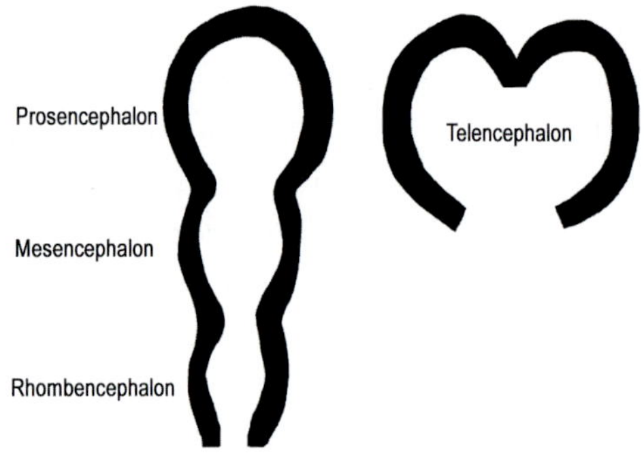

FIGURE 13.9
Schematic drawing of primary cerebral vesicles and cleavage of the prosencephalon.

consumption have been associated with holoprosencephaly. Most infants are stillborn or die in early infancy. Those who survive a few years suffer profound psychomotor retardation, intractable seizures, apneic episodes, temperature irregularities, and diabetes insipidus. Antenatal diagnosis is possible using ultrasonography.

Pathology: Grossly, holoprosencephaly may present under three forms:

- The *alobar* form has no evidence of midline separation (see Fig. 13.10). The small brain displays a markedly simplified convolutional pattern, with broad and abnormally oriented convolutions. The olfactory bulbs and tracts are absent (arhinencephaly). Transverse sections reveal a single large ventricle, severely

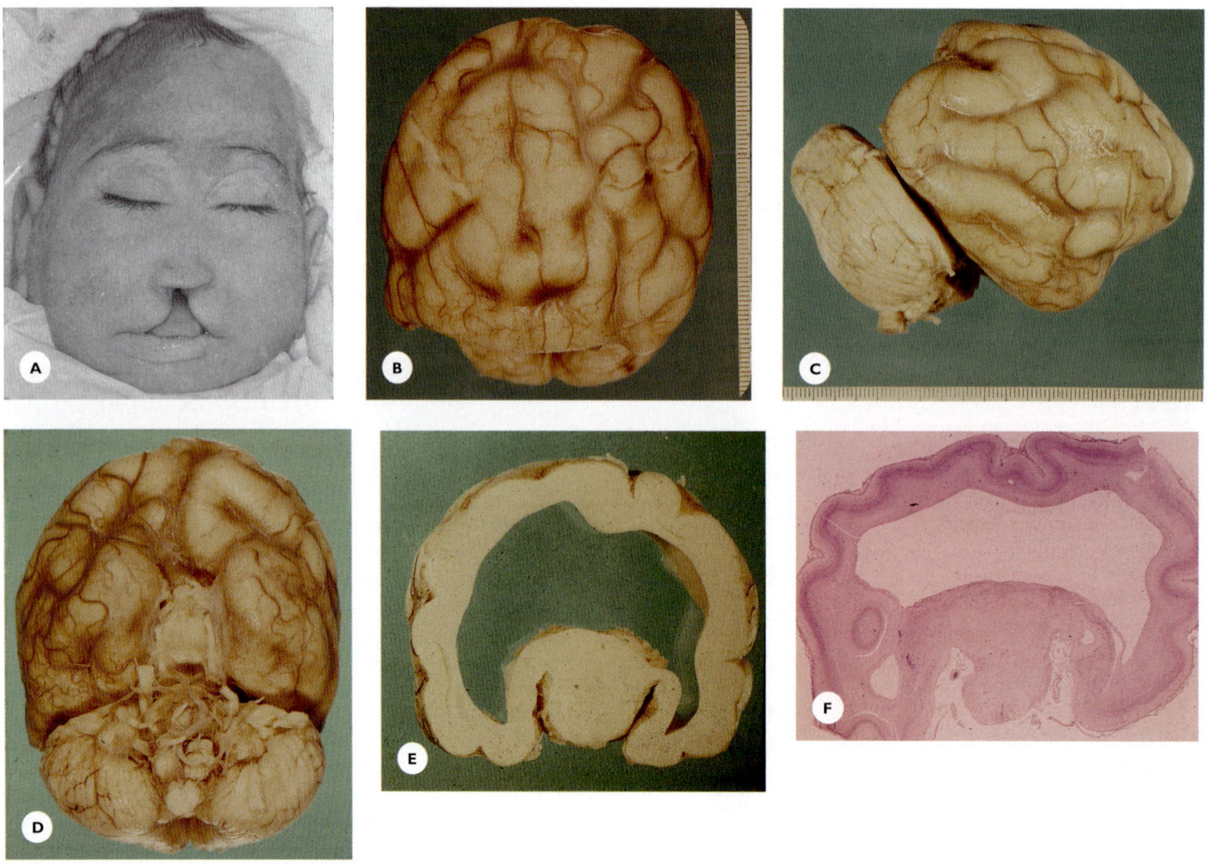

FIGURE 13.10
Holoprosencephaly in a 3-month-old boy. **A.** The head is small and the nose depressed. He has hare lip and cleft palate. Dorsal (**B**), lateral (**C**), and basal (**D**) views display a small alobar brain, undivided into hemispheres. The convolutional pattern is greatly simplified; the convolutions are broad and abnormally oriented. The olfactory bulbs and tracts are absent. **E.** Transverse section reveals a single ventricle. **F.** The cortex displays a four-layer lamination.

reduced white matter, and fusions of the thalami and basal ganglia.

- The *semilobar* form presents partial midline separation and rudimentary lobes.
- The *lobar* form consists of two hemispheres but only a single ventricle.

Histologically, the hippocampus and the pyriform cortex are present and, with the rest of the cerebral cortex, show cytoarchitectonic anomalies. Variable cytoarchitectonic anomalies are also present in the subcortical gray structures, brainstem, and cerebellum.

MALFORMATIONS OF THE CEREBRAL HEMISPHERES

The development of the cerebral hemispheres requires an orderly succession of events beginning with proliferation and differentiation of the periventricular germinal cells into neuroblasts and glial precursors. Then, the neuroblasts and the glial precursors migrate to the cortical plate, laying down the ground for the walls and gray structures of the future hemispheres. Once the neuroblasts, guided by the radiation glia, reach the cortical plate in an inside-to-outside sequence, they grow, mature into neurons, organize into laminae, and eventually establish synaptic connections. Excess neurons are destined to die by the process of apoptosis (programmed cell death). Interference with proliferation, migration, and laminar organization of the neurons results in a broad spectrum of malformations involving (a) the cerebral mantle—that is, the hemispheric wall, and (b) the convolutions and cortical cytoarchitecture.

Malformations of the Cerebral Mantle (Hemispheric Wall)

Schizencephaly or Porencephaly

Both terms denote a *defect* (cavity) in the cerebral wall, but according to one concept they differ regarding the underlying mechanisms. *Schizencephaly* specifically refers to a failure of development due to a defect in the germinal matrix or a failure in the migration of neuroblasts. Mutation in homeobox gene *EMX2* has been reported in familial cases.

Conversely, *porencephaly* specifically refers to a destructive–encephaloclastic cause, probably a vascular insult early during the first half of gestation. Current concept favors a vascular origin for cerebral mantle defects, and the term porencephaly is commonly used.

Pathology: In schizencephaly the defects vary greatly in extent (Fig. 13.11). They may be narrow clefts along the Sylvian fissure or may involve a greater portion of the lateral wall of one or both hemispheres. Large cavities connect the ventricle with the subarachnoid space. In an extreme form, the defects symmetrically involve the lateral and medial walls of both hemispheres (doughnut brain). The leptomeninges over the defects are usually torn, so the ventricles communicate with the subdural space. The convolutions in the walls of the defects are oriented radially and display a polymicrogyric pattern.

Hydranencephaly

In this extreme form of cerebral wall defect, both cerebral hemispheres are transformed into two thin-walled membranous cysts lacking any recognizable gyral pattern (Figs. 13.12 and 13.13). The temporo-basal, occipital, and the orbital regions may be partially present. Histologically, the fibrotic wall of the cyst is lined with glioneuronal tissue: Some areas contain cortical remnants with neurons, glial cells and calcifications. The ependymal layer usually is disrupted, and the deep gray structures may show minor anomalies. Hydranencephaly most likely results from a hypoxic-ischemic insult, but an association with fetal infection, twinning, and maternal gas poisoning have also been suggested.

Malformations of the Convolutions and Cortical Cytoarchitecture

Fissures, sulci, and convolutions appear on the cortical surface in an orderly sequence according to a strict timetable. Up to 12 to 13 weeks' gestation, the cortical surface is smooth. By the 14th week, a shallow indentation appears at the site of the future Sylvian fissure. Secondary and tertiary sulci appear at 7 to 9 months' gestation (Fig. 13.14).

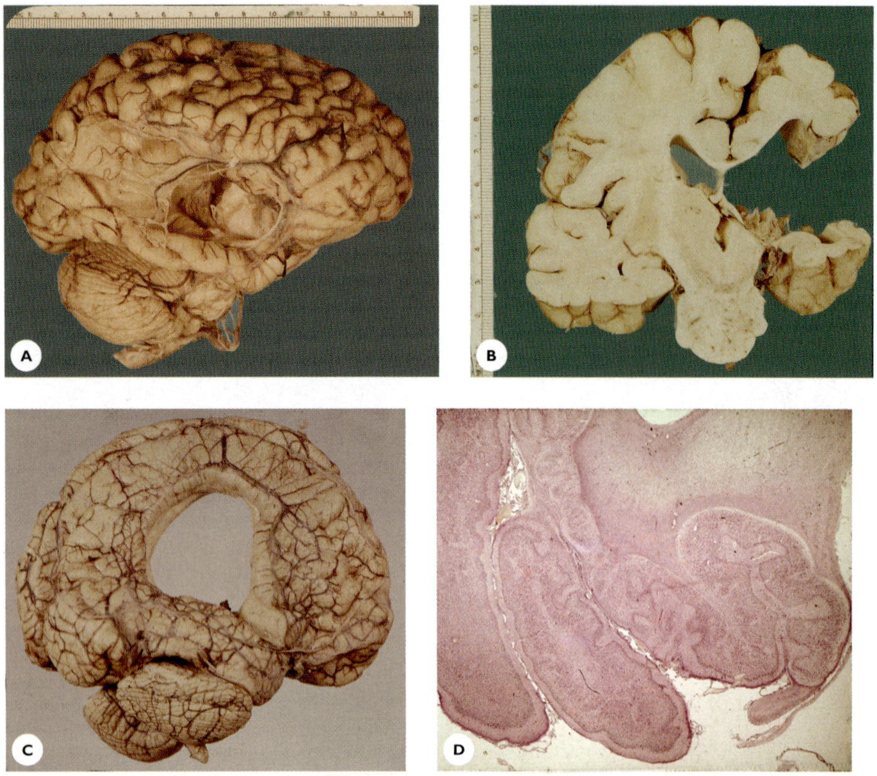

FIGURE 13.11
Schizencephaly or porencephaly. **A** and **B.** A large oval-shaped defect along the Sylvian fissure extends through the entire width of the cerebral wall. The lateral ventricle communicates with the subarachnoid space. **C.** A 5-year-old epileptic, quadriplegic, mentally retarded boy. Symmetrically situated large defects involve the medial and lateral walls of both hemispheres (doughnut brain). **D.** The cortical lamination is abnormal in the lips of the defect.

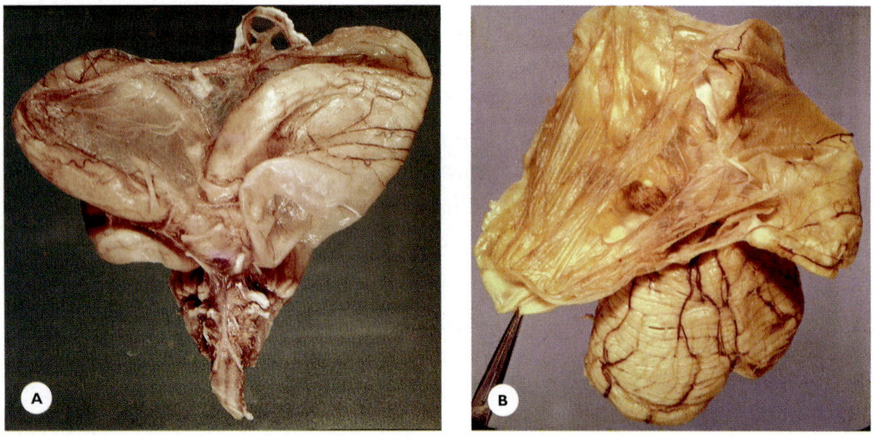

FIGURE 13.12
Hydranencephaly in a 3-year-old, blind, quadriplegic, profoundly retarded epileptic boy. Basal (**A**) and dorsal (**B**) views of the brain; the cerebral hemispheres are transformed into smooth-walled cysts, only the temporobasal lobes have some rudimentary convolution.

Cortical Dysplasia

Cortical dysplasia denotes a large scale of malformations due to disorders of neuronal migration and organization. Seizures, often intractable, mental retardation, and motor deficits of variable severity are common clinical manifestations. Known etiologies are chromosomal aberrations, single gene mutations, hypoxic-ischemic insults, maternal infection with cytomegalovirus, maternal methylmercury poisoning, anticoagulant therapy, and inherited metabolic diseases caused by peroxisomal disorders, such as Zellweger syndrome and neonatal adrenoleukodystrophy. MRI readily demonstrates the convolutional anomalies.

Lissencephaly Type 1 or Agyria

Grossly, the cortical surface is smooth, with no signs of fissures and sulci (Fig. 13.15). Histologically, a thick cortex is densely packed with immature neurons that display a large vesicular nucleus and scanty or no cyto-

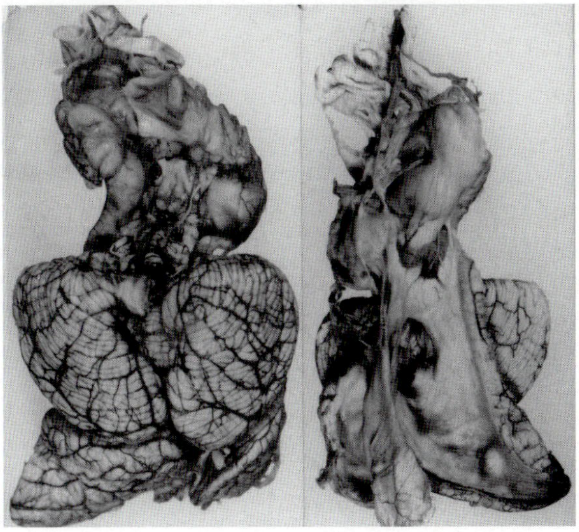

FIGURE 13.13
Hydranencephaly in a 3-year-old, quadriplegic, epileptic girl. **A.** Ventral aspect of the brain shows rudimentary orbital, hippocampal, and occipital convolutions. The rest of the cerebral wall is absent. A paper-thin membrane attached to the dura roofed the interior of the brain.

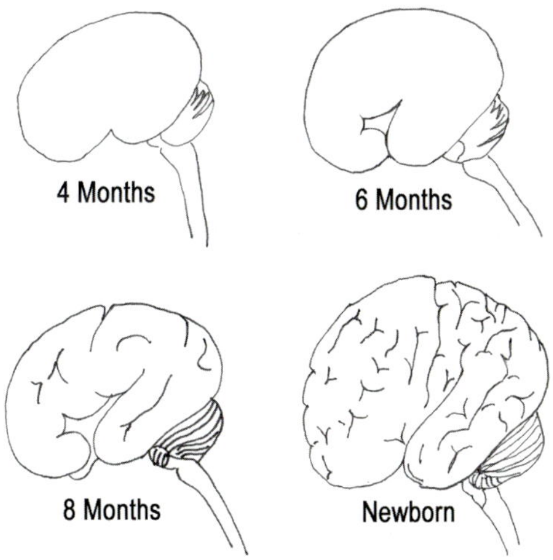

FIGURE 13.14
Schematic drawing of sequences of development of fissures, sulci, and convolutions.

plasm. Various patterns of cortical dysplasias may occur in the same brain.

Lissencephaly type 1 occurs sporadically or is inherited as an autosomal dominant, autosomal recessive, or X-linked trait. Mutations in four different genes have been identified: *LIS1* on chromosome 17; *XLIS* on chromosome X 22.3–23, associated with male occurrence; *RELN*, associated with recessive inheritance and cerebellar hypoplasia; and *ARX* on chromosome X.

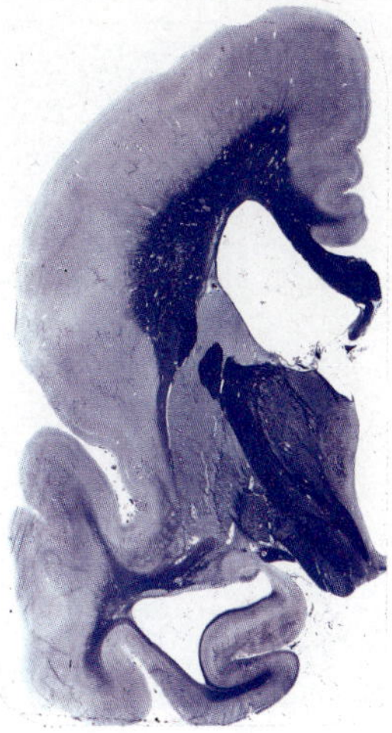

FIGURE 13.15
Lissencephaly. The lateral aspect of the hemisphere is smooth. A shallow Sylvian fissure is present. The temporal sulci are shallow, and the convolutions broad. The cortex is abnormally thick, the white matter is reduced, and the ventricle is enlarged (LFB-CV).

Lissencephaly Type 2

An autosomal recessive disorder, often coexists with cerebellar dysplasia, ocular anomalies, and congenital muscular dystrophy.

Grossly, the cortical surface is uneven (cobblestone) and histologically, the cortical lamination is greatly disorganized. Myelin tracts are intermixed with neurons, which can also be found in the leptomeninges.

Lissencephaly type 2 is a feature of Fukuyama congenital muscular dystrophy (FCMD), Finnish muscle-eye-brain (MEB) disease, and the Walker-Warburg syndrome (WWS) of oculocerebral dysplasia. The FCMD gene, fukutin, maps to chromosome 9; the MEB disease gene maps to chromosome 1p32; and the WWS gene maps to chromosome 9q34.

Macrogyria

The brain has a greatly simplified convolutional pattern with broad, abnormally oriented convolutions (Fig. 13.16).

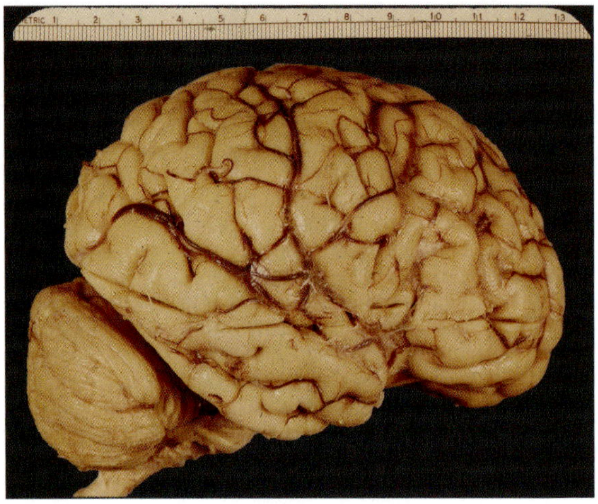

FIGURE 13.16
Macrogyria. Lateral aspect of the hemisphere displays broad convolutions separated by shallow sulci.

Polymicrogyria

Refers to numerous small convolutions, abnormally oriented and separated by shallow sulci (Fig. 13.17). The extent varies from circumscribed areas to total involvement of one or both hemispheres. On cut sections, miniature convolutions are partially fused. The white matter is significantly reduced, and the ventricles are enlarged (colpocephaly). The histologic picture varies from lack of lamination to a four-layered cortex displaying wavy, glandular, or multifoliated patterns (see Fig. 13.17). Familial cases of polymicrogyria have an autosomal dominant, autosomal recessive, or X-linked inheritance. The malformation can be associated with maternal cytomegalovirus infection, Zellweger cerebrohepatic disease, blood loss, and loss of a twin. Polymicrogyria and macrogyria may occur in the same brain (Fig. 13.18).

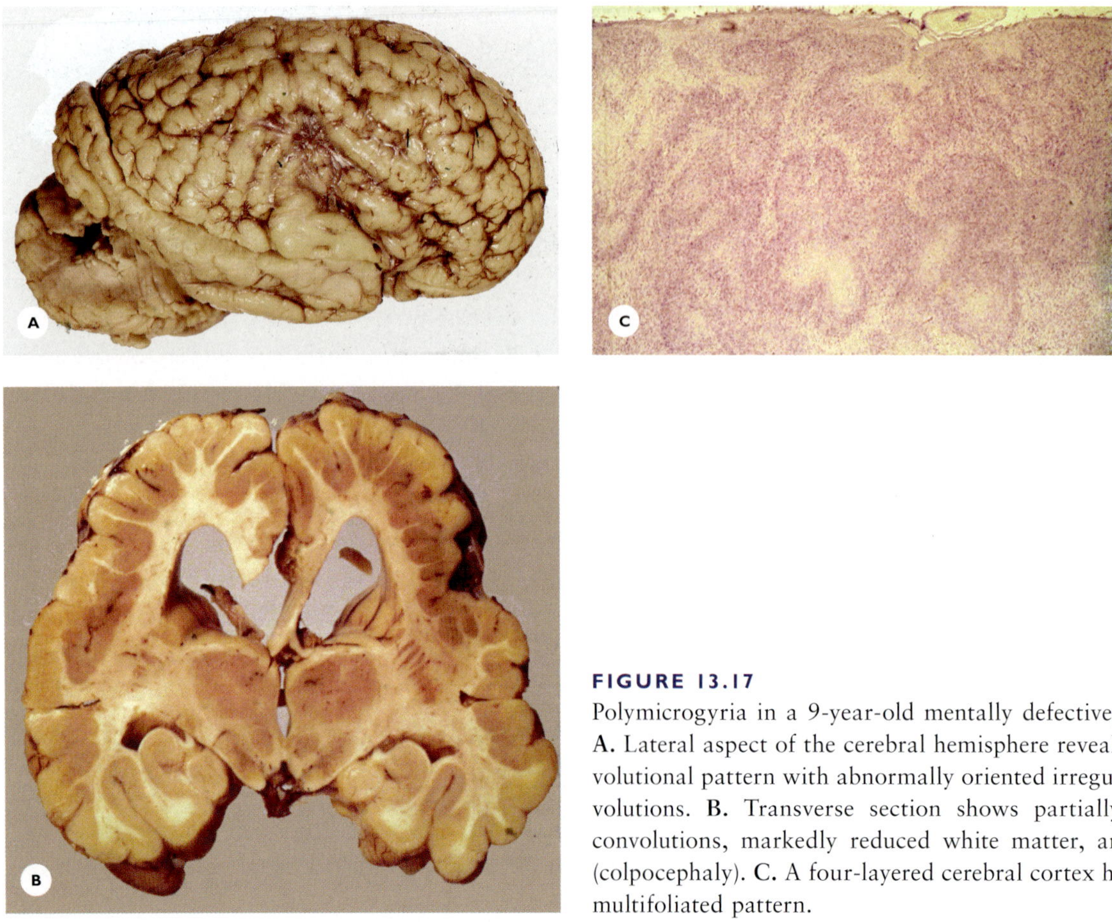

FIGURE 13.17
Polymicrogyria in a 9-year-old mentally defective, quadriplegic girl. **A.** Lateral aspect of the cerebral hemisphere reveals a simplified convolutional pattern with abnormally oriented irregular, embossed convolutions. **B.** Transverse section shows partially fused miniature convolutions, markedly reduced white matter, and large ventricles (colpocephaly). **C.** A four-layered cerebral cortex has a glandular and multifoliated pattern.

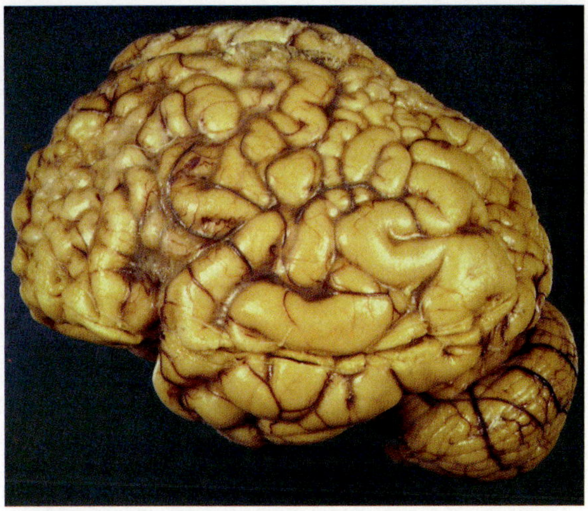

FIGURE 13.18
Polymicrogyria and macrogyria in the same brain.

Intracortical Dysplasia

Grossly, the cortex may be focally thick and poorly demarcated from the white matter. Histologically, the cytoarchitecture is disrupted by abnormal neurons and glial cells haphazardly arranged.

Neuronal Anomalies

Cytomegaly denotes a large neuron with abnormally rich dendritic arborization and argyrophilic tangles. A *balloon cell* has a large eosinophilic cytoplasm that stains positively with both neuronal and glial markers.

Heterotopia

Heterotopia are groups of neurons displaced in the cerebral hemispheric white matter (Fig. 13.19). Common sites are the periventricular zones, centum semiovale, and the subcortical white matter. Rarely, tiny groups of neurons form nodules on the cortical surface (brain warts). Neuroglial nests may also occur in the leptomeninges.

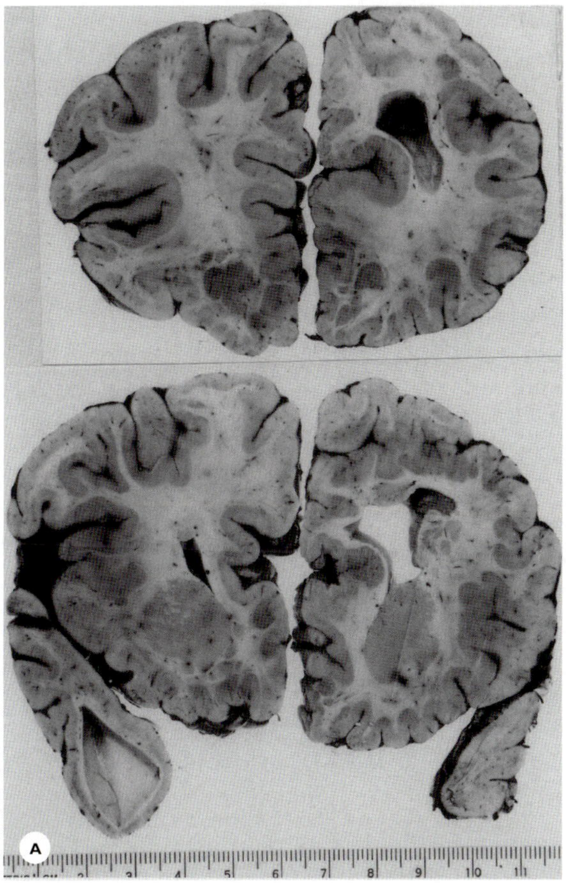

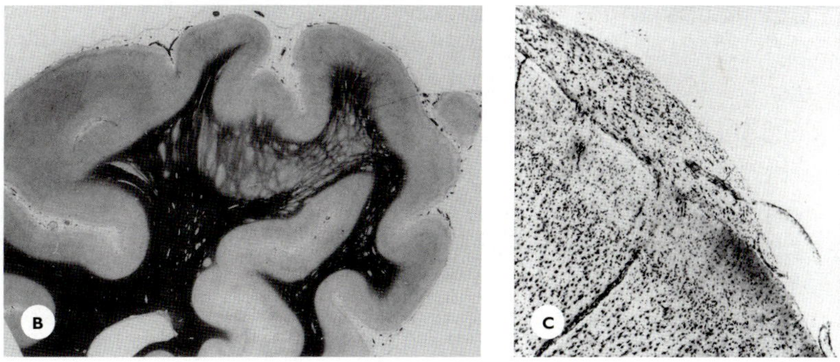

FIGURE 13.19
Heterotopia. A 10-year-old mentally retarded epileptic boy. **A.** Nodular heterotopias in the hemispheric white matter and periventricular zone are associated with agenesis of the corpus callosum. **B.** Laminar heterotopia in the subcortical white matter in a 40-year-old epileptic man (Weil stain). **C.** Neuronal and glial nodule in the leptomeninges (brain wart) (cresyl violet).

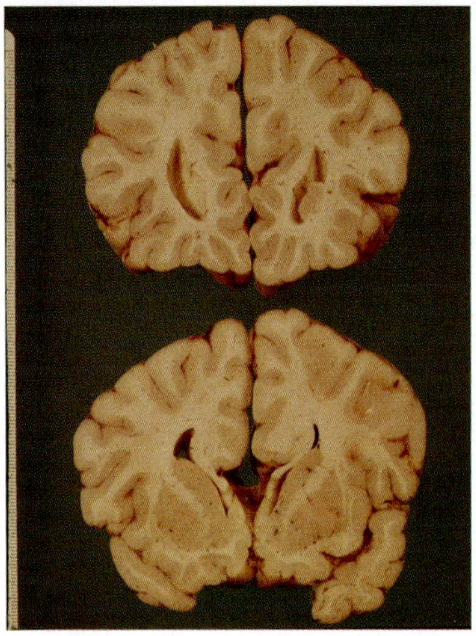

FIGURE 13.20
Agenesis of the corpus callosum and septum pellucidum in a 19-year-old woman. She was the second twin, delivered at 7.5 months' gestation. On transverse sections, thick myelin bundles of Probst extend from the cingular gyri to the rectus gyri to form the medial walls of the lateral ventricles. The ventricles are slit-like with dorsal extensions (bat-wing shape). The septum pellucidum is absent.

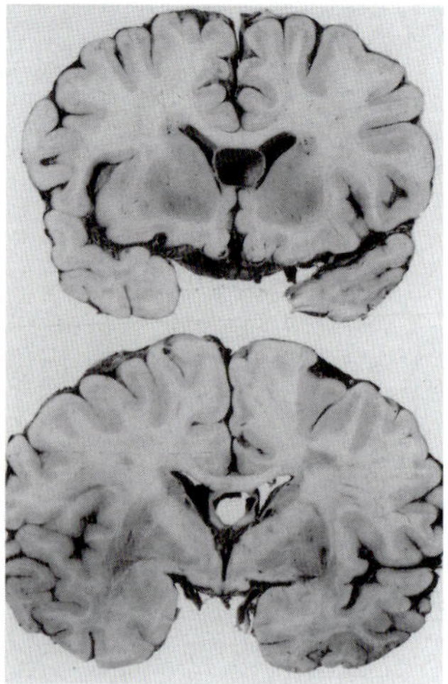

FIGURE 13.21
Cavum septum pellucidum, an incidental autopsy finding.

Hemimegalencephaly

In hemimegalencephaly, one cerebral hemisphere is considerably larger than the other, displaying broad convolutions, a thick cortex, and heterotopia. Histologic anomalies include a disorganized cortical lamination, the presence of cytomegalic and ballooned neurons, and glial proliferation with dysplastic, swollen, and glassy astrocytes.

MALFORMATIONS OF THE MIDLINE STRUCTURES AND VENTRICLES

Agenesis of the corpus callosum (Fig. 13.20). This malformation is characterized by:

- The presence of thick myelin bundles of Probst (uncrossed callosal fibers) extending longitudinally from the lateral ventricles to the fornices
- The absence of cingulate gyri
- A radial arrangement of the convolutions in the medial aspects of the hemispheres
- Widely separated lateral ventricles displaying an angulated dorsal extension (bat-wing shape)
- An enlarged third ventricle with a dorsal extension
- An occasional lipoma, hamartoma, or meningioma in the midlinc

Agenesis of the corpus callosum occurs sporadically and may be associated with chromosomal aberrations and inherited metabolic disorders (see Table 13.2). Usually, it is clinically silent and diagnosed incidentally on MRI or at autopsy. Clinical manifestations, such as seizures and mental retardation, when present, are attributed to associated malformations.

Cavum septum pellucidum, an incidental neuroimaging or autopsy finding, is a cystic cavity bounded by the two membranes of the septum, the crura of the fornices, and the corpus callosum. Its posterior extension is the cavum vergae (Fig. 13.21).

Malformations of the Ventricles

Several forms are distinguished:

- Membranous occlusion of the foramen Monro
- Adhesions between the caudate nucleus and the corpus callosum or between opposite walls of the anterior, temporal, or occipital horns
- Obliteration of the third ventricle by fusion of the thalami

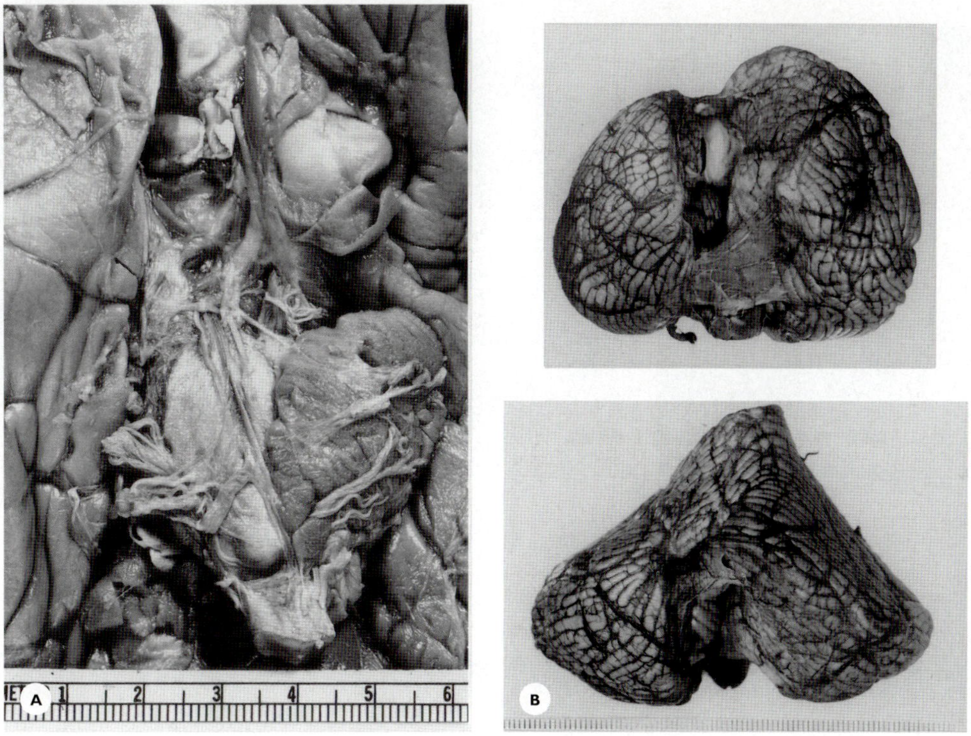

FIGURE 13.22
Cerebellar Malformations. Partial cerebellar agenesis. **A.** The right cerebellar hemisphere is absent. The origin of cranial nerve roots is asymmetrical. The left lower nerve roots emerge through the cerebellar folia. **B.** The inferior vermis is absent. The gap between the hemispheres is covered with leptomeninges. On dorsal aspect, the vermis is fused with the hemispheres. Orientation of convolutions is abnormal.

- Atresia and stenosis of the aqueduct of Sylvius, a leading causes of congenital hydrocephalus
- Membranous occlusions of the foramina Luschka and Magendie of the fourth ventricle, which are inconstant features of the Dandy-Walker malformation

MALFORMATIONS OF THE CEREBELLUM

The spectrum of cerebellar malformations ranges from gross anomalies to discrete histologic derangements. The malformations are conveniently grouped as (a) cerebellar agenesis, hypogenesis, and hypoplasia; (b) minor histologic anomalies; and (c) dysplastic gangliocytoma.

Clinically, gross malformations present with congenital cerebellar ataxia. The symptoms appear in early infancy, with delays and difficulties sitting and standing and a lack of coordination of simple movements. Gait, if it develops, is severely unsteady and broad-based. Speech is impaired.

Agenesis, Hypogenesis, and Hypoplasia

Agenesis of the cerebellum is rare. *Partial agenesis* may involve the hemisphere (neocerebellum) or the vermis (paleocerebellum) (Figs. 13.22 and 13.23). Partial or total absence of the vermis is a feature of the Dandy-Walker malformation (see the section Congenital Hydrocephalus).

Cerebellar hypoplasia refers to underdevelopment of parts or of the whole cerebellum (see Fig. 13.23). Some cases have been reported in nonketotic hyperglycinemia.

Pontoneocerebellar Hypoplasia

This multiple system malformation involves the cerebellar hemispheres and their pontine and medullary connections, resembling the pathology of olivopontocerebellar atrophy. The malformation is associated with a congenital disorder of glycosylation. Grossly, the cerebellar hemispheres are abnormally small, consisting of

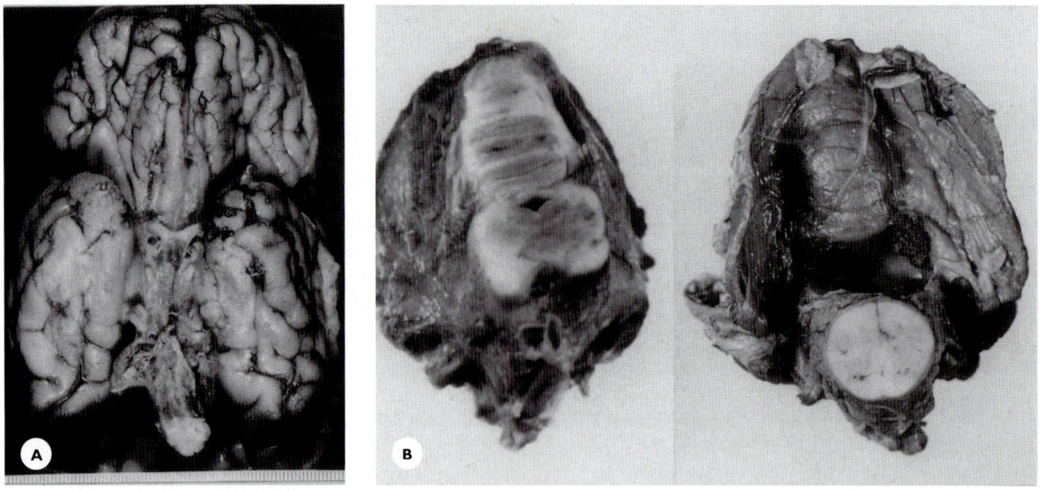

FIGURE 13.23
Cerebellar hypoplasia in a 5-year-old boy who was born during the fifth month of pregnancy following an accident involving the mother. **A.** The cerebellar hemispheres are represented by a few folia. **B.** The vermis is somewhat better developed. The pons is small. (Histologically, there was loss of Purkinje cells and transverse pontine fibers, and of inferior olivary neurons resembling a pontoneocerebellar hypoplasia.)

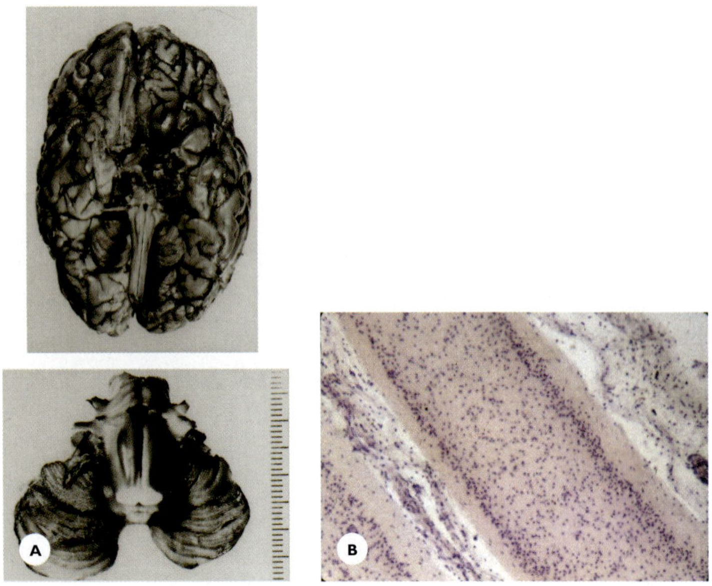

FIGURE 13.24
Aplasia of the granule cell layer in a 6-year-old boy. His development was abnormal from birth: He slept most of the time, was difficult to arouse and feed, and remained bedridden all his life. **A.** The cerebellum is abnormally small, has narrow folia separated by deep sulci. **B.** The cortex is devoid of granule cells, and some folia show Purkinje cells losses (cresyl violet).

merely a few thin folia. The pontine basis is small, and the medullary olives are flat.

Histologically, the cortex reveals a diminished number of Purkinje and granule cells; the dentate nuclei are severely disorganized; the pontine nuclei are hypoplastic and the transverse pontine fibers are reduced in number; the hemispheric white matter and the middle and superior cerebellar peduncles are poorly myelinated; and the olivary neurons are hypoplastic.

Aplasia of the granular cell layer occurs sporadically, although a few familial cases have been reported (Fig. 13.24). Absence of the granule cells is associated

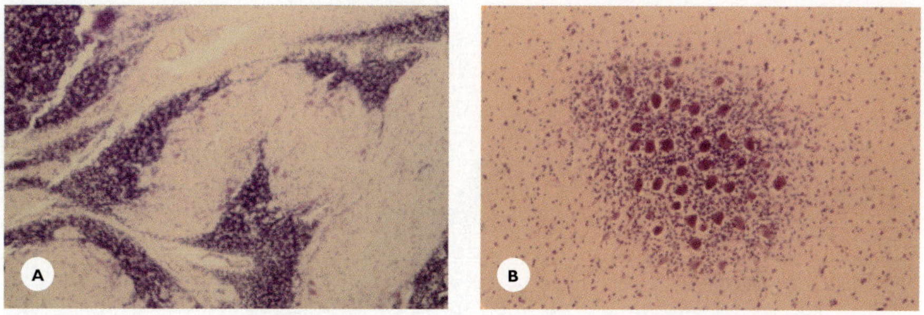

FIGURE 13.25
Cerebellar cortical dysplasia and heterotopia. **A.** Abnormal convolutions show islands of granule cells and scattered Purkinje cells (cresyl violet). **B.** Cluster of Purkinje cells and granule cells in the hemispheric white matter (HE).

with anomalous Purkinje cells, which display a cactus-like dendritic arborization and axonal torpedoes.

Minor Histologic Anomalies

Cortical dysplasia consists of disorganized lamination, often with abnormal neurons (Fig. 13.25).

Heterotopias are nests of Purkinje cells and dentate neurons within the hemispheric white matter (see Fig. 13.25).

Dysplastic Gangliocytoma or Lhermitte-Duclos Disease

The pathology is characterized grossly by focal thickening of the folia and histologically by replacement of the Purkinje and granular cell layers with dysplastic ganglion cells. Abnormally myelinated fibers are present in the molecular layer.

Clinically, cerebellar symptoms and increased intracranial pressure (ICP) may develop at any age, but usually in the third and fourth decades. They gradually progress and often necessitat surgery. T2-weighted MR images reveal focal hyperintense thickening of the folia.

MALFORMATIONS OF THE BRAINSTEM

Stenosis and atresia of the aqueduct of Sylvius are major causes of congenital hydrocephalus. In atresia, tiny channels of ependymal cells indicate the site of the aqueduct.

Syringobulbia is a slit-like cavity in the medulla extending from the floor of the fourth ventricle ventrally, usually between the olives and the hypoglossal nerve roots, or between the olives and the pyramids. It may be associated with syringomyelia and ependymoma of the fourth ventricle. Clinically, it presents with a combination of bulbar palsy, ataxia, and facial sensory deficits.

Other malformations are heterotopia and dysplasia of the inferior olivary nuclei and anomalous crossing of the pyramidal tracts.

TABLE 13.4.
Causes of Secondary Microencephaly and Megalencephaly

Microencephaly	*Megalencephaly*
Fetal/ Perinatal Injuries	Leukodystrophies
Hypoxic-ischemic	Alexander's disease
Infectious	Canavan's disease
Metabolic	Neuronal storage diseases
Traumatic	Tay-Sachs disease
Toxic	Mucopolysaccharidosis
Malformations	Phakomatoses
	Tuberous sclerosis
	Recklinghausen's disease

DISORDERS OF BRAIN WEIGHT

Microencephaly and Microcephaly

The brain volume can be diminished primarily or secondarily to a number of acquired or inherited metabolic disorders (Table 13.4). True or primary microencephaly implies a reduction of brain weight by two standard deviations from the normal for age and sex. It occurs sporadically or is inherited as an autosomal dominant, autosomal recessive, or X-linked trait. Microcephaly is also a feature of several chromosomal defects (trisomy 21, 18, 9, and 13). Clinical manifestation varies from normal intelligence to variable mental retardation.

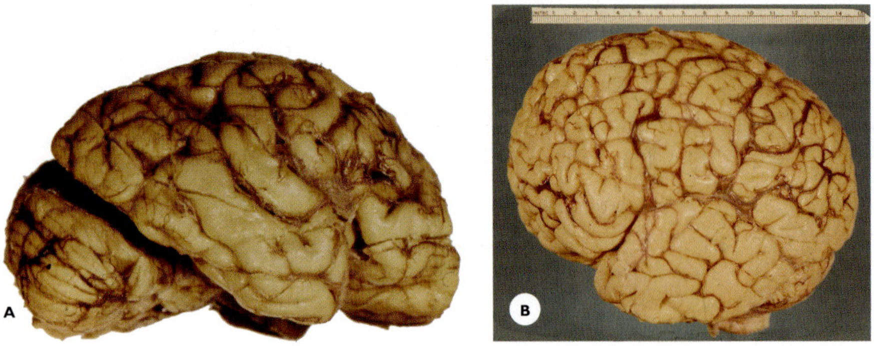

FIGURE 13.26
Brain weight disorders. **A.** Primary micrencephaly in a 70-year-old mentally retarded woman. The 510-g brain displays a greatly simplified convolutional pattern with broad convolutions. **B.** Primary megalencephaly in a 58-year-old mentally severely retarded man. The 1800-g brain displays a richness of haphazardly arranged convolutions.

Grossly, the adult microencephalic brain may weigh from 500 to 900 g and display a simple convolutional pattern of broad convolutions (Fig. 13.26). Histologically, minor cytoarchitectonic anomalies are present in the cortex and deep gray structures. The smallness of the head contrasts with the normal size of the face; the forehead recedes sharply, and the occiput is flat.

Megalencephaly and Macrocephaly

True or primary megalencephaly implies an increase of brain weight by two and a half standard deviations above the normal for age and sex. It occurs sporadically or is inherited as an autosomal dominant or recessive trait. Grossly, the bulky adult megalencephalic brain may weigh from 1,600 to 1,800 g or more (see Fig. 13.26). On section, the cortex is thick, and the volume of the white matter is increased. Histologically, heterotopia and minor cytoarchitectonic anomalies are usually present. The head may be large at birth, or the size increases during early infancy.

MENINGEAL AND VASCULAR ANOMALIES

A *congenital arachnoid cyst* results from a separation of the arachnoid membrane. Common sites are the lateral aspects of the hemispheres, the interhemispheric fissure, the cerebellopontine angle, the posterior fossa, and around the spinal cord. Some cysts remain clinically silent; others enlarge to produce focal symptoms and increased ICP, necessitating surgery.

An *arteriovenous fistula of the vein of Galen* carries serious complications in neonates and infants. The vein of Galen is markedly dilated from draining the blood of the major basal cerebral arteries. Complications include cardiac failure, hydrocephalus, focal neurologic symptoms, seizures, and hemorrhages. Common vascular malformations are covered in Chapter 11.

PHAKOMATOSES: ECTOMESODERMAL DYSGENETIC SYNDROMES

Phakomatosis (Greek *phakos*, birth marks of skin and eyes) refers to a group of syndromes of multisystem malformations. The malformations derive from any of the three germinal layers of the embryonic disc: ectoderm, mesoderm, and entoderm. The nervous system, eyes, and skin are the primary sites of involvement. The visceral and endocrine organs, blood vessels, and skeleton are variably involved. Some malformations are apt to proliferate into neoplasms that may undergo malignant transformation.

Some syndromes occur sporadically, and some are inherited as an autosomal recessive or dominant transmission. The clinical presentation varies greatly from monosymptomatic abortive forms to full-blown syndromes. Symptoms may appear at various ages from infancy through adulthood. Some malformations are identifiable antenatally using ultrasonography and postnatally using MRI.

Tuberous Sclerosis Complex

The syndrome of tuberous sclerosis, or Bourneville-Pringle disease, occurs in 1 to 10,000 births. It presents with cerebral, cutaneous, and ocular malformations; visceral malformations occur with variable frequency. Familial cases are inherited as an autosomal dominant trait. Sporadic cases probably result from spontaneous

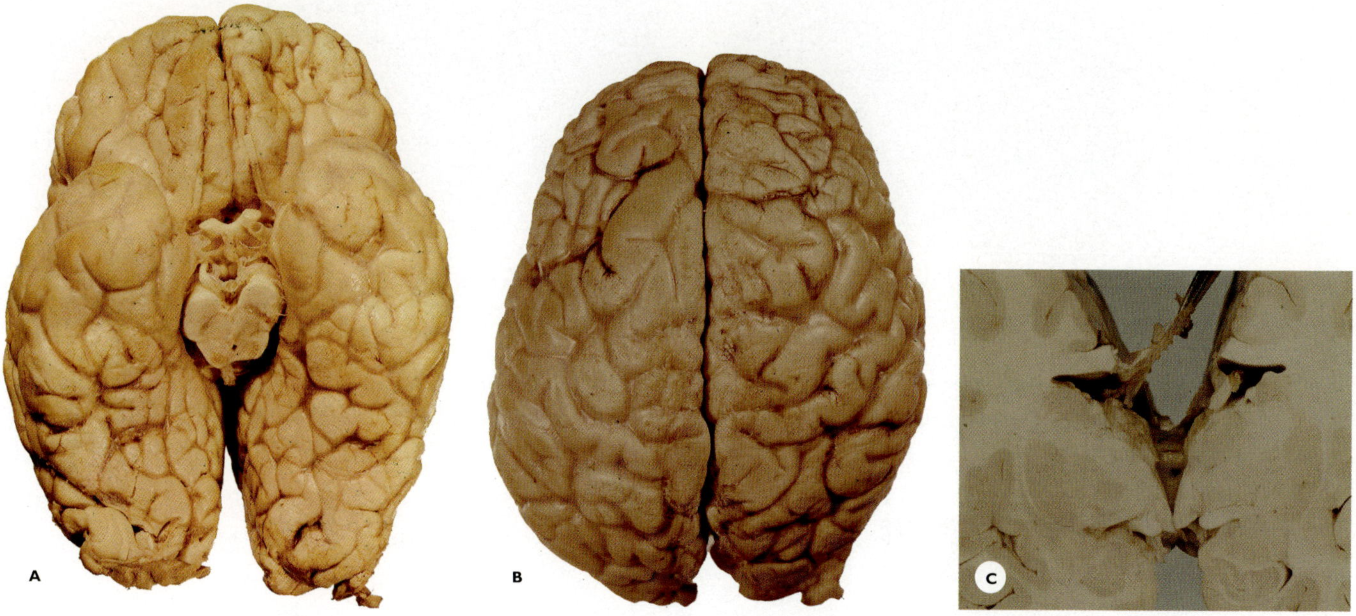

FIGURE 13.27
Tuberous sclerosis in a 20-year-old mentally retarded epileptic man with numerous "warts" on his face. (**A**) Basal and (**B**) dorsal views of the brain show numerous tubers appearing as focal widening of the convolutions; a few have a central dimple. **C.** Small nodules are present in the ventricular walls.

mutations. The defective genes *TSC1* and *TSC2* map to chromosomes 9 and 16, respectively.

Clinical Features

Neurologic manifestations commonly include seizures and mental retardation. The seizures may begin in infancy, and mental retardation may be severe and progressive. Symptoms and signs vary according to the location and size of the lesions. CT scan and MRI demonstrate calcifications, cortical tubers, and heterotopia.

Cutaneous signs are diagnostic and include sebaceous adenomas (angiofibromas) along the nasolabial folds, subungual fibromas, hypomelanotic macules, and Shagreen patches (fibrosis) on the face and trunk.

Ocular sign: Retinal glioma is also characteristic.

Visceral manifestations, important, but often not obvious clinically, include rhabdomyoma of the heart, hamartomas of the kidneys, pheochromocytoma, and cysts and adenomas of various organs (Fig. 13.27).

Pathology

The cerebral malformations are cortical tubers, subependymal ventricular nodules, and heterotopia. These malformations may proliferate into benign or malignant astrocytic tumors, often into a subependymal giant-cell astrocytoma. Ventricular tumors lead to early obstructive hydrocephalus and raised ICP.

Cortical Tubers

Grossly, the tubers appear as nodule-like structures that result from focal broadening and firmness of the convolutions. Some are slightly elevated above the cortical surface, whereas others display a central dimple. Their sizes vary from a few millimeters to 2 to 3 cm, and their number may reach 30 to 40. They are randomly distributed in the cerebral hemispheres, less frequently in the cerebellum (Figs. 13.27 and 13.28).

Histologically, the normal cortical architecture is replaced by dysplastic neurons and glial cells. The neurons display abnormal shapes and orientation; they contain variable amounts of Nissl substance and, occasionally, neurofibrillary tangles. The astrocytes are large, often bizarrely gigantic, and may form clusters. Dense fibrillary astrocytosis and calcifications are common (Fig. 13.29).

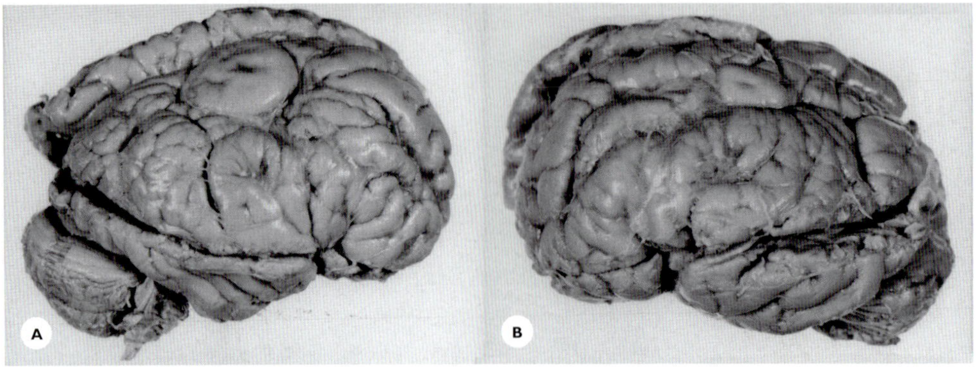

FIGURE 13.28

Tuberous sclerosis in a 15-year-old girl. **A.** Right cerebral hemisphere displays multiple, sharply circumscribed, firm tubers. Some are elevated above the cortical surface and have a central dimple. **B.** The left hemisphere displays abnormally oriented small and broad convolutions.

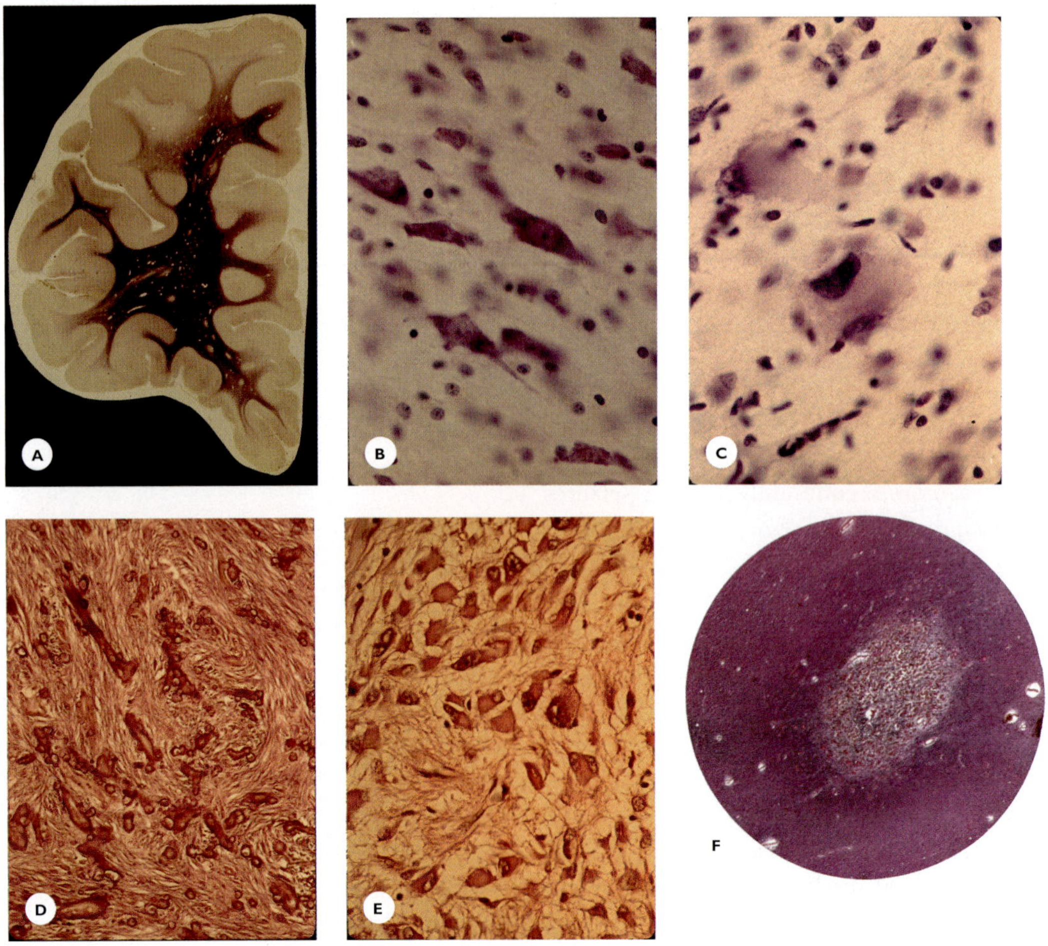

FIGURE 13.29

Tuberous sclerosis. Histology: **A.** Frontal lobe stained for myelin shows myelin loss beneath the cortical tubers. Within the tubers, the cortical cytoarchitecture is disorganized. It consists of (**B**) large, atypical neurons, and (**C**) monstrous astrocytes (cresyl violet). The periventricular nodules consist of (**D**) dense astrocytic fibrosis with numerous calcified capillaries and (**E**) a subependymal astrocytoma (HE). **F.** A heterotopic nodule of glial cells and neuron is present in the hemispheric white matter (LFB-CV).

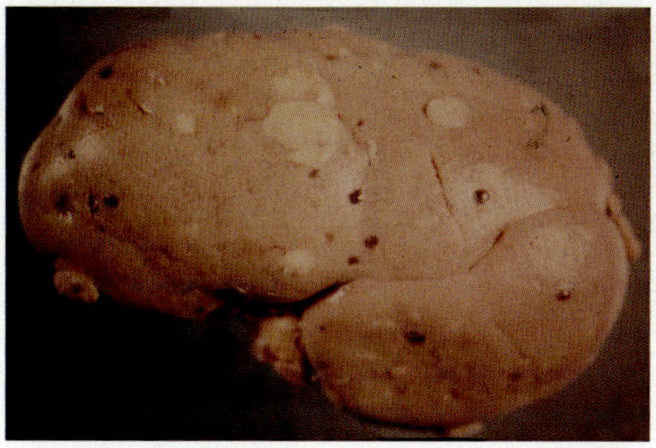

FIGURE 13.30
Tuberous sclerosis. Hamartoma of the kidney consists of fibrous, adipose, and angiomatous nodules.

Subependymal Ventricular Nodules

Subependymal ventricular nodules may occur at any site of the ventricles, often at the foramen Monro, projecting into the lumen like "candle gutterings." They are composed of a mixture of astrocytes, immature glial cells, dysplastic neurons, and calcium deposits (see Fig. 13.29).

Heterotopia

Heterotopia in the hemispheric white matter are clusters of dysplastic neurons and glial cells (see Fig. 13.29).

Encephalofacial Angiomatosis or Sturge-Weber-Dimitri Syndrome

This syndrome is characterized by facial vascular nevus, leptomeningeal angiomatosis, and cortical calcifications on the side of the facial nevus. The syndrome occurs sporadically, and few familial cases are recorded.

Clinical Features

Neurologic manifestations include seizures and focal neurologic deficits; normal intellect or variable degrees of mental retardation are common.

Cutaneous sign, facial vascular nevus (nevus flammeus, port-wine stain) is present at birth, usually confined to the supraorbital region and scalp (Fig. 13.31).

Ocular signs include choroidal angioma, congenital glaucoma, and buphthalmos (abnormal enlargement of the eye).

Radiologic findings: Cortical calcifications, usually demonstrable after 2 years of age, appear on plain radiograph and CT scan as double-contoured (railroad track) curving lines corresponding to the gyral pattern (see Fig. 13.31). Leptomeningeal angiomatosis is readily visible with contrast-enhanced MRI.

Visceral manifestations are angiomas. Bony angiomatosis is an additional feature.

Pathology

The *leptomeningeal angiomatosis*, on the side of the facial nevus, usually in the occipital or occipito-parietal region, is composed of thin-walled small- and medium-sized arteries, veins, and capillaries often showing proliferation, degenerative changes and calcifications (see Fig. 13.31).

Cortical calcifications occur roughly beneath the leptomeningeal angiomatosis. The size of calcific deposits varies from small mulberry-like granules to large coalescent concretions (see Fig. 13.31).

Cortical cytoarchitectonic anomalies and atrophic and dystrophic changes are common.

Encephalofacial angiomatosis may occur in conjunction with angiomatosis osteohypertrophy or the Klippel Trenaunay-Weber syndrome. This consists of cutaneous and bony angiomatosis and hypertrophy of the limbs.

Neurocutaneous Melanosis

This syndrome is characterized by pigmented cutaneous nevi, melanosis of the leptomeninges, and intracerebral melanin pigments (Fig. 13.32). Malignant melanomas may complicate the syndrome. Seizures and mental retardation are common clinical manifestations.

CONGENITAL AND NEONATAL HYDROCEPHALUS

Hydrocephalus may develop *in utero* or during the first few months of life. Congenital hydrocephalus is among the common malformations. The incidence is estimated at 0.5 to 0.8 per 1,000 births. It may be inherited as an autosomal recessive or X-linked trait, or it may be acquired by intrauterine exposure to viral infections

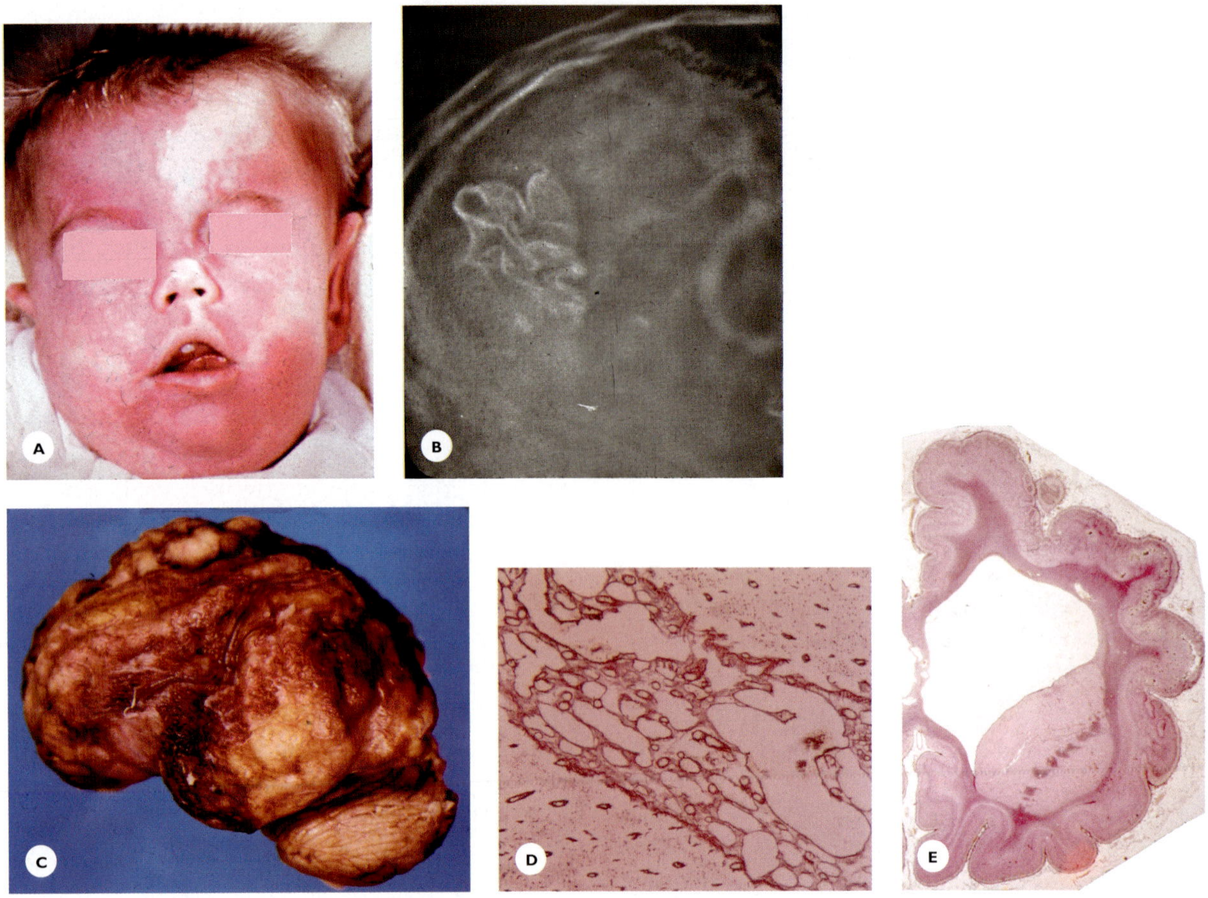

FIGURE 13.31
Sturge-Weber-Dimitri disease. **A.** A 2-year-old boy exhibited extensive vascular nevi of the face, scalp, and extremities. **B.** A skull radiograph shows curvilinear cortical calcifications. **C.** Leptomeningeal angiomatosis covers the lateral aspect of the cerebral hemisphere. **D.** A network of thin-walled vessels fills the subarachnoid space (reticular stain). **E.** Polymicrogyric cortex contains numerous calcospherites (HE).

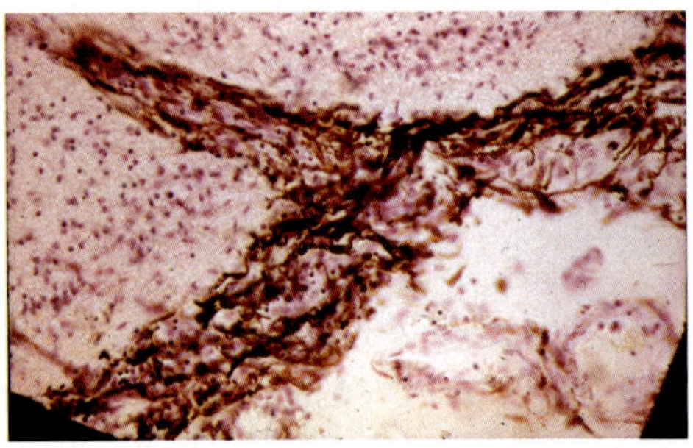

FIGURE 13.32.
Neurocutaneous melanosis in a 16-year-old woman. **A.** Melanocytes infiltrate the leptomeninges and extend into the parenchyma along the Virchow-Robin space (HE).

(cytomegalovirus, rubella, mumps, varicella-zoster viruses), maternal irradiation, and maternal hypo- or hypervitaminosis A.

Clinical Features

Most infants with congenital hydrocephalus are stillborn or die soon after birth, but the lives of some are prolonged. The head, if not enlarged at birth, grows at an abnormal rate. The continuing enlargement of the ventricles is initially compensated by separation of the sutures and distension of the fontanels. As the hydrocephalus progresses, the infant becomes lethargic, devel-

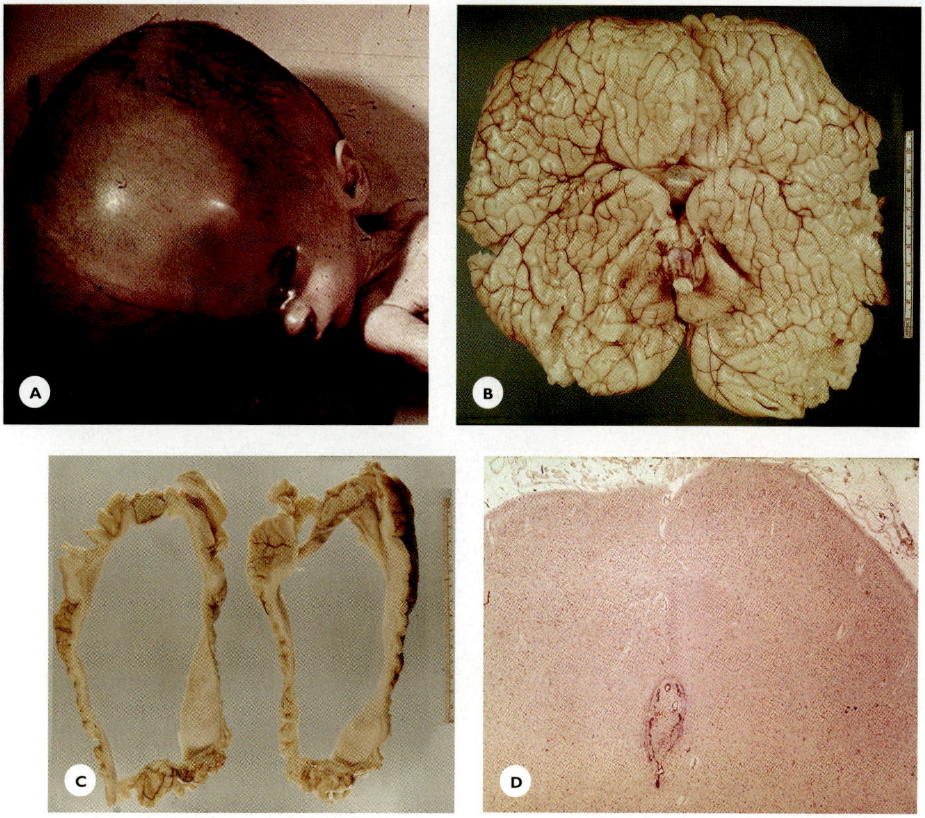

FIGURE 13.33
Congenital hydrocephalus due to occlusion of the aqueduct of Sylvius in a 3-year-old boy. **A.** Enormously enlarged head, small-appearing face, and setting-sun position of the eyeballs. **B.** Basal aspect of the brain shows huge, collapsed cerebral hemispheres; thin, distended floor of the third ventricle; and a small cerebellum. **C.** The cerebral wall is less than 1 cm thick. **D.** Membranous occlusion of the aqueduct (cresyl violet).

ops spasticity of the legs, and abducens palsy, and, if the pressure is not relieved by a shunting procedure, papilledema and optic atrophy develop. The face appears small in relation to the enormously enlarged head, and the eyeballs deviate downward, producing the setting-sun sign (Fig. 13.33). Cranial ultrasound demonstrates the hydrocephalus at 15 to 18 weeks of gestation, and MRI identifies the underlying pathology postnatally.

Pathology

Grossly, the hydrocephalic skull is thin, and the inner table is uneven, resembling digital marking. The cerebral hemispheres are markedly enlarged and soft. The sulci are shallow, and the convolutions appear small. The floor of the third ventricle is thin and distended. On sections, the ventricles are enormously enlarged, and the cerebral wall may be reduced to 1 cm or less. This reduction involves chiefly the white matter, which is unmyelinated and distensible; the width of the cortex is relatively preserved (see Fig. 13.33). Histologically, the ependymal lining is disrupted, and the subependymal astrocytes show focal fibrillary proliferation.

Obstructive congenital hydrocephalus is most often due to cerebral malformations, seldom to cranial anomalies or a congenital neoplasm (Table 13.5).

TABLE 13.5.
Cerebral Malformations That Cause Hydrocephalus

Atresia/Stenosis of aqueduct of Sylvius
Dandy-Walker malformation
Partial/total absence of vermis
Cystic transformation of 4th ventricle
Inconstant atresia of foramina Magendie and Luschka
Large posterior fossa
Arnold-Chiari Type 2 malformation
Displacement of cerebellar tonsils, inferior vermis and elongaged medulla into the spinal canal
Small posterior fossa
Meningomyelocele
Chiari Type 1 malformation
Cerebellar tonsils located below the foramen magnum

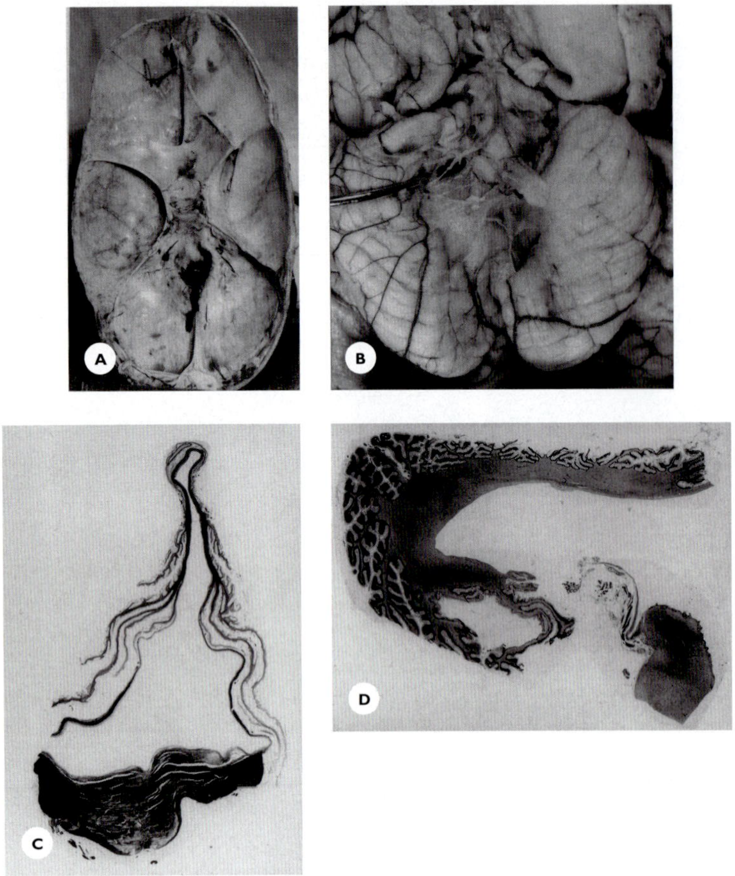

FIGURE 13.34
Dandy-Walker malformation in a 4-year-old boy. At about 2 to 4 weeks of age, it was noticed first that his head was larger than normal. At 2 months of age, the head circumference was 48 cm (normal 40 cm). The sutures were widely separated and the fontanels tense. A ventriculoperitoneal shunt was placed, which 2 months later was replaced with a ventriculocaval shunt. Despite surgical intervention, the infant progressively deteriorated. His head rapidly enlarged. He became blind and paralyzed. **A.** Base of the skull shows a markedly enlarged posterior fossa. **B.** The inferior vermis is absent and a thin membrane roofs the ventricle. **C.** At pontine level, the large cystic fourth ventricle is bounded by severely atrophic cerebellar folia and a thin layer of white matter (myelin stain). **D.** The foramin Luschka is occluded by a fibrous membrane lined with ependymal cells.

Cerebral and Cranial Malformations Associated with Hydrocephalus

Stenosis and atresia (absence) of the aqueduct of Sylvius occur sporadically; a few cases are inherited as a X-linked recessive trait affecting only boys, or as an autosomal recessive trait. In atresia, groups of tiny channels lined with ependymal cells and separated by normal tissue indicate the site of the aqueduct. Rarely, the aqueduct is occluded by a membranous septum (see Fig. 13.33).

The *Dandy-Walker malformation* accounts for 3% to 4% of congenital hydrocephalus. Most cases are sporadic. A few are familial, and some are linked to maternal use of isoretinoid during pregnancy.

In the Dandy-Walker malformation, the vermis is totally or partially absent, mostly its posterior portion. The fourth ventricle is transformed into a large cystic cavity with a thin, glial-vascular membranous roof lined with ependyma. The foramina Luschka and Magendie may fail to open. The posterior fossa is large, and the lateral sinuses and torcular Herophili are elevated (Fig. 13.34).

The *Arnold-Chiari type 2 malformation* is characterized by downward displacement of the cerebellar tonsils, inferior vermis, and the elongated medulla into the spinal canal. Subsequently, the tectum becomes beak-like, the elongated medulla kinked, and the foramen Magendie obstructed (Fig. 13.35). The posterior fossa is small. Meningomyelocele is almost invariably present, preventing the upward movement of the spinal cord, thus reversing the direction of the spinal nerve roots from downward to upward.

Clinically, the hydrocephalus in both Dandy-Walker and Arnold-Chiari type 2 malformations may either be present at birth or manifests in early infancy. If the cerebrospinal fluid (CSF) is not shunted, cerebellar signs, nystagmus, cranial nerve deficits—chiefly sixth nerve palsy—spasticity, and signs of increased ICP develop. The Arnold-Chiari malformation is further aggravated by symptoms of a lumbar or sacral meningomyelocele.

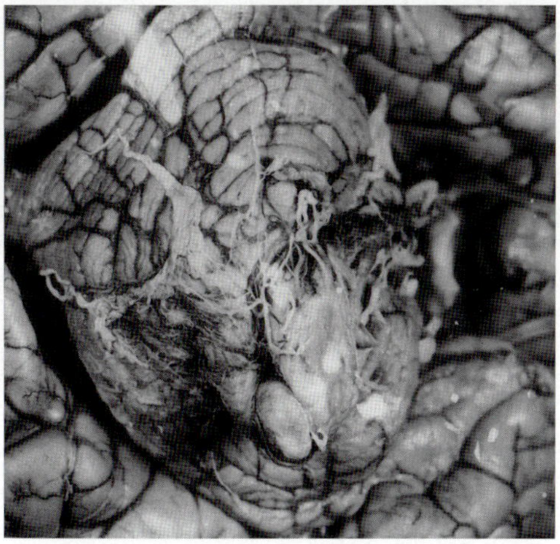

FIGURE 13.35
Arnold-Chiari type 2 malformation in a 1.5-year-old boy. He was delivered by forceps because of his enlarged head. He had a lumbosacral meningomyelocele, club feet, and flaccid paraparesis. By age 2 months, the head circumference increased to 48 cm (normal, 40 cm). Ventral view of the cerebellum shows thickened and partially torn (artifact) basal leptomeninges and elongated tonsils adjacent to the rostral medulla.

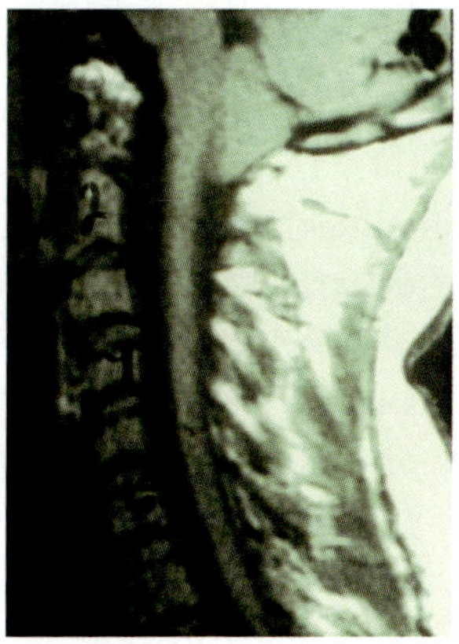

FIGURE 13.36
Chiari type 1 malformation in a 24-year-old man with chronic headache. MRI shows the cerebellar tonsils located below the foramen magnum level.

In the *Chiari type 1* malformation the cerebellar tonsils are located below the foramen magnum (chronic cerebellar herniation), possibly due to smallness of the posterior fossa (Fig. 13.36).

Clinically, infants present with nuchal rigidity and apneic spells, which may culminate in sudden death. Young adults present with headache, cranial nerve deficits, cerebellar ataxia, stridor, sleep apnea, and symptoms of raised ICP.

Craniosynostosis results from a premature closure of the cranial sutures: sagittal, coronal, and lambdoid. The fusion may involve one or several. Subsequently, the head is abnormally shaped and the eyes are proptotic. The patients present with headache, blindness, and mental retardation.

In *achondroplasia*, the hydrocephalus, usually arrested, is associated with an abnormally formed occipital bone and narrow foramen magnum.

TABLE 13.6.
Malformations with Chromosomal Defects

Malformations	*Chromosomal Defects*
Anencephaly	Trisomy 9, 13, 18
Dysraphic disorders	Triploidy
Holoprosencephaly	Trisomy 13, 18
Microencephaly	Trisomy 9, 13, 18, 21 X-chromosome
Dandy-Walker malformations	Trisomy 9, 18, 21
Congenital hydrocephalus	Trisomy 9, 13, 20 Triploidy
Agenesis of corpus callosum	Trisomy 8, 13, 20
Arnold-Chiari type 2 malformations	Trisomy 18 Triploidy

CHROMOSOMAL DISORDERS

Fetal chromosomal aberrations often result in abortions during the first trimester. Trisomies, the most common chromosomal disorders, are frequently implicated in nervous system malformations. Trisomies 13 and 18 are associated with major malformations of the nervous system, eyes, viscera, and skeleton. Affected fetuses are stillborn or short-lived. A larger group of less severe or minor malformations are associated with trisomies 21, 9, and the X chromosome. Affected individuals present with mental retardation, seizures, and variable motor deficits. Cytogenetic studies for suspected chromosomal disorders are performed on amniotic fluid or chorionic villi during the third or fourth month of pregnancy. Major malformations with chromosomal defects are listed in Table 13.6.

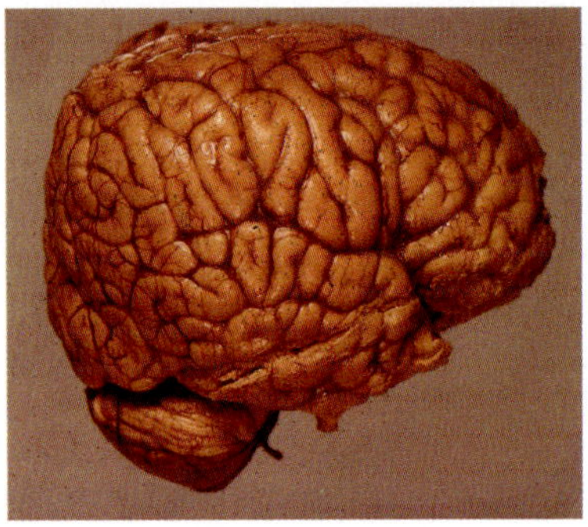

FIGURE 13.37
Down syndrome. The brain of a 4-year-old boy displays a round shape, flattened occipital lobes, and simple convolutional pattern.

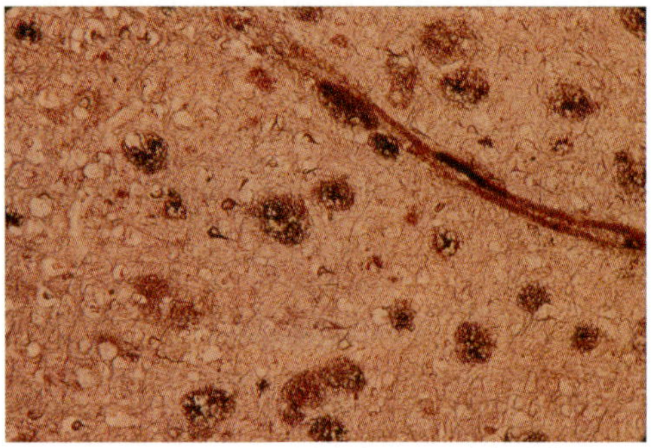

FIGURE 13.38
Down syndrome with Alzheimer's disease. A well-adjusted, neat woman with Down syndrome was easy to get along with and able to perform simple housework until about age 38, when her behavior gradually changed. She neglected her appearance; became irritable with screaming and cursing; and was unable to help with housework. She developed seizures, and her physical and mental condition progressively deteriorated. During the final stage of her illness, she was mute and totally helpless, dying at age 56 years. The cerebral cortex shows numerous neuritic plaques and neurofibrillary tangles (Bodian stain).

Down Syndrome

Down syndrome, a common chromosomal disorder, is associated with trisomy of chromosome 21. Advanced maternal age—35 years or over—is a potential risk for having a child with Down syndrome.

Clinical Features

Somatic characteristics are a square-shaped head; a narrow, upward-slanted palpebral fissure with median epicanthic folds; flat nasal bridge; thick lips and tongue; and low-set ears. The neck, stature, and extremities are short.

Systemic manifestations include congenital heart disease, commonly an atrioventricular septal defect, duodenal stenosis or atresia, umbilical hernia, minor bony anomalies, and abnormal palmar dermogram (simian crease). Patients are at a higher risk of developing acute leukemias and infections.

Neuropsychiatric Manifestations. Mental retardation ranges from mild to severe. The disposition is generally pleasant and happy. Those who reach age 30 or over almost invariably develop a progressive dementia.

Pathologic Features

Grossly, the brain is small and of below average weight. The shape is round with flattened occipital lobes. The convolutional pattern is simple, and the first temporal gyri are narrow (Fig. 13.37).

Histologic findings include minor cortical anomalies, diminished dendritic arborization of the neurons, reduced synaptic density, and calcifications in the basal ganglia. The histology of the dementing process is identical to that of Alzheimer's disease (see Fig. 13.38). The gene of amyloid precursor protein (APP), a basic component of the neuritic plaques in both Down syndrome and Alzheimer's disease, maps to chromosome 21.

BIBLIOGRAPHY

Friede, R.L. (1989). *Developmental neuropathology*, 2nd ed. Berlin: Springer-Verlag.

Golden, J.A. & Harding, B.N. (2004). *Pathology and genetics*. Basel: Developmental Neuropathology ISN Neuropath Press.

Leech, R.W. & Brumback R.A. (1991). *Hydrocephalus: current clinical concepts*. St. Louis: Mosby-Year Book.

Norman, M.G., McGillivray, B.C., Kalousek, D., et al. (1995). *Congenital malformations of the brain*. New York: Oxford University Press.

REVIEW QUESTIONS

1. Maternal diseases that predispose to cerebral malformations in offspring are:
   A. Phenylketonuria
   B. Diabetes mellitus
   C. Wilson's disease
   D. Megaloblastic anemia
   E. Multiple sclerosis

2. Concerning meningomyelocele, all the following statements are correct *except*:
   A. The common site is the lumbosacral region.
   B. It is commonly associated with the Dandy-Walker syndrome.
   C. It is associated with the Arnold-Chiari malformation.
   D. It may be associated with an epidermoid cyst.
   E. It may be associated with an enterogenous cyst.

3. Clinically, syringomyelia is best characterized by:
   A. Loss of vibration and positional sensations
   B. Loss of pain and temperature sensations
   C. Ataxic gait
   D. Loss of positional sense
   E. Urinary incontinence

4. Diastematomyelia refers to:
   A. Two half cords separated by a bony spur
   B. Two whole cords within the dural sac
   C. A cystic cavity within the cord
   D. A dilated central canal
   E. A tube-like cavity in the cervical region

5. Concerning holoprosencephaly, which of the following are correct?
   A. It can be caused by excessive alcohol consumption of the mother during pregnancy.
   B. The brain is not divided into hemispheres.
   C. It can be inherited as an autosomal dominant trait.
   D. It is associated with facial anomalies.
   E. It is associated with trisomy 21.

6. Which of the following characterize hydranencephaly?
   A. The ventricles are dilated due to obstruction of CSF flow at foramen Magendie.
   B. The cerebral hemispheres are transformed into two cystic cavities.
   C. It is caused by an ischemic-hypoxic insult in the carotid territories.
   D. It is caused by an ischemic-hypoxic insult in vertebrobasilar territories.

7. Concerning cortical dysplasia, all the following statements are correct *except*:
   A. It is a complication of hydrocephalus.
   B. It results from a disorder of neuronal migration and organization.
   C. It manifests with seizures.
   D. It manifests as polymicrogyria.
   E. It manifests as lissencephaly.

8. All the following characterize lissencephaly type 1 *except*:
   A. It displays a six-layered cortex.
   B. It is inherited as an autosomal dominant trait.
   C. It is associated with mutations in gene *ARX* on chromosome X.
   D. It is associated with mutations in gene *LIS1* on chromosome 17.
   E. It is sporadic.

9. Common sites of heterotopia are:
   A. Periventricular
   B. Subcortical
   C. Leptomeningeal
   D. All of these
   E. None of these

10. Which of the following characterize dysplastic gangliocytoma, or Lhermitte-Duclos disease?
    A. The cerebellar cortex shows focal thickening.
    B. T2-weighted MRI shows hyperintensity of the cortex.
    C. The cerebellar vermis is malformed.
    D. The cortex is replaced by a dense astrocytic fibrosis.
    E. The granule cell layer is degenerated.

11. Characteristics of the Dandy-Walker malformation include all *except*:

    A. Malformation of the cerebellar vermis
    B. Cystic dilations of the fourth ventricle
    C. Hydrocephalus
    D. Failure of opening of foramen Luschka
    E. Small posterior fossa

12. All the following statements concerning true microencephaly are correct *except*:

    A. The cortex shows lissencephaly.
    B. It can be X-linked inherited.
    C. Autosomal recessive microencephaly is associated with mutation in gene *MCPH1*.
    D. The gene *MCPH1* maps to chromosome 15.
    E. It can be dominantly inherited.

13. Ocular changes that occur in encephalofacial angiomatosis (Sturge-Weber-Dimitri syndrome) are:

    A. Choroidal angioma
    B. Congenital glaucoma
    C. Buphthalmos
    D. All of these
    E. None of these

14. In tuberous sclerosis complex, typical visceral lesions are:

    A. Hamartomas of the kidneys
    B. Rhabdomyoma of the heart
    C. Angioma of the pancreas
    D. Hepatoma
    E. Thymoma

15. Histologic changes that characterize tuberous sclerosis are:

    A. Subependymal ventricular nodules
    B. Heterotopia
    C. Cortical tubers
    D. Four-layered cerebral cortex
    E. Hydromyelia

16. The typical radiologic finding in encephalofacial angiomatosis is:

    A. Periventricular calcification
    B. A small sella turcica
    C. Double-contoured curving lines in the cerebral cortex
    D. Calcification in the globus pallidus
    E. Thinning of the frontal bone

17. Histologic changes commonly encountered in the brains of individuals with Down syndrome who died after age 30–35 years include:

    A. Pick bodies
    B. Neuritic plaques
    C. α-Synuclein positive cytoplasmic inclusions
    D. Neurofibrillary tangles
    E. Amyloid precursor protein (APP) deposits in neuritic plaques

(Answers are provided in the Appendix.)

CHAPTER 14

Fetal and Perinatal Cerebral Pathology

Pathology of Vascular Insults
Late Sequelae of Vascular Insults
Metabolic and Toxic Diseases
Congenital and Neonatal Infections
Sudden Infant Death Syndrome

A number of insults—vascular, infectious, toxic, metabolic, and traumatic—may afflict fetuses and neonates. Vascular insults are especially implicated in a variety of nervous system diseases that can occur during the fetal and perinatal periods. Due to the unique reaction of the immature neural tissue to noxious agents, vascular cerebral injuries occurring during these periods present distinct pathology.

PATHOLOGY OF VASCULAR INSULTS

Fetal Period

Vascular insults during the fetal period, from the seventh or eighth week of gestation to birth, can produce a dual pathology; a destructive lesion associated with a malformation. Two major conditions of this period are (a) *schizencephaly*, often referred to as *porencephaly*, and (b) *hydranencephaly*. (See Chapter 13 on malformations.) (Fig. 14.1)

Schizencephaly is a defect in the cerebral wall, which is surrounded by malformed convolutions. It is associated with a vascular insult in the middle cerebral artery territory.

Hydranencephaly, the replacement of the cerebral hemispheres with two membranous cysts, is attributed to a vascular insult in the carotid artery territory.

Perinatal Period

Pathologic conditions of this period, which roughly encompasses the time from 6 to 8 weeks before birth to 4 weeks after, are (a) intracranial hemorrhages and (b) hypoxic-ischemic parenchymal necrosis. A variety of factors can cause a hemorrhage or induce a hypoxic-ischemic insult and subsequent cerebral perfusion failure (Table 14.1). Prematurity and infection of the mother and/or fetus are major risks for both hemorrhagic and

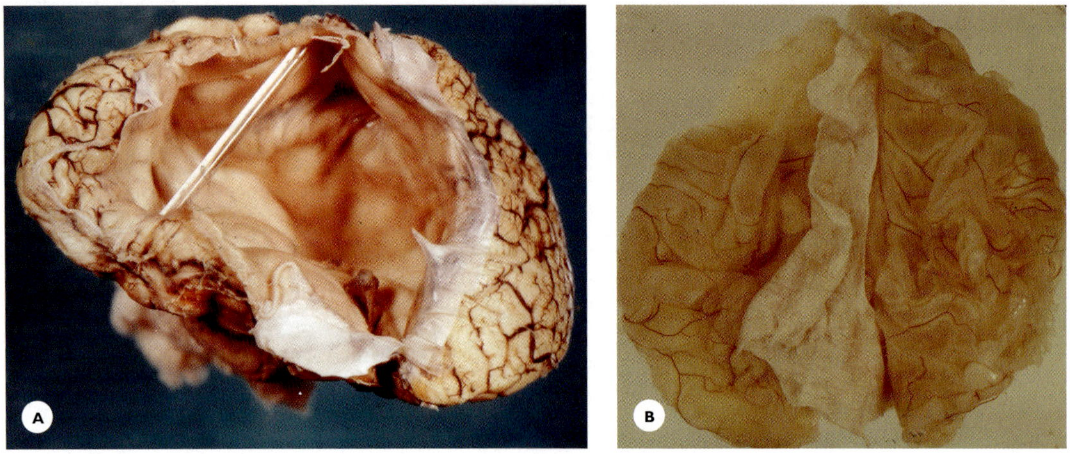

FIGURE 14.1
Malformations of the fetal period. **A.** Schizencephaly or porencephaly in the brain of a 20-year old man with left hemiplegia and hypoplasia of the extremities. A large defect occcupies the lateral wall of the right hemispehere. **B.** Hydranencephaly in a 3-year-old boy. His delivery had been induced because of fetal distress, and the cyanotic newborn needed resuscitation. He showed no awareness of his surroundings during his entire life: he was paralyzed, had cyanotic spells, seizures, and a low temperature. The cerebral surface is smooth; in places, irregular folds represent convolutional remnants.

TABLE 14.1.
Etiologies of Perinatal Vascular Pathology

Intracranial Hemorrhages	*Hypoxic-Ischemic Parenchymal Necrosis*
Prematurity Low birth weight Mechanical injury Neonatal sepsis Cerebral venous/sinus thrombosis Vascular malformation Maternal hematologic diseases Maternal cocaine use	Hyaline membrane disease: (Acute respiratory distress syndrome) Anomalous placenta and umbilical cord Maternal hypertension/ toxemia/anemia Aspiration of amniotic fluid Congenital heart disease Neonatal sepsis Twinning: (feto-fetal transfusion syndrome)

ischemic necroses. About 90% of preterm newborns survive; about 10% to 50% of the survivors will have some motor, cognitive, or behavioral deficits.

Intracranial Hemorrhages

A *germinal matrix zone hemorrhage*, the most typical hemorrhage of the newborn, occurs between the head of the caudate nucleus and the thalamus. This area contains proliferating germinal cells and thin-walled, fragile blood vessels that are prone to rupture and bleed. The hemorrhage may extend into the ventricle or the hemispheric white matter. *Primary ventricular hemorrhage* arises from the choroid plexus. *Subarachnoid hemorrhage*, at the base or over the hemispheres, often is associated with asphyxia or the mother's hematologic disease and sepsis. *Subdural hematoma,* usually traumatic, results from a tearing of bridging or cortical veins (Fig. 14.2).

Hypoxic-Ischemic Parenchymal Necrosis

The lesions of hypoxic-ischemic insult may involve either the cerebral cortex, the white matter, or both.

Periventricular leukomalacia, a typical white matter lesion in neonates, is situated in front of or around the anterior horns; it may extend posteriorly along the ventricular walls. Grossly, the periventricular white matter is yellow, soft, and chalky (Fig. 14.3). Histologically, the necrotic tissue is invaded by macrophages and, in time, is replaced by a glial scar or a small cavity. Diffuse white matter changes interfere with myelination by affecting the premyelinating oligodendrocytes.

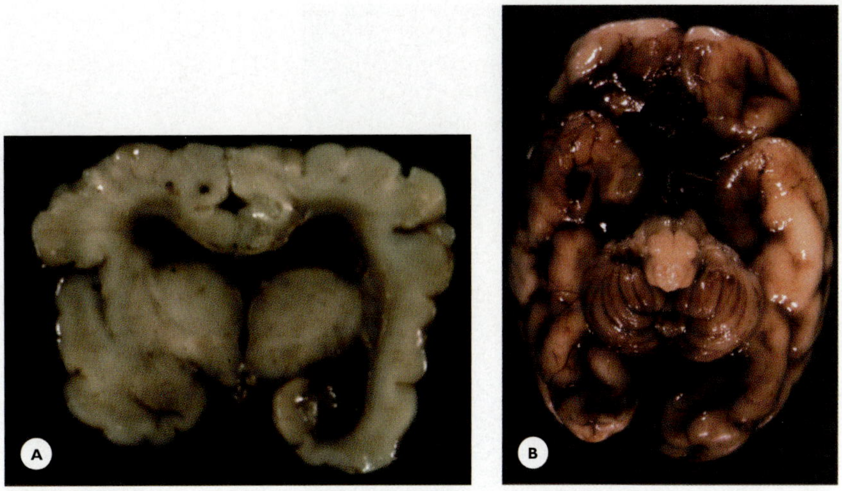

FIGURE 14.2
Intracranial hemorrhages. **A.** Germinal matrix zone hemorrhage extends into the ventricle in a premature infant. **B.** Basal subarachnoid hemorrhage in a premature infant.

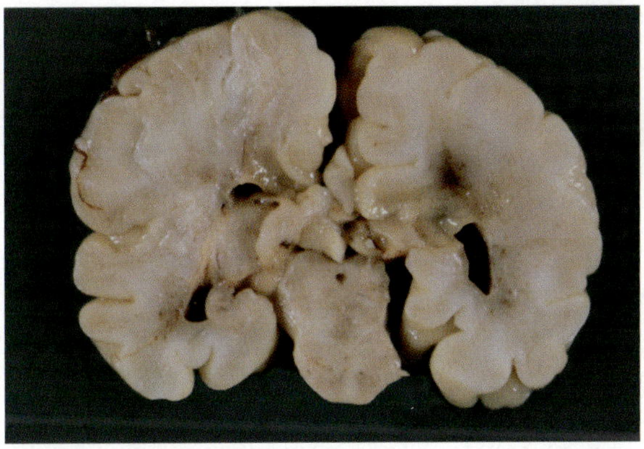

FIGURE 14.3
Periventricular leukomalacia. The periventricular white matter is yellow and soft in this premature infant.

Cortical necrosis, patchy or laminar, varies in extent from small foci to widespread areas. Variable neuronal losses may also occur in deep gray structures and the cerebellum.

LATE SEQUELAE OF VASCULAR INJURIES

Survivors of a severe hypoxic-ischemic episode in the perinatal period display a variety of distinct cerebral lesions. The cerebral cortex, hemispheric white matter, deep gray structures, and cerebellar cortex are affected in varying combinations (Table 14.2). Clinically, the lesions manifest with mental retardation, motor deficits, visual impairment, and seizures, the severity of which vary with the extent and location of the lesions.

TABLE 14.2.
Late Sequelae of Perinatal Hypoxic-Ischemic Insults

Sclerotic microgyria (ulegyria)
Multicystic leukomalacia
Porencephaly
Diffuse sclerosis of white matter
Status marmoratus of deep gray structures
Atrophy and sclerosis of cerebellum

Sclerotic Microgyria or Ulegyria

Grossly, in sclerotic microgyria or ulegyria (Figs. 14.4 through 14.7), the brain is small, and the affected convolutions are severely atrophic and sclerotic. They extend from a few convolutions or one or several lobes to the entire cortex of one or both hemispheres. Any region of the cortex may be involved, but preferentially the frontal and parietal lobes, medial occipital convolutions, and hippocampus. On transverse sections, the affected convolutions display a mushroom shape due to more severe destruction of their walls than of their crests. Histologically, the cortex shows multiple patchy, but more often laminar, neuronal losses involving one or several laminae or the entire width of the cortex. Remaining dead neurons are encrusted with iron and calcium (ferrugination).

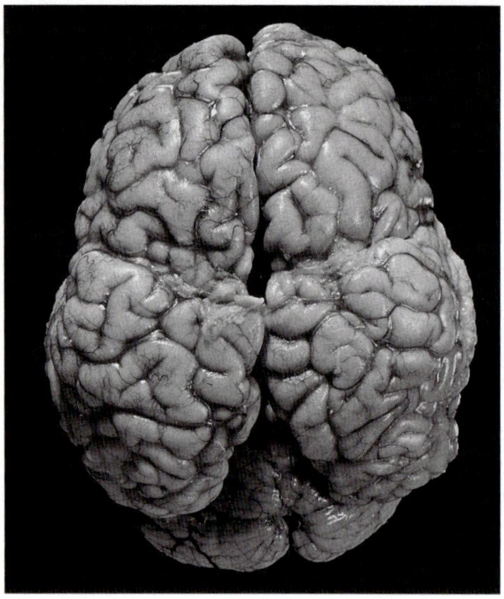

FIGURE 14.4
Bilateral symmetrical sclerotic microgyria in a 2.5-year-old mentally retarded, epileptic, and quadriplegic boy. He had been delivered 2 weeks premature and labor was complicated by premature separation of the placenta. The dorsal aspects of the cerebral hemispheres show sclerotic atrophy of the central convolutions.

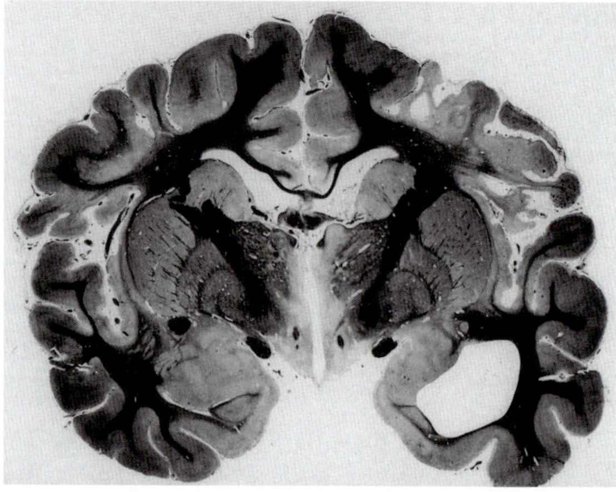

FIGURE 14.5
Multifocal sclerotic microgyria. A 5-year-old boy, severely retarded, quadriplegic, and epileptic was born cyanotic and did not cry for hours. The mother was hypertensive and hemorrhaged during pregnancy, heavily before delivery. Macrosection of the cerebral hemispheres shows multifocal cortical necrosis and diffuse white matter atrophy (Weil stain). Note the mushroom-shaped atrophy of the convolutions.

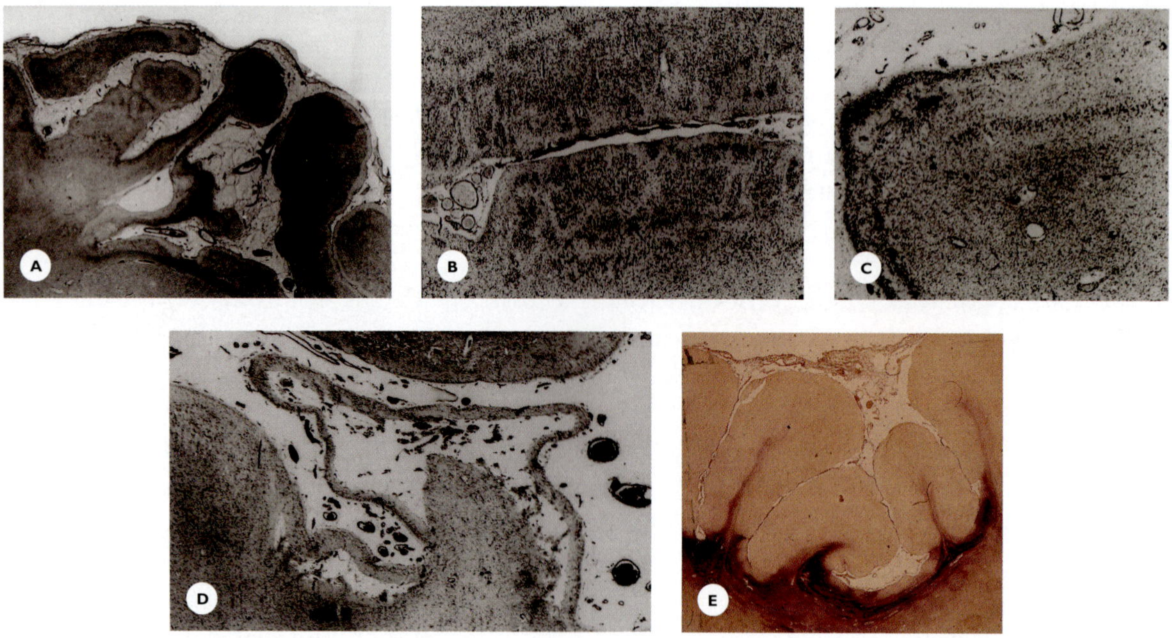

FIGURE 14.6
Histology of sclerotic microgyria. **A.** The necrosis is confined chiefly to the walls and depths of convolutions, giving a mushroom shape. **B.** Multifocal neuronal losses. **C.** Multilaminar neuronal losses, **D.** Necrosis of the entire width of the cortex (cresyl violet). **E.** Dense astrofibrosis in subcortical white matter (Holzer stain).

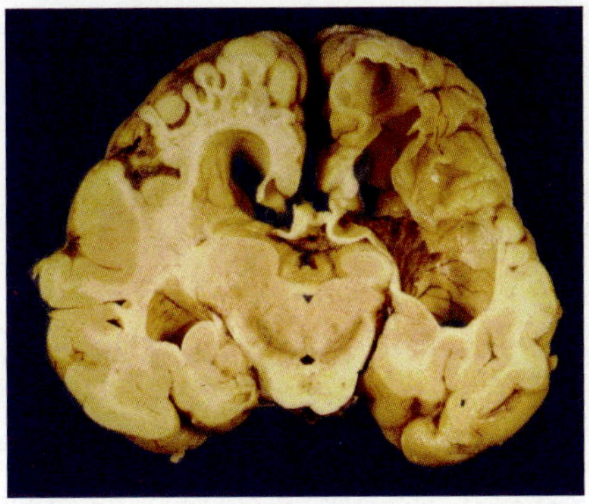

FIGURE 14.7
Porencephaly with sclerotic microgyria. An 8-year-old severely retarded epileptic girl was a twin, delivered second. Transverse section shows a large porencephalic cyst in one hemisphere and sclerotic atrophic convolutions in the opposite hemisphere.

Leukoencephalopathy

In *multicystic leukomalacia*, the cerebral hemispheric white matter is partially or completely replaced with multiloculated cysts separated by strands of fibroglial tissue. Their lumens contain residual macrophages and tissue debris (Fig 14.8).

A porencephalic cyst denotes a large, circumscribed defect in the cerebral wall caused by a vascular insult during the last trimester of gestation. The cyst connects the ventricle with the subarachnoid space. Its wall is lined with gliovascular tissue, and the overlying cerebral cortex may be necrotic but *is not malformed* (Fig. 14.9).

Diffuse gliosis of the white matter is attributed to early ischemic edema.

Status Marmoratus

Status marmoratus (marbling) of the thalamus and basal ganglia results from glial scarring. Bundles of hypermyelinated nerve fibers between glial scars give a marbled appearance (Fig. 14.10).

Cerebellar Sclerosis

In cerebellar sclerosis, grossly, the cerebellar cortex is atrophic and sclerotic, more severely in the depth and

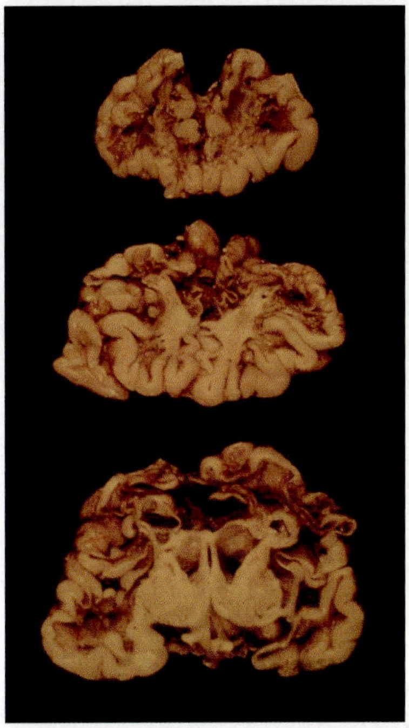

FIGURE 14.8
Multicystic leukomalacia in a 6-year-old quadriplegic, epileptic, and speechless boy. He was delivered by forceps at full term and was cyanotic for 3 days. The mother's pregnancy was complicated by episodes of vaginal bleeding and premature separation of the placenta. Transverse sections of the brain reveal diffuse multicystic necrosis of the white matter extending from the frontal to the occipital lobes. The cortex is necrotic in some areas, and relatively preserved in others.

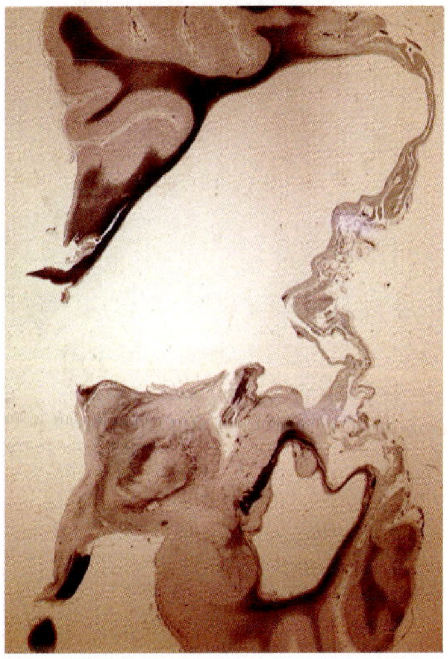

FIGURE 14.9
A porencephalic cyst occupies the entire width of the cerebral wall. The overlying cortex is necrotic (myelin stains).

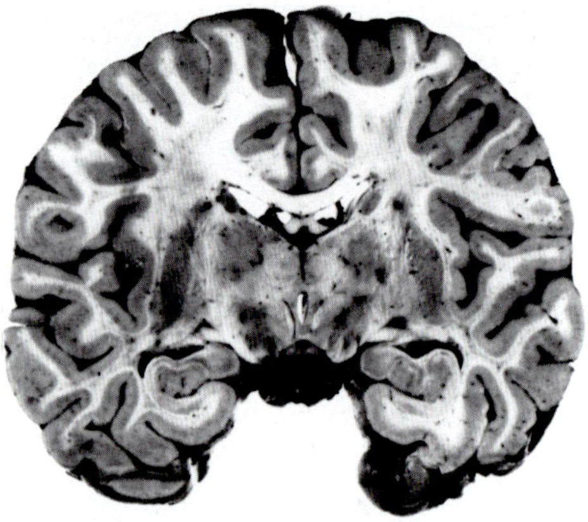

FIGURE 14.10
Status marmoratus. Patchy whitish discoloration in thalamus from bundles of hypermyelinated nerve fibers.

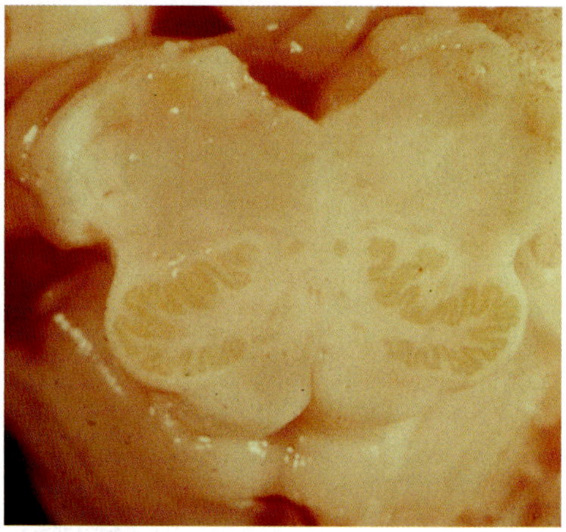

FIGURE 14.12
Bilirubin encephalopathy, acute. Medulla. Deposits of bilirubin pigments stain the inferior olivary nuclei yellow.

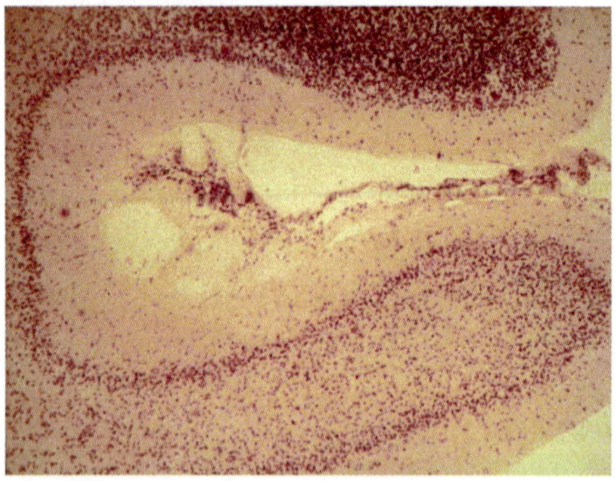

FIGURE 14.11
Cerebellum showing extensive Purkinje cell losses, some granular cell losses, and prominent Bergmann astrocytosis.

walls of folia. Histologically, it displays extensive Purkinje cell and variable granule cell losses. A prominent Bergmann astrocytic layer forms at the site of lost Purkinje cells. The white matter shows astrocytic fibrillary gliosis, and the dentate nuclei show neuronal losses (Fig. 14.11).

METABOLIC AND TOXIC DISEASES

Bilirubin Encephalopathy

Bilirubin encephalopathy or kernicterus results from elevated unconjugated serum bilirubin: 20 mg/100 mL or higher in mature infants, and lower in immature infants.

Hyperbilirubinemia may result from hemolytic anemia due to incompatibility of RH groups; failure of bilirubin conjugation due to liver damage; congenital enzyme (glucuronyl transferase) deficiency; and certain drugs. Unconjugated bilirubin crosses the blood–brain barrier to injure selected neuronal groups.

Clinical manifestations during the neonatal period are lethargy, hypertonia with opisthotonus, loss of Moro reflex, and seizures. Survivors of the encephalopathy are mentally retarded and display choreoathetosis, dystonia, ataxia, gaze palsy, and hearing deficit.

Pathology: the most severely affected regions in a symmetric distribution, are the globus pallidus, subthalamic nucleus and hippocampus. Variably involved structures include the thalamus; mammillary bodies; lateral geniculate bodies; substantia nigra; brainstem reticular nuclei; third, fourth, and eighth cranial nerve nuclei; and the dentate and olivary nuclei. Grossly, during the acute stage, the affected regions, in unfixed preparation, are bright yellow from deposits of bilirubin pigments (bilirubin pigments dissolve in formalin (Fig. 14.12). Histologically, the neurons show chromatolysis, eosinophilia, and vacuolization of the perikaryon. Neurons and glial cells may contain bilirubin pigments. Chronic cases show neuronal losses and replacement astrocytosis in the affected regions (Fig. 14.13).

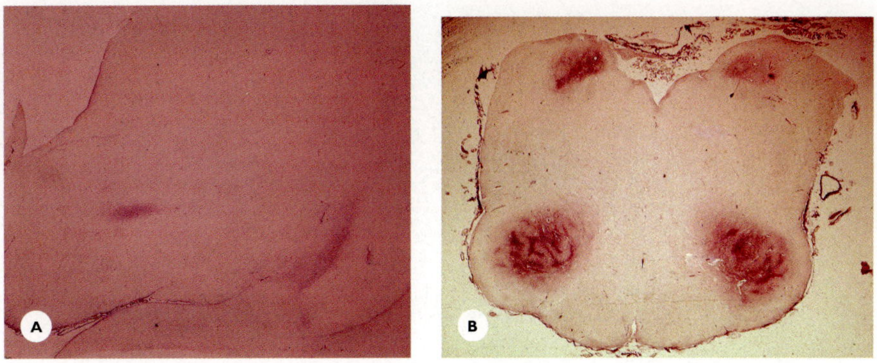

FIGURE 14.13
Bilirubin encephalopathy, late sequelae, in a 14-year-old severely retarded, deaf, spastic-athetotic boy. Dense astrogliosis in (**A**) subthalamic nucleus and (**B**) inferior olivary nuclei and floor of fourth ventricle.

TABLE 14.3.
Fetal Alcohol Syndrome

Craniofacial anomalies:
Small head, narrow palpebral fissure, low nasal bridge, small midface, thin upper lip
Low-birth weight
Growth retardation
Poor motor skills
Hearing deficit
Cognitive deficits
Behavioral disorder

Intrauterine Exposure to Alcohol and Illicit Substances

Regular or episodic excessive maternal drinking results in a spectrum of clinical and pathologic abnormalities in infants ranging from cognitive deficits and behavioral disorders through cerebral malformations to full-blown fetal alcohol syndrome (Table 14.3). The abuse of illicit substances, particularly cocaine and heroine, during pregnancy carries the risk of growth retardation and microcephaly.

Lead Toxicity

Lead toxicity, rare at present, is acquired by exposure to lead-containing paint and dust, and to pica (craving for unnatural food). The toxicity presents with an acute encephalopathy with seizures and signs of raised intracranial pressure (ICP). Protein is elevated in the cerebrospinal fluid (CSF). Anemia and basophilic stippling of red blood cells are hematologic abnormalities. Grossly, the brain is edematous. The histology consists of endothelial swelling, leakage of serum into the perivascular space, and occasional petechial hemorrhages.

CONGENITAL AND NEONATAL INFECTIONS

The most common pathogens of congenital and neonatal infections are viruses and the protozoa *Toxoplasma gondii*. Bacteria and the spirochete *Treponema pallidum* are less common. (See Chapter 6 on infectious diseases.) Fetuses are infected transplacentally, and neonates are infected during delivery through an infected birth canal or by breast feeding with infected milk. The maternal infection may be acutely acquired or more often results from reactivation of a clinically latent infection. Infections during the first trimester produce the most widespread injuries, notably inflammatory destructive lesions in the brain, sensory organs, and viscera, and malformations (Table 14.4). Among the major malformations are hydranencephaly, polymicrogyria, hydrocephalus, and microcephaly. The neurologic sequelae of infections acquired later in gestation are mental retardation; visual, auditory, and motor deficits; and seizures. Maternal infections are diagnosed by serologic tests, and fetal infections are diagnosed using polymerase chain reaction (PCR) assay.

Congenital Cytomegalovirus Infection

Congenital cytomegalovirus infection is the most common fetal infection, affecting an estimated 1% of newborns. It may present at birth with neurologic and

TABLE 14.4.
Major Congenital Infections

Symptoms Signs	*Cytomegalovirus Infection*	*Congenital Rubella Syndrome*	*Congenital Toxoplasmosis*
Ocular	Chorioretinitis Optic atrophy	Pigmentary retinopathy Cataract, microphthalmia	Chorioretinitis
Auditory	Neuronal deafness	Neuronal deafness	
Visceral	Cardiovascular anomalies Pneumonitis Hepatosplenomegaly Thrombocytopenia	Cardiopulmonary anomalies Hepatosplenomegaly Thrombocytopenia	Hepatosplenomegaly Thrombocytopenia Anemia
Cranial	Microcephaly	Microcephaly	Microcephaly
Cerebral	Necrotizing meningoencephalitis with cytomegalic cells Periventricular calcification Polymicrogryria	Proliferative/degenerative vascular changes with mineralization Ischemic necrosis	Granulomatous meningoencephalitis Calcifications in gray and white matter

systemic features or later with mental retardation, motor deficits, and seizures.

Grossly, the brain is small and may display polymicrogyria and porencephaly. The histology is characterized by (a) multifocal necrotizing encephalitis, preferentially in the walls of ventricles; (b) periventricular calcifications, and (c) cytomegalic cells throughout the gray and white matter, which display large intranuclear and small cytoplasmic inclusions.

Congenital Rubella Infection

Since the introduction of rubella vaccine (1969), the rubella syndrome is rare. Grossly, the brain is small and atrophic. The histology is distinguished by (a) vascular changes with necrosis, fibrosis, and mineralization of vessel's walls; and (b) perivascular infiltrations and multifocal inflammatory necrosis. Rarely, the rubella syndrome progresses slowly, presenting several years later as a panencephalitis leading to dementia and severe neurologic deficits. Diffuse demyelination and gliosis are the underlying pathology.

Herpes Virus Infection

Herpes virus infection is more common with herpes virus type 2; about 5% of infections are acquired *in utero* and 85% during parturition. The pathology is a severe necrotizing inflammation of the cerebrum and visceral organs.

Varicella

Congenital varicella infection associated with the varicella/zoster (V2V) virus manifests with systemic features (cutaneous scars, cataract, chorioretinitis, skeletal anomalies) and mental retardation. The cerebral pathology consists of a diffuse chronic inflammatory granulomatous encephalitis. Polymicrogyria may be present.

Congenital and Neonatal HIV Infection

Fetal HIV infections occur in 15% to 40% of untreated maternal infections. The cerebral pathology is characterized by glial nodules of activated microglial cells, macrophages, and multinucleated giant cells; vascular mineralizations in the basal ganglia and white matter; and perivascular lymphocytic infiltrations.

Toxoplasmosis

Congenital toxoplasma infection is estimated at 1 per 1,000 to 1 per 10,000 live births. The infection may manifest at birth with chorioretinitis, hydrocephalus, and intracranial calcifications. Late manifestations are mental retardation and seizures. Grossly, the atrophic brain displays small necrotic granulomas, and necrotic tissue may line the ventricles. The histology is characterized by a granulomatous meningoencephalitis consisting of multiple focal areas of necrosis, granulations, mononuclear cell infiltrations, and mineralization. The *Toxo-*

plasma gondii organisms are enclosed in cysts that may rupture and release the organisms. Obstructive hydrocephalus due to ependymitis is common.

Congenital Neurosyphilis

The neurologic manifestations of syphilis may appear at any age from infancy to adolescence as syphilitic meningitis, meningovascular syphilis, juvenile paresis, and tabes dorsalis. The stigmata of congenital syphilis—hearing loss, chorioretinitis, dental anomalies, and interstitial keratitis—are present in a high percentage of cases.

SUDDEN INFANT DEATH SYNDROME

The death of an infant under 1 year of age that, after an autopsy and clinical review, can not be explained, is called sudden infant death syndrome (SIDS). The incidence is estimated at 0.6 per 1,000 live births, with a male predominance. The etiology is elusive. Both genetic and environmental factors are implicated. The occurrence of SIDS is higher among families with genetic disorders and also subsequent to maternal heavy cigarette smoking and drinking during pregnancy.

Pathologic and experimental studies point to a pathogenetic role of the medullary serotonergic system that controls autonomic functions and arousal. It is suggested that autonomic and respiratory failure due to a prenatal injury to the medullary serotonergic raphe nuclei, and also to some nonserotonergic nuclei, account for the sudden death.

BIBLIOGRAPHY

Folkerth, R.D. (Ed.). (2005). Symposium: perinatal brain injury. *Brain Pathol 15*, 223–260.

Friede, R.L. (1989). *Developmental neuropathology*, 2nd edition (revised). New York: Springer-Verlog.

Golden, J.A., Harding, B.N. (2004). *Pathology and genetics*. Basel: Developmental Neuropathology ISN, Neuropath Press.

Johnson, R.T. (1998). *Viral infections of the nervous system*, 2nd edition. Philadelphia: Lippincott-Raven.

Rorke, L.B. (1982). *Pathology of perinatal brain injury*. New York: Raven Press.

Rorke, L.B. (1992). Anatomical features of the developing brain implicated in pathogenesis of hypoxic-ischemic injury. *Brain Pathol* 3, 211–221.

REVIEW QUESTIONS

1. A cerebral hemorrhage typical in premature infants is:
   - A. Subdural hematoma
   - B. Putaminal hemorrhage
   - C. Pontine hemorrhage
   - D. Epidural hematoma
   - E. Germinal matrix zone hemorrhage

2. Lesions associated with bilirubin encephalopathy typically involve the following structures:
   - A. Substantia nigra and cerebral cortex
   - B. Ammon's horn and frontal cortex
   - C. Occipital cortex and subthalamic nucleus
   - D. Globus pallidus, Ammon's horn, and subthalamic nucleus
   - E. Cerebellum and frontal lobe

3. Histologic changes that occur in congenital cytomegalovirus infection are:
   - A. Polymicrogyria
   - B. Periventricular calcification
   - C. Necrotizing ventriculitis
   - D. All of these
   - E. None of these

4. The lesion that is encountered in the brain of a premature infant who suffered a severe hypoxic insult is:
   - A. Cortical calcification
   - B. Periventricular leukomalacia
   - C. Microgyria
   - D. Necrotizing granuloma
   - E. Cerebellar atrophy

5. Late pathologic sequelae of severe perinatal hypoxic insult are:
   A. Sclerotic microgyria
   B. Heterotopia
   C. Porencephaly
   D. Status marmoratus of the thalamus
   E. Cortical dysplasia

6. Ocular pathology associated with congenital toxoplasmosis includes:
   A. Cataract
   B. Pigmentary degeneration
   C. Glaucoma
   D. All of these
   E. None of these

7. Neurologic manifestations observed in children who suffered a bilirubin encephalopathy during the neonatal period are:
   A. Athetosis
   B. Chorea
   C. Dystonia
   D. Any of these
   E. None of these

8. Risk factors for sudden infant death syndrome (SIDS) include:
   A. Prematurity
   B. Maternal cigarette smoking during pregnancy
   C. Excessive maternal alcohol consumption and illicit substance abuse during pregnancy
   D. All of these
   E. None of these

(Answers are provided in the Appendix.)

APPENDIX

Answers to Review Questions

CHAPTER 1
INTRODUCTION TO CLINICAL NEUROPATHOLOGY

1. D
2. B
3. D
4. D
5. B

CHAPTER 2
BASICS OF NEUROPATHOLOGY

1. E
2. B
3. D
4. C
5. E
6. C
7. A
8. D
9. E
10. D
11. D
12. E

CHAPTER 3
CEREBRAL HYPOXIA

1. C
2. B
3. C
4. D
5. B
6. C
7. A
8. E
9. D
10. E

CHAPTER 4
CEREBROVASCULAR DISEASES

1. E
2. C
3. D
4. B
5. C
6. B
7. D
8. D
9. C
10. D
11. A
12. B
13. D
14. D

CHAPTER 5
NEURODEGENERATIVE DISEASES

1. B, C, D, E
2. B, D, E
3. A, C, D, E
4. B, C, D
5. A, B
6. B, C, E
7. B, C, D, E
8. D
9. A, B, C
10. A, C, D, E

11. A
12. D
13. A, B
14. B, C, E
15. D
16. A, B, C, E
17. D
18. A, D, E
19. D
20. A

CHAPTER 6
INFECTIOUS DISEASES

1. B
2. C
3. D
4. B
5. C
6. B
7. B
8. C
9. B
10. E
11. A
12. D
13. C
14. E

CHAPTER 7
PRION DISEASES

1. B
2. A, D
3. B, C, E
4. A, B, D, E
5. C, D, E
6. A, C, D

CHAPTER 8
DEMYELINATING DISEASES

1. A, B, C, D, E
2. D
3. B
4. B
5. B
6. B
7. A, C
8. C, E
9. B
10. A, B, C, D, E

CHAPTER 9
HEREDITARY NEUROMETABOLIC DISEASES

1. A, B, C
2. B
3. A, D
4. A, B, C, D, E
5. D
6. A, B, C
7. A, B, C
8. B
9. D, E
10. A, C, D
11. B, C, E
12. A, C, D
13. A, B, C
14. A, C, D
15. C, D
16. B, C
17. A, C, D, E
18. A, C, E

CHAPTER 10
ACQUIRED NEUROMETABOLIC DISEASE

1. A
2. B, C
3. B
4. C
5. C
6. E

CHAPTER 11
NEOPLASMS

1. A, C, D
2. A, C
3. B, C, D
4. A, C, D
5. A, B
6. B, D, E
7. A, D, E
8. A, C, E
9. B
10. A, B, D
11. B, C
12. A, B, C, D
13. A, B, D
14. D
15. A, C, D
16. B
17. A, B, E
18. A, C, D
19. D, E
20. D

CHAPTER 12
TRAUMATIC INJURIES OF THE CENTRAL NERVOUS SYSTEM

1. C
2. D
3. D
4. A, C
5. C
6. D
7. D
8. A, B, C, D

CHAPTER 13
CONGENITAL MALFORMATIONS OF THE CENTRAL NERVOUS SYSTEM

1. A, B
2. B
3. B
4. A
5. A, B, C, D
6. B, C
7. A
8. A
9. D
10. A, B
11. E
12. A
13. D
14. A, B
15. A, B, C
16. C
17. B, D, E

CHAPTER 14
FETAL AND PERINATAL CEREBRAL PATHOLOGY

1. E
2. D
3. D
4. B
5. A, C, D
6. E
7. D
8. D

Index

A
Abcess, 137
Abetalipoproteinemia, 110, 195
Acanthamoeba, 142–143
Acanthocytosis, 109
Acetylcholine (ACh), 88, 103
Achondroplasia, 295
Acoustic schwannoma, 238
Acquired immune deficiency syndrome. *See* AIDS
Acquired obstructive hydrocephalus, 27
Acromegaly, 236
Activated microglia, 17
Active chronic plaque, multiple sclerosis, 159–161
Acute hemorrhagic leukoencephalitis, 167
Acute radiation effect, 255
Acute respiratory distress syndrome, 300
Addison disease, 181
Adenomas, pituitary, of, 235–236
AD-PEO, Autosomal dominant progressive external ophthalmoplegia, 188
Adrenal insufficiency, 180
Adrenoleukodystrophies (ALDs), 186, 181, 280
Adrenomyeloneuropathy (AMN), 181
Adult NCL, Neuronal ceroid lipofuscinosis, 175
Adult Refsum's disease (ARD), 181–182
AFP (α-fetoprotein), 111
African trypanosomiasis, 142, 144
Agenesis of the corpus callosum, 284
Aging, cerebral changes in, 27–29
Aging, premature, 111
Agyria, 280–281
AIDS, 119, 131
  lymphomas and, 246
  opportunistic infections in, 133
  trypanosomiasis, and, 144–145
Air and gas embolization, injuries, from, 270
Akinetic rigidity, extrapyramidal diseases with, 101–107
Akinitic mutism, locked-in syndrome and coma compared, 59
Alcohol, 110
  abuse, 205–210
  methyl, 209
  syndrome, fetal, 305
ALDs (adrenoleukodystrophies), 186
Alexander's disease, 185–186, 287
Alexander's leukodystrophy, 14
α-1–4-glucosidase deficiency, 179
α-fetoprotein, 111, 237
α-galactosidase deficiency, 174
α-keto-acid dehydrogenase, 189
α-L-iduronidase deficiency, 178
α-lipoprotein, 196
α-synuclein, 11, 84, 91, 101, 115
α-tocopherol, 200
α-tocopherol transfer protein gene, 111
ALS, 97–99
Alsin, 98
Aluminum, 90, 209
Alzheimer type 1 and 2 astrocytes, 14, 192, 203
Alzheimer's disease, 68, 84, 85–91
Amaurosis fugax, 73
Amebiasis, 143
Amenorrhea, 236
American trypanosomiasis, 142, 144
Amino acid metabolic diseases, 188–189
Amino acids, 170
Aminoacidurias, 110
Ammon's horn sclerosis, 40–41
AMN (adrenomyeloneuropathy), 181
Amnesia, 268
Amniotic fluid, 120
  aspiration of, 300
Amoebiasis, 142
Amphetamine, 75
Amyelia, 276
Amylacea, corpora, 14, 15
Amyloid angiopathy, 68, 87
Amyloid precursor protein (APP), 90, 265
Amyotrophic CJD, 154
Amyotrophic lateral sclerosis (ALS), 97–99
Anaplastic astrocytoma, 252
Anaplastic meningioma, 232, 233
Anaplastic oligodendroglioma, 226
Anaplastic pontine astrocytoma, 220
Androgen receptor, 110
Anemia, 33
  maternal, 300
  anemic hypoxia, 33
Anencephaly, 275, 276
Aneurysms, subarachnoid hemorrhage and, 64, 69
Angiitis, primary central nervous system, 68
Angiofibromas, 289
Angiomas, 70
Angiomatosis, 250
Angiomatous meningioma, 233
Angiomatosis osteohypertrophy, 291
Angiosarcoma, 244, 245
Animal prion disease, 152
Anterograde (wallerian) degeneration, 19–20
Anterograde amnesia, 268
Anthrax meningoencephalitis, 121–122
Anticardiolipin antibody, 73
Anticoagulants, 75, 280
Antiphospholipid antibody syndrome, 66, 67, 72–75

Antithrombin-III deficiences, 72
Anti-yo antibodies, 256
Antoni types A and B schwannomas, 239
Aortic arch syndrome, 67–68
Anaplastic astrocytoma, 217–219
Aplasia of the granular cell layer, 286–287
APOE4 (apoliprotein E4), 90
Apoliprotein E4 (APOE4), 90
Apoptosis, 84, 279
  neurons, of, 12–13
APP (amyloid precursor protein), 90, 265
Aqueduct of Sylvius, 16, 26, 293–294
  stenosis and atresia of, 287, 294
Arachnoid, 18–19
  cysts, 243, 288
  villi, 18–19
Arboviruses (arthropod borne), 126, 127
ARD (Adult Refsum's disease), 181
Area cerebrovasculosa, 275
Argyll-Robertson pupils, 141
Argyophilic fibrils, 8
Argyrophilic astrocytic plaque, 15
Argyrophilic grain dementia, 16
Argyrophilic inclusions, 14
Arhinencephaly, 278
Arnold-Chiari malformation, 26, 275, 277
  type 2, 293, 294
Arrhythmias, cardiac, 33, 65
Arsenic, 209
Arterial dissection, 66, 76–77
Arteries
  basal cerebral, 70–71
  cerebral, 19
  cervicocranial, 44–47
Arteriopathies, heriditary, 68
Arteriosclerosis, 44–47, 77–79
  atherosclerosis, 44
  arteriolosclerosis, 44, 61, 77
Arteriovenous angioma, 245
Arteriovenous fistula of the vein of Galen, 288
Arylsulfatase A (ASA), 183
Aseptic encephalitis, 125
Aseptic meningitis, 125, 130
Aseptic myelitis, 125
Aspartylglucosaminuria, 177, 179
Asperillosis, 138
Asperillus fumigatus, 138
Astrocytes, 13–14
Astrocytic fibrillary gliosis, 35
Astrocytic gliosis, 89
Astrocytic tumors, 216, 222
  children, in, 252
Astrocytoma, 250, 254, 255
Ataxia
  episodic, 112
  isolated witamin E deficiency
  telangiectasia, 109, 111
Ataxic CJD, 154
Ataxin, 110
Atherosclerosis, 44
Atherothrombosis, 66
Atresia of the aqueduct of Sylvius, 287, 294
Atrial fibrillation, chronic, 45
Atrophin-1, 110
Autoimmune pathogenesis, 157–167
Autolysis, *in vivo*, 37
Autosomal dominant progressive external ophthalmoplegia (AD-PEO), 188
Axonal spheroids, 12
Axonal torpedo, 12
Axons, 8, 11–12
  multiple sclerosis, in, 159
  trauma, in, 265

B
B cell lymphoma, 134
B cells, 125
B. streptococcus, 120
Bacillus anthracis, 121
Bacteria, 68
Bacterial infection, 120–124
Bailey, 216
Balloon cell, 283
Ballooned achromatic neurons, 10
Balo's concentric sclerosis, 165
Basal cerebral arteries, anomalies of, 70–71
Basal ganglia hemorrhage, 63
Bassen-Kornzweig disease, 195
Batten-Vogt-Spielmeyer disease, 175
Battered children, 267. *See also* Shaken baby syndrome
BBB (blood-brain barrier), 19
B-cell lymphoma, 130
Benedikt syndrome, 58
Benign meningiomas, 232
Bergman astrocytes, 15, 35, 114, 256, 305
Berry aneurysm. *See* Saccular aneurysm
β-amyloid, 91
β-amyloid precursor protein (β-APP), 159
β-APP (β-amyloid precursor protein), 159
β-hemolytic streptococci, 121
Bielschowsky stain, 3
Bilirubin encephalopathy, 304
Binswanger's disease, 77, 78
Birth defects, 273–298
Bland infarct, 46
Blastomyces dermatitidis, 137
Blood vessels, 19
  tumors of, 244
Blood-brain barrier (BBB), 19
Blue cell tumor, 229
Blues (pyribenzamine), 75
Bodian stain, 3
Bone marrow transplants, 119
Bony erosions, 25
Border-zone infarct, 47–50
Borrelia burgdorferi, 68, 147
Bourneville-Pringle disease, 288
Bovine spongiform encephalopathy, 152
Boxing injuries, 270
Brain abcess, 122
Brain death, 37–39
Brain warts, 283
Brain weight disorders, 287–288
Brainstem (Düret) hemorrhage, 25
Brainstem, malformations of, 287
Breast carcinoma, 251, 255
Bronchogenic carcinomas, 75
BSE, Bovine spongiform encephalopathy, 152, 154
BSMA (bulbospinal muscular atrophy), 99, 100
Bulbar palsy, 98
Bulbospinal muscular atrophy (BSMA), 97, 99, 100, 109, 110
Bunina bodies, 11, 99
Buphthalmos, 291
Burnt-out plaque Alzheimer's disease, 87
Buscaino bodies, 29

C
CACNA1A, 110
Cactus formation dendrites, of, 11
CADASIL, cerebral autosomal dominant arteriopathy with subcortical infarcts and leukoencephalopathy, 68
Café-au-lait pigmentations, 254
Cajal stain, 3
Calcium metabolic disorders, 205–207
California encephalitis virus, 126, 127
Canavan's disease (Spongy degeneration), 183, 185, 287
Candidiasis, 138
Capillaries, 19
Capillary hemangioblastoma, 244, 250, 254
Capillary telangiectasis, 70, 245
Carbamazepine, 275
Carbohydrate, 170
  lysosomal diseases, 175
  metabolic diseases, 190–192
Carbon monoxide, 34, 104, 209
Carcinoembryonic antigen, 111
Carcinomas, 247–249, 251
  breast, of the, 257
  testes, of the, 256
Carcinomatous meningitis, 249
Cardiac arrest, 33
Cardiac arrhythmias, 33, 65
Cardiac valvular diseases, 73
Cardiomyopathy, 66
Caseation necrosis, 123
Caudate hemorrhage, 63
Cavernous angioma, 245
Cavitation stage of infarct, 46–47
Cavum septum pellucidum, 284
CBD (corticobasal degeneration), 96
CBS, cystathionine-β-synthase deficiency, 190
CD4⁺ T lymphocytes, 131, 163
CDG (congenital disorders of glycosylation), 195
Cell body, 8
Cellular (cytoxic) edema, 14, 21–22, 52
Central neuroblastoma, 230

Central neurocytoma, 228
Central pontine myelinosis, 207–208
CERAD (Consortium to Establish a Registry of Alzheimer's Disease), 86
Cerebellar ataxia, 109, 111, 112
Cerebellar cortical atrophy, 40–41
Cerebellar degenerations, 109–112
Cerebellar hemorrhage, 63
Cerebellar hypoplasia, 285
Cerebellar sclerosis, perinatal, 303–304
Cerebellar stroke syndromes, 59
Cerebellum congenital malformations of, 185–287
Cerebral arteries/infarcts, and 55–59
Cerebral atrophy, 85
  from alcohol abuse, 209
Cerebral calcification, 205, 207, 254
Cerebral candidiasis, 140
Cerebral changes, artificial, 29
Cerebral defects, 275
Cerebral edema, 21–22
Cerebral hemispheres, malformations of, 279–284
Cerebral mycoses, 133
Cerebral neoplasms, 75
Cerebral perfusions pressure (CPP), 37
Cerebral sinovenous thrombosis, 75
Cerebrohepatorenal syndrome, 180
Cerebrosides, 171
Cerebrospinal fluid (CSF), 18–19
Cerebrotendinous xanthomatosis, 196
Cerebrovascular diseases, 43–81
Ceruloplasmin, 192
Chagas disease, 142, 144
Chamarro tribe of Guam, 107
Charcot, 159
Charcot classic type MS, 165
Charcot joints, 141, 277
Chemotherapy complications, 255–256
Chiari malformations, 275–276, 293
Chiasma glioma, 254
Chickenpox. *See* Varicella zoster virus
Children, battered, 267. *See also* Shaken baby syndrome
Chiropractic manipulation, 75
Cholesterol lowering drugs, 91
Choline actyltransferase deficiency, 88
Cholinergic deficiency, 88, 91
Chondroma, 251
Chondrosarcoma, 251
Chordoid glioma of the third ventricle, 227
Chordoma, 237, 251
Choreic movements, 107
Choriocarcinoma, 75, 237, 238
Choristoma, 236
Choroid angioma, 291
Choroid plexus papilloma, 226–227, 251, 252
Christmas disease, 72
Chromatolysis, 9
Chromosomal disorders, fetal, 295–296
Chromosome 17-linked dementia, 104
Chronic basal meningitis, 138
Chronic wasting disease, 152
Cingulate gyri, absence of, 284
Circle of Willis, 69, 70
CJD (Creutzfeldt-Jakob disease), 152–154
Clear-cell meningioma, 233
Clotting factor VIII and IX, 72
CMV. *See* Cytomegalovirus
Coagulation factor V gene, 72
Coagulation, disorders of, 72
Coagulative leukoencephalopathy, 255
Coarctation of the aorta, 66
Cobalamine (Vitamin B_{12}), 200, 201–202, 203
Cocaine, 75
Coccidioides immitis, 137
Cockayne syndrome, 195
Coiled bodies, 16
Colloid cysts of the third ventricle, 243
Colpocephaly, 282
Coma, 37
  conditions resembling, 55, 59
  locked-in syndrome and akinitic mutism compared, 59
  persistent vegetative state *vs.*, 39
Compact plaque, 87
Concussion, 265, 268
Congenital arachnoid cyst, 288
Congenital cytomegalovirus infection, 305–306
Congenital disorders of glycosylation (CDG), 195
Congenital glaucoma, 291
Congenital heart disease, 66, 300
Congenital herpes virus infection, 306
Congenital HIV infection, 306
Congenital hydrocephalus, 285
Congenital immunodeficiency syndrome, 246
Congenital malformations. *See* Malformations, congenital
Congenital neurosyphilis, 142, 307
Congenital obstructive hydrocephalus, 26
Congenital rubella infection, 306
Congenital toxoplasmosis, 143, 306–307
Congenital tumors, 251–252
Congenital varicella infection, 306
Conjunctival telangiectasia, 111
Consortium to Establish a Registry of Alzheimer's Disease (CERAD), 86
Contraceptives, oral, 75
Contre-coup contusions, 265
Contusions, 264–266
Convolutions, malformations of, 279–284
Copper, 170
Copper metabolic diseases, 192–193
Corpora amylacea, 14, 15, 29, 78–79
Cortical atrophy, generalized, 91
Cortical calcifications, 291
Cortical cytoarchitecture
  anomalies, 291
  malformations of, 279–284
Cortical dysplasia, 280, 287
Cortical laminar pan-necrosis, 35
Cortical necrosis, perinatal, 301
Cortical tubers, 289–290
Corticobasal bodies, 96
Corticobasal degeneration (CBD), 96
Corticobasal dementia, 16, 104
Corticosteroids, 119
Coup contusions, 265
Cowden syndrome, 228
Cowdry inclusions, 125
Coxsackie virus, 126
CPP (cerebral perfusions pressure), 37
Crack, 75
Cranial defects, 275
Cranial nerves, tumors of, 238–240
Cranial ultrasound, 293
Craniopharyngioma, 237, 240–241, 252, 253
Craniosynostosis, 295
Cranium, tumors of, 251–253
Creutzfeldt-Jakob disease (CJD), 152–154, 156
  sporadic, 110
Cribriform state, 77, 78
Cryptococcosis, 137–138
Cryptococcus neoformans, 137–138
CSF (cerebrospinal fluid), 18–19
Cushing, 216
Cushing syndrome, 236
Cutaneous neurofibromas, 239
Cutaneous telangiectasia, 111
CWD, chronic wasting disease of deer, 152
Cyanide, 209
Cystadenoma of epididymis, 244
Cystathionine-β-synthase (CBS) deficiency, 190
Cystatin C amyloid angiopathy, 69
Cysticerosis, 143
Cysts, 240–244
Cytoarchitectonic anomalies, 279
Cytomegalovirus (CMV), 16, 128, 130, 132, 133, 280
  congenital infection, 305–306
  hydrocephalus, and, 292
Cytomegaly, 283
Cytoplasm. *See* Perikaryon
Cytoplasmic inclusions, 14–16
Cytoplasmic processes, 8
Cytoskeletal organelles, 8
Cytotoxic (cellular) edema, 21–22, 52, 120

D

DAI (diffuse axonal injuries), 265
Dandy Walker malformation, 26, 285, 294
Dawson's fingers, 164
Degeneration, types of, 19–20
Delayed radiation effect, 255
Dementia, 84–97
  Alzheimer's disease, 85–91
  corticobasal, 16
  corticobasal degeneration, with, 96

Dementia (*continued*)
  diffuse cortical, 85–92
  distinctive-histologic features, without, 97
  frontotemporal, 92–96, 99
  HIV infection, in
  Lewy bodies (DLB), with , 84, 91–92
  motor neuron disease, with, 96–97
  neuritic plaque-only, 92
  paralytica, 139
  Parkinsonism linked to chromosome 17, with, 96
  pugilistica, 104, 270
  rare pathologic forms, 92
  tangle-only, 92
  ubiquitin-only-positive inclusions, with, 97
  vascular, 77–79
Demyelinating diseases, 157–168
Dendrites, 8, 11
Dentatorubro-pallidoluysial atrophy (DRPLA), 109, 110, 111–112
Dermoid cyst, 251, 237, 243
Desmoplastic infantile astrocytoma ganglioglioma, 228
Desmoplastic medulloblastomas, 230
Devic's disease, 165
Diabetes mellitus, 110, 119
  congenital malformations and, 275
Dialysis encephalopathies, 204
Diastematomyelia, 276
DIC (disseminated intravascular coagulation), 75
Diffuse astrocytoma, 216–219, 252
Diffuse axonal injuries (DAI), 265
Diffuse gliosis, 303
Diffuse plaque, Alzheimer's disease, in, 86
Diffuse poliodystrophy, 131, 132
Diffuse vasogenic edema, 267–268
Diffusion-perfusion-weighted imaging, 214
Dilantin, 75
Diplomyelia, 276–277
Disequilibrium syndrome, 204
Disseminated intravascular coagulation (DIC), 75
Distended storage neurons, 10
DLB. *See* Dementia, Lewy bodies, with
Dolichoectasia, 70, 71
Doughnut brain, 279
Down syndrome, 90, 296
DRPLA. *See* Dentatorubro-pallidoluysial atrophy, 111
Drug abuse. *See* substance abuse
Dumbbell schwannoma, 238
Dumbbell tumor, 251, 239
Dura mater, 18
Dural fibroma, 234
Dural fibrosarcoma, 234
Dural sinus thrombosis, 26
Dürck nodules, 144
Düret (brainstem) hemorrhage, 25, 263
Dutch familial cerebral amyloid angiopathy, 68
Dwarfism, 111, 178
Dysautonomia of the Shy-Drager syndrome (SDS), 112–113
Dying-back degeneration, 20
Dysembryoplastic neuroepithelial tumor, 228
Dyslipoprotenemia, 66
Dysostosis multiplex, 178
Dysplastic gangliocytoma, 287
  cerebellum, of, 228
Dysraphic disorders, 274–277
Dystonias, 109
Dystrophic axonal spheroids, 12

E
EAE (experimental allergic encephalomyelitis), 163
Early delayed radiation effect, 255
Eastern encephalitis virus, 126, 127
EBV. *See* Epstein-Barr virus
Echinococcosis, 143, 145–146
Echovirus, 126
Ectomesodermal dysgenetic syndromes, 288–291
Edema
  cerebral, 21–22
  trauma, due to, 267–268
  schemic stroke, in, 52
  types of, 21–22
EDH (epidural hematoma), 262
EEG in
  Creutzfeldt-Jakob disease, 153
  herpes simplex-1 infections, 128
  human prion diseases, 152
EGFR (epidermal growth factor receptor), 213
Ehlers-Danlos syndrome, 66, 69
EIBT (enzyme-limited immunoelectrotransfer blot), 145
Electrical injuries, 270
Electroencephalogram. *See* EEG
Electromyogram (EMG), 97
ELISA. *See* enzyme linked immunosorbent assay
Elk, 152
EMA (epithelial membrane antigen), 232
Embolic stroke, 54
Embolization, air and gas, injuries, from, 270
Embryonal carcinoma, 237, 238, 253
Embryonal choriocarcinoma, 253
Embryonal malignant teratoma, 253
Embryonal tumors, 228, 253
EMG (electromyogram), 97
Encephalitis, HIV related, 11, 131
Encephalitis, limbic, 256
Encephalitis viruses, 126, 127
Encephalitis with microglial nodules, 130
Encephalofacial angiomatosis, 291–292
Encephalomyelitis, 256
  postinfectious and postvaccination, 166
Encephalomyopathies/mtDNA, and, 187–188
Encephalopathy, hypertensive, 64
Encephalopathy, metabolic, 202–205
Encephalopathy, hypoxic and ischemic, 36
Endarteritis, 138
Endocarditis, 120
  verrucous, 67, 73
Endocrine dysfunction, 230
Endodermal sinus tumor, 237, 238
Entamoeba histolyca, 142–143
Enterogenic cyst, 277
Enteroviruses, 126
Enzyme assay, 169–170, 236
Enzyme single deficiencies peroxisomal diseases, in, 181
  generalized peroxisomal diseases in, 180
Enzyme-limited immunoelectrotransfer blot (EIBT), 145
Enzyme linked immunosorbent assay, 137, 145
Eosinophilic granuloma, 246
Eosinophilic viral inclusions, 127
Ependymal glia, 16
Ependymal tumors, 225–227
Ependymitis, 16
Ependymoblastoma, 230
Ependymoma, 226, 249, 252, 254
Epidermal growth factor receptor (EGFR), 213
Epidermoid cysts, 237, 241–243
Epidural abcess, 123
Epidural hematoma (EDH), 262
Epilepsy pathology
  chronic, 37
  temporal lobe, 40
Epithelial membrane antigen (EMA), 232
Epstein-Barr virus (EBV), 128, 130, 134, 214
  lymphomas and, 246
Erosions, bony, 25
Escherichia coli, 120
Ethanol. *See* Alcohol abuse
Evolving stroke, 54
Examination, 1–5
Exanthem subitum, 130
Excitotoxicity, ischemic stroke, in, 53–54
Experimental allergic encephalomyelitis (EAE), 163
Extraocular muscle palsy, 64
Extrapyramidal diseases, 100–109
Eye, abnormal enlargement of, 291

F
Fabry's disease, 66, 76, 170, 174
Factor Leiden, 72
Fahr's disease, 205
Falx meningioma, 232
Familial cerebral amyloid angiopathy, 68
Familial hepatocerebral degeneration, 192
Farber's disease, 174
Fat embolization, injuries, from, 270

Fatal familial insomnia (FFI), 152, 154
FCMD (Fukuyama congenital muscular dystrophy), 281
Ferrugination of neurons, 9
Fetal alcohol syndrome, 209–210, 305
Fetal and perinatal cerebral pathology, 299–308
  infections, 305–307
  metabolic and toxic diseases, 304–305
  sudden infant death syndrome, 307
  vascular injuries, 301–304
  vascular insults, 299–301
Feto-fetal transfusion syndrome, 300
Fetoprotein (α-fetoprotein), 111
FFI (fatal familial insomnia), 152, 154
Fibrillary astrocytoma, 217
Fibrillary astrogliosis, 15
Fibrils, argyophilic, 8
Fibrinoid necrosis, 45
Fibrohyalinosis, 78–79
Fibromuscular dysplasia, 66, 68
Fibrinolytic agents, 75
Fibrous astrocytes, 15
Fibrous meningioma, 232
Finnish muscle-eye-brain (MEB) disease, 281
FLAIR (fluid-attenuated inversion recovery), 214
Fluid-attenuated inversion recovery (FLAIR), 214
Focal pontine leukoencephalopathy, 205
Folic acid, 200
Forebrain, 277
Frataxin, 110
Friedreich's ataxia, 109, 110
Frontal lobe dementia, 96
Frontotemporal dementia, 99
Frontotemporal lobar dementia, 92–96
  ubiquitin-only pathology, with, 96–97
Fucosidosis, 177, 179
Fukutin, 281
Fukuyama congenital muscular dystrophy (FCMD), 281
Fulminant meningococcus meningitis, 121–122
Fungus, 68. *See also* Mycotic infections
Fusiform aneurysm, 64

G

GABA, 103, 108
Ganglioglioma, 250
GAGs (glycosaminoglycans), 177
Galactorrhea, 236
Galactose-1-phosphate uridyl transferase (GALT), 190
Galactosemia, 190
Galactosyl ceramidase deficiency, 183
Galen, vein of, 25
Gallyas stain, 3
GALT (galactose-1-phosphate uridyl transferase), 190
γ-aminobutyric acid (GABA), 103, 108
Gangliocytoma, 228, 250
Ganglioglioma, 250
Gangliosides, 171
Gas and air embolization, 270
Gaucher's disease, 173–174
GCS (Glasgow coma scale), 268
Gemistocytic astrocytes, 14, 15
Gemistocytic astrocytoma, 217–218
General paresis, 139
Genetic anticipation, 109
Genetic testing, 83
Germ cell tumors, 237–238
  children, in, 253
German measles. *See* Rubella virus
Germinal matrix zone hemorrhage, 300
Germinoma, 237, 251
  children, in, 253
Gerstmann-Sträussler-Scheinker disease (GSS), 110, 152, 154
GFAP (glial fibrillary acidic protein), 13, 185
Giant cell temporal arteritis, 67
Giant cells, multinucleated, 17
Glasgow coma scale (GCS), 268
Glaucoma, congenital, 291
Glees and Marsland stain, 3
Glia, ependymal, 16
Glial cells, 13–17
Glial cytoplasmic inclusions, 104
Glial fibrillary acidic protein (GFAP), 13–14, 185
Glial tumors, rare variants of, 227
Glioblastoma, 75, 219–222, 251, 255
  congenital, 251
Glioma, 13
  children, in, 252
  neuroepithelium, of, 216–228
  neurohypophysis, of, 236
Gliomatosis, 227
Gliosarcoma, 222
Gliosis
  diffuse, 303
  subendymal, 16
Globoid cell leukodystrophy, 183
Glucuronyl transferase deficiency, 304
Glue sniffing, 209
Glutamate, 36, 103
Glutamate decarboxylase, 108
Glycogenoses, 179
Glycoproteinoses, 177, 179
Glycoproteolipids, 174
Glycosaminoglycans (GAGs), 177
Glycosphingolipids, 171
Glycosylation, congenital disorders of (CDG), 195
GM1 gangliosidosis, 173, 177
GM2 gangliosidosis, 171
Golgi types 1 and 2 axons, 8
Gömöri stain, 3
Gorlin syndrome, 255
Gram-positive bacilli, 148
Granular cell myoblastoma, 236
Granular cell tumor, pituitary, of, 236
Granular cortical atrophy, 77, 78–79
Granular ependymitis, 16
Granuloma, 137
Granulomatous angiitis, 130
Granulomatous inflammatory diseases, 123
Granulomatous meningitis, 137
Granulo-vacuolar degeneration, 10, 87, 89
GSS (Gerstmann-Sträussler-Scheinker disease), 152, 154
Guam. *See* Parkinsonism-dementia complex of Guam
Guillain-Barré syndrome, 130
Gumma, 141

H

HAART (highly active antiretroviral therapy), 131, 133
Haemophilus influenzae, 120, 121
Hair cells, 222
Hallervorden-Spatz disease, 104, 193
Haltia-Santavuori disease, 174
Hamartomas of the iris, 254
Hamartin, 254
Hamartoma, 237
  kidneys, of, 254, 289
  hypothalamic, 244
Hand-Schüler-Christian disease, 246
Hartnup disease, 110
HbA, 71
HbS, 71
HD. *See* Huntington's disease
Heat shock proteins, 186
Heat stroke, 110, 205
Heidenhain disease, 154
Helminth, 142–143, 145–147
Hemangioblastoma, capillary, 244
Hemangioma, 244–245, 251
Hemangiopericytoma, 233, 244
  spinal dura, of, 251
Hematologic diseases, 71–75
Hematoma, spontaneous intracerebral, 61
Hematopoietic diseases, 254
Hematoxylin-eosin stain, 3
Hemimegalencephaly, 284
Hemispheric wall, 279
Hemodynamic stroke, 54
Hemoglobin A (HbA) and S (HbS), 71
Hemophilia, 66, 72
Hemopoietic metastases, 249
Hemopoietic tumors, 245–247
Hemorrhage
  brainstem (Düret), 25
  cerebral, 62
  injuries, from, 270
Hemorrhagic infarct, 46
Hemorrhagic leukoencephalitis, acute, 167
Hemorrhagic stroke, 61–66
Hepatic encephalopathy, 202–203
Hereditary neurofibromatosis syndromes, 238
Hereditary spastic paraparesis, 97, 100

Herniation, 22–25
  central diencephalic-rostral midbrain, 26
  cerebellar, 23, 26
  hippocampal, 23, 26
  subfalcial, 23
  tonsillar, 62
  transtentorial uncal, 23, 26
Heroine, 75
Herpes infections, 128–130
Herpes simplex encephalitis, 14
Herpes simplex virus (HSV-1 and HSV-2), 128, 129
Herpes virus infection, congenital, 306
Herpes zoster, 68
Heterotopia, 254, 283, 287, 291
Heubner endarteritis, 138
Hexacarbon, 209
HHV 6 and 7. *See* Human herpes viruses 6 and 7
Highly active antiretroviral therapy (HAART), 131
Hippel-Lindau syndrome, 250
Hirano bodies, 10, 11, 87, 89
Histocompatibility complexes, major (MHC), 162
Histoplasma capsulatum, 137
Histotoxic hypoxia, 33
HIV, 75, 130–135, 138
  children, in, 134
  congenital and neonatal infection, 306
  encephalitis, 11, 131
  HIV-associated cognitive motor complex, 131
  HIV-associated dementia, 131
  HIV-associated vasculitis, 68
  immunosuppression-related diseases, 132–135
  leukoencephalopathy, 131
  nervous system diseases related to, 131–132
  neuropathy, 132
  p24 antigen, 132
  transmission routes, 131
  vacuolar myelopathy, 132
HLA-A3 -B7 and -DR2, 162
Hodgkin disease, 249, 256
Holmes stain, 3
Holoprosencephaly, 277–279
Holzer stain, 3
Homocysteine, 90
Homocystinuria, 66, 76, 190
Horner syndrome, 70, 77
Hortega stain, 3
Hourglass schwannoma, 238
HSV-1 and HSV-2. *See* Herpes simplex virus
Human chorionic gonadotrophin, 237
Human herpes viruses 6 and 7 (HHV 6 and 7), 128, 130
Human prion diseases, 152–156
Human prion protein gene (PRNP), 151
Human T-cell leukemia/lymphotropic virus-1, 134–135
Hunter's disease, 177–179
Huntingtin, 107, 110
Huntington's disease, 107–108, 109, 110
Hurler's disease, 179
Hurst's disease, 167
Hyalin bodies, 99, 102
Hyalin platelet thrombus, 74
Hyaline membrane disease, 300
Hydatoid disease, 145–146
Hydranencephaly, 279, 299, 305
Hydrocephalus, 26–27, 138, 305
  congenital and neonatal, 291–295
  ex vacuo (passive hydrocephalus), 27, 85
  normal pressure, 27
  strokes and, 66
Hydromyelia, 276–277
Hyperammonemia, 190
Hyperbilirubinemia, 304
Hypercoagulability, inherited, 72
Hyperglycemia, 34
Hyperleukocytosis, 72
Hypertension, 45
  benign intracranial, 75
  maternal, 300
Hypertensive encephalopathy, 64
Hyperthermia, 205
Hypertrophied astrocytes, 14
Hyper/hypo-vitaminosis A, 26
  hydrocephalus, and, 292
Hypoglycemic encephalopathy, 203–204
Hypogonadism, 236
Hypomelanotic macules, 289
Hypothalamic dysfunction, 65, 230
Hypothalamic hamartomas, 244
Hypothermia, 34
Hypothyroidism, 110
Hypo-vitaminosis A. *See* Hyper/hypo-vitaminosis A
Hypoxemic hypoxia, 33
Hypoxia, cerebral, 33–42
Hypoxic encephalopathy, 36
Hypoxic-ischemic leukoencephalopathy, 35–36
Hypoxic-ischemic neuronal necrosis, 36
Hypoxic-ischemic parenchymal necrosis, perinatal, 300–301

I

Iatrogenic complications, stroke etiology, 75
Icelandic familial cerebral amyloid angiopathy, 68–69
I-cell disease, 177
ICP. *See* Intracranial pressure
ICSCA. *See* Inherited cerebellar and spinocerebellar ataxias
Idiopathic cerebellar ataxia, 109
Idiopathic Parkinson's disease, 101–103
IgA and IgE, 111
Immune mechanism, defective, 111
Immune-mediated vasculitis, 67
Immunofluorescent stain, 128
Imunoglobulin A and E, 111
Inactive chronic plaque multiple sclerosis, 159–161
Inclusion bodies, neuronal, 10–11
Inclusion bodies, glial, 104, 115
Infantile neuroaxonal dystrophy, 193
Infantile Refsum disease (IRD), 180–181
Infarct, 25
  stages of, 46–47
  stroke syndromes from, 55–59
Infection
  fetal and perinatal, 305–307
  injury, due to, 268
Infectious diseases, 119–149
  assessment of, 119
  bacterial, 120–124
  mycotic infections, 136–138
  parasitic, 142–147
  risk factors for, 120
  syphilitic, 138–142
  viral, 124–136
Infectious mononucleosis, 166
Infectious (mycotic) aneurysm, 64
Infectious vasculitis, 68
Inflammation, 119
  ischemic stroke, in, 52
Inflammatory demyelinating polyradiculopathy, 166
Inflammatory vascular diseases, 67
Infundibulum, 124
Inherited cerebellar and spinocerebellar ataxias (ICSCA), 109
Injuries, 261–271
  blunt head, 261–267
  clinical presentation of, 268
  missile head, 267
  secondary, 267–268
  spinal cord, 269–270
In-situ hybridization, 125
Intergenomic communication, 188
Interstitial edema, 22
Intracortical dysplasia, 283
Intracranial hemorrhage, 262–264
  perinatal, 300
Intracranial pressure (ICP), 21, 33, 37
Intracranial tumors in children, 251–253
Intradermal neurinomas, 240
Intramedullary tumors, 249–250
Intraneural perineurinomas, 240
Intraparenchymal schwannoma, 238
Involuntary movements, extrapyramidal diseases with, 107–109
IRD (infantile Refsum disease), 180–181
Irradiation, hydrocephalus, and, 292
Ischemia, 33
  events related to, 50–52
  permanent global, 37–39
Ischemic demyelination, 78–79
Ischemic encephalopathy, 36, 73
Ischemic hypoxia, 33
Ischemic-hypoxic encephalopathy trauma, with, 267
Ischemic necrosis, 50–52

Ischemic stroke, 43–61, 73
presentation of, 54
Isolated abducens nerve palsy, 26

J
Jansky-Bielchowsky disease, 175
Japanese encephalitis virus, 126, 127
JC virus, 16, 135
Juvenile paresis, 307

K
Kayser-Fleischer ring, 192
Kearns-Sayre syndrome, 187–188
Kennedy's disease. *See* Bulbospinal muscular atrophy
Kernicterus, 304
Kernohan's notch, 23–24
Kinky hair (Menkes) disease, 11, 193
Klippel-Trenauny-Weber syndrome, 291
Klüver-Barrera stain, 3
Klüver-Bucy syndrome, 92, 96
Knife-blade atrophy, 93–94
Korsakoff amnestic syndrome, 200–201
Korsakoff syndrome, 128
Krabbe's disease, 183
Kuf disease, 175
Kugelberg-Welander disease, 99
Kuru, 152, 153, 154
Kyphoscoliosis, 277

L
Lacerations, 265
Lactic acid, 33
Lactic acidosis, ischemic stroke, in, 54
Lacunar infarct, 45, 47
Lacunar state, 77, 78–79
Lacunar syndromes, 79
Lafora bodies, 11, 192
Lafora disease, 11
with myoclonic epilepsy, 192
Lambert-Eaton syndrome (LES), 257
Langerhans' histiocytosis, 251, 246
Langhan's-type multinucleated giant cells, 123, 124
Large cell anaplastic medulloblastomas, 230
Latent viruses, 125
LA test, 137
Latex agglutination (LA) test, 137
Lead, 110, 209, 305
Leber's hereditary optic neuropathy, 188
Leigh syndrome (LS), 188–189
Leptomeningeal angiomatosis, 291
Leptomeningeal sarcoma, 234
Leptomeningitis, purulent, 120–121
Leptomeninges, 18–19
LES (Lambert-Eaton syndrome), 257
Lesions, distribution of, 34
Lesions, vascular, 22
Letterer-Siwe disease, 246
Leukemia, 66, 255
Leukemic meningitis, 249
Leukencephalopathy, HIV related, 132
Leukoaraiosis, 77, 85
Leukodystrophies, 182–186
Leukoencephalopathy
hypoxic-ischemic, 35–36
perinatal, 303
progressive multifocal, 16
Leukostasis, 249
Lewy bodies, 10, 11, 84, 91–92, 102
Lhermitte-Duclos disease, 228, 287
Li-Fraumeni syndrome, 255
Lightning injuries, 270
Limbic encephalitis, 256
Lipase deficiency, 174
Lipofuscin accumulation, 9
Lipofuscin (wear-and-tear pigment), 29
Lipoma, 237, 243, 251
congenital, 251
Lipomatous medulloblastomas, 230
Liquefaction stage of infarct, 46–47
Lisch nodules, 254
Lissencephaly, 280–281
Lithium, 110
Livedo reticularis, 73
Locked-in syndrome, 55, 58
coma and akinetic mutism compared, 59
Locus ceruleus, 88
Lorenzo's oil, 181
Louis-Bar syndrome, 111
Low-grade diffuse astrocytoma, 252
Loyez stain, 3
LS (Leigh syndrome), 188–189
Lumbar puncture, 120
Lupus anticoagulant, 73
Lupus erythematosis, 73
Lyme disease, 68, 75, 147
Lymphomas, 245–247, 249, 251
B and T cell, 246
Lysosomal carbohydrate diseases, 175–179
Lysosomes, 170
Lysteria monocytogenes, 120

M
Machado-Joseph desease, 110
Macroadenoma, 236
Macrocephaly, 288
Macrogyria, 281–283
Macrophage, 17
activation, 52
Macula, red spot at, 171, 179
Mad cow disease, 152
Magnetic resonance angiogram (MRA), 61
Magnetic resonance imaging. *See* MRI
Magnetic resonance spectroscopy (MRS), 131, 164, 214
Magnetization transfer imaging, 214
Malaria, 142–144
Malformations, congenital, 273–298
brainstem, of, 287
brain weight disorders, 287–288
cerebellum, of, 185–287
cerebral hemispheres, of, 279–284
chromosomal disorders, 295–296
ectomesodermal dysgenetic syndromes, 288–291
hydrocephalus, 291–295
meningeal anomalies, 288
midline structures, of, 284–285
neural tube defects, 274–277
phakomatoses, 288–291
prosencephalon, of, 277–279
vascular anomalies, 288
ventricles, of, 284–285
Malformations, vascular, 69–71
Malignant fibrous histiocytoma, 234
Malignant HIV leukoencphalopathy, 131
Malignant meningioma, 233
Malignant peripheral nerve sheath tumors, 240
Maltase deficiency, 179
Maltese cross pattern, 86
Manganese toxicity, 209
Manganese poisoning, 104
Mannosidosis, 177, 179
Maple syrup urine disease (MSUD), 189–190
Marbling, 303
Marburg type MS, 165
Marchiafava-Bignami disease, 208
Marfan syndrome, 66, 69
Mass lesions, intracranial expanding, 22–26
Masson stain, 3
Mastoiditis, 120
MCA aneurysm, 69
Measles, 166
associated diseases, 135–136
inclusion body encephalitis, 136
virus, 126, 127
MEB (Finnish muscle-eye-brain disease), 281
Medullary stroke syndromes, 58
Medulloblastoma, 228–230, 251, 253, 255
Medulloepithelioma, 230
Medullomyoblastomas, 230
Megalencephaly, 287–288
Megaloblastic anemia, 201–202
Melanocytoma, 235
Melanoma, 75
Melanotic medulloblastomas, 230
MELAS, 66, 75–76, 188
Meningeal anomalies, 288
Meningeal carcinomatosis, 249
Meningeal mesenchymal tumors, 232–235
Meningeal sarcomas, 234
Meningeal tumors, 250–251
Meninges, 18–19
tumors of, 231–235
Meningioma, 232–233, 237, 251, 254
children, in, 253
Meningitis, 133
Meningocele, 276
Meningococcus meningitis, 121
Meningoencephalitis, 91, 130, 137
Meningoencephalocele, 275
Meningomyelocele, 276
Meningothelial meningioma, 232
Meningothelial tumors, 232–233

Meningovascular syphilis, 133, 138, 140, 307
Menkes (kinky hair) disease, 11, 193
Mercury, 110, 209, 210, 280
MERRF (myoclonus epilepsy with ragged-red fibers), 188
Mesial temporal infarct, 25
Mesolimbic cortex, 105
Metabolic diseases. *See also* Neurometabolic diseases, acquired; Neurometabolic diseases, hereditary
  fetal and perinatal, 304–305
  hereditary, 75–76
Metabolic encephalopathies, 202–205
Metachromatic leukodystrophy (MLD), 107, 182–184
Metastatic tumors, 247–249
Methanol, 209
Methotrexate, 209
Methotrexate leukoencephalopathy, 256
Methyl alcohol, 209
Methyl mercury poisoning, 280
Meynert, nucleus of, 88
MHC (major histocompatibility complexes), 162
Microatheroma, 44–45
Microcephaly, 130, 287–288, 305
Microencephaly, 287–288
Microgemistocytic oligodendroglioma, 226
Microglia, 17
Microglial nodules, 17
Microcystic meningioma, 233
Microsomal triglyceride transfer protein (MTP), 195
Midbrain stroke syndromes, 58
Mineralization
  aging related, 71
  cerebral arteries, in, 67
Missile head injuries, 267
Mitochondria, 170
Mitochondrial diseases, 110, 186–189
Mitochondrial neurogastrointestinal encephalopathy (MNGIE), 188
Mitral valve prolapse, 66
Mixed meningioma, 232
MLD (metachromatic leukodystrophy), 107
  multiple sulfatase deficiency, with, 177
MLII and MLIII, 177
MNDs. *See* Motor neuron diseases
MNGIE (mitochondrial neurogastrointestinal encephalopathy), 188
Morquio B disease, 173
Motor neuron diseases (MNDs), 96
Moyamoya disease, 66, 68
MPS (mucopolysaccharides), 177
MPTP poisoning, 104, 101
MRA (Magnetic resonance angiogram), 61
MRS (magnetic resonance spectroscopy), 131
  single-enzyme deficiencies, and, 181
  subacute necrotizing encephalomyopathy, and, 189
MS. *See* Multiple sclerosis
MSD (Multiple sulfatase deficiency), 183
MSUD (maple syrup urine disease), 189–190
MTP (microsomal triglyceride transfer protein), 195
Mucolipidosis, 177, 179
Mucopolysaccharides (MPS), 177
Mucopolysaccharidosis, 27, 177–179, 287
Mucoraceae species, 137
Multicystic leukomalacia, 303
Multifocal necrotizing leukoencephalopathy, 205, 206
Multinucleated giant cells, 17
Multiple disseminated embolic microabcesses, 122
Multiple sclerosis (MS), 157–166
  clinical presentation, 163–165
  geographic distribution of, 163
  pathology, 157–163
  remitting-relapsing vs. progressive, 164
  variants of, 165–166
Multiple sulfatase deficiency (MSD), 183
Multiple system atrophy, 104, 112–116
Mumps, 166
  hydrocephalus, and, 292
  virus, 126, 127
Mycobacterium tuberculosis, 123, 133
Mycoses, 136
Mycotic infections, 136–138
Mycotic (infectious) aneurysm, 64, 123
Myelin, 17–18
Myelin basic protein, 158
Myelocytic leukemia, 74
Myocardial infarct, 33, 45–46
Myoclonus epilepsy with ragged-red fibers (MERRF), 188
Myxoma, 66
Myxopapillary ependymoma, 249

N

N-acetyl-transferase (NAA), 131
Naegleria fowleri, 142–143
NALD (neonatal adrenoleukodystrophy), 180–181
N-aspartoacylase deficiency, 183
Necrosis, ischemic, 50
Necrosis, neuronal, 12–13
  cortical laminar, 35
  hypoxia, in, 34
  hypoxic-ischemic, 36
Necrosis, pituitary, of, 25
Necrosis stage of infarct, 46–47
Necrotizing vasculitis, 137
Negri bodies, 127
Neisseria meningitidis, 120, 121
Neonatal adrenoleukodystrophy (NALD), 180–181
Neonatal sepsis, 300
Neoplastic transformation, 11, 14
  glial cells, of, 16
Nerve root tumors, 250
Neural tissue reaction to diseases, 7–19
Neural tube defects (NTDs), 274–277
Neurenteric cyst, 277
Neurinomas, 254
Neuritic plaque-only dementia, 92
Neuritic (senile) plaques (NP), 85, 86
Neuroacanthocytosis, 104, 109
Neuroaxonal dystrophies, 170, 193–194
Neuroblastomas, 11
Neurocutaneous melanosis, 235, 291
Neurocysticercosis, 145
Neurocytomas, 11
Neurodegenerative diseases, 83–118
  categories of, 84
  cerebellar degenerations, 109–112
  dementias, 84–97
  extrapyramidal, 100–109
  motor neuron, 97–100
  multiple system atrophy, 112–116
  spinocerebellar degenerations, 109–112
Neuroepithelium, tumors of, 216–231
Neurofibrillary tangles (NFT), 11 , 10, 85, 87, 89, 91
Neurofibromas, 239–240, 250
Neurofibromatosis, 239
  type 1 (NF1), 222
  types 1 and 2 (NF1 and NF2), 253–254
  children, in, 253
Neurofibromin, 254
Neurogenic sarcoma, 240
Neuroglial nests, 283
Neurohypophysis, tumors of, 235, 236
Neuroleptic malignant syndrome, 205
Neurometabolic diseases, acquired, 100–211
  alcohol abuse, 205–210
  calcium metabolic disorders, 205–207
  metabolic encephalopathies, 202–205
  toxic disorders, 209–210
  vitamin deficiencies, 199–202
Neurometabolic diseases, hereditary, 169–198
  amino acid metabolic, 188–189
  carbohydrate metabolic, 190–192
  categories of, 170
  copper metabolic, 192–193
  leukodystrophies, 182–186
  lysosomal, 170–179
  miscellaneous, 194–196
  mitochondrial, 186–189
  peroxisomal, 179–182
Neuromyelitis optica, 165
Neuronal ceroid lipofuscinosis, 174–175
Neuronal cytoplasmic inclusions, 104
Neuronal degeneration, 104
Neuronal glial tumors, 227–228
Neuronal lipidoses, 170–174
Neuronal tumors, 227–228
Neuronophagia, 125
Neurons
  ballooned achromatic, 10
  death of, 12–13
  described, 7–8
  distended storage, 10

ferrugination of, 9
pathology of, 8–10
red, 9
Neurosarcoidosis, 147
Neurosyphilis, 68, 138
congenital infection, 307
Neurotransmitters, 8
Nevus flameus, 291
New-variant CJD (nv CJD), 152, 154–155
NF1 and NF2 (neurofibromatosis types 1 and 2), 222, 253–254
NFT. *See* Neurofibrillary tangles
Niacin, 200
Nicotinic acid, 200
Niemann-Pick disease, 173
type c (NPC), 194
Nigropallidostriatal system, 105
Nipah virus, 126, 127
Nissl bodies, 8
dissolution of, 9
Nissl stain, 3
Nodular medulloblastoma, 229
Nodules, microglial, 17
Non-Hodgkin's lymphoma, 249
Nonketotic hyperglycinemia, 190
Nonobstructive hydrocephalus, 27
Nonsteroidal anti-inflammatory agents, 91
Normal pressure hydrocephalus (NPH), 27
Northern epilepsy syndrome, 175
NP (neuritic plaques), 85
NPC (Niemann-Pick type c disease), 194
NPH (normal pressure hydrocephalus), 27
NTDs (neural tube defects), 274–277
Nucleus, 8
Nucleus of Meynert, 88
Null-cell adenomas, 236
nv CJD (new-variant CJD), 152, 154–155

O
Obstructive hydrocephalus, 26, 289
Occipital infarct, 25
Occipitotemporobasal stroke syndromes, 57
Oculocerebral dysplasia, 281
Oligoastrocytoma, 226
Oligodendrocytes, 13, 15
Oligodendroglioma, 75, 224–226, 250, 251
children, in, 253
Olives, inferior, 21
Olivopontocerebellar atrophy (OPCA), 109, 112
Oncogenes, 213
Oncogenic viruses, 125
Opalski cells, 192
OPCA, 109, 112
Opportunistic infections, 132–134
Opsoclonus, myoclonus, 257
Opthalmic zoster, 129
Optic atrophy, 100
Optic nerve glioma, 254
Optic neuropathy, 208
Ornithine transcarbamylase, 190
Osteoma, 251
Osteomyelitis, 120
skull, of the, 123
Osteosarcoma, 251
Otic zoster, 129
Otitis media, 120
Otorrhea, 262
Ovarian dysgenesis, 111
Owl's eye, 130
Oxidative phosphorylation (OXPHOS), 186, 188

P
Palsy, isolated abducens nerve, 26
Pancreatic cysts, 66
Pancreatic islet cell tumor, 244
Panencephalopathic CJD, 154
Papillary meningioma, 233
Papilledema, 25
Papovavirus SV40, 214, 226
Papp-Lantos inclusions, 115
Paraganglioma, 251
Parainfluenza virus, 126, 127
Paramyxoviruses, 126, 127
Paraneoplastic diseases, 256–257
Parasagittal meningioma, 232
Parasitic infections, 142–147
Paratyphoid vaccination, 166
Parenchymal hemorrhages traumatic (PH), 245, 264
Parenchymal injuries, 264–267
Parenchymal neurosyphilis, 139–142
Parinaud syndrome, 230
Park1 and Park2, 101
Parkinsonian syndrome, 103
injuries, from, 270
Parkinsonism, 103
dementia complex of Guam, 99, 104, 107
linked to chromosome 17, 96
Parkinson's disease, 91
dementia, plus, 103
ideopathic, 101–103
Lewy bodies and, 10
PAS-positive bacilli, 148
Passive hydrocephalus (hydrocephalus ex vacuo), 27
PBD (peroxisomal biogenesis disorders), 180
PCNSLs (primary central nervous system lymphomas), 246
PCR (polymerase chain reaction), 119
PCR assay, 125, 305
PCR/herpes infections, 128
PD (Pick's disease), 93–96
PDGF (platelet-derived growth factor receptor), 213
Pearly tumor, 241
Pelizaeus-Merzbacher disease, 186
Pelvic infections, 120
Penfield stain, 3
Penumbra, 50
Perikaryon, 8
Perinatal cerebral pathology. *See* Fetal and perinatal cerebral pathology
Perinatal vascular insults, 299–301
Perineurinomas, 240
Periodic sharp wave complexes (PSWC), 152, 153
Peripheral nerve neurinoma, 240
Periventricular leukomalacia, 300
Pernicious anemia, 201–202
Peroxisomal biogenesis disorders (PBD), 180
Peroxisomal diseases, 179–182
Peroxisomes, 170
PNET (primitive neuroectodermal tumors), 255
PH (parenchymal hemorrhage), 264
Phakomatoses, 288–291
Phenylalanine hydroxylase, 189
Phenylketonuria (PKU), 189
Phenytoin, 110, 209
Pheochromocytoma, 244, 254, 289
Phosphomannomutase, 195
Phosphotungstic acid/hematoxylin (PTAH) stain, 3
PHYH (Phytanoyl coenzyme A-hydroxylase), 182
Phytanoyl coenzyme A-hydroxylase (PHYH), 182
Pia mater, 18–19
Pica, 305
Pick bodies, 10, 11
Pick's disease (PD), 11, 93–96
Pilocytic astrocytoma, 222, 254
children, in, 252
Pineal gland
parenchyma, tumors of, 230
tumors, children, in, 253
Pineal region, tumors of, 231
Pineoblastoma, 230–231
children, in, 253
Pineocytoma, 230–231
Pituicytoma, 236
Pituitary
apoplexy, 236
chromophobe adenoma, 236
hyperthyroidism, 236
necrosis, 25
necrosis, injuries, from, 270
large bizarre cells in, 111
PKU (phenylketonuria), 189
Placenta, anomalous, 300
Plaque in multiple sclerosis
active *vs.* inactive, 159–161
remyelinating, 162
Plaque meningioma, 232
Plasmacytoma, 246
Plasmodium falciparum, 142–144
Platelet-derived growth factor receptor (PDGF), 213
Platelets, disorders of, 72
Pleomorphic cystic xanthoastrocytoma, 224, 252
Plexiform neurofibromas, 239
Plexus papilloma, 26
congenital, 251

PML (progressive multifocal leukencephalopathy), 135
PNET. *See* Primitive neuroectodermal tumor
Pneumocystis carnii pneumonia, 134
PNLs. *See* Polymorphonuclear leukocytes
Poliovirus, 126
Polyarteritis nodosa, 67
Polycystic kidneys, 66
Polycythemia, secondary, 244, 254
Polycythemia vera, 72, 74
Polyglucosan diseases, 191–192
Polyglutamine disease, 83, 109
Polymerase chain reaction (PCR), 119, 120
Polymicrogyria, 282–283, 305
Polymorphonuclear leukocytes (PNLs), 120
Polyneuropathic CJD, 154
Pompe's disease, 179
Pontine hemorrhage, 63
Pontine raphe nuclei, 88
Pontine tegumentum and basis syndrome, 58
Pontomedullary separations, 265
Pontomesencephalic separations, 265
Pontoneocerebellar hypoplasia, 285–286
Porencephalic cyst, 303
Porencephaly, 279, 299, 303
Port-wine stain, 291
Postencephalitic Parkinsonism, 104, 107
Posterior subcapsular cataract, 254
Postherpetic neuralgia, 129
Post polio syndrome, 126
Postradiation neoplasms, 256
Posttraumatic syringomyelia, 269
Polycythemia vera, 74
Presenilin 1 and 2, 90
Pressure cone syndrome. *See* Herniation, cerebellar tonsilar
Pressure, intracranial, 21
Primary central nervous system angiitis, 68
Primary central nervous system lymphomas (PCNSLs), 246
Primary cerebral lymphomas, 134
Primary lateral sclerosis, 97, 100
Primary meningeal melanocytic tumors, 235
Primary meningeal sarcomatosis, 234
Primary torsion dystonia, 109
Primary ventricular hemorrhage, perinatal, 300
Primitive neuroectodermal tumors (PNET), 228, 255
  supratentorial, 230
Primitive plaque, 86
Prion diseases, 151–156
  dendritic processes, and, 11
Prion protein, 151
PRNP, 151
Probst fibers, 284
Programmed cell death, 84
Progressive dementia, injuries, from, 270
Progressive multifocal leukencephalopathy (PML), 16, 135
Progressive rubella panencephalitis, 136
Progressive supranuclear palsy, 16, 103–107
Prosencephalon, 277
Prostate carcinoma, 251
Prosthetic heart valve, 66
Protein-C and -S deficiencies, 72
Prothrombin time, 73
Protoplasmic astrocytoma, 217
Protozoal infections, 142–145
PrPc, 151
PrPsc, 151
Psammoma body, 232
Psammomatous meningioma, 233
Pseudobulbar palsy, 98
Pseudohypertrophic degeneration of the inferior olives, 21
Pseudohyphae, 138
Pseudomyasthenia, 257
PSWC (periodice sharp wave complexes), 152, 153
PTAH stain, 3
P-type ATPase, 193
Pulseless disease, 67–68
Punch-drunk syndrome, 270
Purulent encephalitis, 122, 123
Purulent inflammatory diseases, 120
Purulent leptomeningitis, 120–121, 122
Putaminal hemorrhage, 63
Pyocephalus, 122
Pyribenzamine, 75
Pyridoxine, 200
Pyruvate dehydrogenase complex, 188

Q

Quaternary neurosyphilis, 133

R

Rabies, 11
  vaccination, 166
  virus, 126, 127
Radiation
  complications, 255–256
  hydrocephalus, and maternal, 292
Radiculoganglionitis, 127, 130
Radiculomyelitis, 130
Radiculoneuropathy, 130
Ragged-red fibers (RRF), 187
Rasmussen's encephalitis, 147–148
Rathke pouch, 241
rCBF (regional cerebral blood flow), 43
Recklinghausen's disease, 254, 287
Red neurons, 34, 50
Reflexes, pathologic, 37
Refsum's disease, 180–181
Remyelinating plaque, 162
Renal carcinoma, 75, 244
Resident microglia, 17
Respirator brain, 37
Respiratory arrest, 33
Retardation, mental, 130
Retinal angioma, 254
Retinal angiomatosis, 244
Retinal glioma, 289
Retinitis, 130
Retinopathy, 257
Retrograde amnesia, 268
Retrograde axonal transport, 125
Retrograde trans-synaptic degeneration, 20
Reye's disease, 129
Reye's syndrome, 204–205
Rhabdomyoma of the heart, 289
Rhabdovirus, 126, 127
Rhabdomyoma of the heart, 254
Rhaboid tumors, 230
Rhesus factor incompatibility, 304
Rheumatic valvular disease, 66
RH incompatibility, 304
Rhinorrhea, 262
Rhombencephalon, 277
Rickettsial infections, 147
RNA viral infections, 126–128
Rocky Mountain spotted fever
Rod cells, 17
Romberg sign, 141
Rosenthal fibers, 14, 15, 186–186
Roseola, 130
RRF (ragged-red fibers), 187
Rubella
  congenital infection, 306
  hydrocephalus, and, 292
  virus, 126, 128

S

S-100 protein, 232
Saccular (berry) aneurysm, 64, 69
Sacrococcygeal teratoma, 251
SAH (subarachnoid hemorrhage), 64–66, 264
Satellitosis, 15
Sandhoff disease, 171
Sarcoidosis, 147
Sarcoma, 255
Scarlet fever, 166
Schilder's disease, 166
Schindler's disease, 179
Schistosomiasis, 143, 147
Schizencephaly, 279, 299
Schwann cells, 238
Schwannomas, 238, 250, 254
Sclerose en plaque. See Multiple sclerosis
Sclerotic microgyria, 301, 303
Scrapie, 151, 152
Scrub typhus, 147
SDH (subdural hematoma), 262–264
SDS (Shy-Drager syndrome), 112–113
Sebacious adenomas, 289
Secretory meningioma, 233
Seizures, 25, 37
Sellar region, nonpituitary tumors in, 237
Senile (neuritic) plaques, 86
Sepsis, neonatal, 300
Septic hemorrhagic necrosis, 137
Serotonin deficiency, 88
Shadow plaque, 162
Shagreen patches, 289
Shaken baby syndrome, 262, 265

Shingles. *See* Varicella zoster virus
Shy-Drager syndrome (SDS), 112–113
SIADH (syndrome of inappropriate antidiuretic hormone secretion), 65
Sialuria, infantile, 177
Sickle cell disease, 66, 71
Sick sinus syndrome, 45
Siderocalcinosis, 71–72
SIDS, 307
Silicon toxicity, 90
Single photon emission computed tomography (SPECT), 85
Sinopulmonary infection, 111
Sinusitis, 120
Skein-like inclusions, 11
Skin-fold freckling, 254
Skull fractures, 262
SLE. *See* Systemic lupus erythematosus
Sleeping sickness, 142, 144
SMA (Spinal muscular atrophy), 99–100
Small-cell carcinoma of the lung, 256, 257
Smallpox vaccination, 166
SMN1 (survival motor neuron gene), 99
SND. *See* Striatonigral degeneration
Soft-tissue perineurinomas, 240
Sommer's sector, 34
SPECT (Single photon emission computed tomography), 85
  hypometabolism, 93
  ideopathic Parkinson's disease, 101
  lymphomas, 246
  striatal dopamine uptake, 101
Spheroids, axonal, 12
Sphingolipids, 171
Sphingomyelin, 171
Spina bifida occulta, 276
Spinal and spinal cord defects, 276–277
Spinal cord, section of, 3
Spinal enterogenous cyst, 250
Spinal epidural abcess, 123
Spinal muscular atrophy (SMA), 97, 99–100
Spinal nerves, tumors of, 238–240
Spine, tumors of, 251–253
Spinocerebellar ataxias, 109, 110
  adult-onset inherited, 112
Spinocerebellar degenerations, 109–112
Spirochetes, 68
Spiroplasma infection, 151
Spongiform encephalopathies, transmissible, 151–156
Spongy degeneration (Canavan's disease), 183, 185
Spontaneous intracerebral hematoma, 61
SSPE (subacute sclerosing panencephalitis), 135–136
St. Louis encephalitis virus, 126, 127
Staghorn vessels, 234
Stagnant hypoxia, 33
Stains for histologic examination, 1–5
Staphylococcus aureus, 120, 122
Stars, 125
Status epilepticus, 33, 37
Status marmoratus, 303–304
Status spongiosis, 89
Steele-Richardson-Olszewski disease, 103–107
Stenosis of the aqueduct of Sylvius, 287, 294
Stercoralis, 143
Sterol, 196
Streptococcus pneumoniae, 120, 122
Striatonigral degeneration (SND), 104, 105–107, 112
Striatopallidodentate calcification, 205
Stroke, 43–77
  hemorrhagic, 43, 61–66
  ischemic, 43–61
  mortality, 55
  neuroimaging, 59, 61, 64
  risk factors, 54
  syndromes, 55–59
  young, in the, 66–79
Strongyloidiasis, 143, 147
Sturge-Weber-Dimitri syndrome, 291–292
Subacute cerebellar degeneration, 256
Subacute combined degeneration of the spinal cord, 201
Subacute necrotizing encephalomyopathy, 188–189
Subacute sclerosing panencephalitis (SSPE), 135–136
Subarachnoid hemorrhage (SAH), 64–66, 70, 245, 264
  perinatal, 300
Subclavian steal syndrome, 57
Subcortical arteriosclerotic encepalopathy, 77
Subcortical dementia, 77, 101
Subdural abcess, 123
Subdural hematoma (SDH), 262–264
  perinatal, 300
Subdural hygroma, injuries, from, 270
Subependymal giant cell astrocytoma, 222–224, 252
Subependymal gliosis, 16
Subependymal ventricular nodules, 291
Subependymoma, 226
Subhyaloid hemorrhage, 64
Substance abuse, 75
  strokes, and, 66
Substantia nigra, 34
Subungual fibromas, 289
Sudden infant death syndrome, 307
Sulfatide lipidosis, 182–184
Superior cerebellar infarct, 25
Supranuclear palsy, progressive, 16
Supratentorial primitive neuroectodermal tumor (PNET), 230
Survival motor neuron gene (SMN1), 99
SV40 virus, 135
Synapses, 8
  loss of, 87
Syncope, 36
Syncytial meningioma, 232
Syndrome of inappropriate antidiuretic hormone secretion (SIADH), 65
Synucleinopathies, 84
Syphilitic granuloma, 141
Syphilitic infections, 138–142
Syphilitic meningitis, 307
Syphilitic optic atrophy, 141
Syringobulbia, 287
Syringomyelia, 250, 276–277
Syrinx, 276–277
Systemic lupus erythematosus (SLE), 66, 67

T

T's (Talwin), 75
Tabes dorsalis, 139–140, 307
Taenia echinococcus, 143, 145
Taenia solium, 143, 145
Takayasu's arteritis, 66, 67–68
Talwin (T's), 75
Tangier disease, 196
Tangle-only dementia, 92
Tau gene, 103
Tauopathies, 14, 84
Tau positive inclusions, 14
Tau protein, 10, 11, 84, 91, 153
Tay-Sach's disease, 9, 171–173, 287
Telangiectasis, capillary, 70
Temporal lobe epilepsy, 40
Teratogenic viruses, 125
Teratogens, 273–274
Teratoid tumors, atypical, 230
Teratoma, 237–238
  children, in, 253
  congenital, 251
Testicular dysgenesis, 111
Tethered spinal cord, 276
Thalamic stroke syndromes, 57
Thalamus hemorrhage, 63
Thallium, 110
T-helper cells, 125
Thiamine pyrophosphate (TPP), 199–200
Third nerve palsy, 64
Thrombotic stroke, 54
Thrombotic thrombocytopenia, 66
Thromboangiitis obliterans, 68
Thrombocythemia, 72
Thrombocytopenia, 72, 73, 74
Thrombophlebitis, 123
Thromboplastin time, 73
Thrombotic thrombocytopenic purpura, 72, 74
Thymus, hypoplasia of, 111
TIA (Transient ischemic attack), 54
Ticks, 127
Toga virus, 126, 128
Tonsillar herniation, 62
Top of the basilar syndrome, 58
Torpedo, axonal, 12
Torulosis, 137–138
Touraine syndrome, 235
Toxemia, maternal, 300
Toxic diseases, perinatal, 304–305

Toxic disorders, 209–210
Toxoplasma gondii, 142, 305, 306–307
Toxoplasmosis, 133, 142
  congenital infection, 306–307
TPP (thiamine pyrophosphate), 199–200
Transfusions, 119
Transient ischemic attack (TIA), 54, 73
Transitional meningioma, 232
Translation initiation factor eIF2B, 195
Transmissible spongiform encephalopathies, 151–156
Transplacental transmission of infection, 120
Trans-synaptic degeneration, 19–20
Treponema pallidum, 68, 133, 138, 305
Trichinella spiralis, 143, 146
Trichinosis, 143, 146
Trigeminal artery, persistence of, 71
Trigeminal neuralgia, 71
Trigeminal schwannoma, 238
Trinucleotide repeat diseases, 109
Triplet-repeat diseases, 109
Tropical spastic paraparesis, 135
Trypanosomiasis, 142, 144–145
TSC (tuberous sclerosis complex), 254
T-suppressor/cytotoxic cells, 125
Tuberculous granulomatous meningitis, 123–124
Tuberin, 254
Tuberous sclerosis, 287
  syndrome, 224
  complex (TSC), 254, 288–289
Tubers, cortical, 289–290
Tumor supressor genes, 213
Tumors, 213–259
  age-related distribution of, 214
  chemotherapy complications, 255–256
  cranial nerves, of, 238–240
  cranium, of, 251–253
  germ cell, 237–238
  grading, 214
  hemangiomas, 244–245
  hemopoietic, 245–247
  hereditary syndromes, 253–254
  lymphomas, 245–247
  maldevelopmental and cysts, 240–244
  meninges, of, 231–235, 249–251
  metastatic, 75, 247–249
  nerve roots, of, 249–251
  neuroepithelium, of, 216–231
  oligodendroglial, 224–226
  paraneoplastic diseases, 256–257
  pituitary gland, of, 235–237
  proliferation capacity, 215
  radiation complications, 255–256
  sellar region, of, 235–237
  spinal cord, of, 249–251
  spinal nerves, of, 238–240
  spine, of, 251–253
  stains for diagnosing, 215
Turcot syndrome, 255
Twin, loss of, 282
Twinning, 300
Typhoid vaccination, 166
Typhus, 147

U
Ubiquitin, 11, 84, 91
Ubiquitin c terminal hydroxylase-L1 (UCH-L1), 101
Ubiquitin-only dementia pathology, 96–97
UCH-L1, 101
Ulegyria, 301, 303
Umbilical cord, anomalous, 300
Uremic encephalopathy, 204

V
Vaccination, autoimmune pathogenesis, as, 166
Valproate, 190
Valproic acid, 75, 275
van Gieson stain, 3
Vanishing white matter disease (VWD), 195
Varicella, 166
  congenital infection, 306
  vasculopathy, 68
  -zoster virus (VZV), 128, 129, 292
Vascular anomalies, 288
Vascular dementia, 77–79
Vascular diseases, inflammatory, 67
Vascular injuries
  fetal and perinatal, 301–304
  of the spinal cord, 269
Vascular insults, fetal and perinatal, 299–301
Vascular lesions malformative, 22, 245
Vascular malformation, 66, 69–71
Vascular tumors, 244, 249, 277
Vasculitis
  HIV-associated, 68
  immune-mediated, 67
  infectious, 68
Vasculopathy, 130
  noninflammatory, 68
Vasogenic edema, 21, 22, 52
Vegetative state, persistent, 38
  coma *vs.*, 39
Vein of Galen, 25
  fistula of, 288
Venezuelan encephalitis virus, 126, 127
Venous angioma, 245
Venous thrombosis, 66
Ventilation, mechanical, 37
Ventricle, colloid cysts of, 243
Ventricular puncture, 120
Ventricular tumors, 289
Ventriculitis, 130
Ventriculoperitoneal shunt, 120
Verhoeff stain, 3
Verocoy bodies, 239
Verrucous endocarditis, 67, 73
Vertical gaze palsy, 230
Vessels, blood, 19
Vimetin, 232
Vincristine, 209
Viral infections, 124–136
  chronic, 135–136
  neural inclusions in, 11
Viral nuclear inclusions, 14, 16
Virchow-Robin space, 18–19, 292
Vitamin B_1, 199–200
Vitamin B_6, 200
Vitamin B_{12}, 200, 201–202, 203
Vitamin deficiencies, 199–202
Vitamin E deficiency, 109, 111, 200
Volume, brain, increase in, 21–22
von Economo encephalitis lethargica, 107
von Hippel Lindau syndrome, 244, 254
VZV. *See* Varicella zoster virus

W
Walker-Warburg syndrome (WWS), 281
Wallerian (anterograde) degeneration, 18–20, 159
Waterhouse-Friderichsen syndrome, 121
Watershed infarct, 47–50
Wear-and-tear pigment (lipofuscin), 29
Weber syndrome, 58
Wegener's granulomatosis, 67
Werdnig-Hoffman disease, 99
Wernicke's encephalopathy, 199–202
Wernicke-Korsakoff encephalopathy, 200–202
Western encephalitis virus, 126, 127
West Nile virus, 126, 127
Whipple's disease, 148
Wilson's disease, 14, 104, 192
Woelcke stain, 3
Wolman's disease, 174
World Health Organization, 216
WWS (Walker-Warburg syndrome),281

X
X-irradiation, 255
X-linked recessive adrenoleukodystrophies (X-ALDs), 181

Y
Yeast, 138
Yolk sac tumor, 238

Z
Zellweger cerebrohepatic disease, 282
Zellweger's disease (ZS), 180
Zellweger syndrome, 280
Zinc toxicity, 90
Zoster. *See* Varicella zoster virus
ZS (Zellweger's disease), 180